Medical Neuroscience

Second Edition

Kevin D. Alloway, Ph.D.
Professor of Neural & Behavioral Sciences
Milton S. Hershey Medical Center
Pennsylvania State University
Hershey, Pennsylvania

Thomas C. Pritchard, Ph.D.
Associate Professor of Neural & Behavioral Sciences
Milton S. Hershey Medical Center
Pennsylvania State University
Hershey, Pennsylvania

HB
HAYES • BARTON
RALEIGH, NORTH CAROLINA

11 10 09 08 07 1 2 3 4 5

First edition, *Medical Neuroscience,* was published in 1998 by Fence Creek Publishing, Inc., and reissued by Hayes Barton Press in 2003. Hayes Barton Press published the second edition, *Medical Neuroscience,* in 2007.

ISBN 1-59377-200-9 (soft cover)
ISBN 1-59377-220-3 (e-book)

Queries and book orders: 919.755.8110 (voice) or nlucas@vitalsource.com

Cover design by Linda de Jesus, Wing and Prayer Design, Springfield, Massachussetts
Illustrations by Dave Carlson, Visible Productions
Page design and composition and art revisions by ICC Macmillan, Portland, Oregon
Soft cover printed and bound on demand by Lightning Source, LaVergne, Tennessee
Electronic edition produced by ICC Macmillan, Portland, Oregon

The authors and publishers have made every effort to ensure that the methods of treatment and drug recommendations are correct at the time of publication. However, new research and new therapies alter approaches constantly and usually there are several methods of diagnosis and treatment available for every condition. We have offered our best approach and advice. Nevertheless, we recommend consulting other sources (textbooks, package inserts, *Physicians' Desk Reference,* and so on) before deciding on treatment.

Hayes Barton Press
A division of VitalSource Technologies, Inc.
234 Fayetteville St., Suite 300
Raleigh North Carolina 27601-1300
USA

Table of Contents

To my family, whose steadfast love and affection
have enriched my life
— KDA

To Chris, for her love and support
— TCP

Preface

As stated in the preface to the first edition of *Medical Neuroscience,* this text is intended to provide basic knowledge about the nervous system to students in the health sciences. In addition to describing the anatomy and fundamental physiologic principles of the nervous system, we emphasize clinically relevant information and concepts. Our goal is to make the second edition of *Medical Neuroscience* a bridge between the basic science curriculum and clinical practice. For this reason, we have expanded the coverage of clinical topics in neuroscience by adding two new chapters. Chapter 16, Life Span Development of the Brain, describes neural development beginning with the embryo and continuing through the subsequent stages of childhood, adolescence, and adulthood, as well as the pathologic changes that often accompany aging. Chapter 17, Neural Basis of Anxiety and Depression, describes the neural correlates of depression and other mood disorders that afflict a large portion of the general population. Virtually all of the remaining chapters include new clinical topics and have been updated to keep students abreast of clinical developments in the neurosciences. To this end, we retained the clinical case and reconciliation format, and included a new section on Internet resources. In addition to listing Web sites that are instructive to students, we also list sites that contain valuable information for both patients and practitioners. As the second edition goes to press, all of the Web links work, but some require an institutional subscription in order to gain access. For students who would like to study certain topics in more detail, we expanded the list of research articles that provide the scientific foundation for the content in each chapter. Some of these references provide an historical perspective, whereas others are landmark research articles. Finally, we increased the number of questions at the end of each chapter and have formatted most of them so that they are compatible with the guidelines developed by the National Board of Medical Examiners.

We hope that instructors and students find the content in this text to be relevant, interesting, and challenging. The authors, as well as Hayes Barton Press, welcome your comments and suggestions for improving future editions of *Medical Neuroscience.* We are especially interested in reader feedback about the Web sites that we provided, and suggestions for new Web sites to include in the next edition. Because the anatomical sciences rely so heavily upon illustrations, we will consider using photographic materials, including MRI and CT scans, that are submitted to us to illustrate the normal or pathologic structure of the nervous system.

KEVIN D. ALLOWAY AND THOMAS C. PRITCHARD
HERSHEY, PENNSYLVANIA
AUGUST 2007

Acknowledgments

We are especially thankful to editor Nancy Gable Lucas, of Hayes Barton Press for supervising the overall production of this book, for smoothing out many unanticipated wrinkles, and for giving us encouragement at critical points in the book's development. Winifred Sanchez, our project manager at ICC Macmillan, as well as Crystal Thomas, copy editor, ensured a consistent and readable style. We also thank the indexer, Marilyn Anderson, whose efforts make the content more accessible to our readers. In addition, the staff at ICC Macmillan made numerous improvements to the line drawings and other illustrations that were originally produced by Dave Carlson of Visual Productions for the first edition. We thank Matt Harris at Vital Source Technologies for making the second edition of this book possible.

Several individuals provided photographs that appear in many figures. In addition to those who contributed to the first edition, we thank Edward Bixler, William Cantore, Shubhodeep Chakrabarti, Timothy Mosher, Javad Towfighi, and the late Ronald Cranford for providing photographs and other material for the second edition.

We are especially indebted to those individuals who read drafts of selected chapters and made numerous suggestions for improving the quality and accuracy of the final text. For this purpose, we thank our colleagues at Pennsylvania State University including William Cantore, Matthew McEchron, Thyagarajan Subramanian, and Thomas Uhde. In addition, we received constructive advice from Glenn Giesler (University of Minnesota), Michael Graziano (Princeton University), and Hui-Lin Pan (University of Texas). We are also indebted to Michael Quick (University of Southern California) for providing valuable feedback on the first edition. In a similar vein, the second edition benefited enormously from comments and other suggestions given to us by the Penn State students who used our book the last few years. Nonetheless, even though all of these individuals deserve substantial credit for their contributions, the ultimate responsibility for ensuring the accuracy of this text is ours alone. In this respect, Kevin Alloway took primary responsibility for writing Chapters 1, 2, 4, 5, 7, 11, 14, 15, and 17, while Thomas Pritchard was the lead author for the remaining chapters.

Finally, we wish to express our gratitude to Malcolm Carpenter, who passed away in 1999, shortly after publication of the first edition. After retiring from the Uniformed Services University in 1992, Dr. Carpenter resided in Hershey and helped us teach Penn State's course in Human Neurobiology for several years. He not only instructed the students, but he also helped develop our teaching skills in many ways. Furthermore, he donated substantial histologic and photographic material to Penn State that continues to be used for the instruction of our medical and graduate students. While writing the first edition, Dr. Carpenter kindly gave us permission to use items from his unpublished collection. Several of these appear in figures throughout the book, and we acknowledge him for these invaluable contributions.

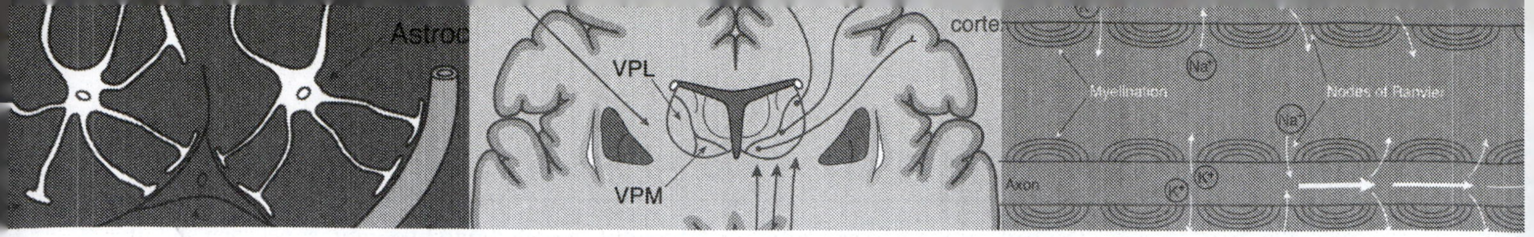

CHAPTER 1

Cellular Neuroscience

INTRODUCTION OF CLINICAL CASE

A female patient, age 30, complained of blurred vision. The clinical exam revealed weakness of the medial rectus of each eye when attempting to gaze to the contralateral side. When she was asked to fixate on an object that slowly moved toward her nose, both of her eyes showed a normal convergence response. When she was asked to fixate on objects with one eye closed, the blurriness disappeared and vision appeared normal in each eye. Further examination revealed slight weakness in the lower face on the right side. All other findings were normal, but review of the patient's history indicated that she had experienced a mild urinary disturbance a few months earlier, although the basis for this complaint was never determined. A subsequent MRI scan revealed multiple small lesions in both the periventricular region and the brainstem.

INTRODUCTION TO CELLULAR NEUROSCIENCE

Neurons process information and communicate with other neurons.

Glia support the metabolic functions of neurons.

The cells of the nervous system are broadly classified into two groups: neurons and glia. Neurons are highly specialized cells that use electrochemical signals to convey information from one brain region to another. Groups of neurons are organized into circuits that perform computations and mediate a variety of integrative functions ranging from simple reflexes to complex processes such as perception, cognition, and purposeful behavior. By comparison, glial cells do not transmit electrochemical signals but support the metabolic and information processing functions of neurons.

Neurons

Neurons are distinct from other cells in the body because of their unique ability to transmit information rapidly over long distances. This functional attribute is directly related to their geometric structure, the biophysical properties of their membranes, and their functional interactions with other groups of neurons.

Most neurons have four distinct components: a soma, dendrites, an axon, and synaptic terminals. The dendrites receive inputs from other neurons and then convey these signals to the soma. The soma integrates the inputs from multiple dendrites and determines whether an action potential should be initiated. These electrochemical impulses are conducted the entire length of the axon to synaptic terminals that contact other neurons or effectors, such as muscles or glands. In response to each action potential, the terminal releases a chemical substance that diffuses across the narrow gap or synapse that separates a neuron from other neurons or effectors.

Types of Neurons. The cell body of a neuron is called the soma or perikaryon. All dendritic and axonal processes originate from the soma; therefore, neurons are classified into multipolar, bipolar, or pseudounipolar groups according to the number of these processes (Figure 1.1).

Multipolar, bipolar, and **unipolar** indicate the number of processes arising from the soma.

Multipolar neurons have multiple dendrites extending from a polygonal-shaped cell body. Although several primary dendrites may arise from its soma, a multipolar neuron has only one axon. Most neurons in the central nervous system (CNS) are multipolar and can be subdivided into many categories, the most common being pyramidal cells, stellate cells, and basket cells.

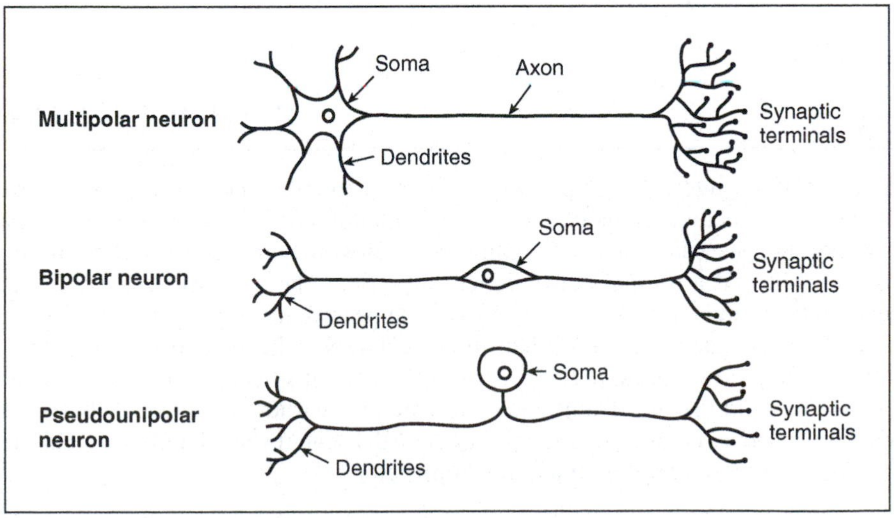

FIG. 1.1. Neuronal Classifications. Neurons are classified according to the number of dendritic and axonal processes that originate from the soma of the neuron.

Bipolar neurons have two processes that extend from opposite sides of a round or oval-shaped cell body. One process acts as a dendrite and receives synaptic contacts from other neurons; the other process acts as an axon and sends signals away from the cell body. Most bipolar neurons are in sensory structures such as the retina or olfactory epithelium, where they transmit sensory signals from the periphery to the CNS.

A pseudounipolar neuron has a large, round cell body with a single process that bifurcates shortly after leaving the soma. By dividing into two branches, the single process of a pseudounipolar neuron functions as both a dendrite and an axon. Most pseudounipolar neurons are located in the peripheral nervous system (PNS) where they send somatosensory signals from the skin, muscles, and joints to the CNS.

Soma. Neurons are among the most metabolically active cells in the body. This is due, in part, to their structural complexity and the need to assemble an extensive cytoskeleton and cellular membrane. In addition, neuronal function depends on concentrating several types of ions against a concentration gradient, and this requires that neurons manufacture different types of ion channels and other molecular complexes that facilitate ion movement.

As the metabolic center of the neuron, the soma contains a variety of organelles that mediate the essential functions of the neuron. A large nucleus in the soma usually contains at least one prominent nucleolus. The soma also contains an extensive endoplasmic reticulum (ER), Golgi apparatus, ribosomes, and mitochondria to meet the metabolic demands of the neuron (Figure 1.2).

The **soma** is the metabolic center of the neuron.

Most neurons have a high concentration of ribonucleic acid (RNA) in the nucleus and in ribosomes associated with the rough endoplasmic reticulum (RER). The nucleic acids in these structures make the soma highly basophilic and, consequently, the soma can be stained by basic dyes. Neuroanatomists frequently stain the Nissl substance of the cell (i.e., organelles that contain nucleic acids) with basic dyes to differentiate brain regions according to the density and distribution of their neuronal soma.

Dendrites. Most neuronal soma give rise to a number of slender dendrites that resemble the arborizations of a tree. Those dendrites that extend directly from the soma are

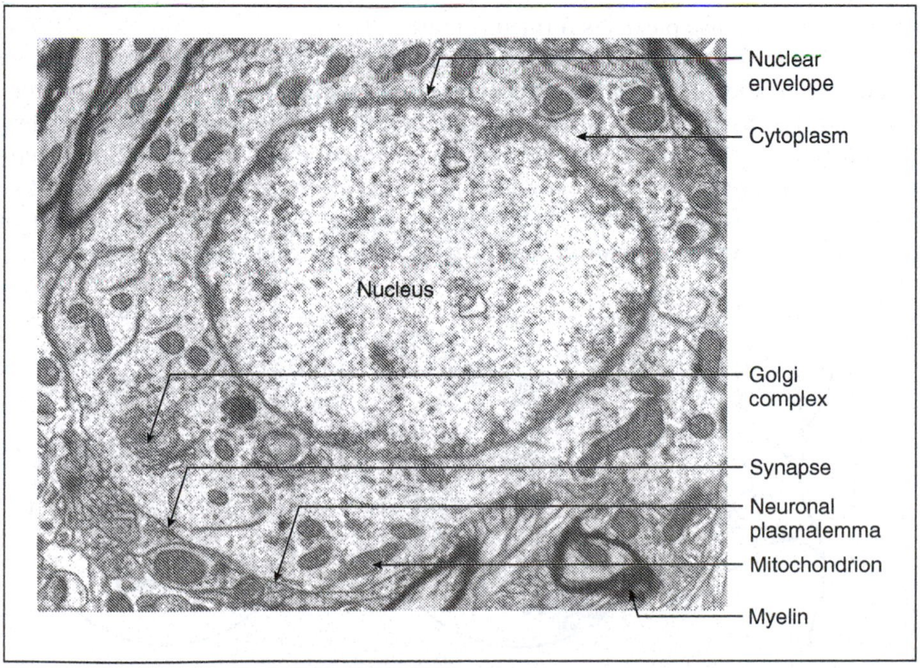

FIG. 1.2. Neuronal Soma. This electron micrograph illustrates the subcellular organelles in the soma of a neuron. (Photograph provided courtesy of Mr. Roland Myers, Pennsylvania State University.)

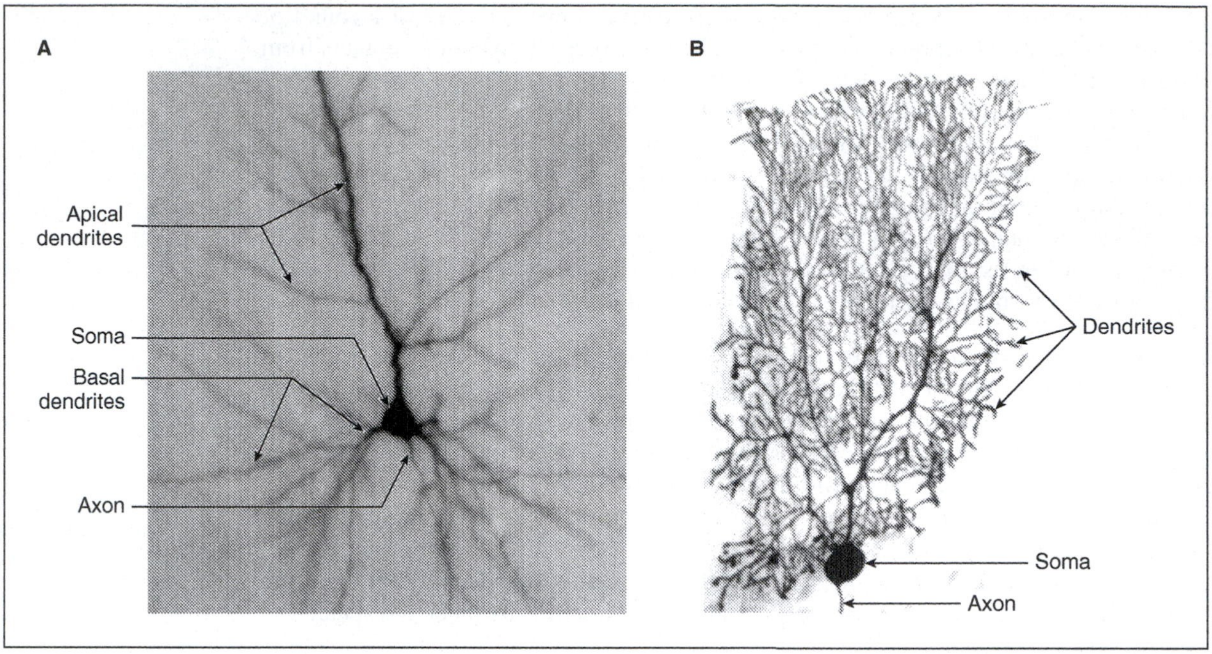

FIG. 1.3. Dendritic Arborizations. (A) Pyramidal neurons have a single apical dendrite and a few basal dendrites. (Photomicrograph provided courtesy of Shubhodeep Chakrabarti, Penn State University). (B) A dense plexus of dendrites extend from the soma of a Purkinje neuron located in cerebellar cortex. (Photomicrograph provided courtesy of Dr. Linda Larson-Prior, Washington University.)

called primary dendrites, and the typical neuron has only a few of these processes. Primary dendrites branch into secondary dendrites, which then subdivide into smaller tertiary dendrites, and so on. The number, density, and spatial patterns of dendrites often define different neuronal subtypes. Thus, pyramidal neurons have one apical dendrite and a few basal dendrites. Purkinje neurons, by contrast, have a dendritic tree that branches repeatedly until a dense plexus is formed (Figure 1.3).

Dendrites are tree-like processes that receive inputs from other neurons and convey this information to the soma

Dendrites provide a receptive area for integrating signals from other neurons. Neuronal communication occurs at specific sites called synapses, many of which are located on the dendrites. Synapses are small, often no more than a few microns or less in length, and the dendrites of a typical neuron may have thousands of synapses. Some neurons have smooth dendrites, and others have dendrites that are studded with hundreds of small bud-like protrusions called spines, which are specialized for receiving signals from other neurons (see Figure 1.4). Dendritic spines tend to be located on secondary, tertiary, or

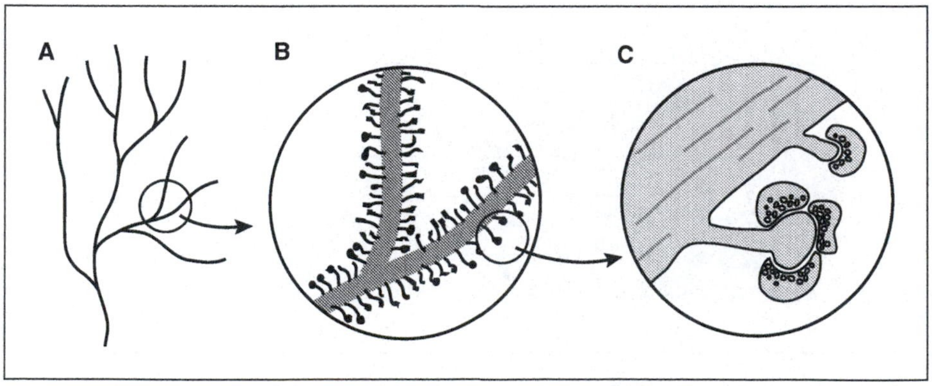

FIG. 1.4. Dendritic Spines. (A) Drawing of a dendritic arborization at low magnification. (B) Drawing of spiny processes protruding from a dendrite viewed at high magnification. (C) Drawing of dendritic spines and their synaptic connections as seen through an electron microscope.

more distal dendritic branches. Primary dendrites rarely contain any spines, but they may receive many synapses. The soma may also have synapses, but these generally comprise a small fraction of the synapses on a typical neuron.

Dendrites contain cytoplasm and an elaborate cytoskeletal system that maintains its complex structure. Large dendrites near the soma contain many neurofilaments and microtubules, some of which extend into the smaller, more distal dendrites. The primary dendrites also contain mitochondria, ribosomes, and saccules of ER.

Axons. The term "axon" is derived from the phrase "axial propagation." As this phrase implies, the axon is an elongated process that may extend for long distances before contacting other neurons. Each neuron has only one axon, and it usually originates from a small protrusion of the soma called the axon hillock. Axons contain bundles of neurofilaments and microtubules that provide structural support as well as a mechanism for transporting complex molecules and vesicular structures to and from the synaptic terminals. In contrast to dendrites, axons do not contain ribosomes and are not involved in protein synthesis (see Figure 1.5).

After leaving the soma, an axon may split into collateral branches that terminate in different brain regions. Many axons bifurcate close to the axon hillock so that a local collateral branch may innervate nearby neurons while the main branch projects to more distant targets. The main axonal branch may also subdivide to enable communication with multiple brain regions. Upon entering the target region, an axon usually forms a plexus of multiple endings that terminate on many postsynaptic neurons. The number of synaptic contacts that a neuron makes on a target neuron is highly variable, but it is not unusual for one neuron to form dozens of synaptic contacts on another neuron. Because a single synapse has little effect on the activity of a postsynaptic neuron, many synapses are usually needed to influence a target cell.

The main function of an axon is to conduct action potentials (electrochemical impulses) from the soma to the synaptic terminals. Axons are electrically excitable because of the biophysical properties of their membranes and the differential concentration of specific ions in the cytoplasm and extracellular space. The conductive properties of the axon are discussed later in this chapter.

Axons conduct electrochemical impulses from the soma to the synaptic terminals.

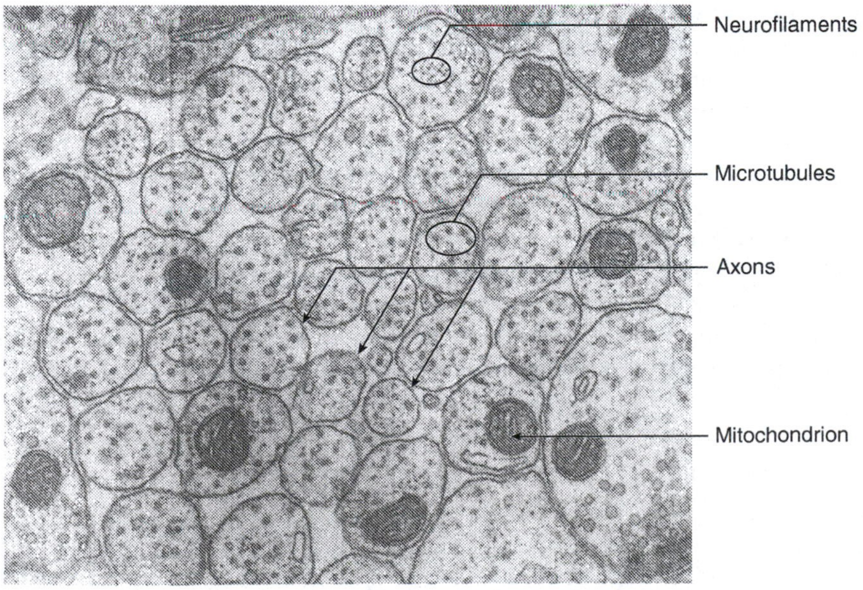

FIG. 1.5. Microtubules and Neurofilaments. Several groups of microtubules and neurofilaments can be seen in this bundle of axons. (Photograph provided courtesy of Mr. Roland Myers, Pennsylvania State University.)

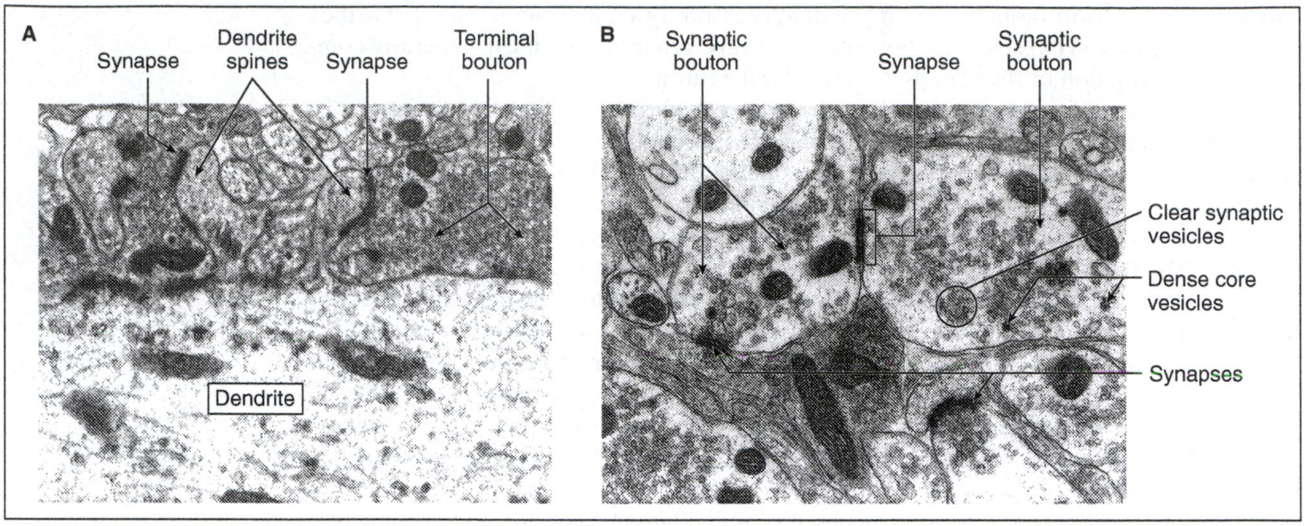

FIG. 1.6. Axodendritic or Axoaxonic Synapses. (A) Two dendritic spines receive contacts from axonal terminals packed with synaptic vesicles. (B) An axon terminal makes a synaptic contact onto another axon terminal. Both terminals contain clear and dense core vesicles. (Photograph provided courtesy of Mr. Roland Myers, Pennsylvania State University.)

Synaptic Terminals. Synaptic terminals are specialized structures that allow one neuron to communicate with other neurons, muscles, or glands. The terminal ending of an axon forms a distinct structure, the synaptic bouton, which lies in close apposition to the plasma membrane of the target cell. Synaptic boutons are slightly larger in diameter than the axon and are filled with synaptic vesicles, mitochondria, enzymes, and other neurochemicals. Synaptic vesicles contain neurotransmitter molecules that are released from the synaptic terminal in response to incoming action potentials. Thus, after one of these impulses invades the synaptic terminal, a neurotransmitter substance is rapidly released so that it will alter the excitability of the target cell (see Chapter 2).

Synaptic terminals release neurotransmitters to communicate with other neurons.

The synaptic terminals of an axon may contact the dendrites or soma of a postsynaptic neuron (Figure 1.6). Such "axodendritic" or "axosomatic" synapses are the most common type of synapse in the CNS. Although axons never form synaptic contacts on the conductive or long part of another axon, they may form "axoaxonic" synapses on other axon terminals. Finally, in some brain regions, "dendrodendritic" synapses have been observed between the dendrites of neighboring neurons.

Although it is common for an axonal ending to form a synapse on a postsynaptic neuron, many axons form synapses at multiple points along their terminal arbors. These synaptic contacts are known as en passant ("in passing") synapses because they appear as a series of axonal enlargements or varicosities that contain vesicles filled with neurotransmitter molecules (Figure 1.7). Consistent with their presynaptic function, each axonal varicosity is apposed to a postsynaptic site on the dendrite, soma, or terminal ending of another axon. En passant synapses allow neurons to have large numbers of synaptic contacts without the biologic expense of building and maintaining an axon collateral for each synapse.

FIG. 1.7. Synaptic Terminals. Axonal terminals may contain single boutons at the end of the axon or a series of "en passant" synapses.

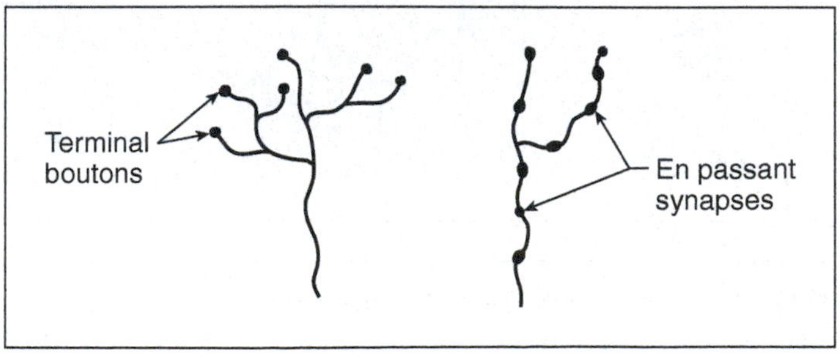

TABLE 1.1 Properties of Axoplasmic Transport

Direction	Rate (mm/d)	Transported Material
Anterograde		
Fast	200–400	Vesicles, neurotransmitters, membrane proteins, lipids
Medium	50–100	Mitochondria
Slow-a	0.2–1.0	Protein subunits for neurofilaments and microtubules
Slow-b	2–8	Clathrin, calmodulin, metabolic enzymes
Retrograde		
Fast	150–300	Lysosomal packaged enzymes, neurotrophic factors

Axoplasmic Transport. Many proteins and subcellular organelles are transported through the axon, either to maintain the axon's structure or to supply its synaptic terminals with essential molecules. This process, known as axoplasmic transport, is necessary because axons do not contain ribosomes or RER. Axoplasmic transport was demonstrated in 1948 when Paul Weiss observed the gradual accumulation of material in the axoplasm after ligating the sciatic nerve with a slender thread. Time-elapsed videomicroscopy and the analysis of transported radioactive amino acids have shown that a variety of particles are transported at different rates and in both directions through the axon (Table 1.1).

Anterograde Movement. Anterograde transport is an axoplasmic process that moves material from the soma to the synaptic terminals. Proteins and lipids synthesized by the RER and Golgi apparatus are assembled into organelles, moved into the axon, and then conveyed by fast or medium transport through the axon (Table 1.1). This process is mediated by a series of kinesin molecules that alternately attach themselves to an organelle and move it a short distance along a microtubule before releasing it (Figure 1.8). Kinesin is a microtubule-associated adenosine triphosphatase (ATPase) molecule that requires oxidative metabolism for its functions.

Compared to fast or medium anterograde transport, the cytoskeletal components and their associated proteins move very slowly in the anterograde direction. As neurofilaments and microtubules are assembled in the soma, the resulting scaffold moves continuously through the axon at a slow rate (0.2-1 mm/d) that matches the depolymerization of the cytoskeleton in the synaptic terminal. Macromolecules such as clathrin, calmodulin, microfilaments, and several enzymes are also transported slowly through the axon (2-8 mm/d), but this mechanism of anterograde transport is poorly understood.

Microtubules provide a conduit for transporting vesicles and other macromolecules through the axon.

Retrograde Movement. Many subcellular organelles, enzymes, and membrane fragments are partially degraded and packaged into lysosomal vesicles for retrograde transport to the soma. This process allows these materials to be recycled and used in the synthesis of new cellular components. Retrograde transport occurs rapidly and is mediated by dynein, another microtubule-associated ATPase that operates like kinesin but in the reverse direction.

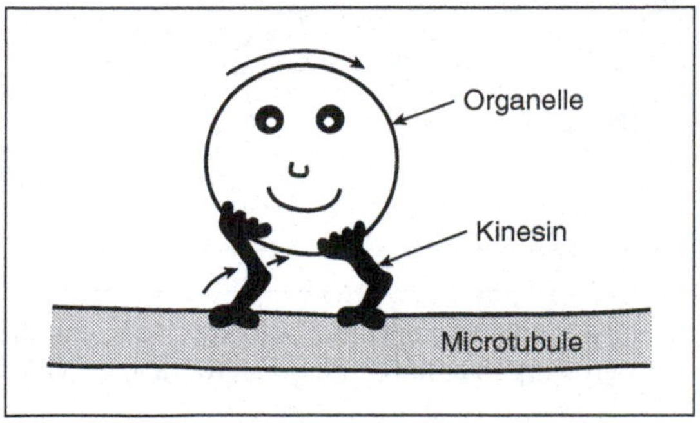

FIG. 1.8. Kinesin. Axoplasmic transport in the anterograde direction is mediated by a series of kinesin molecules. Each kinesin molecule has a fan-tailed end that attaches to the organelle and a globular end that binds to the microtubule. Movement of the organelle occurs as one end of the kinesin molecule pivots around the center hinge.

In addition to its role in transporting cellular fragments, retrograde transport plays an important role in development and certain regulatory mechanisms. In the growing embryo, for example, the terminals of developing axons find their appropriate cellular targets by taking up chemicals, such as nerve growth factor, that are released by the target cells. Nerve growth factor is retrogradely transported to the soma where it regulates the synthesis of material that is subsequently transported to the tip of the growing axon. Even in the adult, the integrity of the neuron depends on the presence of neurotrophic factors released from postsynaptic targets. If postsynaptic targets are damaged or degenerate, the loss of the neurotrophic factor often causes the presynaptic terminals to retract.

Unfortunately, retrograde transport provides a mechanism for the spread of viruses and toxins. For example, herpes simplex, rabies, polio, and tetanus toxin enter the axons or synaptic terminals of peripheral nerves and are shuttled into the CNS by retrograde axoplasmic transport. After these viruses find their way to the soma, they exploit the metabolic functions of the nucleus to replicate themselves.

Glia

Glial cells do not transmit electrochemical signals but are essential for maintaining the biochemical environment for neural functions. Thus, glia maintain the pH and osmolarity of the extracellular fluid within normal physiologic limits. In addition, glial cells increase the conduction velocity of action potentials, modulate neurotransmission at synaptic junctions, and assist nerve regeneration following peripheral nerve injury. The importance of glia for supporting neuronal functions is underscored by the fact that they account for 70%–80% of all cells in the nervous system.

Based on their structural and functional features, neuroglial cells in the CNS are classified as astrocytes, oligodendrocytes, and microglia. Similar types of glial cells exist in the PNS and serve equivalent functions. Schwann cells represent the most common type of glia in the PNS and perform the same functions as the oligodendrocytes of the CNS.

Astrocytes. Astrocytes have numerous branching processes that give them a stellate or star-like appearance. These radiating processes terminate as "end feet" on the free surfaces of neuronal dendrites, cell bodies, and other structures. In addition to the meninges, astrocytic end feet may join to form a secondary barrier that isolates the CNS from other tissues (Figure 1.9). Thus, the outer surfaces of the brain and spinal cord are lined by astrocytic end feet that form the glial limitans membrane located below the pia mater (the inner layer of the meningeal membranes; see Chapter 3). Astrocytic end feet also cover the endothelial cells of blood vessels in the CNS and provide an ancillary membrane in the blood-brain barrier.

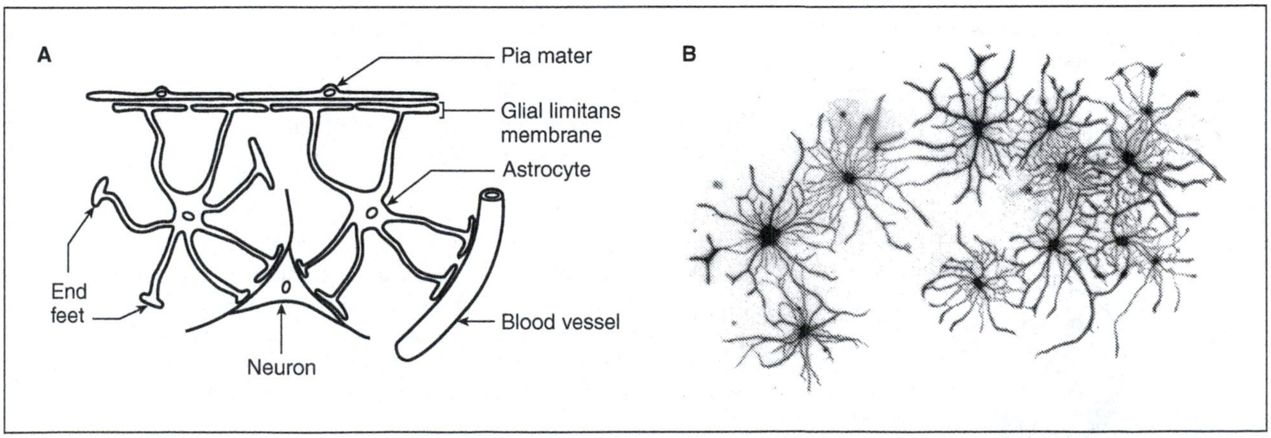

FIG. 1.9. Astrocytes. (A) Astrocytes have elongated processes that terminate as end feet on neurons, blood vessels, and the pia mater. (B) This photomicrograph shows the radiating processes of astrocytes growing in culture. (Photomicrograph provided courtesy of Dr. Robert Milner, Pennsylvania State University.)

Astrocytes control the molecular composition of the extracellular fluid in several ways. For one, astrocytes remove ions discharged into the extracellular fluid during the conduction of action potentials along the axon. Furthermore, astrocytes participate in the uptake and metabolism of glutamate, which is the major excitatory neurotransmitter in the CNS. Thus, after glutamate is released from a synaptic terminal and diffuses through the extracellular space, it is transported into neighboring astrocytes and converted into glutamine. The astrocytes release glutamine into the extracellular fluid where it is recovered by the nerve terminals and converted back to glutamate for subsequent use as a neurotransmitter.

Astrocytes:
- Isolate neurons from blood vessels
- Metabolize the neurotransmitter glutamate
- Provide structural support during development or injury

Astrocytes also provide structural support during development and in response to injury. The developing neocortex contains a specific type of astrocyte, the radial glial cell, which provides a cellular substrate for migrating neurons. Finally, damage to the adult CNS often produces cell loss that leads to pockets of space that become filled by the proliferation of astrocytes. Because astrocytes are one of the few cell types that maintain their ability to proliferate in the mature brain, they are more susceptible to chemical agents that alter cellular replication, which may explain why most tumors in the CNS have an astrocytic origin.

Oligodendrocytes. Oligodendrocytes are highly specialized glial cells that form the myelin insulation around the axons in the CNS. Myelination is the result of a cell-cell interaction in which surface proteins on the oligodendrocyte react to the presence of an axon by producing a sheet-like process that repeatedly grows around the axon. The cytoplasm is squeezed from the glial process as it wraps around the axon; eventually, the axon is insulated from the extracellular fluid by multiple layers of myelin.

Oligodendrocytes are located in all of the major fiber tracts of the CNS. Each oligodendrocyte has multiple processes, each of which insulates a small segment of a single axon. Thus, multiple processes emerge from an oligodendrocyte like the tentacles of an octopus to wrap around short segments of a group of axons (Figure 1.10).

Oligodendrocytes form myelin insulation around axons in the CNS.

The myelination surrounding a single axon is formed by many oligodendrocytes. Thus, each myelinated axon consists of a series of myelin segments that are separated from each other by short intervals called nodes of Ranvier. The myelinated segments insulate the axonal membrane from ions in the extracellular fluid except at the nodes of Ranvier. For this reason, action potentials "jump" from one node of Ranvier to the next. This process, called saltatory conduction, greatly increases the rate of action potential propagation and allows myelinated nerves to conduct impulses at velocities that are several times faster than the velocities recorded from unmyelinated nerves of a similar diameter.

Multiple Sclerosis (MS). Multiple sclerosis causes demyelination at multiple sites of the CNS, as shown in Figure 1.11. Initially, focal lesions of demyelination may appear and then disappear in multiple brain regions, including the corona radiata, and in the major fiber tracts that traverse the brainstem, cerebellum, and spinal cord. The transient and widespread nature of the lesions is reflected by a range of neurologic symptoms that follow a pattern of relapse and remission. Both sensory and motor functions are usually affected, but symptoms vary among individuals because of variations in the location of lesions within different fiber tracts.

Although the initial loss of myelination slows down the propagation of action potentials, neuronal communication is eventually disrupted because the disease destroys both the axons and their myelin covering. The exact cause of MS is unknown, but its pathogenesis is influenced by several factors, including genetic susceptibility, autoimmune mechanisms, and environmental conditions. Multiple sclerosis causes degeneration of myelin sheaths in the major fiber tracts of the CNS, but does not affect myelination in the peripheral nervous system.

Microglia. Microglia, which comprise approximately 1% of the cells in the CNS, originate from the mesoderm and migrate into the CNS during embryologic development. Microglial cells are small cells that function chiefly as scavengers. When CNS tissue is injured, microglial cells migrate to the injured region where they proliferate and devour

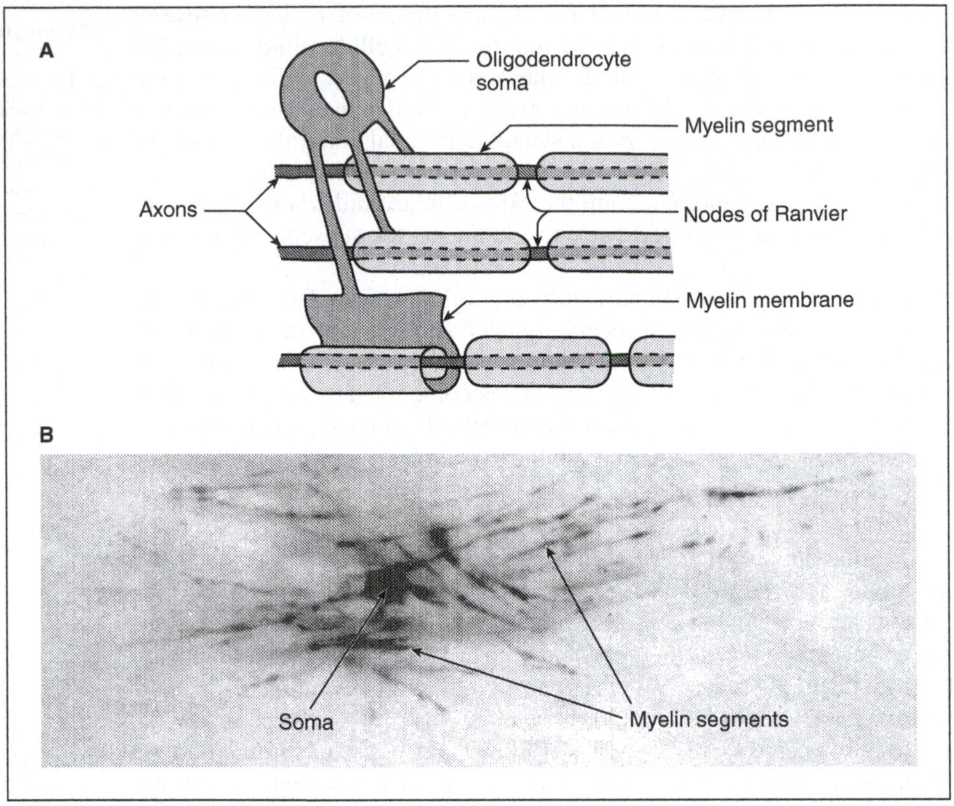

FIG. 1.10. Oligodendrocytes. (A) Fiber tracts in the CNS contain axons wrapped by myelin sheaths extending from a single oligodendrocyte. Nodes of Ranvier represent sites between the myelin segments where ions can flow more easily across the axonal membrane. (B) This photomicrograph illustrates a myelinating oligodendrocyte in the corpus callosum of an 8-month-old rat. The myelin segments of this oligodendrocyte envelop several axons having different orientations. (Photomicrograph provided courtesy of Dr. Steven Levison, University of Medicine & Dentistry of New Jersey.)

FIG. 1.11. Multiple Sclerosis. Magnetic resonance image of a patient with multiple sclerosis. This T2-weighted parasagittal image was enhanced by using the fluid-attenuated inversion recovery (FLAIR) method, which suppresses signals from the cerebral spinal fluid. The small arrows indicate focal lesions in multiple brain regions including the corpus callosum (CC), corona radiata (CR), occipital lobe (OC), internal capsule (IC), and at the base of the cerebellum (CB). (Image provided courtesy of Dr. Timothy Mosher and Dr. Dan Ngyen, Pennsylvania State University.)

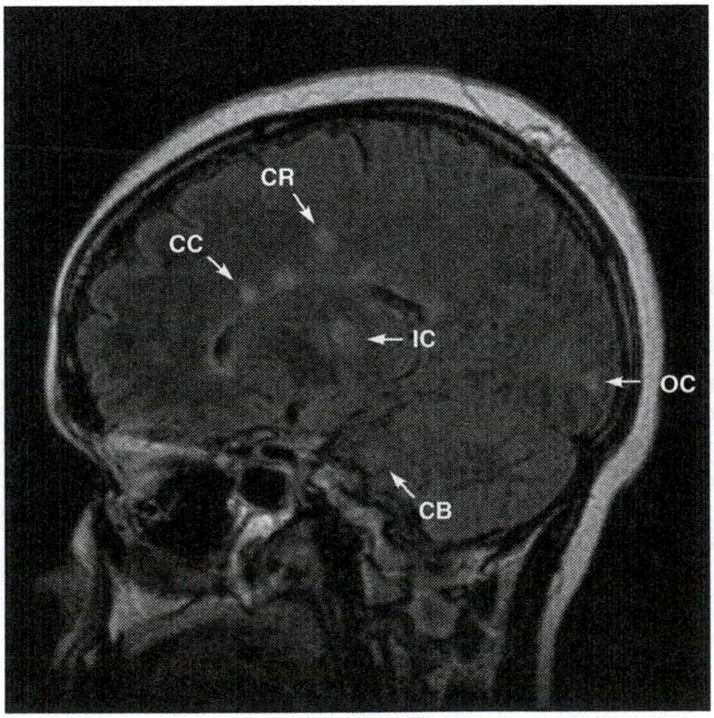

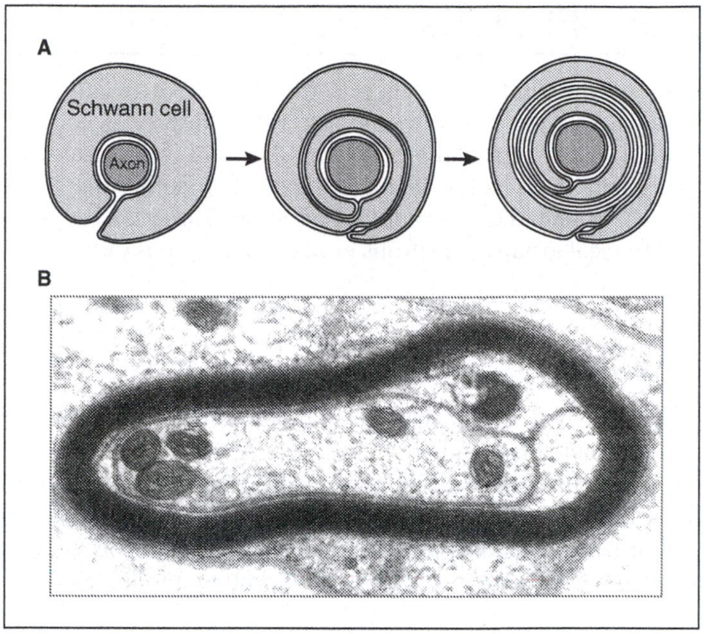

FIG. 1.12. **Schwann Cells.** (A) Myelin growing around the axon of a peripheral neuron. The Schwann cell surrounds the axon and then spirals around the fiber repeatedly. The cell membranes fuse together as the cytoplasm is squeezed from each layer. (B) Electron micrograph illustrating multiple layers of myelin around a peripheral axon. The axon appears to be oval in shape because it was sectioned obliquely. (Photograph provided courtesy of Mr. Roland Myers, Pennsylvania State University.)

the cellular debris. This mechanism of action and other evidence have prompted the view that microglia may participate in certain autoimmune disorders.

Schwann Cells. Schwann cells are structurally and functionally similar to the oligodendrocytes in the CNS but are located exclusively in the PNS. Schwann cells produce multiple layers of myelin sheaths that wrap around all but the smallest nerve fibers (Figure 1.12). As with an oligodendrocyte, cytoplasm is expelled from a Schwann cell as it repeatedly grows around the axon during development. In contrast to oligodendrocytes, however, Schwann cells give rise to a single process that encircles a solitary axon.

The smallest axons in a peripheral nerve are not encircled by layers of myelin, but occupy invaginations in the plasmalemma of a Schwann cell (Figure 1.13). By encapsulating small axons in this way, a single Schwann cell may provide support to approximately 20 unmyelinated axons.

Schwann cells form myelin around axons in the PNS.

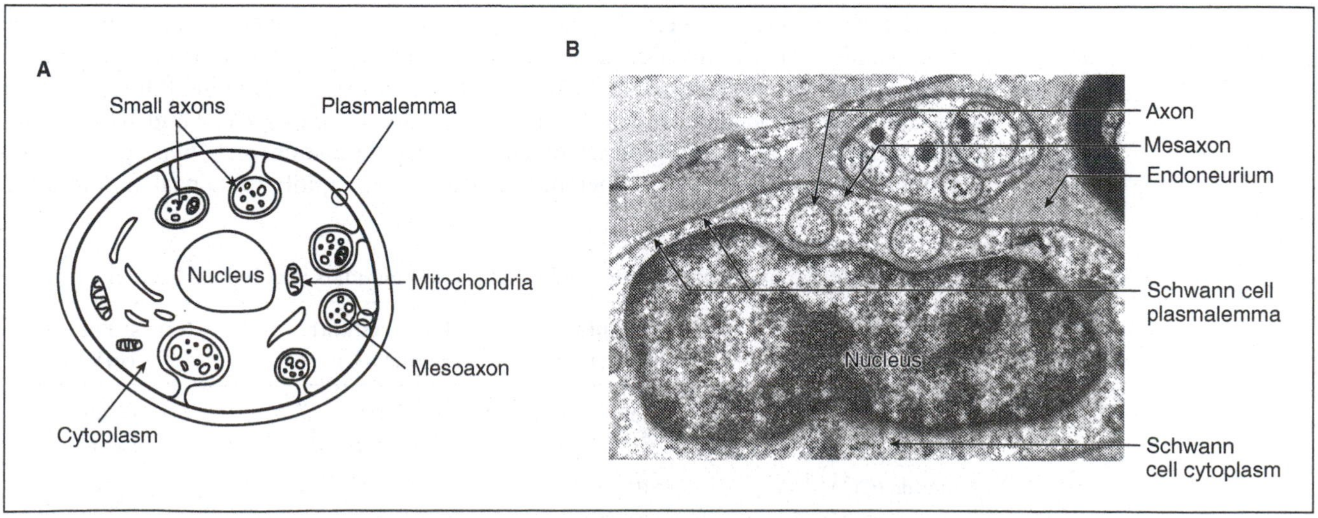

FIG. 1.13. **Unmyelinated Axons.** (A) Small diameter fibers occupy canal-like invaginations in the Schwann cell plasmalemma. (B) The electron micrograph shows two unmyelinated axons ensheathed by a nearby Schwann cell. (Photograph provided courtesy of Mr. Roland Myers, Pennsylvania State University.)

ELECTROCHEMICAL PROPERTIES OF NEURONS

Virtually all mammalian cells have a slight imbalance in the number of positive and negative ions that are distributed across the plasma membrane. Hence, nearly all cells are electrically charged with respect to the surrounding extracellular fluid. Nerve cells are unique, however, because their membranes endow them with special properties that allow them to use changes in membrane potential to represent information. These electrochemical signals can be transmitted to local groups of neurons or to distant regions of the nervous system.

Neuronal Membranes

The membrane of a neuron is a physical barrier that prevents molecules from diffusing freely into or out of the cell. Constructed from a lipid bilayer that acts as an insulator, the neuronal membrane contains ionic pumps that differentially concentrate specific ions in the cytoplasm and extracellular fluid. Neurons maintain high concentrations of potassium (K^+) and negatively charged protein molecules in the cytoplasm; ions such as sodium (Na^+), chloride (Cl^-), and calcium (Ca^{2+}) are more highly concentrated in the extracellular fluid (Table 1.2).

The separation of positive and negative charges across a neuronal membrane results in a membrane potential or voltage. The membrane potential does not remain constant, however, but fluctuates in response to synaptic inputs from other neurons. In the absence of synaptic input, the typical neuron has a resting membrane potential that is approximately −65 millivolts (mV), which means that the cytoplasm is slightly more negative than the extracellular fluid. The membrane potential of a neuron changes whenever ions such as K^+, Na^+, Ca^{2+}, or Cl^- flow through specialized pores or ion channels in the membrane. When the difference in charge across the membrane is reduced, either because positive ions enter the cytoplasm or negative ions escape, the reduction in membrane potential is called a "depolarization." By comparison, an increase in membrane potential that is produced by an influx of negative ions or an efflux of positive ions is called a "hyperpolarization."

Graded Potentials

Graded potentials are monophasic waveforms of variable amplitude that spread passively through the dendrites and soma.

The release of neurotransmitter molecules from a synaptic terminal produces changes in the membrane potential of the postsynaptic neuron. Synaptic transmission may cause either depolarization or hyperpolarization in the postsynaptic neuron, depending on the neurotransmitter that is released and the types of ion channels that are activated (i.e., become opened). Local changes in the postsynaptic membrane potential of the dendrite or soma are called graded potentials because they vary in amplitude. Graded potentials are always monophasic and consist of either a depolarization or a hyperpolarization that spreads passively across the membrane. After rising rapidly to its peak amplitude, a

TABLE 1.2 Ionic Concentrations and Equilibrium Potentials in a Typical Neuron

Ions	Intracellular (mM/L)	Extracellular (mM/L)	Nernst Potential (mV)
Potassium (K^+)	150	5.5	−86
Sodium (Na^+)	15	150	+60
Chloride (Cl^-)	10	125	−66
Calcium (Ca^{2+})	0.0001	2	+180
Organic anions[a]	130	1–2	.....

[a] Organic anions do not cross the plasma membrane because they are too large.

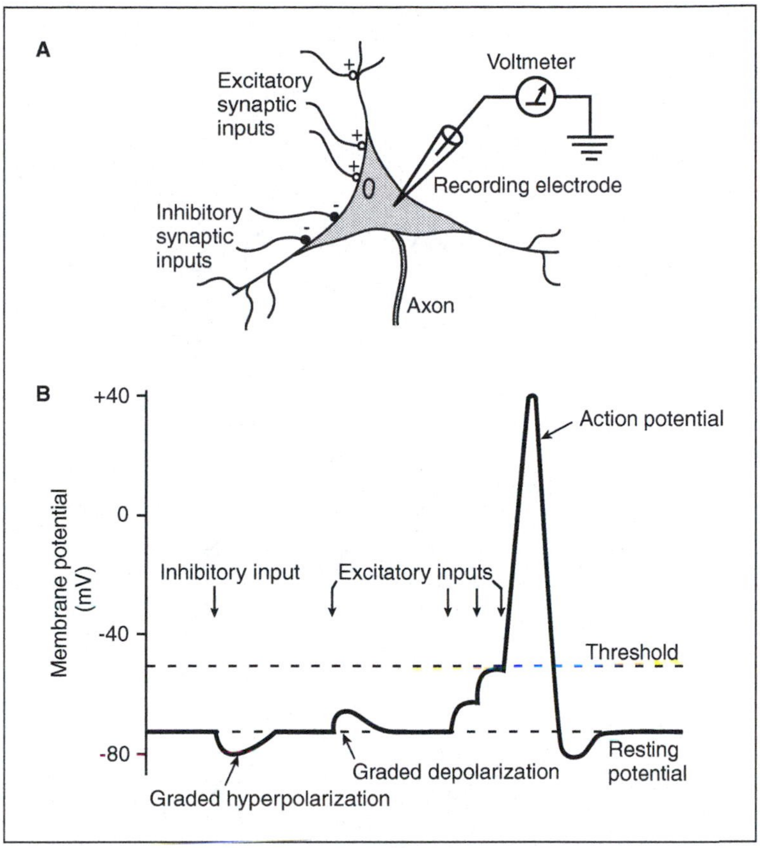

FIG. 1.14. Neuronal Membrane Potentials. (A) An intracellular electrode records the membrane potential of a neuron that receives both inhibitory and excitatory inputs. (B) Release of an inhibitory neurotransmitter causes a graded hyperpolarization; release of an excitatory neurotransmitter causes a graded depolarization. Activation of several excitatory synapses in a brief time period depolarizes the membrane to threshold and produces an action potential.

graded potential gradually decays to the neuron's resting membrane potential (Figure 1.14). Graded depolarizations are called excitatory postsynaptic potentials (EPSPs); graded hyperpolarizations are called inhibitory postsynaptic potentials (IPSPs).

Action Potentials

When a graded depolarization at the axon hillock exceeds a specific threshold level, the neuron produces a special electrochemical impulse known as an action potential (Figure 1.14). Action potentials consist of biphasic changes in membrane potential that are actively propagated along the entire length of the axon. Unlike graded potentials, action potentials are all-or-none signals that remain constant in amplitude as they travel from the axon hillock to the synaptic terminal. Upon reaching the synaptic terminal, an action potential initiates a series of chemical events that culminates in the release of neurotransmitters from the presynaptic membrane. Neurons often produce a rapid series of action potentials, and changes in the timing of these impulses are important for coding specific types of information.

Action potentials are biphasic waveforms of constant amplitude that are actively conducted along a neuron's axon.

Pumps and Channels

The flow of charged ions across a neuronal membrane is controlled by two basic mechanisms. Ion pumps actively transport certain ions through the membrane against their concentration gradients. Ion channels, by contrast, allow passive diffusion of ions across the membrane according to their concentration gradients.

FIG. 1.15. Na^+-K^+ Pump. The Na^+-K^+ pump removes three Na^+ ions from the cytoplasm for every two K^+ ions transported into the cytoplasm. (A) Three Na^+ ions leave the intracellular fluid and bind to specific sites on the Na^+-K^+ pump. (B) The Na^+-K^+ pump is phosphorylated by the conversion of ATP to ADP and releases three Na^+ ions into the extracellular fluid as two 2 K^+ bind to the Na^+-K^+ pump. (C) Dephosphorylation of the Na^+-K^+ pump causes the release of the two K^+ ions into the cytoplasm.

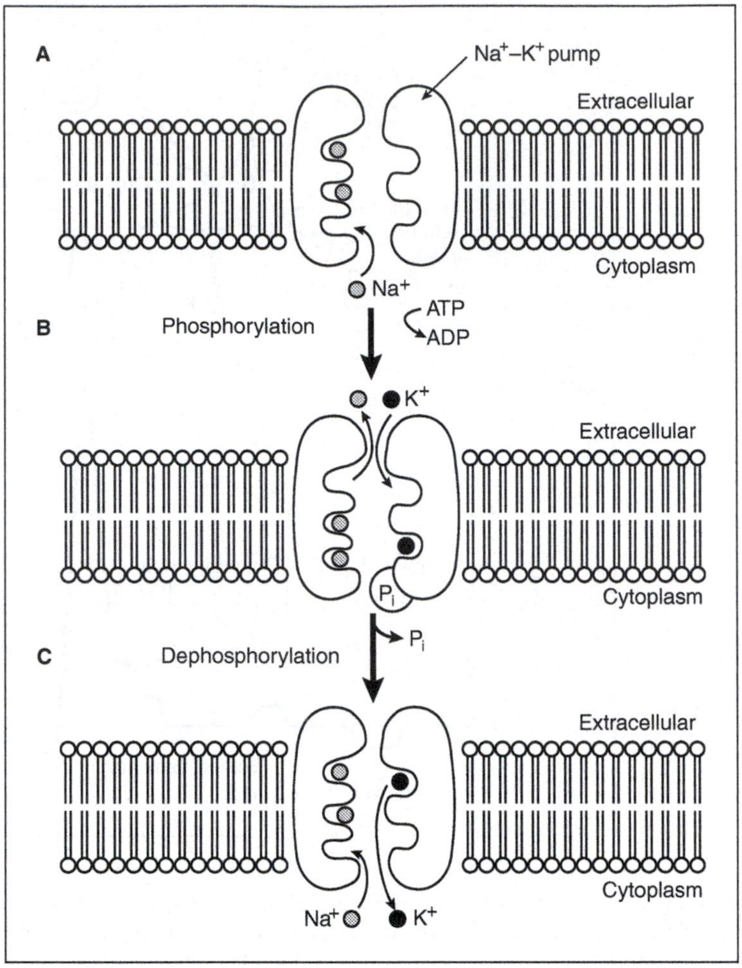

Ion pumps are transmembrane macromolecules that require energy to transport ions against their concentration gradient.

Ion channels are transmembrane macromolecules that allow ions to flow down their concentration gradient.

Ion Pumps. An ion pump is any protein molecule that has the ability to concentrate a specific ionic species in the neuronal cytoplasm or in the surrounding extracellular fluid. Several types of ion pumps have been identified, and all of them require chemical energy to move ions against their concentration gradient. Because some ion pumps depend on the hydrolysis of adenosine triphosphate (ATP) to transport ions across a membrane, these pumps are called ATPase pumps.

Na^+/K^+ Pump. The most important pump for understanding neuronal membrane properties is the Na^+/K^+-ATPase pump. Like many other pumps, the Na^+/K^+ pump relies on ion exchange to transport ions across the neuronal membrane. Thus, it moves Na^+ from the cytoplasm to the extracellular fluid while moving K^+ in the opposite direction (Figure 1.15). These ionic movements are mutually dependent; removing K^+ from the extracellular fluid occurs simultaneously with the removal of Na^+ from the cytoplasm. If K^+ is not present in the extracellular fluid, Na^+ cannot be pumped out of the cytoplasm.

The Na^+/K^+ pump is called an electrogenic pump because it produces an electric potential across the neuronal membrane. A small voltage potential develops across the membrane as the Na^+/K^+ pump removes three Na^+ ions from a neuron for every two K^+ ions that are transported into the cell. Although the cytoplasm becomes more negative with respect to the extracellular fluid, the Na^+/K^+ pump has only a small influence on the resting membrane potential and absolutely no role in generating action potentials. Selective inhibition of the Na^+/K^+ pump with ouabain, a plant glycoside, does not prevent the generation of action potentials. After applying ouabain, the concentration gradients for Na^+ and K^+ eventually dissipate, but only after thousands of action potentials have occurred. The importance of the Na^+/K^+ pump lies in its ability to generate large concentration gradients

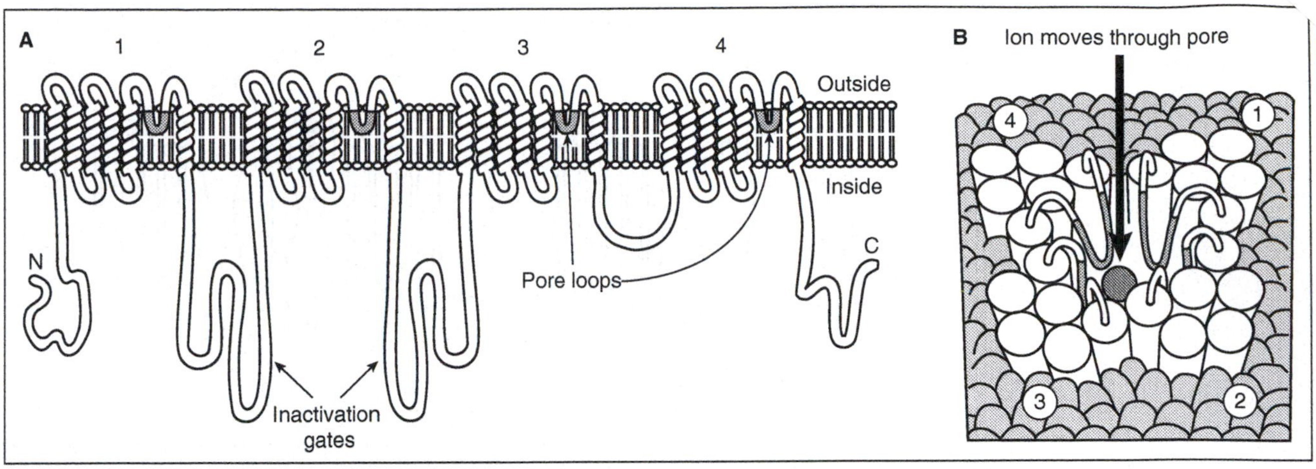

FIG. 1.16. Ion Channels. (A) An example of an ion channel constructed from four protein subunits, each of which has six membrane-spanning regions. The extracellular and intracellular loops act as gates that block ions from passing through the pore. (B) The protein subunits encircle a central, water-filled pore.

that provide the driving force for the diffusion of Na^+ and K^+ when the membrane becomes selectively permeable to these ions during the conduction of action potentials.

Ion Channels. Neuronal membranes contain many ion channels that provide stable openings for the diffusion of specific ions. Although most channels are selective for only one type of ion (e.g., K^+ channels), some channels permit diffusion of more than one ionic species.

Ion channels consist of multiple protein subunits that are bound to the lipid plasma membrane by uncharged lipophilic amino acid residues. Each subunit is a glycoprotein molecule that is composed of several transmembrane segments linked to each other by intracellular and extracellular loops of amino acids. When grouped together, the subunits form a cylindrical structure that encircles a water-filled channel through the plasma membrane (Figure 1.16).

The selectivity of an ion channel is determined by its geometric structure, the diameter of its pore, and the distribution of charged groups of amino acids within the pore. Ions can be blocked from passing through a channel by small loops of amino acid residues that project into the aqueous pore from the transmembrane subunits. These intrapore loops act as "gates" that control the flow of ions through the channel. Electrostatic forces across the membrane may alter the conformational structure of the gate, thereby causing the channel to open or close.

Voltage-Gated Channels. Voltage-gated ion channels are located in all parts of a neuron's membrane, including the axon, and are essential for the propagation of action potentials. The ability of an ion to pass through a voltage-gated ion channel is controlled by the magnitude and polarity of the potential difference across the plasma membrane. The amino acid loops within the channel pore contain electrical charges and, depending on the polarity of those charges, the loops either open or close the channel according to the polarity of the ionic charges that line the two sides of the neuronal membrane. In addition, because of the polarity of the channel "gate," it may rapidly switch between the open and closed states when the membrane potential reverses its polarity.

Some ion channels, such as the voltage-gated K^+ channel, have only a single gate (Figure 1.17), while others, such as the voltage-gated Na^+ channel, have multiple gates (Figure 1.18). If all the gates of a voltage-gated Na^+ channel are in the open position, the channel permits the flow of hydrated sodium ions. If one or more gates are closed, however, sodium ions cannot pass through the channel. Ion channels that have more than

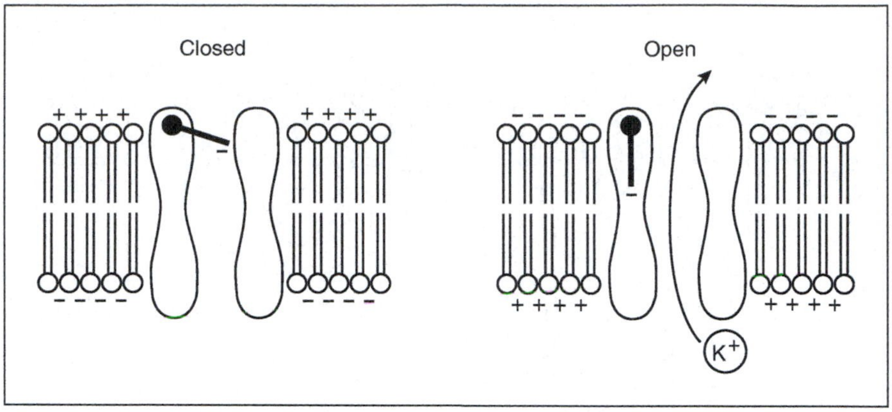

FIG. 1.17. Voltage-Gated K^+ Channel. A single gate determines whether a voltage-gated K^+ channel is in the open or closed state.

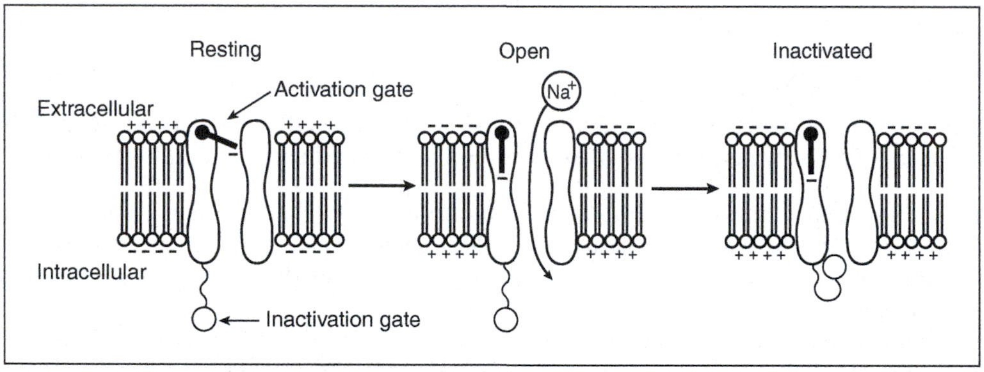

FIG. 1.18. Voltage-Gated Na^+ Channel. Two gates control ion flow through a voltage-gated Na^+ channel. The combination of opened and closed positions allows voltage-gated Na^+ channels to exist in three different states. The activation gate is controlled exclusively by membrane voltage. The inactivation gate closes in a time-dependent manner soon after the membrane is depolarized.

one gate have special biophysical properties because different mechanisms may control each gate (see Ionic Basis of Action Potentials, later in this chapter).

Ligand-Gated Channels. Ligand-gated ion channels are physically linked to receptors that are activated by specific neurotransmitters or other ligands that have a similar molecular structure. When a neurotransmitter molecule binds to the receptor of a ligand-gated channel, the conformational structure of the ion channel changes and the gate opens.

Ligand-gated channels mediate the local EPSPs and IPSPs initiated by synaptic transmission. Consequently, ligand-gated channels are very dense at synaptic sites located on the soma, dendrites, or synaptic terminals. In contrast to voltage-gated channels, ligand-gated channels are not located along the axon.

Ionic Basis of Membrane Potentials

Membrane potentials are determined by ion concentration gradients and by the ionic permeability of the membrane.

The membrane potential of a neuron is determined by the differential concentration of ions across the membrane and by the permeability of specific ion channels. The intracellular and extracellular concentrations of K^+, Na^+, Ca^{2+}, and Cl^- usually stay in a narrow range, but the permeability of the voltage-gated and ligand-gated ion channels may vary tremendously. By opening just a few ion channels, the resulting flow of ions can

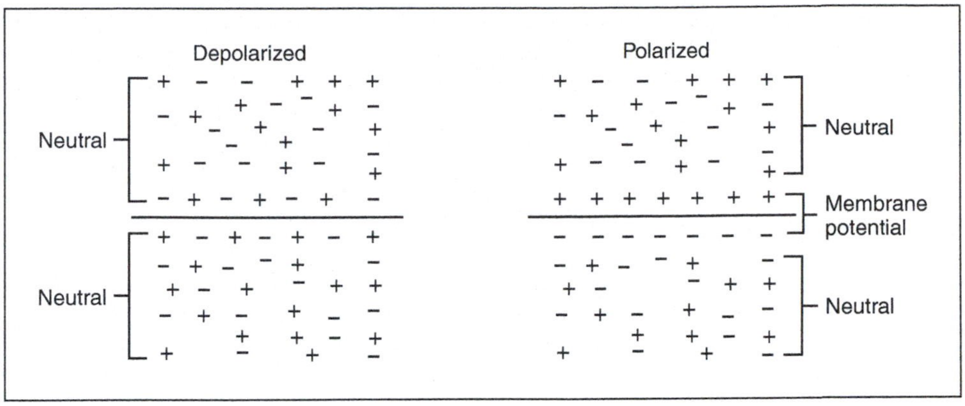

FIG. 1.19. Membrane Potentials. Most of the extracellular fluid and neuronal cytoplasm is electrically neutral. Only a small fraction of the ions move across the membrane and produce a membrane potential; the charges contributing to the membrane potential line each side of the membrane.

produce noticeable changes in the membrane potential. Large shifts in membrane potential may accompany small ionic currents because most of the cytoplasm and extracellular fluid are electrically neutral. Only the ions lining the surfaces of the membrane contribute to the magnitude and polarity of the membrane potential (Figure 1.19).

Resting Membrane Potentials

Most neurons have resting membrane potentials between −60 and −70 mV. The negative polarity of the resting membrane potential is due largely to leaky voltage-gated K^+ channels. To understand this phenomenon, consider what would happen if a neuron had a membrane potential that was neutral and the membrane was only permeable to K^+ (Figure 1.20). Under these conditions, K^+ would flow out of the neuron because K^+ is 30 times more concentrated in the cytoplasm than in the extracellular fluid (see Table 1.2). As K^+ leaves the cytoplasm, a potential difference develops across the membrane because negative charges accumulate inside the cell. In time, K^+ efflux would gradually slow down

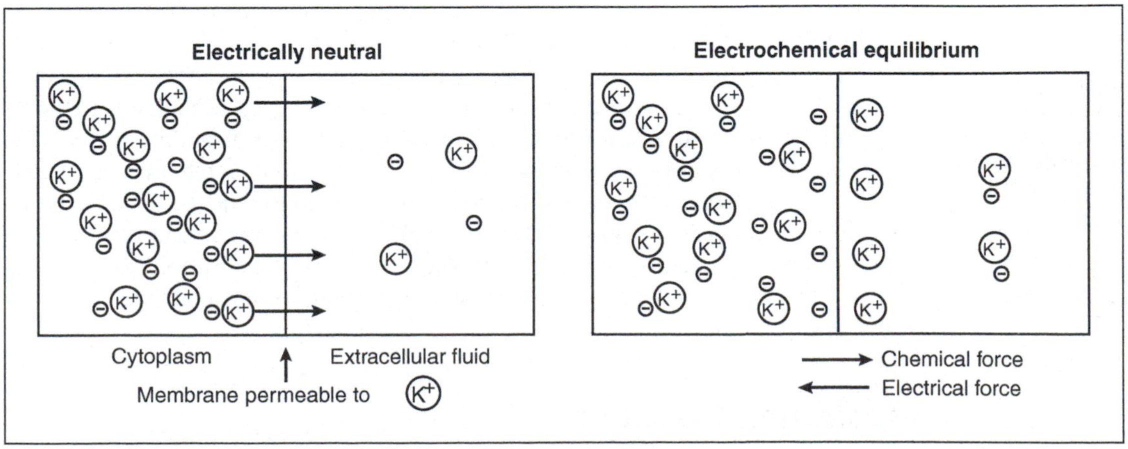

FIG. 1.20. Ionic Basis for Resting Membrane Potentials. A negative membrane potential develops if the membrane is selectively permeable to K^+. The membrane potential is initially zero but becomes negative as K^+ flows down its concentration gradient. Equilibrium is reached when the force of the chemical concentration gradient is counterbalanced by an electrical force acting in the opposite direction.

because of the increasing electrostatic attraction between the negatively charged cytoplasm and the positively charged K^+ ions. Eventually, K^+ influx and efflux would attain a state of equilibrium because the chemical force of the concentration gradient would be opposed by an electrical force of equal strength. Hence, although K^+ ions would still move across the neuronal membrane, K^+ would flow in both directions at equal rates.

Nernst Equation

The membrane potential at which equilibrium occurs for an ionic species is called the equilibrium potential for that ion. The equilibrium potential for K^+ (E_{K^+}), Na^+ (E_{Na^+}), Ca^{2+} ($E_{Ca^{2+}}$), or Cl^- (E_{Cl^-}) can be calculated from the Nernst equation, which assumes that the chemical and electrical gradients are equal:

$$\text{electric potential gradient} = \text{chemical concentration gradient} \quad (1)$$

In the Nernst equation, the magnitude or driving force of the electric potential gradient is the product of the valence of the ion (z), Faraday's constant (F), and the membrane potential at that ion's equilibrium point (E):

$$\text{electric potential gradient} = zFE \quad (2)$$

The driving force of the chemical concentration gradient is the product of the gas constant (R), the absolute temperature (T), and the natural logarithm of the ratio of the ionic concentrations in the extracellular and intracellular compartments:

$$\text{chemical concentration gradient} = RT\ln[\text{ion}]_{out}/[\text{ion}]_{in} \quad (3)$$

By substituting the expressions from equations 2 and 3 into equation 1, we get:

$$ZFE = RT\ln[\text{ion}]_{out}/[\text{ion}]_{in} \quad (4)$$

The equilibrium potential (E) is the only unknown value and is expressed as the Nernst equation:

$$E = (RT/zF)\ln[\text{ion}]_{out}/[\text{ion}]_{in} \quad (5)$$

The Nernst equation can be simplified by substituting standard values for body temperature and the other physical constants, and by converting to base 10. For ions with a valence of 1, the Nernst equation is expressed as:

$$E = 60(\log_{10}[\text{ion}]_{out}/[\text{ion}]_{in} \quad (6)$$

Using the concentrations in Table 1.2, the equilibrium potential for K^+ is approximately −86 mV. By comparison, the equilibrium potential for Na^+ is +60 mV and the equilibrium potential for Cl^- is −66 mV.

An ion's **equilibrium potential** is the membrane potential that results when a membrane is permeable to only one ionic species.

The equilibrium potential is a key concept because a selective increase in the permeability of one type of ion channel shifts the entire membrane potential toward the equilibrium potential of that ion. If a neurotransmitter increases the permeability of Na^+ channels, for example, the concentration gradient for Na^+ compels it to flow into the cell, thereby shifting the membrane potential toward the equilibrium potential for Na^+ (+60 mV). By contrast, an increase in the permeability of K^+ channels shifts the membrane potential toward the equilibrium potential for K^+ (−86 mV). An increase in the permeability of Cl^- channels has little effect because the resting potential and the equilibrium potential for Cl^- are nearly identical (see Table 1.2).

Goldman Equation

The Nernst equation indicates how the membrane potential is affected if the membrane is permeable to only one ionic species, but this assumption is rarely true. In most neurons, some fraction of each type of ion channel is always open, and the membrane potential at any moment in time reflects the relative permeability of the membrane to ions that diffuse through different ligand-gated and voltage-gated channels. For this reason, the Goldman equation was developed to provide a general account of the relationship between membrane potential (V) and the relative permeability (P) of each population of ion channels:

$$V = 60\log\frac{P_{K^+}[K^+]_{out} + P_{Na^+}[Na^+]_{out} + P_{Cl^-}[Cl^-]_{in}}{P_{K^+}[K^+]_{in} + P_{Na^+}[Na^+]_{in} + P_{Cl^-}[Cl^-]_{out}} \quad (7)$$

The Goldman equation is similar to the Nernst equation, but it applies whenever the membrane is permeable to more than one ion. If the permeability for two of the ions approaches zero, the Goldman equation is virtually equivalent to the Nernst equation. The only difference is that the Goldman equation does not contain a valence factor, and therefore, the ratio of intracellular and extracellular concentrations must be inverted for Cl^- ions.

The Goldman equation is important because it illustrates how the membrane potential is determined by both ionic concentration and membrane permeability. If the membrane becomes permeable to only one ion, the membrane potential will shift toward the equilibrium potential for that ion. If the membrane becomes permeable to more than one ion, the Goldman equation indicates that the membrane potential varies according to the relative permeability of the membrane to different ions. During a sudden increase in the permeability of one type of ion channel, the membrane potential rapidly shifts toward the equilibrium potential of that ion.

Given the factors that influence the membrane potential, it is possible to understand why most neurons have a negative resting membrane potential between −60 and −70 mV. Because the resting membrane is permeable to K^+, an efflux of K^+ down its concentration gradient causes an accumulation of negative charges in the cytoplasm. Intracellular recordings have confirmed this explanation by showing how relative changes in the extracellular concentration of K^+ affect the resting membrane potential. When extracellular K^+ is experimentally increased, the resting membrane potential shifts to a depolarized level. When the extracellular and intracellular concentrations of K^+ are made equal, the resting membrane potential is 0 mV. By comparison, changing the extracellular concentrations of Na^+ or Cl^- has negligible effects on resting membrane potential. These findings indicate that the resting membrane potential is negative mainly because the resting membrane is more permeable to K^+ than to Na^+ or Cl^-. The resting membrane potential is not identical to equilibrium potential for K^+, however, because the resting membrane is slightly permeable to Na^+ and Cl^-.

> The **resting membrane potential** of most neurons is between −60 and −70 mV because the resting membrane is leaky to K^+.

Passive Membrane Properties of Neurons

Neurons are relatively poor conductors of passive ionic currents. To illustrate this fact, consider an experiment in which a micropipette is filled with a concentrated NaCl solution, and then its tip is carefully placed inside an axon. As the axon is depolarized by injecting Na^+ into the cytoplasm, the change in membrane potential is monitored by electrodes placed at regular intervals along the axon (Figure 1.21). Assuming the depolarization is too weak to evoke an action potential, the change in membrane potential is greatest at the site of Na^+ injection and declines exponentially along the axon.

The magnitude of depolarization is not equal at all points along the neuron's membrane for two reasons. First, the axon cytoplasm impedes ionic diffusion, especially in small-diameter axons, because the resistance to flow varies inversely with the cross-sectional area of the conductor. Cytoplasmic resistance also increases with axon length because ions are more likely to collide with each other as they travel a longer route through the axon. Second, even though the neuronal membrane is a formidable barrier, some of the Na^+ ions injected into the cytoplasm will leak through the plasma membrane into the extracellular space. This efflux of Na^+ allows the depolarization to dissipate with increasing distance from the injection site because fewer Na^+ ions are available to charge the inner surface of the membrane.

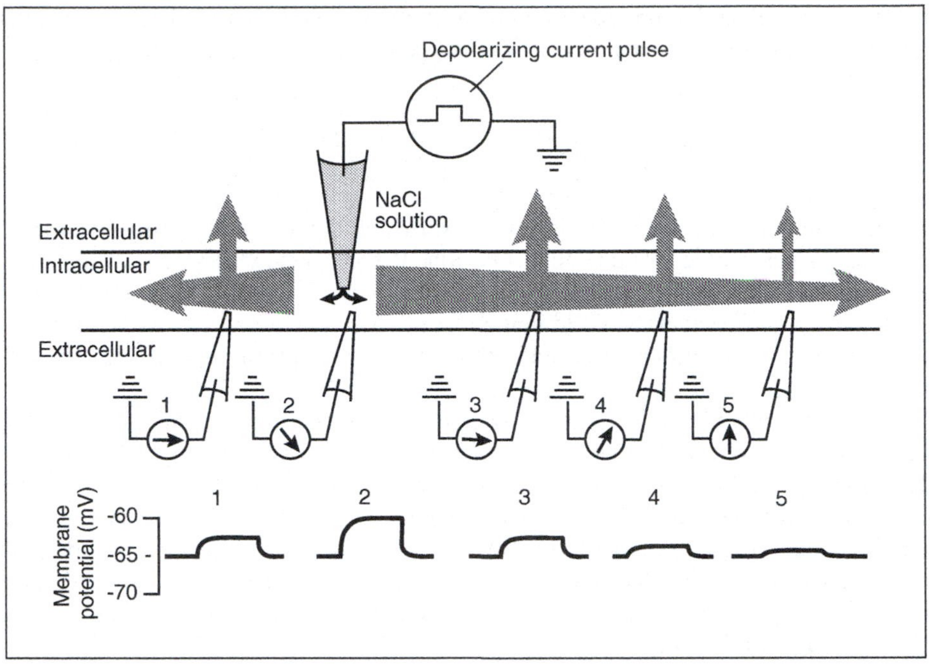

FIG. 1.21. Passive Current Flow. When small amounts of Na^+ are injected into a neuron, the level of depolarization is greatest at the injection site. The level of depolarization declines with distance as Na^+ flows back to the extracellular space.

Membrane Time Constants

A **membrane time constant** indicates how long a charge is held by a membrane before dissipating.

When Na^+ enters the cytoplasm, either experimentally or during neuronal activity, the change in membrane potential does not occur instantaneously. It takes time for membrane depolarization to develop because some of the Na^+ ions entering the cytoplasm return immediately to the extracellular fluid. Only Na^+ ions that remain in the cytoplasm contribute to the depolarization of the membrane potential. Eventually, as Na^+ continues to enter the cytoplasm, the membrane attains a steady state or peak amplitude of depolarization. The time it takes for the membrane to reach 63% of the peak depolarization is called the membrane time constant τ_m (tau). The magnitude of the time constant is proportional to the resistance (R_m) and capacitance (C_m) of the membrane:

$$\tau_m = R_m \times C_m \tag{8}$$

Membrane resistance (R_m) indicates how well the membrane prevents the passage of charged ions, and it is inversely proportional to the conductance of its ion channels. Hence, a membrane in which the ion channels are closed has a higher membrane resistance than one in which the ion channels are open. The capacitance of a membrane (C_m) indicates the capacity of the membrane to hold positive and negative charges. Thin membranes hold charges much better than thick membranes because electrostatic attraction decreases with increasing distance between the charged ions.

Neurons with long time constants have membrane properties that enhance their ability to integrate multiple inputs. Because the membrane resistance is high in neurons with a long time constant, a given amount of Na^+ influx produces a large depolarization that dissipates slowly. Both of these characteristics increase the probability that inputs from neighboring synapses may sum together to produce a larger graded potential. By comparison, neurons with shorter time constants have a lower membrane resistance that permits the return of Na^+ to the extracellular space before the graded potentials have an opportunity to be summed.

Membrane Length Constants

Sodium ions entering the cytoplasm at one region either return to the extracellular space immediately or travel through the axon's cytoplasm for some distance before exiting the neuron. The standard unit for measuring the passive spread of Na^+ current through the axon is the membrane length constant λ (lambda). The length constant represents the distance between the point of peak depolarization produced by Na^+ influx and the point where depolarization has declined to 37% of the peak value. Because Na^+ ions either flow through the cytoplasm or through the membrane, the length constant is related to the resistance offered by these two routes. Thus, λ is expressed as the square root of the ratio of the membrane resistance (R_m) to the internal resistance of the cytoplasm (R_i):

$$\lambda = (R_m/R_i)^{1/2} \tag{9}$$

This equation for the length constant indicates that Na^+ current is more likely to spread farther along the axon if the membrane resistance (R_m) is higher than the internal resistance (R_i) of the cytoplasm. The resistance offered by these routes is determined not only by their inherent conductivity but also by the diameter of the axon. As the axon diameter increases, both R_m and R_i decrease. For a given length, a thicker axon has a larger membrane area and more channels through which Na^+ may pass. Similarly, a thicker axon allows Na^+ current to pass more easily through the cytoplasm, just as water encounters less resistance when passing through a wide hose than through a narrow hose. Because of differences in the relative growth of volume and surface area, R_i decreases more rapidly than R_m as axons become larger in diameter. Thus, when all other factors are equal, the length constant is longer for large-diameter axons than for small-diameter axons.

A **membrane length constant** indicates the distance that a graded potential spreads passively before dissipating.

Passive Spread of Graded Potentials

The passive movement of graded potentials through the dendrites and soma is determined largely by the length and time constants of the neuron. In general, a subthreshold stimulus spreads further and persists longer in neurons that have large length and time constants. Neurons with these properties are more likely to discharge because the subthreshold depolarizations produced by multiple synaptic inputs are more likely to sum together to produce a membrane potential that exceeds the threshold for generating an action potential.

Ionic Basis of Action Potentials

If the membrane potential at the axon hillock depolarizes to a critical threshold level, the neuron produces an action potential. In contrast to graded potentials, which vary in amplitude and may dissipate after traveling a short distance, action potentials propagate the entire length of the axon without any decrement in amplitude and, therefore, are often called "all-or-none" potentials. Unlike graded potentials, which have monophasic shapes, action potentials have biphasic waveforms that reflect underlying changes in membrane permeability (or conductance) to Na^+ and K^+ (Figure 1.22).

Action potentials are generated when the axonal membrane becomes permeable to Na^+ and the resulting influx of Na^+ is sufficient to depolarize the membrane to threshold. When this critical value has been reached, Na^+ permeability increases dramatically and the electrochemical gradient for Na^+ forces it into the cell. The tremendous influx of Na^+ further depolarizes the membrane potential toward the equilibrium potential for Na^+ (+60 mV). Subsequently, this strong depolarization of the membrane potential activates the voltage-gated K^+ channels and K^+ begins to flow out of the neuron (see "open" state in Figure 1.17). Eventually, Na^+ influx ceases because the voltage-gated Na^+ channels become inactivated during maintained depolarization (see "inactivated" state in Figure 1.18). The efflux of K^+ shifts the membrane potential toward the equilibrium potential for K^+ and re-establishes the resting membrane potential.

Action potentials are mediated by an influx of Na^+ and a delayed efflux of K^+.

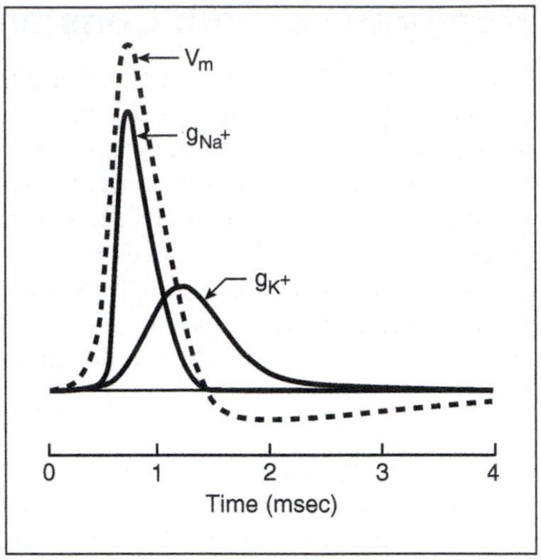

FIG. 1.22. Ionic Basis of Action Potentials. Changes in the membrane conductance of Na^+ (g_{Na^+}) and K^+ (g_{K^+}) determine the action potential waveform (V_m). Note that the initial depolarization is mediated by an increase in sodium conductance, whereas the subsequent hyperpolarization is mediated by an increase in potassium.

Voltage-Dependent Ion Currents

Action potentials are triggered when the membrane is depolarized to a critical level. This finding suggests that the changes in membrane permeability during an action potential are controlled by the ionic charges on the membrane. In the 1940s, Alan Hodgkin and Andrew Huxley tested this hypothesis by using the voltage-clamp technique to hold (i.e., clamp) the membrane voltage of an axon at a constant level. By clamping the membrane potential at a constant voltage, they could study time-dependent changes in membrane permeability independent of the secondary shifts in potential that accompany each change in membrane permeability.

The voltage-clamp experiments by Hodgkin and Huxley demonstrated that transmembrane ionic currents are voltage-dependent. Clamping the membrane at a constant level of depolarization causes an initial inward current that is followed by a later outward current (Figure 1.23). The magnitude of the inward current varies with the clamped voltage, gradually increasing as the membrane potential is clamped at voltages ranging from

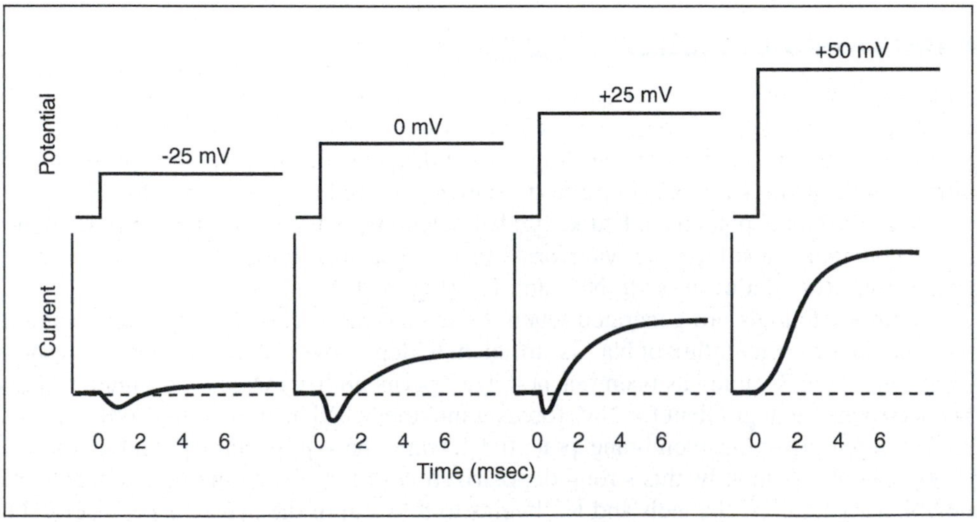

FIG. 1.23. Ionic Currents during Voltage Clamp. These graphs show changes in current flow when clamping the membrane potential at successively higher levels of depolarization. At moderate levels of depolarization, current initially flows inward and then outward. When the membrane is clamped near the equilibrium potential for Na^+ (+50 mV), all current flows outward.

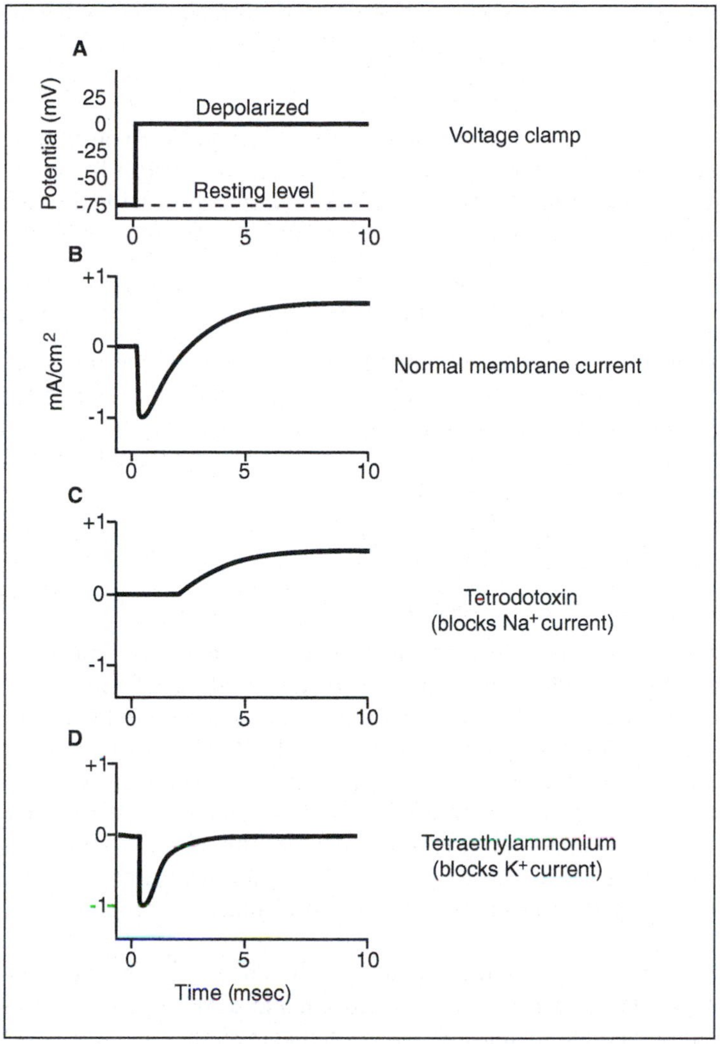

FIG. 1.24. Ionic Basis of Early and Late Currents. (A) The change in membrane potential is recorded when a neuron is clamped at a constant voltage level during different pharmacologic manipulations. (B) The membrane potential normally shows an early inward and a late outward current during depolarization. (C) When Na^+ channels are blocked by tetrodotoxin, only the late outward current is present. (D) When K^+ channels are blocked by tetraethylammonium, only the early inward current is present.

−40 to 0 mV. Inward current is maximal at depolarizations maintained between 0 and +20 mV but is weaker when the membrane is clamped above +20 mV. If the membrane potential is clamped at the equilibrium potential for Na^+ (+60 mV), the initial inward current disappears, and this suggests that Na^+ influx must mediate the early inward current. By comparison, the late outward current increases as the membrane potential is clamped at progressively higher voltage levels. When the membrane voltage is clamped at the equilibrium potential for K^+ (−86 mV), the late outward current disappears, suggesting that K^+ efflux mediates the late outward current.

Pharmacologic manipulations confirm that the inward and outward currents of action potentials are mediated by Na^+ and K^+, respectively (Figure 1.24). Application of tetrodotoxin, a neurotoxin emitted by the puffer fish, selectively blocks Na^+ channels and prevents the early inward current regardless of the membrane potential. Application of tetraethylammonium, which selectively blocks K^+ channels, prevents the late outward current without affecting the early inward current.

Ion Channel Conductance

After establishing that action potentials are mediated by Na^+ influx followed by K^+ efflux, Hodgkin and Huxley used Ohm's law to calculate the changes in Na^+ and K^+ ion channel conductance as a function of membrane voltage. Ohm's law is a mathematical expression of current (I) as it relates to voltage (V) and resistance (R):

$$I = V/R \qquad (10)$$

In terms of the ionic current flow across a neuronal membrane, Ohm's law is expressed:

$$I = (V_m - E_{ion})/R \qquad (11)$$

Ionic conductance indicates the relative ease with which an ion passes through a channel.

where the difference between the resting membrane potential (V_m) and the equilibrium potential (E_{ion}) is the driving force that compels the ion across the membrane. Ion channel conductance (g_{ion}) indicates the permeability or relative ease of passing an ion through a channel. In mathematical terms, conductance is the reciprocal of resistance and, after substitution, equation 11 becomes:

$$I_{ion} = g_{ion}(V_m - E_{ion}) \qquad (12)$$

In the voltage-clamp experiments by Hodgkin and Huxley, a series of current measurements were taken in the presence and absence of extracellular Na^+ to establish the flow of I_{Na^+} and I_{K^+} at different membrane potentials. When the membrane voltage (V_m) is experimentally controlled and the equilibrium potentials for Na^+ and K^+ are known, it is possible to calculate the conductances for these ions:

$$g_{Na^+} = I_{Na^+}/(V_m - E_{Na^+}) \qquad (13)$$

$$g_{K^+} = I_{K^+}/(V_m - E_{K^+}) \qquad (14)$$

Hodgkin and Huxley's calculation of Na^+ and K^+ conductances at different membrane potentials indicates that ion conductance is proportional to the level of depolarization. This relationship between ionic conductance and membrane potential indicates the presence of voltage-gated ion channels that are controlled by the polarity of ionic charges on the plasma membrane. Loops of amino acids in the channel's pore and groups of amino acids in the membrane-spanning domains have electrical charges that cause them to change their conformational position when the membrane polarity is altered. These changes in the physical structure of a channel explain why shifts in membrane potential can selectively control ion flow through the channel (see Figures 1.17 and 1.18).

When a membrane is depolarized, the time course of the change in channel conductance is not identical for Na^+ and K^+ voltage-gated channels. While the onset of depolarization produces an immediate increase in Na^+ conductance, the increase in K^+ conductance is delayed. This timing difference allows Na^+ influx to precede K^+ efflux; otherwise, the membrane potential would never depolarize. If depolarization is prolonged over several milliseconds, however, Na^+ conductance quickly reaches a peak and then declines as the voltage-gated Na^+ channels start to close, thereby reducing the rate of Na^+ flow into the cytoplasm. This suggests that voltage-gated Na^+ channels become inactivated even if the membrane remains in a constant state of depolarization. By comparison, depolarization causes a gradual increase in K^+ conductance that reaches an asymptotic level and persists for the duration of the depolarization (Figure 1.24C). This indicates that K^+ channels remain open indefinitely when the membrane is depolarized.

In summary, action potentials are mediated entirely by changes in the permeability of Na^+ and K^+ voltage-gated channels (see Figure 1.22). The rising phase of the action potential is due to the rapid influx of Na^+ produced by an increase in Na^+ conductance. The rate of Na^+ influx slows as the difference between the membrane potential and the equilibrium potential for Na^+ is reduced. Subsequently, even before the membrane potential reaches the equilibrium potential for Na^+, the action potential reaches its peak amplitude when the Na^+ channels become inactivated. The falling phase of the action potential is mediated by the delayed increase in K^+ conductance. Consequently, K^+ efflux is greatest just after the peak of the action potential and declines as the membrane potential approaches the equilibrium potential for K^+. The membrane is briefly hyperpolarized because K^+ conductance only returns to resting levels after the membrane voltage has declined below the normal resting potential.

Threshold

The threshold for initiating action potentials may vary but is usually around −50 mV for most mammalian neurons, or approximately 10–15 mV above the resting potential. If a synaptic input does not activate enough voltage-gated Na^+ channels, a subthreshold excitatory potential is produced. At resting potentials, K^+ normally leaks out of most neurons and K^+ conductance is generally higher than Na^+ conductance. Because K^+ permeability is higher than Na^+ permeability at the resting potential, the tonic efflux of K^+ slows depolarization and provides enough time to activate additional K^+ channels that restore the membrane potential to resting levels. Consequently, small depolarizations are easily countered by the efflux of K^+. As graded excitatory potentials become larger, however, Na^+ influx and K^+ efflux act as competing influences, and the membrane potential may briefly linger at a constant level of depolarization before returning to the resting potential. If Na^+ influx exceeds K^+ efflux, the exponential increase in Na^+ conductance cannot be offset by the delayed activation of additional K^+ channels. Hence, the threshold for generating an action potential is the membrane potential at which the rate of Na^+ influx surpasses the rate of K^+ efflux.

The **threshold** for an action potential is the membrane potential at which Na^+ influx exceeds K^+ efflux.

Axonal Propagation of Impulses

After an action potential has been generated at the axon hillock, it propagates the entire length of the axon without stopping or losing amplitude. This feature is related to the active and passive conduction properties of the membrane. When an action potential occurs, the influx of depolarizing current is passively conducted through neighboring parts of the axoplasm. Although the amount of current declines rapidly with distance (see Figure 1.21), it is strong enough to depolarize adjacent parts of the axon to threshold. At these neighboring sites, the voltage-activated Na^+ channels allow even more Na^+ to enter the axoplasm and spread passively to the next axonal segment. Thus, the passive and active membrane properties cooperate with each other to generate an action potential in successive regions of the axon. As this process is repeated continuously along the axon, the action potential propagates without any decrement in its amplitude (Figure 1.25).

Refractory Periods

Immediately after an action potential has occurred, the neuron is unable to discharge again for a brief time period. This interval, known as the absolute refractory period, occurs because voltage-gated Na^+ channels are inactivated during the falling edge of the action potential waveform (see "inactivated" state in Figure 1.18). The neuron is unable to discharge an action potential during this period, regardless of the intensity of the depolarizing stimulus. As Na^+ channels gradually recover from their state of inactivation, the neuron enters a relative refractory period and can discharge only in response to large, suprathreshold depolarizations. The duration of the refractory period varies across neurons as a function of density of ion channels along the axonal membrane.

The refractory period imposes an upper limit on the discharge rate that can be sustained by a neuron. This upper rate (in discharges/sec) can be calculated by dividing 1 second of time (1000 msec) by the duration (in msec) of the refractory period. Another consequence of the refractory period is that action potentials travel in only one direction after leaving the axon hillock. After an action potential propagates down the axon, inactivation of voltage-gated Na^+ channels at the trailing edge of the waveform prevents a reversal in the direction of propagation.

The **refractory period** is the time interval during which Na^+ channels are inactivated.

Conduction Velocity and Saltatory Propagation

Each axon conducts action potentials at a constant velocity, but a wide range of conduction velocities have been recorded from different axons because the speed of propagation is proportional to axon diameter and myelin thickness. Large-diameter axons are heavily

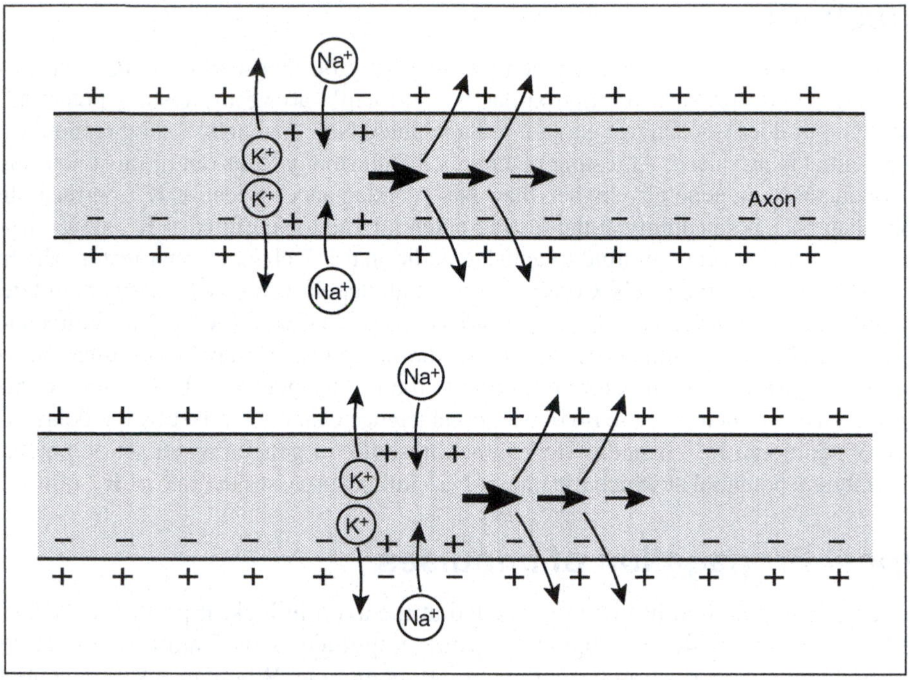

FIG. 1.25. Propagation of an Action Potential. An action potential requires active and passive flow of depolarizing current in the axoplasm. Where the voltage-gated sodium channels are open, Na^+ actively flows into the axon. Incoming Na^+ flows passively in both directions of the axon, but Na^+ channels are inactivated at the trailing edge of the action potential. By contrast, Na^+ channels located at the leading edge of the action potential are activated and allow more Na^+ to enter the axoplasm. As the action potential propagates through the axon, the membrane potential returns to resting levels as K^+ flows into the extracellular fluid at the trailing edge of the action potential. Thin arrows represent the direction of ion movements; thicker arrows represent the direction of the action potential.

myelinated and have fast conduction velocities; small-diameter axons are thinly myelinated and have moderate conduction velocities. The thinnest axons are unmyelinated and have the slowest conduction velocities.

Axon diameter and myelination dictate conduction velocity as a consequence of their effects on the length constant of the membrane. As discussed earlier, the length constant varies as a function of the resistive properties of the neuron's membrane and axoplasm. Large-diameter axons have a low axoplasmic resistance that allows depolarizing currents to spread rapidly in a passive manner. Thus, when compared to small-diameter axons, passive Na^+ currents travel more efficiently through the axoplasm of large-diameter axons, and this enhances the conduction velocity of their action potentials.

Myelination:
- Increases membrane resistance.
- Increases the membrane length constant.
- Increases axonal conduction velocity.

Conduction velocity also increases as the resistance of the axon membrane increases. Myelination increases membrane resistance by adding another barrier that prevents the flow of ions from the axoplasm to the extracellular space. Because ionic currents do not pass easily through myelination, incoming Na^+ is more likely to flow through the axoplasm until it reaches the next node of Ranvier, which is unmyelinated. Nodes of Ranvier are spaced at regular intervals along the axon and contain a higher density of voltage-gated Na^+ channels than the myelinated parts of the axon. Consequently, depolarizing current at one node of Ranvier flows passively through the axoplasm to the next node of Ranvier, thereby driving the membrane potential to threshold so that the voltage-activated Na^+ channels produce another action potential. As this process is repeated, action potentials essentially jump from one node of Ranvier to the next. This rapid form of propagation is called saltatory conduction (Figure 1.26).

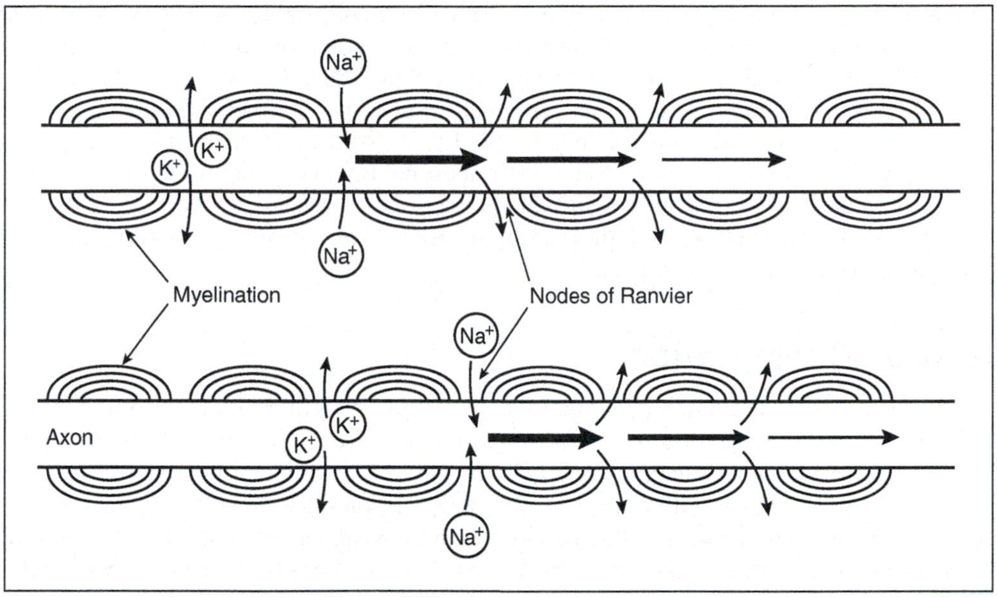

FIG. 1.26. Saltatory Conduction. Myelination increases the resistance of the axonal membrane and prevents Na^+ from leaving the axon except at the nodes of Ranvier. Current flows passively through the axoplasm and depolarizes the axon to threshold at the next node of Ranvier. This process causes the action potential to propagate more quickly than in unmyelinated axons.

NEURONAL INTERACTIONS

One of the major functions of the CNS is to integrate information from different sources. For this reason, the brain and spinal cord are organized into nuclei that process sensory, motor, autonomic, or cognitive information.

Definition of a Nucleus

A nucleus is a compact group of neurons that perform a specific function or neural computation. The function of a nucleus depends on the type of information that it receives from its afferent connections, the layout of its intrinsic neuronal circuits, and the pattern of its output projections to other brain regions. The main purpose of most nuclei is to perform some transformation on the input signals so that information useful to the organism can be extracted and sent to other brain regions for further processing. Nuclei that process similar information and have direct connections with each other are frequently grouped together into neural systems such as the visual system, the auditory system, and so on.

All nuclei are composed of three basic components: (1) incoming axons and their synaptic terminals, (2) intrinsic neurons, and (3) principal neurons. Intrinsic neurons are called local circuit neurons or interneurons because all of their processes, including their axons, reside within the nucleus. By comparison, the axon of a principal neuron is longer and projects beyond the nucleus to other brain regions. Principal neurons are sometimes called projection neurons because their axons comprise the projection fibers of the brain and spinal cord.

Intrinsic neurons project locally.
Principal neurons project to distant targets.

The specific interconnections between intrinsic and principal neurons determine how information is processed in a nucleus. These interconnections can be extremely complex, and few rules govern the types of neuronal connections that may exist within a nucleus. For example, axons may terminate on all neurons in a nucleus or only on certain subsets of neurons. Thus, incoming axons may synapse on intrinsic neurons, principal neurons, or both sets of cells. Within a nucleus, intrinsic neurons may send local projections to other interneurons, to principal neurons, or to both sets of cells. Although principal neurons must project beyond the boundaries of the nucleus, it is not uncommon for principal neurons to have local collaterals that terminate on interneurons or principal neurons within the nucleus.

The physiologic interactions that occur between neurons, either within a nucleus or across different brain regions, cannot be predicted from their neuronal connections. Although most principal neurons excite their neuronal targets, some inhibit their postsynaptic targets. The diversity of neuronal interactions is related to the wide range of different neurotransmitters and the variations in neurotransmitter receptors that are present on the postsynaptic targets.

Neuronal Integration

Each neuron is a miniature computational unit that integrates inputs from multiple sources. The dendrites and soma of most neurons receive excitatory and inhibitory inputs from thousands of synaptic terminals. In general, excitatory inputs from several synapses must summate within a short time period to produce an action potential. The membrane potential of a neuron fluctuates continuously, and action potentials are evoked only when the membrane potential at the axon hillock reaches the threshold level of depolarization. When compared to other parts of the soma, the axon hillock has the highest density of voltage-gated Na^+ channels and, consequently, the lowest threshold level for evoking an action potential. Therefore, much larger changes in membrane potential are needed at the dendrites and soma to produce a graded potential that can travel to the axon hillock and evoke an action potential.

The dendrites and soma constantly integrate numerous excitatory and inhibitory inputs to determine when the neuron should discharge an action potential. The timing of discharges at the axon hillock is determined by several factors, including the number of EPSPs and IPSPs at a given moment, the spatial configuration of these inputs, and the passive membrane properties of the dendrites and soma. The passive membrane properties of a neuron, which are defined by the length and time constants, have predictable effects on the probability that a neuron will integrate synaptic inputs at separate sites or points in time.

Excitatory inputs to a single synapse rarely produce action potentials. Instead, a neuronal discharge usually occurs when the summation of multiple EPSPs exceeds the threshold for an action potential. Synaptic inputs to separate dendrites are unlikely to summate, however, unless the dendritic membrane has a long length constant (Figure 1.27). Long length constants allow EPSPs produced at one dendritic site to spread toward the soma where they may summate with EPSPs produced in other dendrites. This integrative process is known as spatial summation.

Consecutive subthreshold inputs to the same synaptic site may evoke action potentials by means of temporal summation. To integrate a sequence of inputs at the same synapse, the postsynaptic membrane must have a long time constant so that the first EPSP will persist long enough to summate with subsequent EPSPs (Figure 1.27). Otherwise, if the time constant is short and the graded potentials dissipate quickly, a series of impulses arriving at the same synapse would have exactly the same impact on postsynaptic responsiveness as a single EPSP.

As indicated by equations 8 and 9 (in the preceding sections), time constants and length constants are related to the resistive properties of the membrane. Membrane resistance fluctuates, however, because ion channels constantly open and close in response to synaptic inputs. Therefore, time constants and length constants are not static qualities for a given neuron but vary continuously as the neuron receives different excitatory and inhibitory inputs. Hence, antecedent synaptic events may alter a neuron's response to a particular set of inputs by changing the neuron's passive membrane properties.

Synaptic Circuits

The spatial configuration of synaptic connections is extremely important for determining how neurons process information received from multiple sources. Certain synaptic arrangements occur frequently in the CNS and are identified by specific terms (Figure 1.28).

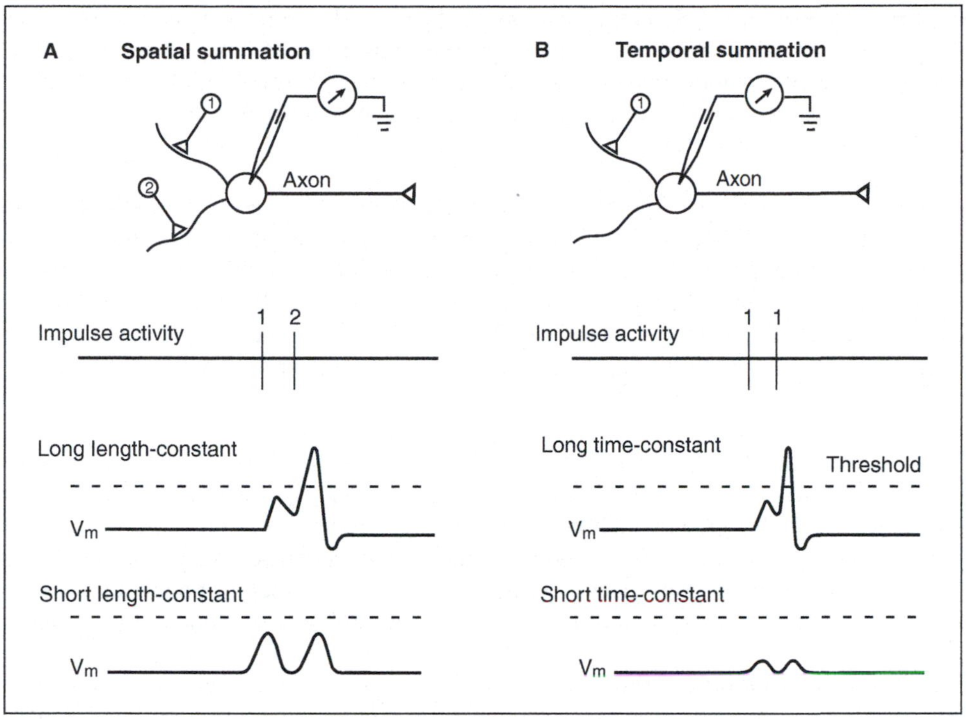

FIG. 1.27. Spatial and Temporal Summation. (A) Two EPSPs produced by neurons 1 and 2 are more likely to combine if the postsynaptic neuron has a long length constant. (B) Two EPSPs produced by consecutive impulses in neuron 1 are more likely to combine if the postsynaptic neuron has a long time constant.

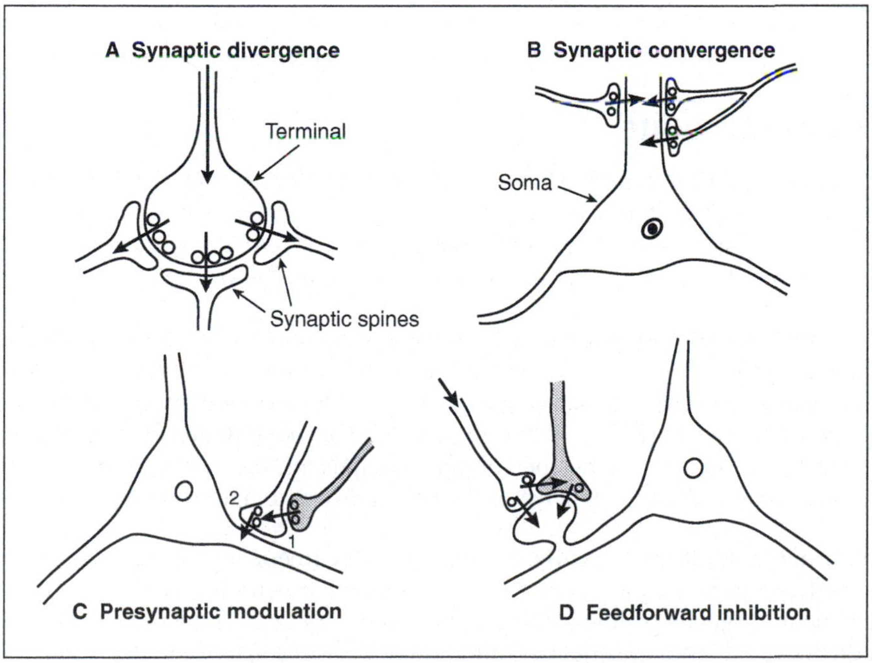

FIG. 1.28. Synaptic Circuits. (A) Synaptic divergence allows incoming signals to activate multiple postsynaptic neurons. (B) Synaptic convergence increases the likelihood that a postsynaptic neuron will discharge. (C) Presynaptic modulation is mediated by an axoaxonic synapse (1) that modulates the efficacy of an axodendritic synapse (2). (D) Synaptic feedforward inhibition occurs when a synaptic terminal simultaneously activates a postsynaptic dendrite and a nearby inhibitory terminal (shaded). This synaptic arrangement produces an EPSP-IPSP sequence in the postsynaptic dendrite.

Synaptic Divergence. Synaptic divergence occurs when one synaptic terminal has functional connections with two or more postsynaptic neurons. By contacting multiple dendrites, the presynaptic neuron can activate multiple neurons simultaneously. Thus, synaptic divergence is a physical arrangement that amplifies the physiologic influence of an incoming action potential.

Synaptic Convergence. Synaptic convergence occurs whenever multiple terminals synapse on the same neuron. The synaptic terminals may originate from the same presynaptic neuron or from several different neurons. In either case, simultaneous activation of a group of convergent synapses increases the size and strength of the postsynaptic potential, thereby increasing the probability that an action potential will be generated. One form of synaptic integration, spatial summation, requires the presence of synaptic convergence.

Presynaptic Modulation. Presynaptic modulation is mediated by a combination of axoaxonic and axodendritic synapses. When one axon terminates on another terminal, neurotransmitter release from the first terminal alters the Ca^{2+} conductance of the second terminal. This process alters the amount of neurotransmitter that the second neuron releases in response to an action potential that propagates down its axon. Hence, presynaptic modulation may temporarily strengthen (or weaken) the efficacy of neurotransmission at axodendritic synapses.

Feedforward Synaptic Inhibition. In some synaptic circuits, synaptic excitation is quickly followed by inhibition. This sequence of events is mediated by three synaptic processes in which an excitatory terminal contacts a postsynaptic dendrite and a neighboring inhibitory terminal (Figure 1.28D). Neurotransmitter release from the excitatory terminal simultaneously depolarizes the postsynaptic dendrite and the neighboring inhibitory terminal. Subsequently, the inhibitory terminal releases its neurotransmitter, and the net effect in the postsynaptic dendrite is a rapid sequence of excitation followed by inhibition. By restricting the duration of EPSPs, feedforward inhibition prevents the prolonged excitation that causes seizures and glutamate-induced neurotoxicity (see Chapter 2). As shown by Figure 1.28, feedforward synaptic inhibition is mediated by a combination of synaptic divergence, synaptic convergence, and presynaptic modulation.

Neuronal Circuits

Basic patterns of neuronal connections are repeated throughout the CNS to process information in specific ways. As shown in Figure 1.29, most neural circuits consist of combinations of the following types of connections: (1) feedforward excitation, (2) feedforward inhibition, (3) lateral inhibition, (4) recurrent inhibition, and (5) disinhibition.

Feedforward Excitatory Circuits. Most principal neurons in the CNS are excitatory, and they frequently project to target neurons that are also excitatory. These neurons, in turn, may excite neighboring neurons in the nucleus or two different groups of excitatory neurons that are reciprocally connected. In addition to providing an opportunity for neuronal convergence and divergence, the combination of monosynaptic and disynaptic excitation alters the timing of excitatory inputs and increases the probability of temporal summation.

Feedforward Inhibitory Circuits. Afferent fibers frequently branch into collaterals that simultaneously activate excitatory and inhibitory neurons. Activation of the inhibitory neuron suppresses the activity in the excitatory neuron. Hence, this mechanism of feedforward inhibition restricts the duration of neuronal activity in the target nucleus.

Lateral Inhibitory Circuits. Lateral inhibition is a specific form of feedforward inhibition that restricts excitation to a small population of neurons. Lateral inhibitory connections are often, but not always, mediated by interneurons that enhance the disparity in activity between neighboring populations of neurons. Lateral inhibition is a common neural mechanism that is used in the visual and somatosensory systems to enhance the perception of edges and boundaries of sensory stimuli when they are encoded in the CNS.

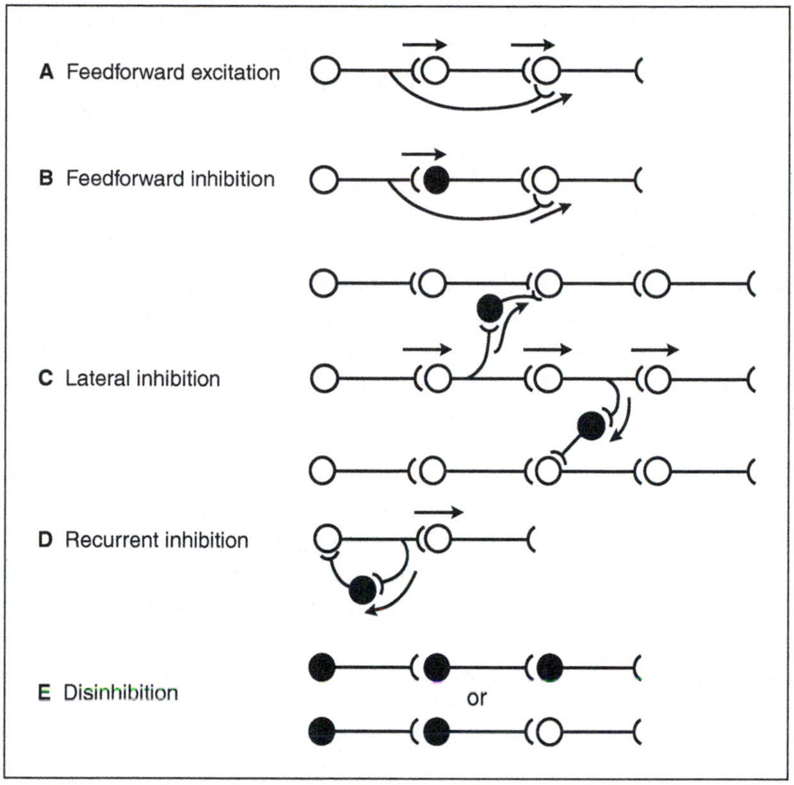

FIG. 1.29. Neuronal Circuits. Diagrams depict basic circuits found in many nuclei. Excitatory and inhibitory neurons are represented by open and solid soma, respectively. Arrows illustrate the flow of excitatory activity. (A) Feedforward excitation alters the timing of excitatory transmission and provides an opportunity for synaptic divergence and convergence. (B) Feedforward inhibition limits the duration of excitatory activity in the third neuron. (C) Lateral inhibition restricts excitatory activity to a select population of neurons. (D) Recurrent inhibition, which is mediated by a local interneuron, limits the duration of activity in the first neuron of the series. (E) Disinhibition involves serial connections between two inhibitory neurons. The third neuron is spontaneously active, and its output is regulated by the preceding inhibitory connections.

Recurrent Inhibition. Recurrent inhibition is common throughout the CNS and is characterized by neurons whose collateral axons activate local inhibitory neurons that project back to the original neuron. Recurrent inhibition restricts the duration of repetitive discharges and enhances the temporal resolution of the excitatory neuron.

Disinhibition. Disinhibition occurs when at least two inhibitory neurons are serially connected with a third neuron. Activity in the first inhibitory neuron inhibits the second neuron, and this prevents the second neuron from inhibiting the third neuron. Consequently, the third neuron is released from inhibition and its discharge rate increases. Disinhibition gradually modulates the discharge rate of the third neuron and thus maintains its discharge rate in a narrow physiological range.

Synaptic Locations

The effectiveness of a synapse depends on its postsynaptic location. Synaptic terminals on distal dendrites may exert less influence on a postsynaptic neuron than synapses near the soma or the axon hillock. Inhibitory neurons often exploit this situation by forming the majority of their synapses near trigger sites on the soma and axon hillock. Because the axon hillock has the lowest threshold for producing an action potential, inhibitory transmission at this site hyperpolarizes the membrane potential and may prevent the

Excitatory synapses form the majority of synapses on the dendrites.

Inhibitory synapses form the majority of synapses on the soma and axon hillock.

neuron from discharging in response to excitatory inputs on the dendrites. For the same reason, inhibitory synapses on the dendritic tree are often located at branch points where they can block excitation at either branch from reaching the soma and axon hillock.

RESOLUTION OF CLINICAL CASE

Most patients will present a constellation of signs and symptoms during the clinical exam. To be competent, the physician must recognize the clinical profiles that characterize specific neurologic disorders. The case in this chapter provides an illustration of multiple sclerosis, an autoimmune disease of unknown etiology that is characterized by demyelination of multiple sites in the central nervous system.

There is no "classic" form of MS, nor is there a specific test for detecting this disease. Accurate diagnosis requires the presence of multiple signs and symptoms, evidence of multiple lesions in the CNS, and a history of remissions and relapses. Onset of MS usually occurs in young adults between the ages of 20 and 40, and the incidence of this disease has a female-to-male ratio of 2:1. Because numerous brain systems can be affected by MS, a wide range of neurologic symptoms have been correlated with the plaques of demyelination. The optic chiasm as well as fiber tracts in the brainstem, cerebellum, and spinal cord are often involved. Consequently, MS is often accompanied by visual field defects, disturbances in eye movements, muscle weakness, spasticity, impaired somatosensory sensations, pain, ataxia, tremor, and autonomic problems. When obvious signs of MS are first present, the patient often remembers previous manifestations of the disease that were ignored because of their mild and transient nature. Additional evidence for MS includes MRI findings of multiple white matter lesions and a decrease in conduction velocities of evoked potentials. Analysis of the cerebral spinal fluid also reveals a large increase in the amount of gamma immunoglobulins because of alterations in the immune system.

Presently there is no cure for MS. The disease follows a relapsing-remitting pattern and may gradually become progressive over the course of several years. Treatments for MS usually rely on repeated administration of steroids or other immunomodulators to manage the acute symptoms and to delay progression of the disease.

REVIEW QUESTIONS

Directions: For each of the following questions, choose the **one best** answer.

1. What biophysical events would hyperpolarize a typical neuron?
A. A decrease in Cl^- conductance
B. An increase in K^+ conductance
C. An increase in Na^+ conductance
D. An increase in Ca^{2+} conductance
E. Inhibition of the Na^+-K^+ pump

2. Why does myelination increase axonal conduction velocity?
A. It increases membrane capacitance
B. It decreases the axon's refractory period
C. It increases the equilibrium potential for Na^+
D. It decreases the membrane resistance
E. It increases the axon's length constant

3. What biophysical changes are associated with the leading edge of an action potential?
A. A decrease in potassium conductance
B. An increase in sodium conductance
C. An increase in chloride conductance
D. An increase in membrane resistance
E. An increase in axoplasmic conductance

4. What sequence of biophysical events characterizes an action potential?
A. An EPSP followed by an IPSP
B. A passive depolarization followed by an active depolarization
C. An influx of potassium followed by an influx of chloride
D. An influx of sodium followed by an efflux of potassium
E. An influx of potassium followed by an efflux of chloride

5. Which type of synaptic connection is absent in the central nervous system?
   A. Axoaxonic synapses on axon terminals
   B. Dendrodendritic synapses
   C. Axodendritic synapses
   D. Axoaxonic synapses on myelinated axons
   E. Axosomatic synapses

6. What effect does an increase in diameter have on an axon's biophysical properties?
   A. It decreases the axon's cytoplasmic resistance
   B. It decreases the axon's length constant
   C. It decreases the axon's conduction velocity
   D. It decreases the axon's time constant
   E. It increases the axon's time constant

7. What structural or functional property defines the nodes of Ranvier?
   A. They contain a high density of voltage-gated sodium channels
   B. They represent regions of thick myelination
   C. They impede the velocity of action potentials
   D. They increase membrane resistance
   E. They contain a high density of ligand-gated potassium channels

8. Which neuronal function is most strongly facilitated by a long length constant?
   A. Axoplasmic transport in the retrograde direction
   B. Maintenance of potassium equilibrium potential
   C. Spatial summation of postsynaptic potentials
   D. Inhibitory neurotransmission
   E. Axoplasmic transport in the anterograde direction

9. Multiple sclerosis is characterized by what neurological changes?
   A. Proliferation of myelin in multiple brain regions
   B. Hardening of multiple cerebral blood vessels
   C. Motor weakness and sensory impairment
   D. Imbalance of Na^+ and K^+ channels
   E. Glial proliferation

10. What type of synaptic interaction is mediated by an axo-axonic synaptic contact?
   A. Temporal summation
   B. Feedback inhibition
   C. Spatial summation
   D. Presynaptic inhibition
   E. Postsynaptic excitation

ADDITIONAL READING

Classic Literature

Hodgkin AL: *The Conduction of the Nervous Impulse*. Springfield, IL: Charles C Thomas, 1967.

Hodgkin AL, Huxley AF: Currents carried by sodium and potassium ions through the membrane of the giant squid axon of *Loligo. J Physiol* 116:449–472, 1952.

——: The components of membrane conductance in the giant axon of *Loligo. J Physiol* 116:473–496, 1952.

——: The dual effect of membrane potential on sodium conductance in the giant axon of *Loligo. J Physiol* 116:497–506, 1952.

Hodgkin AL, Huxley AF, Katz B: Measurements of current-voltage relations in the membrane of the giant axon of *Loligo. J Physiol* 116:424–448, 1952.

Katz B: *Nerve, Muscle, and Synapse*. New York, NY: McGraw-Hill, 1966.

Reviews and Landmark Research Articles

Armstrong CM, Hille B: Voltage-gated ion channels and electrical excitability. *Neuron* 20:371–380, 1998.

Catterall WA: Structure and function of voltage-sensitive ion channels. *Science* 242:50–61, 1988.

Jan LY, Jan YN: Voltage-gated and inwardly rectifying potassium channels. *J Physiol* 505:267–282, 1997.

Neher E: Ion channels for communication between and within cells. *Science* 256:498–502, 1992.

Owens T: The enigma of multiple sclerosis: inflammation and neurodegeneration cause heterogeneous dysfunction and damage. *Curr Opin Neurol* 16:259– 265, 2003.

Rothman JE: Mechanisms of intracellular protein transport. *Nature* 372: 55–63, 1994.

Vanderberg CA, Bezanilla F: A sodium channel model based on single channel, macroscopic ionic, and gating currents in the squid giant axon. *Biophys J* 60: 1511–1533, 1991.

Yang NA, George AL, Horn R: Molecular basis of charge movement in voltage-gated sodium channels. *Neuron* 16:113–122, 1996.

Zhang J, Hutton G: Role of magnetic resonance imaging and immunotherapy in treating multiple sclerosis. *Ann Rev Med* 56:273–302, 2005.

INTERNET RESOURCES

Colorado College
http://www.coloradocollege.edu/idprog/Neuroscience/Cellular1-21.html

Multiple Sclerosis Foundation
http://www.msfacts.org/

National Multiple Sclerosis Society
http://www.nationalmssociety.org/prc.asp

Neurobiology Animations by Gary G. Matthews
http://www.blackwellpublishing.com/matthews/animate.html

Neuroscience for Kids
http://faculty.washington.edu/chudler/introb.html

The Multiple Sclerosis Association of America
http://www.msaa.com/

University of Minnesota Neurohistology Atlas
http://vanat.cvm.umn.edu/neurHistAtls/

University of Newfoundland
http://www.med.mun.ca/anatomyts/nerve/neuron.htm

University of Utah—Multiple Sclerosis
http://medstat.med.utah.edu/kw/ms/

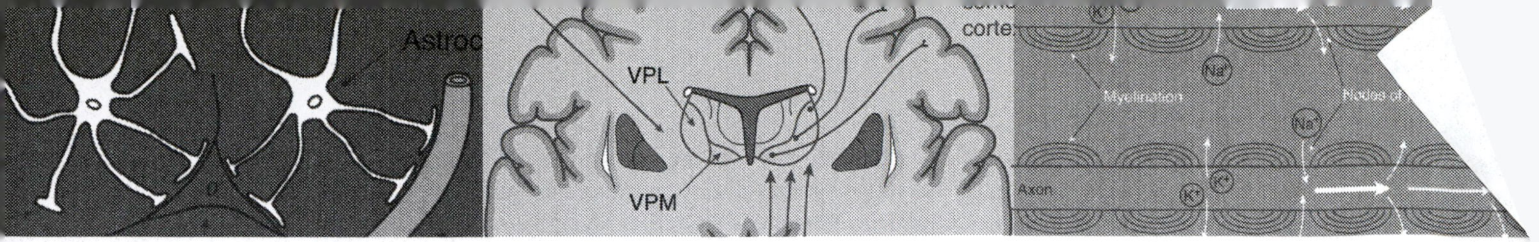

CHAPTER 2

Chemical Neurotransmission

INTRODUCTION OF CLINICAL CASE

A 34-year-old woman was brought to the emergency room because she had difficulty swallowing and breathing. Her face was expressionless, and speaking was problematic because of weakness on both sides of her tongue and mouth. Both eyelids showed ptosis; the right eyelid was elevated 6 mm, and the left eyelid was elevated only 4 mm. The patient said that her eyelids started drooping a few weeks earlier, but this problem seemed to disappear after a good night's sleep. The patient had normal pupillary light reflexes in both eyes but experienced double vision when gazing laterally. Her arms were weak and unable to maintain position when tested against resistance. Despite this weakness, deep tendon reflexes were present at the wrist and elbow of both arms and at the knee and ankle of both legs. Breathing was shallow, but regular; inspiratory and expiratory pressures were both below normal. Blood pressure and heart rate were normal, but body temperature was elevated. Prior to this the woman had been in excellent health, she exercised regularly, and she had never suffered from fatigue. Her 60-year-old mother had rheumatoid arthritis, but all other family members were in good health.

INTRODUCTION TO CHEMICAL NEUROTRANSMISSION

In the early 1900s, researchers thought that neurons were physically continuous with each other and that the nervous system was an elaborate syncytium. This view of the nervous system was eventually disproved by the discovery of the synaptic cleft, a narrow space that separates axonal terminals from the postsynaptic membrane. But if neurons did not directly contact each other, how did they communicate? We now know that most neurons in the central nervous system (CNS) communicate with each other by secreting minute quantities of chemical substances from their synaptic terminals. These chemical messengers produce electrochemical changes in the postsynaptic membranes of neurons and muscles. Although synaptic transmission between neurons is more complicated than transmission at the neuromuscular junction, the two types of neurochemical transmission are similar. In fact, the neuromuscular junction was used extensively to study neurochemical transmission because this preparation provides a simple and accessible model for neural mechanisms in the brain and spinal cord of all vertebrates.

The presence of chemical transmitters in the nervous system was first demonstrated in a classic experiment performed by Otto Loewi in 1920. In this experiment, Loewi placed two frog hearts in separate chambers and electrically stimulated the vagus nerve innervating one of the hearts to slow its rate of contraction. He then collected a sample of the perfusate that bathed this heart and injected it into the chamber containing the second heart. Application of the perfusate caused the second heart to beat slower even though its vagus nerve had been removed. Loewi deduced that the perfusate contained a substance that was released from the vagus nerve of the first heart, and that this substance was responsible for slowing the rate of contraction in both hearts. This substance or "vagus stuff" was later identified as acetylcholine (ACh), the first chemical substance to be recognized as a neurotransmitter.

Criteria for Defining a Neurotransmitter

A neurotransmitter is any chemical released from a neuron that changes the electrical activity of other neurons or muscles. Although this definition is conceptually simple, it is not easy to identify which chemicals are neurotransmitters. The following criteria have been developed to determine whether a chemical compound should be classified as a neurotransmitter:

1. *The chemical must be present in the presynaptic neuron.* The chemical must be located in the vesicles of the presynaptic terminal. As part of this criterion, the presynaptic neuron must also contain the precursor molecules and synthetic enzymes for manufacturing the neurotransmitter.
2. *The chemical must be released from the presynaptic neuron during depolarization.* The chemical must be released from the synapse when the axon and its terminal are invaded by action potentials or when they are electrically stimulated. Furthermore, this process should occur in a Ca^{2+}-dependent manner.
3. *Application of the chemical to a postsynaptic neuron must mimic the physiologic response produced by presynaptic stimulation.* The postsynaptic neurons should exhibit identical responses when the chemical is released from the presynaptic terminal or applied exogenously. This criterion is also satisfied by showing that application of an antagonist blocks the synaptic response as well as the response to exogenous application of the substance.
4. *There must be a mechanism for inactivating the chemical at the synapse.* Neurotransmitters usually have brief effects on the postsynaptic neuron because they are inactivated by degradative enzymes, selective reuptake into the presynaptic nerve terminals, or uptake into adjacent glial cells. Diffusion of the neurotransmitter through the extracellular space may augment these inactivating mechanisms.

When all of these criteria are satisfied, the chemical's function as a neurotransmitter is firmly established. The identity of many neurotransmitters is still uncertain, however, because many experiments are required to satisfy these criteria. More than 100 neurochemicals meet some of these criteria; these are called putative neurotransmitters.

Neurotransmitters are divided into two main groups: small-molecule neurotransmitters and neuropeptides. Small-molecule neurotransmitters include substances such as ACh, biogenic amines (e.g., dopamine), and small amino acids (e.g., glutamate). Neuropeptides,

TABLE 2.1 Neurotransmitters in the Nervous System

Small Molecules	Neuropeptides
Acetylcholine	**Opioid peptides**
	Leucine enkephalin
Biogenic amines	Methionine enkephalin
Dopamine	α-Endorphin
Norepinephrine	β-Endorphin
Epinephrine	Dynorphins
Serotonin	
Histamine	**Pituitary peptides**
	Adrenocorticotropic hormone
Amino acids	Oxytocin
Aspartate	Thyroid-stimulating hormone
γ-Aminobutyric acid	Vasopressin
Glutamate	
Homocysteine	**Other neuropeptides**
Taurine	Angiotensin-II
	Bombesin
Nucleotides	Bradykinin
Adenosine	Cholecystokinin
Adenosine triphosphate	Gastrin
	Glucagon
Retrograde	Insulin
Nitric oxide	Neuropeptide Y
	Neurotensin
	Somatostatin
	Substance P
	Vasoactive intestinal peptide

on the other hand, are composed of 3-35 amino acids and include opioid peptides, pituitary peptides, and peptides that are also found in the gastrointestinal tract. A partial list of neurochemicals that have been identified as neurotransmitters is provided in Table 2.1.

Small-Molecule Neurotransmitters. Small-molecule neurotransmitters are produced by short biosynthetic pathways involving substrates derived from carbohydrate metabolism. The enzymes for synthesizing these neurotransmitters are produced by free polysomes in the soma's cytoplasm. These enzymes and the neurotransmitter precursor are transported to the synaptic endings by slow axoplasmic transport. After arriving in the synaptic cytosol, the enzyme converts the small precursor molecule into a neurotransmitter. When this synthetic reaction is completed, the small-molecule neurotransmitter is transported from the cytosol into synaptic vesicles by an ATP-dependent pump (or transporter) located in the vesicular membrane.

Neurotransmitters are sequestered in vesicles to protect them from enzymatic degradation and to provide a mechanism for releasing precise quantities of neurotransmitter into the synaptic cleft during neurotransmission. Most of the small-molecule neurotransmitters are contained in small (40-60 nm), translucent vesicles, but some, especially the biogenic amines, are packaged in dense-core vesicles that vary from small (40-60 nm) to medium (90-120 nm).

Small-molecule neurotransmitters are synthesized in the cytosol of synaptic terminals.

Neuropeptides are synthesized in the soma and then transported in vesicles through the axon.

Neuropeptides. Neuropeptide synthesis occurs within the soma and involves genetic transcription. Large polypeptide molecules are synthesized by a series of reactions that take place in the rough endoplasmic reticulum (RER). Newly synthesized polypeptides are transported to the Golgi apparatus, which packages the polypeptides into vesicles. Subsequently, the polypeptides are broken into several smaller molecules by a series of steps involving proteolytic cleavage, glycosylation, phosphorylation, and other chemical reactions. Vesicles containing neuropeptides are rapidly transported through the axon by microtubules until they reach the synaptic terminal. In the synaptic terminals, neuropeptide neurotransmitters are packaged in medium (90-120 nm) vesicles or in large (200-250 nm) vesicles that have a granular or electron-dense core.

Colocalization of Neurotransmitters

Small-molecule neurotransmitters are in small (40-60 nm), clear vesicles.

Biogenic amines are in small (40-60 nm) and medium (90-120 nm) vesicles with a dense core.

Neuropeptides are in medium (90-120 nm) and large (200-250 nm) vesicles with a dense core.

Neurons may synthesize more than one neurotransmitter, and it is not unusual to observe different types of synaptic vesicles in the same synaptic terminal (Figure 2.1). Although many neurons contain a small-molecule neurotransmitter and at least one type of neuropeptide it is extremely rare for a neuron to synthesize more than one type of small-molecule neurotransmitter. Small-molecule neurotransmitters are usually located in the small, clear vesicles, whereas neuropeptides are located in larger, dense-core vesicles. The small vesicles are generally docked closest to the active sites on the presynaptic membrane, whereas the dense-core vesicles are located further away from the presynaptic membrane. Because of this differential location, small vesicles release their contents sooner than the dense-core vesicles. Furthermore, small vesicles fuse with the presynaptic membrane in response to slow neuronal discharge rates, whereas the dense-core vesicles require higher rates of neuronal activity before they release their neuropeptides into the synaptic cleft. Thus, co-localization of small-molecule neurotransmitters and neuropeptides in the same synaptic terminal provides many neurons with two modes of neurochemical transmission.

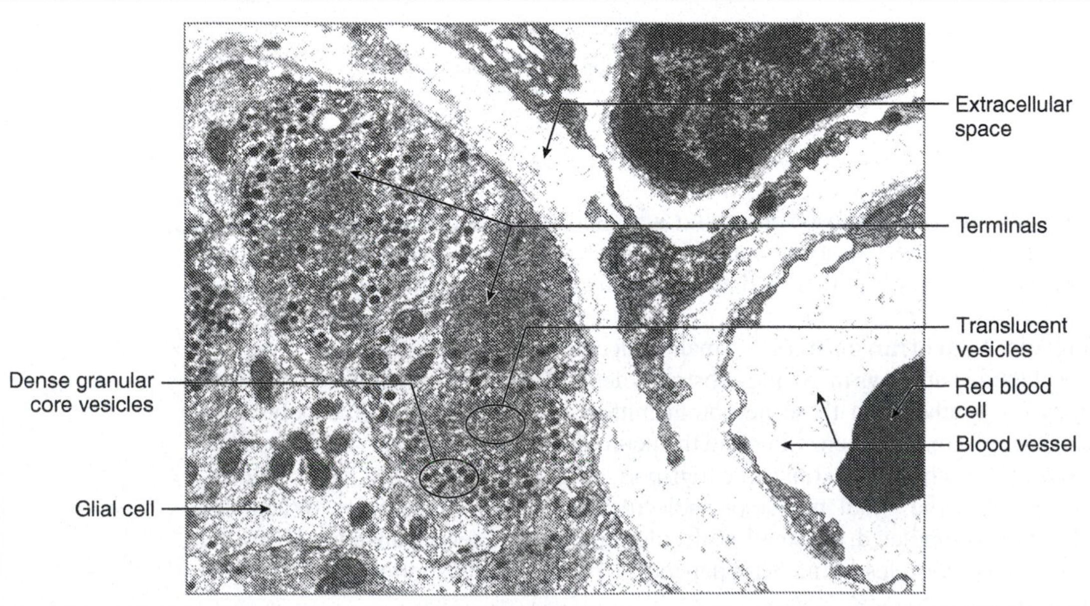

FIG. 2.1. Co-localization of Translucent and Dense-Core Vesicles. Synaptic terminals in the hypothalamus contain small translucent vesicles and large vesicles with a dense granular core. The former contain small molecule transmitters; the latter contain neuropeptides. Unlike most synapses, many hypothalamic terminals release neurotransmitters into the extracellular space for diffusion into nearby blood vessels. (Electron micrograph provided courtesy of Ms. Tina Rutherford and Dr. Robert Page, Pennsylvania State University.)

Properties of the Major Neurotransmitters

Although many different neurotransmitters are used by the nervous system, some are more prevalent and have been studied more intensively. This section briefly describes some of the major neurotransmitters, their distribution and functional importance, and their biosynthetic and inactivation pathways.

Acetylcholine. Acetylcholine, the main neurotransmitter in the peripheral nervous system (PNS), is present at all neuromuscular junctions, in the preganglionic neurons of the sympathetic system, and in the preganglionic and postganglionic neurons of the parasympathetic system. In addition, ACh is present in the CNS, especially in the brainstem tegmentum and in the ventral forebrain. Experimental studies have shown that ACh is an excitatory neurotransmitter at the neuromuscular junction and at most synapses in the CNS and PNS.

The synthesis of ACh from acetyl coenzyme A (acetyl CoA) and choline is catalyzed by the enzyme choline acetyltransferase (Figure 2.2). Acetyl CoA is derived from pyruvate generated during glycolysis; the choline precursor is transported across the presynaptic membrane by a transporter molecule. After ACh is released into the synaptic cleft, its effect on the postsynaptic receptors is terminated by a hydrolytic enzyme, acetylcholinesterase (AChE). The synaptic cleft contains high concentrations of AChE, which catalyzes ACh into acetate and choline. The choline molecules in the synapse and extracellular fluid are returned to the synaptic ending where they are used to synthesize more ACh.

Acetylcholine is found in neuromuscular junctions, sympathetic and parasympathetic ganglia, the brainstem tegmentum, the ventral forebrain, and the cerebral cortex.

Numerous chemical compounds have been developed that interact at cholinergic synapses in the neuromuscular junction to produce muscular paralysis. Organophosphates, such as mustard gas and many insecticides, produce muscular paralysis by binding irreversibly to AChE. By preventing the degradation of ACh, these compounds allow ACh to accumulate in the neuromuscular junction. Consequently, the postsynaptic membrane is maintained in a constant state of depolarization and the muscle becomes unresponsive to additional release of ACh from the motor neuron terminal. Acute exposure to sufficient quantities of these chemicals leads to death because of respiratory paralysis.

Glutamate. Regarded as the main excitatory neurotransmitter in the CNS, glutamate is present in virtually every brain region and is released from about half of the brain's synapses. In fact, glutamate is the neurotransmitter that is used by most principal neurons for sending excitatory signals from one region to another in the CNS.

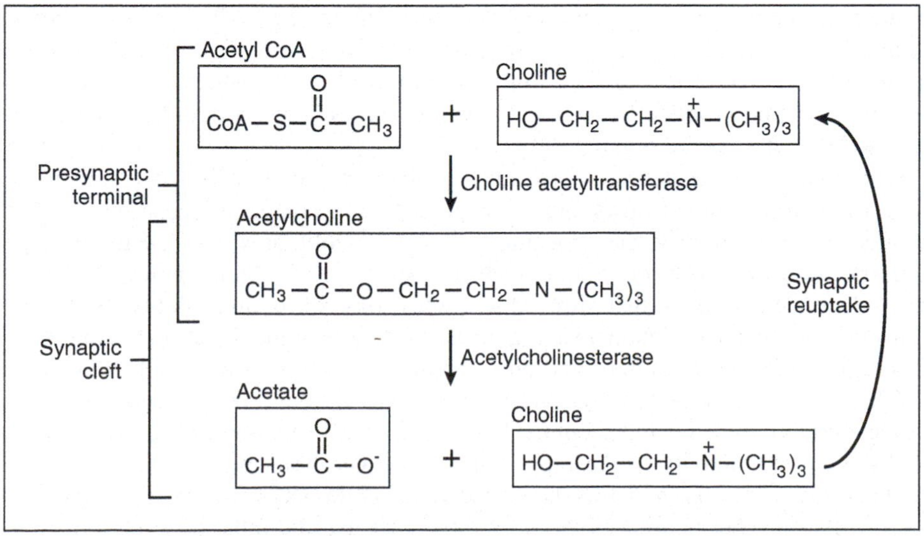

FIG. 2.2. Acetylcholine Metabolism. Acetylcholine (ACh) is synthesized from acetyl CoA and choline in the presynaptic terminal. After its release into the synaptic cleft, ACh is metabolized into acetate and choline. The choline is transported into the synaptic terminal and recycled into ACh.

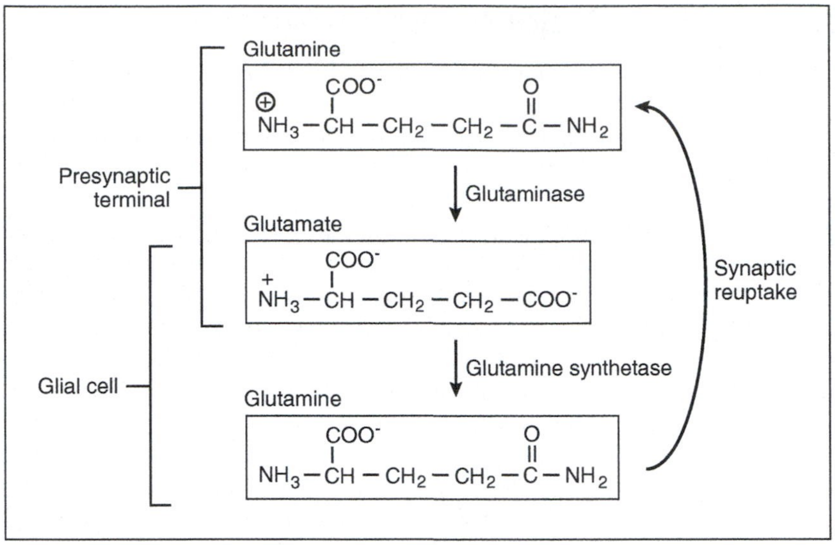

FIG. 2.3. Glutamate Metabolism. Glutamate is synthesized from glutamine in the presynaptic terminal. Following synaptic release, glutamate is transported into surrounding glial cells where it is converted into glutamine.

Glutamate is a fast-acting excitatory neurotransmitter that is found in virtually every part of the CNS.

Glutamate is an amino acid that is synthesized in synaptic terminals from glutamine (Figure 2.3). The conversion to glutamate is catalyzed by the mitochondrial enzyme glutaminase. After glutamate is released from a presynaptic terminal, it is quickly removed by high-affinity dicarboxylic acid transporters located mainly on glial cells and, to a lesser extent, on presynaptic glutamatergic terminals. Glutamate that is transported into the presynaptic terminal can enter the synaptic vesicles. Alternatively, glutamate that enters an astrocyte is metabolized by glutamine synthetase into glutamine. Subsequently, the glutamine is released into the extracellular space so that it can be transported into glutamatergic terminals and recycled into another glutamate molecule.

Glutamate Excitotoxicity, Ischemia, and Epilepsy. Excessive levels of extracellular glutamate can overstimulate neurons and cause them to die. In animals, a diet high in glutamate is correlated with neuronal degeneration in the retina and in other brain regions. Glutamate toxicity results from excessive activation of postsynaptic receptors that open Ca^{2+} channels. The Ca^{2+} influx activates Ca^{2+}-dependent proteases in postsynaptic cells that produce free radicals, which may damage a neuron's plasma membrane and its cytoplasmic organelles.

High concentrations of glutamate have toxic effects on neurons.

Glutamate-induced neurotoxicity may explain the relationship between ischemia (i.e., a reduction in blood flow) and subsequent brain damage. When a blood vessel is occluded, even transiently, the concentration of extracellular glutamate increases. This occurs because the transport of glutamate into synaptic terminals or into the glia is an energy-dependent process that slows down when oxygen is unavailable. Experimental studies have shown that glutamate antagonists, which block the receptors mediating Ca^{2+} influx, can reduce the amount of neuronal damage that occurs during ischemia.

Glutamate neurotoxicity may contribute to the repetitive seizures seen in epilepsy. In essence, epileptic seizures represent the behavioral manifestation of excessive and uncontrollable neuronal activity in the hippocampus and cerebral cortex. Excessive neuronal activity in these regions increases the extracellular glutamate concentration, and this has toxic effects on other neurons, especially those that use the inhibitory neurotransmitter, γ-aminobutyric acid (GABA). Samples of cerebral cortex from animals or individuals suffering from epilepsy indicate a significant loss of GABAergic neurons. Synaptic release of GABA normally inhibits neuronal activity, and any loss of GABAergic neurons during an epileptic episode increases the probability and severity of subsequent seizures. For this reason, most anticonvulsant drugs act by enhancing GABAergic inhibition, thereby suppressing the excitatory actions of glutamatergic neurons.

GABA and Glycine. GABA and glycine are the main inhibitory neurotransmitters in the CNS. Most brain areas contain GABAergic neurons, but glycine is distributed primarily in the spinal cord. Neurons that use GABA or glycine play an important role in preventing recurrent or excessive neuronal excitation. GABAergic terminals often form "baskets" or "pericellular nests" of inhibitory synapses around the soma of certain types of neurons. By opening Cl^- channels in the postsynaptic membrane, GABAergic transmission holds the membrane potential of the soma and axon hillock at subthreshold levels. Hence, inhibitory synapses located near the axon hillock can effectively prevent EPSPs in the distal dendrites from initiating action potentials in the axon.

GABA is a fast-acting inhibitory neurotransmitter that is used mainly by intrinsic neurons in virtually every part of the CNS

GABA is synthesized from glutamate by glutamate decarboxylase (GAD), an enzyme found only in GABAergic neurons (Figure 2.4). Pyridoxal phosphate, a vitamin B6 derivative, is an essential co-factor for GAD activity. Insufficient amounts of vitamin B6 in the diet cause a decrease in GABA synthesis, which can lead to seizures. Many types

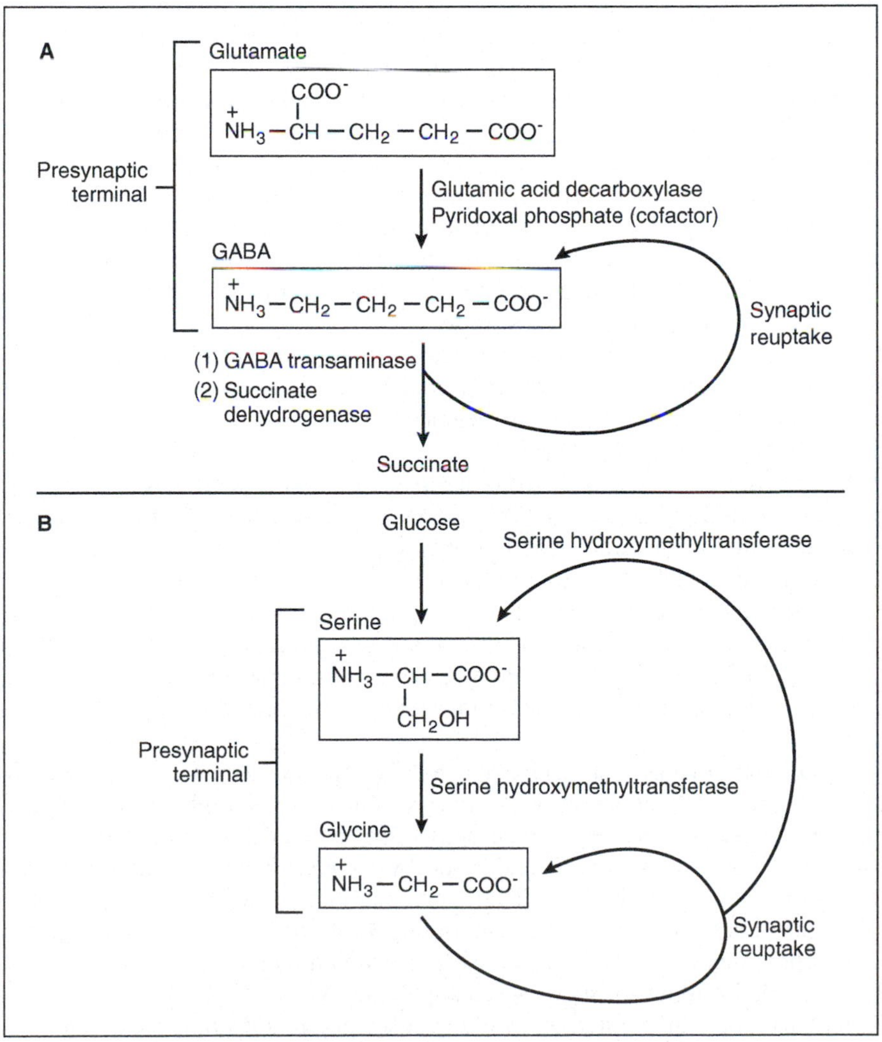

FIG. 2.4. GABA and Glycine Metabolism. (A) γ-Aminobutyric acid (GABA) is synthesized from glutamate in the presynaptic terminal. After synaptic release, GABA is either transported back into the terminal or metabolized into succinate via the tricarboxylic acid cycle. (B) Glycine is synthesized from serine by mitochondrial enzymes. After synaptic release, glycine is transported into the synaptic terminal for recycling.

of neurons and glial cells contain specific transporter molecules that remove GABA from the synaptic cleft. Extracellular GABA that is transported into GABAergic terminals is recycled for subsequent synaptic transmission. By comparison, GABA transported into other neurons or into glial cells is converted into succinate as part of the tricarboxylic acid cycle, which produces adenosine triphosphate (ATP). In this latter pathway, GABA is degraded by GABA transaminase into succinic semialdehyde, which is then metabolized by succinic semialdehyde dehydrogenase. Both of the enzymes in this metabolic pathway are in mitochondria located in GABAergic terminals. Inhibiting these enzymes increases extracellular GABA, especially in the synaptic cleft; inhibitors of GABA transaminase are widely used as anticonvulsants.

Glycine is synthesized from serine by a mitochondrial enzyme, serine hydroxymethyltransferase. After its synaptic release, glycine is removed from the synaptic cleft by glycine transporters on the synaptic terminals. After glycine enters the synaptic terminal, it is recycled into synaptic vesicles.

Catecholamines. Dopamine, norepinephrine, and epinephrine are called catecholamines because they contain an amine group attached to a catechol, which is a six-carbon ring with two hydroxyl groups. These three neurotransmitters are similar in their molecular structure, and all are derived from the same dietary amino acid, tyrosine, which is converted by tyrosine hydroxylase to dihydroxyphenylalanine, or L-dopa (Figure 2.5). Tyrosine hydroxylase, the rate-limiting enzyme in catecholamine production, is present in all catecholaminergic neurons. The L-dopa is converted to dopamine by aromatic amino acid decarboxylase (AAAD). In noradrenergic neurons, dopamine is converted to norepinephrine by dopamine-β-hydroxylase. The conversion of dopamine to norepinephrine is unusual because it represents the only case in which a small-molecule neurotransmitter is synthesized within the synaptic vesicles rather than in the cytosol. Finally, a small percentage of catecholaminergic neurons convert norepinephrine into epinephrine by means of phenylethanolamine-*N*-methyltransferase.

Catecholaminergic transmission is inactivated by synaptic reuptake involving high affinity transporters that are Na^+-dependent ATPases. After being transported into the synaptic terminal, catecholamines are degraded by monoamine oxidase (MAO) or by catechol *O*-methyltransferase (COMT).

> Dopamine neurons are located in the substantia nigra and ventral tegmental area.
>
> Noradrenergic neurons are located in the locus ceruleus.

Most dopamine-containing neurons are located in two midbrain nuclei, the substantia nigra and ventral tegmental area. The axons of these neurons terminate in the basal ganglia and medial frontal cortex. Additional dopamine-containing neurons are located in the hypothalamus and a few other regions. By comparison, the cell bodies of virtually all noradrenergic neurons are located in a single brainstem nucleus, the locus ceruleus. The locus ceruleus sends its axons throughout the neuraxis, especially to the telencephalon and the brainstem. Compared to dopamine and norepinephrine, few nuclei use epinephrine as a neurotransmitter, and those that do are located in the rostral part of the medulla.

> **Catecholamines** modulate neuronal responsiveness to other neurotransmitters and regulate the forebrain circuits that control mood, arousal, and sleep.

One function of catecholamines is to modulate the overall tone of neural activity in selected brain regions. Consistent with their projections to the limbic forebrain and other parts of the telencephalon, the level of activity in the catecholamine pathways plays a critical role in regulating psychological mood. A decrease in catecholamine transmission may cause depression, a serious psychiatric disorder that can lead to suicide if not treated. Some classes of antidepressants act by inhibiting MAO or by blocking synaptic reuptake of the catecholamines. Conversely, excessive catecholaminergic stimulation may produce mania or psychotic illnesses such as schizophrenia. Most antipsychotic drugs interfere with catecholamine transmission by blocking postsynaptic dopamine receptors.

Parkinsonism. Parkinson's disease is a neurodegenerative disorder associated with severe loss of dopaminergic neurons in the substantia nigra. Behaviorally, this disease is characterized by a general poverty in locomotor activity, muscular rigidity, and oscillating tremors of the head and forelimbs. Although the precise role that dopamine plays in regulating motor activity is poorly understood, knowledge of the biosynthetic pathway

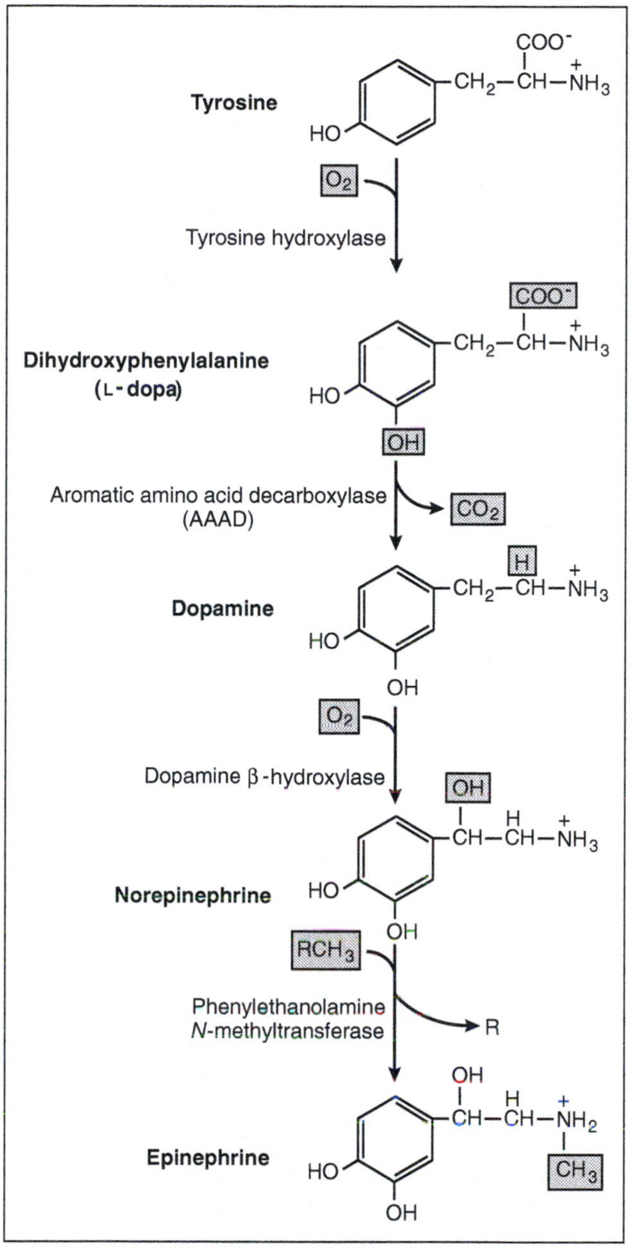

FIG. 2.5. Catecholamine Metabolism. Tyrosine is the necessary amino acid precursor for the biosynthesis of dopamine, norepinephrine, and epinephrine. Tyrosine hydroxylase is the rate-limiting enzyme for synthesizing these catecholamines. AAAD = aromatic amino acid decarboxylase.

has been used to develop pharmacologic treatments that ameliorate the symptoms of parkinsonism. Dopamine does not pass through the blood-brain barrier, but its precursor does. For this reason, L-dopa is administered to Parkinson's disease patients so that it can be transported into the brain, where it eventually is transported into the terminals of all neurons that contain AAAD, including serotonergic neurons as well as the remaining dopamine neurons that have not yet been destroyed by the disease. The L-dopa is then converted into dopamine. Because AAAD is also located in the periphery and may metabolize L-dopa before it crosses the blood-brain barrier, L-dopa is usually administered with an AAAD inhibitor, carbidopa, that does not cross the blood-brain barrier.

Serotonin. Serotonin (5-hydroxytryptamine, 5-HT) is synthesized from tryptophan, a common amino acid that is obtained in the diet. Tryptophan is selectively transported into serotonergic neurons where it is converted into serotonin by the rate-limiting enzyme, tryptophan hydroxylase (Figure 2.6). Serotonin is found in the raphe nuclei located along the midline of the brainstem. The raphe nuclei have diffuse ascending projections that

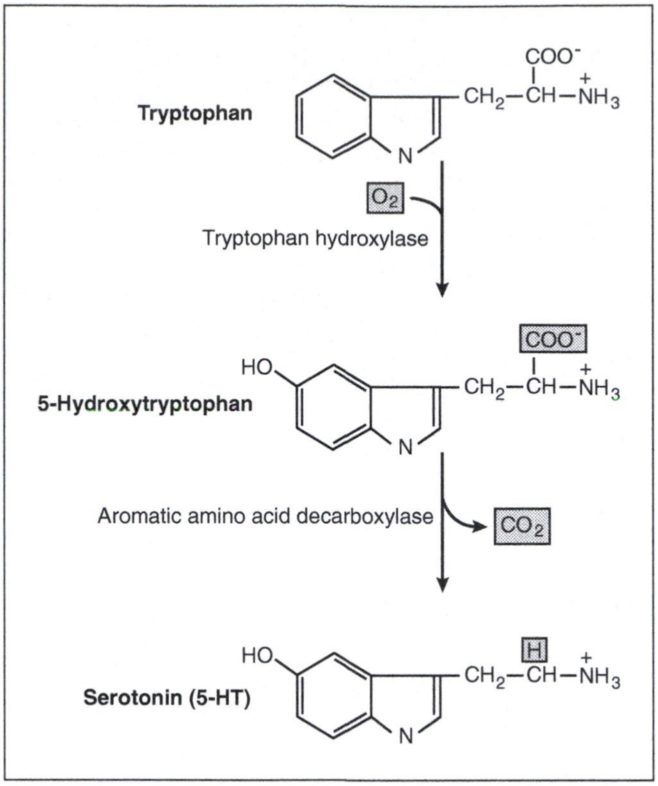

FIG. 2.6. Serotonin Metabolism. The amino acid tryptophan is converted into serotonin by tryptophan hydroxylase and aromatic amino acid decarboxylase (AAAD). 5-HT = hydroxytryptamine.

innervate the telencephalon and diencephalon, as well as descending projections to the spinal cord. Consistent with its innervation of the limbic system, serotonin has been implicated in the regulation of mood and arousal; for this reason, serotonergic agonists have been developed to treat depression and related mental states.

Peptide Neurotransmitters. Many peptides are hormones that are released from endocrine cells or endocrine regions of the brain such as the hypothalamus and pituitary gland. In addition to functioning as a hormone on target organs located some distance from the brain, some peptides act as neurotransmitters in specific regions of the PNS and CNS.

> One prepropeptide molecule is a precursor for many neuropeptides.

Peptide neurotransmitters consist of specific sets of amino acids that are synthesized in the neuronal soma. Instead of developing a specific biosynthetic pathway for each neuropeptide, neurons produce several neuropeptides from a much larger protein molecule that contains a long series of peptides (Figure 2.7). The original protein precursor, called a prepropeptide, is cleaved into a propeptide that undergoes further proteolytic processing to form several classes of neuropeptides.

Substance P and the opioid peptides are among the most studied neuropeptides in the nervous system. Substance P is located in peripheral nerves and is released from synaptic terminals in the spinal cord, where it transmits nociceptive information in response to peripheral tissue damage. Opioid peptides in the spinal cord antagonize substance P neurotransmission, thereby suppressing the transmission of nociceptive information. There are at least two dozen opioid peptides that are grouped into three major classes: endorphins, enkephalins, and dynorphins. All of the opioid peptides have central effects that, to a greater or lesser degree, are mimicked by morphine and other narcotic drugs. The opioid peptides are distributed throughout the brain and play a major role in the behavioral response to pain and other forms of stress.

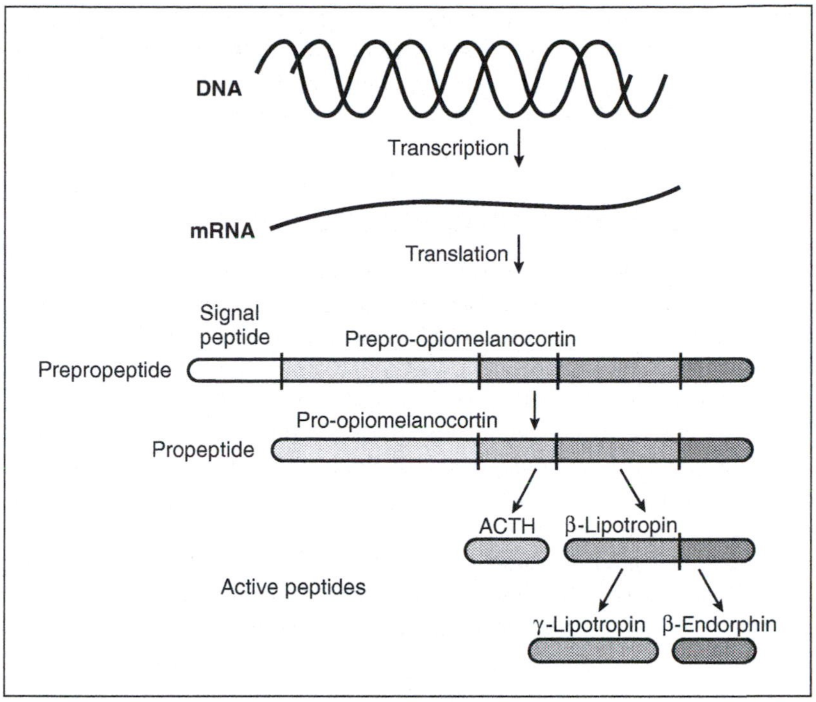

FIG. 2.7. Neuropeptide Synthesis. Genetic transcription and translation in the soma give rise to large polypeptides that act as precursor molecules. Subsequent cleavage of the prepropeptide leads to the production of several smaller neuropeptides including opioids. ACTH = adrenocorticotropic hormone.

Synaptic Transmission

Synaptic transmission is a complex process initiated by the arrival of action potentials at the synaptic terminal. The terminal responds by releasing one or more neurotransmitters into the synaptic cleft. After diffusing across the synaptic cleft, the neurotransmitter causes an excitatory or inhibitory response in the postsynaptic membrane. Although some details in this process are not completely understood, the basic mechanisms of synaptic transmission have been elucidated.

Synaptic Morphology

Synapses are characterized by structures that are essential for a variety of synaptic functions. For example, synaptic terminals usually contain mitochondria that provide energy for the synthesis of a large number of neurochemicals used in neurotransmission. Synaptic boutons also contain many vesicles that maintain a ready supply of releasable neurotransmitter molecules. These vesicles tend to aggregate near active sites in the presynaptic membrane and release their contents into the synaptic cleft immediately following the arrival of an action potential. Because synaptic clefts are narrow (20-50 nm wide), neurotransmitter molecules can diffuse across this space in a fraction of a millisecond. Finally, the postsynaptic membrane is often characterized by a thick, dense region that contains specific receptors for binding the neurotransmitter molecules released from the presynaptic neuron.

Synapses are classified according to their ultrastructural appearance. Asymmetric synapses have clear round vesicles and a prominent postsynaptic density, which is noticeably thicker than the presynaptic membrane. By comparison, the presynaptic and postsynaptic membranes of symmetric synapses are the same thickness, and the synaptic vesicles tend to be oval or flattened. Although most asymmetric synapses are excitatory and most symmetric synapses are inhibitory, physiologic studies have shown that excitatory

> The effects of a neurotransmitter are determined by the postsynaptic receptor.

or inhibitory effects exerted by a neurotransmitter are determined by the types of receptors that are activated in the postsynaptic neuron. Furthermore, there is no correlation between the presence of dense-core vesicles or small translucent vesicles and the physiologic response produced in the postsynaptic neuron. Thus, the structure of a synaptic vesicle is not a reliable indicator of its synaptic function.

Mechanism of Neurotransmitter Release

Depolarization of the synaptic terminal causes Ca^{2+} influx, which is necessary for vesicle docking and neurotransmitter release.

The general sequence of events occurring during synaptic transmission is shown schematically in Figure 2.8. When an action potential reaches the synaptic terminal, the incoming depolarization activates voltage-gated Ca^{2+} channels located throughout the presynaptic membrane. Opening these channels allows Ca^{2+} to enter the terminals by flowing down its concentration gradient. The influx of Ca^{2+} activates several Ca^{2+}-sensitive proteins in the synaptic terminal, many of which cause the vesicular membrane to fuse with "active sites" in the presynaptic membrane. Many of the proteins involved in this process have been identified, but the mechanism by which Ca^{2+} mediates vesicular fusion with the presynaptic membrane is not precisely known. After the vesicle releases its contents into the synaptic cleft, the neurotransmitter molecules diffuse across the synaptic cleft and bind to specific receptors in the postsynaptic membrane. Activation of the postsynaptic receptors causes a change in the permeability of specific ion channels. The resulting change in ionic current alters the membrane potential of the postsynaptic neuron; this increases or decreases the probability that an action potential will be initiated.

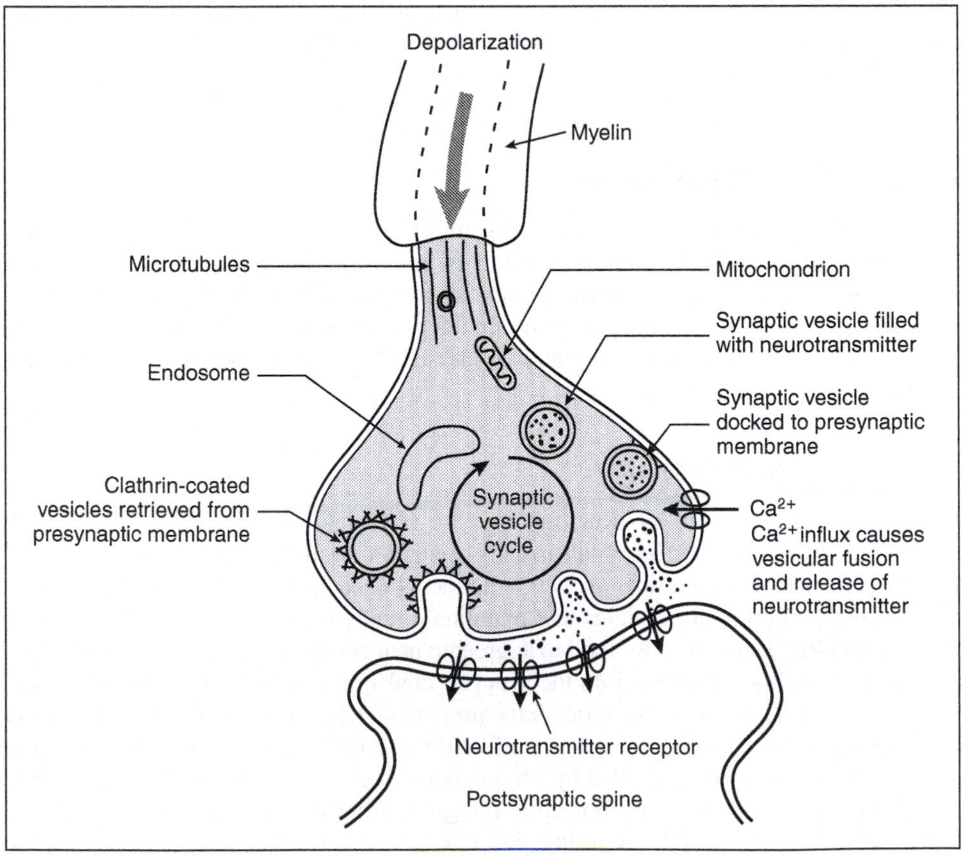

FIG. 2.8. Neurochemical Transmission. Depolarization causes synaptic vesicles to fuse with the presynaptic membrane and release their neurotransmitters. Although vesicles are originally produced in the soma and transported to the terminal by microtubules, segments of the presynaptic membrane are retrieved and recycled into synaptic vesicles by endosomes.

Recycling of Synaptic Vesicles

When synaptic vesicles fuse with the presynaptic membrane, there is a temporary increase in the amount of membrane in the synaptic terminal. The surface area of a synaptic terminal fluctuates within certain limits but is prevented from unlimited expansion because the presynaptic membrane is used to form new synaptic vesicles (Figure 2.8). On the lateral edge of the synaptic terminal, away from the active sites near the synaptic cleft, small segments of the plasma membrane invaginate and are pinched off from the presynaptic membrane to form clathrin-coated vesicles. Subsequently, the coated vesicles merge into an intracellular organelle, the endosome, which recycles the segments of presynaptic membrane into new vesicles. When a newly formed vesicle emerges from the endosome, neurotransmitter molecules are pumped into the vesicle from the cytosol by specific transporter molecules. When loaded with neurotransmitter, the vesicle migrates to active sites in the synapse and docks with the presynaptic membrane until fusion occurs. This recurring sequence of events is called the synaptic vesicle cycle.

Neuromuscular Junctions

A neuromuscular junction is a special type of synapse formed between the terminals of a peripheral motor neuron and a skeletal muscle fiber (Figure 2.9). Motor nerves have beaded synaptic terminals called motor end-plates because they resemble a collection of saucers. Unlike central synapses, which employ a variety of different neurotransmitters, all motor neurons release ACh from their terminal end-plates to depolarize a muscle fiber's membrane potential and thereby contract the skeletal muscle. Because ACh is the only neurotransmitter that is released at the neuromuscular junction, there is no mechanism by which peripheral nerves may directly inhibit a muscle fiber.

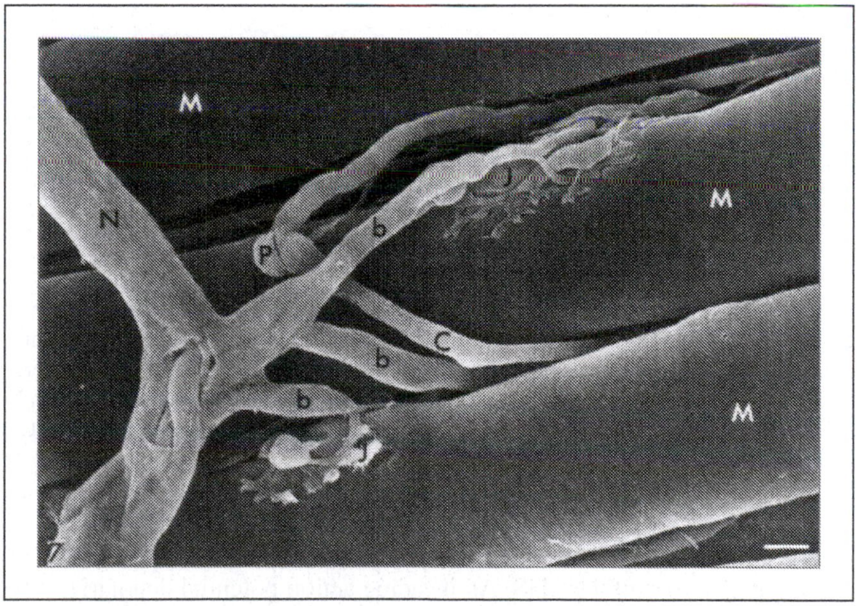

FIG. 2.9. Neuromuscular Junctions. This scanning electron micrograph depicts neuromuscular junctions in the sternothyroid muscle of a hamster. The peripheral nerve fiber (N) has collateral branches (b) which form junctions (J) with individual motor nerve fibers (M). A capillary (C) and pericyte (P) are also present. (This electron micrograph appeared originally in an article by Desaki J and Uehara Y: The overall morphology of neuromuscular junctions as revealed by scanning EM, *J Neurocyto* 10:107, 1981, and is reprinted here with the kind permission of Springer Science and Business Media.)

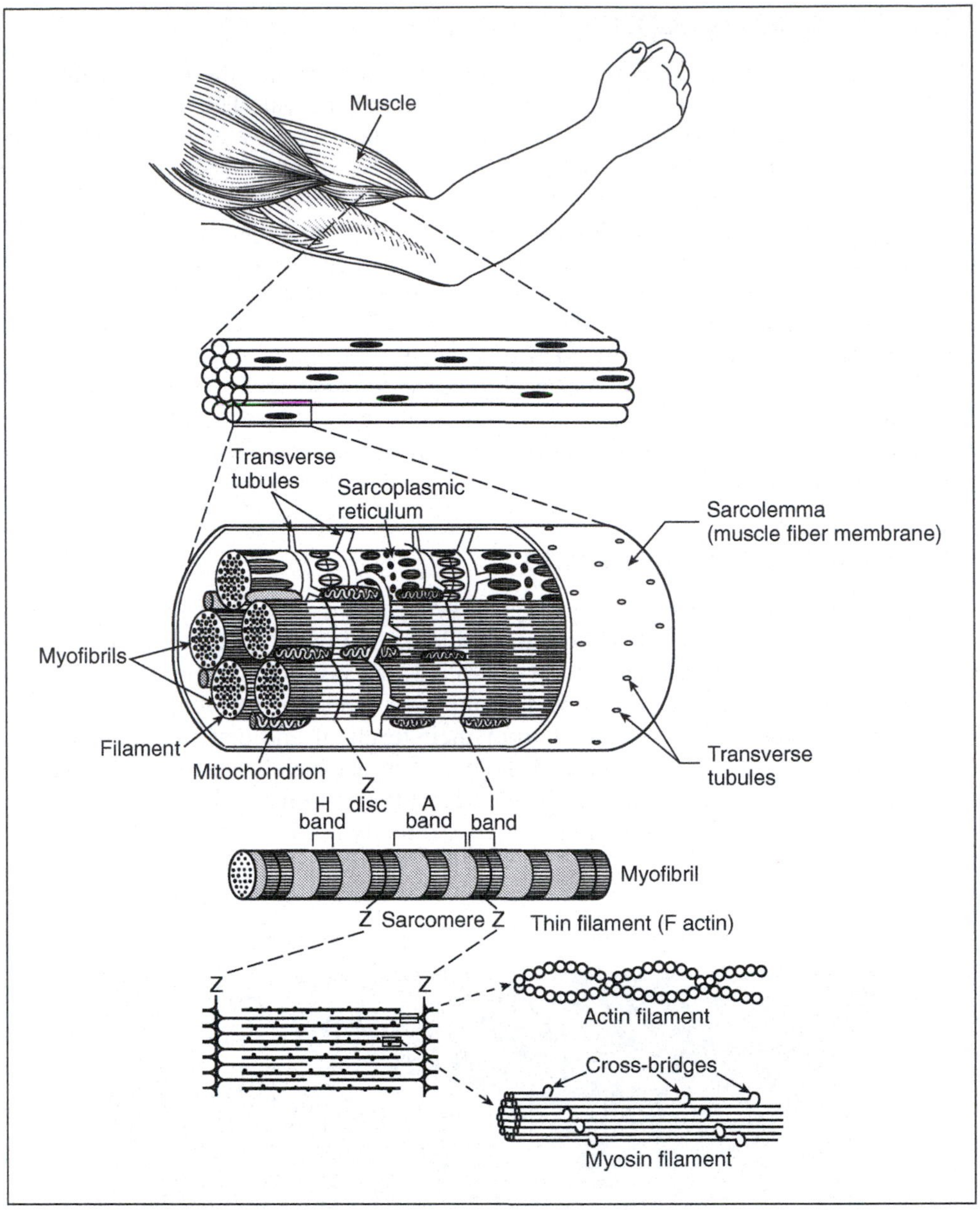

FIG. 2.10. Muscle Fibers. Muscles are composed of actin and myosin filaments. Cross-bridges between the actin and myosin fibers are activated by Ca^{2+} released from the lateral sacs of the sarcoplasmic reticulum (shown in the upper myofibril). Muscle contraction is driven by small, ratchet-like movements of the cross-bridges, which force the actin and myosin filaments to move in opposite directions.

Motor end-plates are motor neuron terminals at the neuromuscular junction.

Release of ACh at the neuromuscular junction resembles the process of chemical transmission at synapses in the CNS. An invading action potential depolarizes the motor end-plate, and this opens the voltage-gated Ca^{2+} channels that line the presynaptic membrane. The immediate influx of Ca^{2+} causes the synaptic vesicles to fuse with the presynaptic membrane and release ACh into the cleft separating the motor end-plate from the muscle fiber.

Cholinergic transmission at the neuromuscular junction triggers a rapid sequence of events that leads to muscular contraction (Figure 2.10). First, ACh molecules diffuse across the neuromuscular junction to activate cholinergic receptors lining a delicate postsynaptic membrane, the sarcolemma, which surrounds all striated muscle. Cholinergic receptor activation increases the permeability of both Na^+ and K^+ channels, but K^+ flow is usually small unless the postsynaptic membrane of the muscle is depolarized above 0 mV. If the membrane potential of the muscle fiber is at rest (near −90 mV), the resulting influx of Na^+ produces a local depolarization of the muscle known as an end-plate potential. The end-plate potential opens more voltage-gated Na^+ channels and, because of the electrochemical concentration gradient for Na^+, this ion flows rapidly into the muscle fiber and produces an action potential similar to those in a neuronal axon. When initiated, the action potential travels across the surface of the muscle cell and into transverse tubules, which perforate the muscle at regular intervals. Propagation of the action potential through the transverse tubules stimulates Ca^{2+} release from the lateral sacs of the sarcoplasmic reticulum, a cylindrical network of membranous tubules that envelop each myofibril. The sudden release of Ca^{2+} into the myofibrils initiates muscle contraction by activating movements of the cross-bridges that link the myosin and actin filaments.

Quantal Release of Acetylcholine

A synaptic vesicle releases a discrete quantity or "quantum" of neurotransmitter.

Microelectrode recordings from individual muscle fibers have revealed extremely small end-plate potentials when the motor nerve fiber is inactive. These potentials, called miniature end-plate potentials, occur spontaneously but are too weak to generate action potentials in the sarcolemma of the muscle fiber. Miniature end-plate potentials have extremely small amplitudes that are remarkably constant across different muscle fibers. Careful measurements of the larger end-plate potentials indicate that their amplitudes are integer multiples of the amplitude of a miniature end-plate potential. This suggests that a miniature end-plate potential represents the effect of a single synaptic vesicle releasing its reservoir of ACh. In fact, synaptic vesicles in the motor end-plates are nearly identical in size, and each one contains about 10,000 molecules of ACh. Hence, the miniature end-plate potential represents the effects of an incremental volume or "quantum" of neurotransmitter.

Neurotransmitter Receptors

Neurotransmitter receptors are transmembrane macromolecules that alter ionic flow across the plasma membrane in response to activation by a specific neurotransmitter molecule. In addition to being activated by endogenous neurotransmitters released by a presynaptic terminal, they are also activated by exogenous chemical compounds (e.g., drugs) that have a molecular structure similar to the neurotransmitter. In contrast to voltage-gated ion channels, which exist on all parts of a neuron's membrane including the axon, neurotransmitter receptors are present only on the soma, its dendrites, and on the synaptic terminals. In addition, whereas voltage-gated ion channels generally permit the flow of only one type of ion, a neurotransmitter receptor may permit several different ions to flow through the channel when the receptor is activated.

One major difference between neurotransmission at neuromuscular junctions and neuronal synapses is the diversity of postsynaptic responses that can be mediated by neurotransmitters in the CNS. Whereas the presynaptic neuron at a neuromuscular junction always uses ACh to produce rapid depolarization and contraction of the postsynaptic muscle fiber, different presynaptic terminals in the CNS use different neurotransmitters to produce a variety of postsynaptic effects. Moreover, when a neurotransmitter binds to a postsynaptic receptor in the CNS, the change in ionic conductance may shift the membrane potential closer or farther away from the action potential threshold.

Many types of postsynaptic receptors have been identified for each neurotransmitter. In many cases, different receptor subtypes for the same neurotransmitter produce different postsynaptic responses. This is an important functional property of the CNS because a neuron must release the same neurotransmitter from all of its axonal collaterals. Hence, different types of postsynaptic receptors enable collateral branches of a neuron to produce divergent responses in different brain regions.

Many drugs used to treat psychiatric illnesses achieve their therapeutic effects by binding to receptors as an agonist, which mimics a specific neurotransmitter, or as an antagonist, which prevents the neurotransmitter from activating the receptor. As more is learned about the pharmacokinetics of different receptor subtypes, this information can be used to design drugs that act with greater receptor specificity. Thus, it may be possible to develop drugs that ameliorate certain symptoms yet produce fewer side effects.

Two major classes of neurotransmitter receptors are recognized based on their mechanisms for changing the postsynaptic membrane potential: ionotropic and metabotropic. In the case of ionotropic or ligand-gated receptors, the ligand binding site and the ion channel are a single entity, and the bound ligand causes the channel to open. In the case of metabotropic receptors, however, the ligand binding site is physically separated from the ion channel. Ligand binding at a metabotropic receptor initiates a series of internal biochemical reactions that eventually open the separate ion channel. Because of these additional steps, metabotropic receptors take longer, sometimes several seconds or minutes, to alter ionic conductance. Some neurotransmitters may activate both ionotropic and metabotropic receptors to produce immediate and delayed postsynaptic changes at the same synapse.

Ionotropic Receptors. Ionotropic receptors are usually composed of five elongated protein subunits that extend across the plasma membrane to form a pentameric structure that encircles a central water-filled pore or channel (Figure 2.11). One end of each protein subunit extends into the synaptic cleft, and at least one of these extracellular domains contains a site for binding a neurotransmitter molecule or an exogenous ligand. When a neurotransmitter or agonist binds to the receptor, the resulting conformational change in the protein subunit alters the ionic conductance of the encircled channel. For most ionotropic receptors, the change in ionic conductance occurs independently of the pre-existing membrane potential. When the ion channel is open, however, the electrochemical gradients produce an ionic flux that alters the local membrane potential.

Ionotropic receptors:
- Neurotransmitter receptor and ion channel are directly linked.
- Receptor activation alters channel conductance rapidly.

Neurotransmitter binding at an ionotropic receptor produces a direct alteration in ion channel conductance, which leads to a rapid change in membrane potential. This postsynaptic change usually begins within a fraction of a millisecond, and the entire postsynaptic response is generally brief, extending over an interval of perhaps 100 milliseconds.

The molecular structure and distribution of many ionotropic receptors have been fully characterized. Consistent with their rapid response to neurotransmitter binding, ionotropic receptors are located at synapses where a quick postsynaptic response is

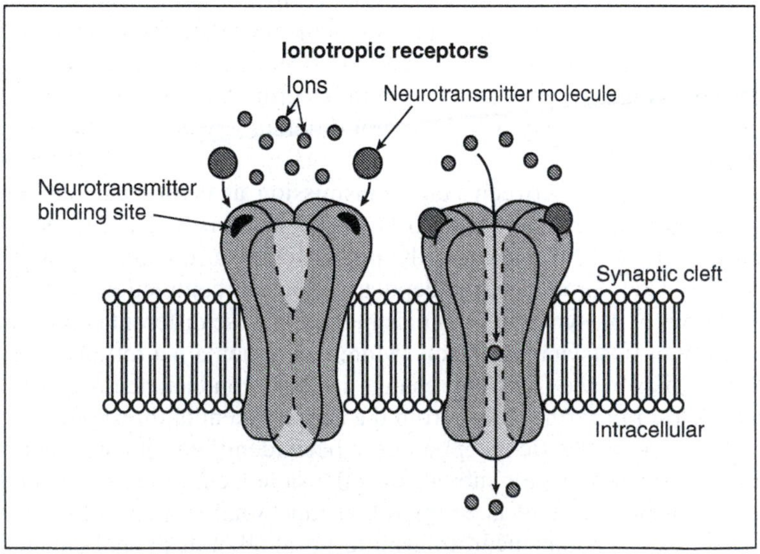

FIG. 2.11. Ionotropic Receptors. A typical ligand-gated ionotropic receptor consists of five protein subunits that surround a central pore. In this case, binding of two neurotransmitter molecules to the binding site causes the ion channel to open.

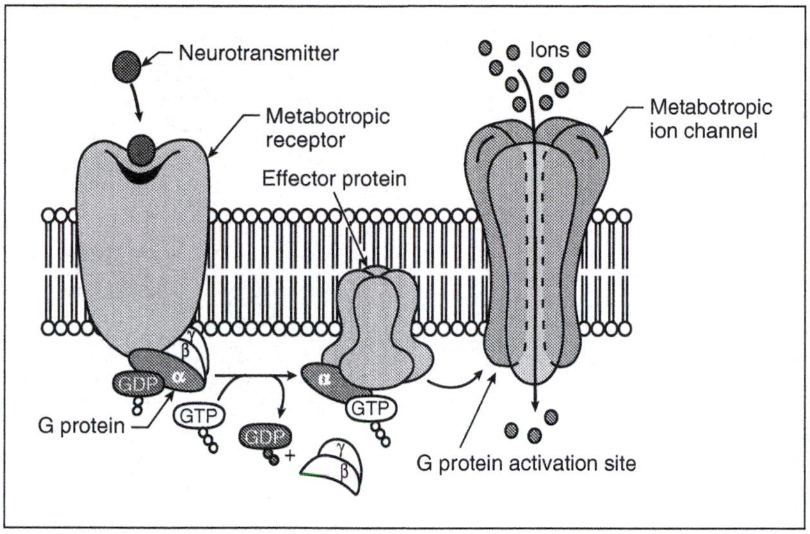

FIG. 2.12. Metabotropic Receptors. Metabotropic receptors control ion channels through a series of intermediate steps involving activation of G-proteins. In some metabotropic receptors, the G-proteins activate a cascade of intracellular enzymes or cause long-lasting changes in genetic expression. GTP = guanosine triphosphate; GDP = guanosine diphosphate.

required. Among the ionotropic receptors that have been characterized are the cholinergic receptors at the neuromuscular junction, the glutamatergic receptors that mediate fast EPSPs, and the GABAergic receptors that mediate fast IPSPs.

Metabotropic Receptors. Metabotropic receptors are physically separated from their ion channels and, therefore, must activate a series of intermediate proteins to regulate channel conductance (see Figure 2.12). Because these metabolic steps take time, synaptic transmission that involves metabotropic receptors is relatively slow. Postsynaptic responses mediated by metabotropic receptors may last for hundreds of milliseconds or much longer, even minutes or hours. There are many types of metabotropic receptors, but each type responds to only one of the neurotransmitters, including ACh (muscarinic receptor), glutamate, GABA, norepinephrine, dopamine, serotonin, histamine, or one of the neuropeptides.

Unlike ionotropic receptors, each metabotropic receptor is a single protein that has seven membrane-spanning regions. Metabotropic receptors are also called G-protein receptors because they activate proteins associated with guanosine triphosphate (GTP) or guanosine diphosphate (GDP). The extracellular domain of a metabotropic receptor has a neurotransmitter binding site, whereas the intracellular domain has a site for binding G-protein molecules.

> **Metabotropic receptors:** Neurotransmitter receptor and ion channel are separate.
>
> Receptor activation alters intermediate proteins.
>
> Change in ionic conductance occurs slowly.

When the receptor is inactive, the G-proteins that are bound to the intracellular domain contain three subunits (α, β, γ) of which the α-subunit is linked to GDP. When a neurotransmitter molecule binds to the receptor, the GDP is exchanged for GTP, and the α-GTP subunit dissociates from the $\beta\gamma$-subunits. The α-GTP and the $\beta\gamma$-subunits may activate other effector proteins in the neuron that control ion channel conductance. Most of the effector proteins are enzymes, such as adenylyl cyclase, guanylyl cyclase, and phospholipase C, that produce a variety of second messengers such as cyclic adenosine monophosphate (cAMP), diacylglycerol (DAG), and inositol triphosphate (IP_3). These second messengers activate different protein kinases that in turn regulate the degree of phosphorylation of different ion channels to increase or decrease their conductance.

Activated G-proteins may act directly at certain ion channels to produce a postsynaptic response. Direct interaction with the ion channel allows G-proteins to mediate postsynaptic responses in a few milliseconds, but these responses do not occur as quickly as

FIG. 2.13. Autoreceptors. Presynaptic receptors that respond to neurotransmitter molecules released from the same synaptic terminal are called autoreceptors. As indicated in this diagram, many autoreceptors activate G-proteins that close calcium channels. This mechanism provides negative feedback to the terminal and reduces the amount of neurotransmitter released in response to subsequent action potentials.

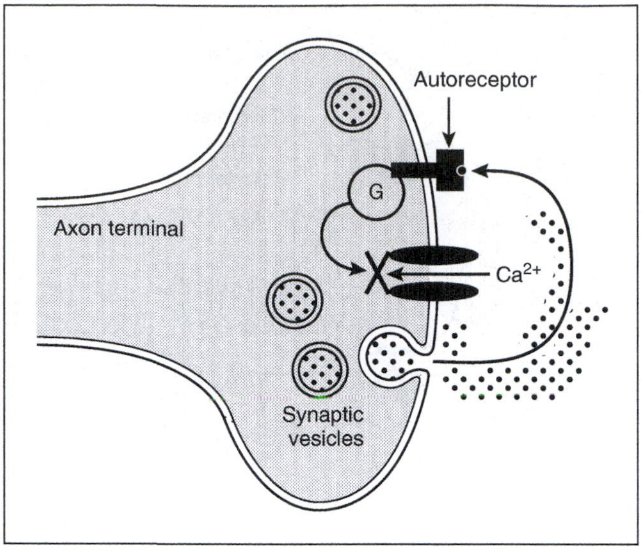

responses mediated by ionotropic receptors. In other cases, the G-proteins activate a cascade of multiple biochemical reactions that requires even more time. Metabotropic receptors may also alter gene expression to regulate the synthesis of enzymes or other proteins involved in synaptic transmission. Protein synthesis requires substantial time and probably mediates the long-lasting changes in synaptic structure that increase or decrease synaptic efficacy during learning and memory.

Autoreceptors:
Presynaptic receptors activated by neurotransmitter released from the same neuron provide a homeostatic mechanism for reducing neurotransmitter release.

Autoreceptors. Neurotransmitter receptors are located not only on the postsynaptic soma and dendrites, but also on the presynaptic terminals (Figure 2.13). Presynaptic receptors that respond to the neurotransmitter released from the same neuron on which they reside are called autoreceptors. Virtually all autoreceptors are metabotropic receptors that have homeostatic functions in regulating neurotransmission. When a neurotransmitter binds to an autoreceptor, the activated G-protein initiates a sequence of biochemical events that alter the amount of neurotransmitter that is released in response to an incoming action potential. In most but not all cases, autoreceptors represent a negative feedback mechanism for modulating synaptic transmission. For example, autoreceptor activation at an excitatory synapse reduces subsequent release of the neurotransmitter, thereby preventing excessive excitation of the postsynaptic neuron. By reducing the number of neurotransmitter molecules that are released into the synaptic cleft, autoreceptors also prevent the postsynaptic receptors from becoming desensitized (i.e., less responsive) to the neurotransmitter.

Different types of autoreceptors use different mechanisms to regulate synaptic transmission. In most cases, autoreceptor activation stimulates a G-protein, which binds directly to the calcium channel, thereby reducing the flow of calcium into the synaptic terminal. This prevents synaptic vesicles from docking with the presynaptic membrane and reduces the neurotransmitter release that is evoked by subsequent action potentials.

Autoreceptors on catecholamininergic or serotonergic neurons reduce neurotransmission by decreasing neurotransmitter synthesis. On dopamine neurons, for example, autoreceptors stimulate G-protein inhibition of adenyly cyclase, which decreases the cystolic concentration of cyclic adenosine monophosphate (cAMP). The decline in cAMP prevents the active form of tyrosine hydroxylase from being phosphorylated by protein kinase A. Given that tyrosine hydroxylase is the rate-limiting enzyme for dopamine synthesis, a decrease in its activity reduces dopamine synthesis.

Many drugs act selectively at specific receptor subtypes, including autoreceptors. Hence, autoreceptors are clinically significant because they provide a potential site for pharmacologic intervention in the treatment of neurologic disorders. In cases in which an increase in synaptic transmission is desired, drugs that block autoreceptors can increase neurotransmitter release. In fact, some psychoactive drugs enhance synaptic transmission by acting both as an autoreceptor antagonist and as a postsynaptic agonist.

Nicotinic Acetylcholine Receptors. Cholinergic receptors at the neuromuscular junction are called nicotinic receptors because nicotine is an agonist that opens the ionic channel. The isolation and purification of nicotinic receptors has revealed that each receptor consists of five protein subunits that form a pentamer around a central pore. Each subunit contains four transmembrane amino acid sequences that are coiled into a helical structure. The nicotinic ACh receptors at the neuromuscular junction contain two α-subunits, a β-subunit, a γ-subunit, and a δ-subunit. Each α-subunit has a single ACh binding site that may bind nicotine or other cholinergic ligands.

The five subunits form a funnel-shaped pore that has a large entrance and a small lumen near the cytoplasmic side of the channel. The channel opens when two ACh molecules bind to the receptor: one ACh molecule at each of the binding sites in the two α-subunits. Receptor activation by two ACh molecules causes a conformational change in the subunits that allows both Na^+ and K^+ ions to flow through the channel. If the muscle fiber is hyperpolarized, the respective concentration gradients for Na^+ and K^+ produce an influx of Na^+ that is much greater than the efflux of K^+. The net effect is that muscle fiber becomes depolarized.

Venoms and Toxins That Alter Cholinergic Transmission. Given the vital importance of ACh for mediating neuromuscular responses throughout the animal kingdom, it is not surprising that many species of plants and animals synthesize toxins and venoms that alter cholinergic transmission, either as a defense mechanism or to capture prey. Cholinergic receptors are classified as nicotinic or muscarinic because they are differentially sensitive to toxic alkaloids that are synthesized by plants. Nicotine is produced by the tobacco plant, *Nicotinia tabacum,* and muscarine is present in a red mushroom, *amanita muscaria*. Nicotine and muscarine are both cholinergic agonists that can produce nausea, vomiting, and convulsions. Moreover, muscarine poisoning poses a significant risk by interfering with circulatory functions, an effect that can lead to coma and death.

Some plant toxins interfere with cholinergic transmission by acting as nicotinic receptor antagonists. The alkaloid δ-tubocurarine, which is derived from the plant *chondodendron tomentosum,* blocks nicotinic receptors at the neuromuscular junction and causes death by paralyzing the respiratory muscles. Indeed, South American Indian tribes exploited this potent pharmacologic effect by dipping their arrowheads in curare.

The deadly effect of cholinergic antagonists is further illustrated by several animal species whose venoms act at the neuromuscular junction. Thus, the venoms of snakes such as the cobra (i.e., α-neurotoxin) and the branded krait (i.e., α-bungarotoxin) are lethal because they block nicotinic receptors on muscles. Interestingly enough, nicotinic receptors in the CNS differ from those at the neuromuscular junction. In contrast to nicotinic receptors on muscles (see above), nicotinic receptors in the CNS contain three α-subunits and two β-subunits. This small change renders CNS nicotinic receptors insensitive to α-bungarotoxin.

Glutamate Receptors. Several families of glutamate receptors have been identified, but the functional properties of the different receptor subtypes are not completely understood. In general, glutamate receptors are represented by one family of metabotropic receptors (mGluR), which are activated by quisqualate and related compounds, and by a larger family of ionotropic receptors, which are activated by α-amino-3-hydroxyl-5-methyl-4-isoxazole-propionate (AMPA), kainic acid (kainate), or *N*-methyl-D-aspartate (NMDA). The postsynaptic effects of glutaminergic transmission vary widely throughout the brain because some glutamate synapses have one glutamate receptor subtype, whereas other synapses contain many glutamate receptor subtypes.

Different protein subunits may combine to form specific receptor subtypes that possess unique physiologic characteristics.

The AMPA and kainate receptor subtypes are formed by five subunits that are assembled around a central pore. Six different protein subunits can be used to form the pentameric structure of a specific AMPA or kainate receptor. Hence, there are dozens of AMPA or kainate receptor subtypes that can be constructed from different combinations of these subunits, and each subtype may differ in its functional properties. Glutamate-induced activation of an AMPA or kainate receptor usually causes a rapid increase in Na^+ and K^+ conductance. Hence, if the postsynaptic membrane is in a hyperpolarized state, a rapid influx of Na^+ would evoke an EPSP.

The NMDA receptor is formed by a family of five subunits that can combine in different permutations to form dozens of NMDA receptor subtypes. These receptors differ from the AMPA and kainate receptors, however, in that glutamate activation of an NMDA receptor increases the conductance of Ca^{2+} as well as Na^+ and K^+. As a result, NMDA receptor activation increases the intracellular concentration of Ca^{2+}. The NMDA receptors are unique because Mg^{2+} ions are strongly attracted to the Ca^{2+} channel when the membrane is hyperpolarized, and the presence of Mg^{2+} prevents Ca^{2+} from passing through the channel. Therefore, NMDA receptors are activated by glutamate only if the Mg^{2+} block has been removed by previous depolarization of the membrane. This is significant because it means that NMDA receptors are both ligand gated and voltage dependent. Current flow through an NMDA-controlled ion channel is more likely to occur when the postsynaptic neuron is depolarized by convergent excitatory synapses from a large number of presynaptic neurons. Hence, NMDA receptors represent a mechanism for detecting strong excitation from multiple convergent pathways, a property that contributes to the strengthening of synaptic efficacy that takes place during learning and memory. This view is based, in part, on the fact that Ca^{2+} influx is needed for protein synthesis and other metabolic responses required for altering synaptic morphology.

GABA Receptors. There are two main categories of GABA receptors: $GABA_A$ and $GABA_B$. The $GABA_A$ receptors are ionotropic, whereas the $GABA_B$ receptors are metabotropic receptors. $GABA_A$ receptors have a pentameric structure similar to the ligand-gated ion channels described for glutamate and ACh. There are five different protein subunits (α, β, γ, δ, ρ) that can combine to produce several different $GABA_A$ receptor subtypes. Activation of any of these $GABA_A$ receptors causes a rapid increase in Cl^- membrane conductance. Because the equilibrium potential for Cl^- is close to the resting membrane potential of most neurons, Cl^- influx usually produces very small changes in the membrane potential. Nonetheless, when Cl^- conductance is increased, the membrane potential becomes less responsive to excitatory inputs arriving from other synapses, which reduces the probability of a neuronal discharge.

Numerous drugs interact with GABAergic synapses by binding with one of the subunits of the $GABA_A$ receptor. Tranquilizers such as diazepam (i.e., valium) bind to the α- and β-subunits, whereas barbiturates such as phenobarbital bind to the γ-subunits. Many of the GABAergic agonists do not directly alter ionic conductance but promote the inhibitory effects of GABAergic transmission by enhancing the affinity of GABA for its binding site. The clinical effectiveness of these drugs is based on their ability to suppress neuronal activity in specific brain regions. Alcohol also acts at GABA receptors, which explains why combining alcohol with tranquilizers or barbiturates has a powerful synergistic effect on cognitive processing and behavior.

Muscarinic Acetylcholine Receptors. Perhaps the best-characterized example of a metabotropic receptor is the muscarinic ACh receptor found in the heart and the CNS. Muscarine is a cholinergic agonist that slows cardiac output and reduces the frequency of action potentials in many neurons in the CNS. These responses occur because muscarinic receptors activate G-proteins that open K^+ channels; the resulting efflux of K^+ causes rapid hyperpolarization. This effect can be mimicked by injecting the $\beta\gamma$-subunits into the cell. Furthermore, muscarinic activation of the α-subunit causes rapid closing of both Ca^{2+} and Na^+ channels, an effect that increases the inhibitory actions of the βγ-subunits.

Catecholamine Receptors. All of the catecholamines activate metabotropic receptors. The adrenergic receptors, which can be activated by either epinephrine or norepinephrine, are classified into three families, α1, α2, and β, each of which can be further subdivided into three subclasses. The α2 and β1 receptor classes represent the main adrenergic receptors in the brain that are well characterized. Thus, the α2 subtype is an autoreceptor on adrenergic terminals that inhibits the production of adenylate cyclase. By contrast, all of the β receptor subtypes activate adenylate cyclase. Many adrenergic agonists and antagonists act on smooth muscles, and selective activation of the different receptor subtypes is used to treat high blood pressure, asthma, and other symptoms associated with the cardiovascular and respiratory systems.

Dopamine receptors are subdivided into five subtypes that are grouped into two main classes, the D1-like and D2-like receptors. The vast majority of dopamine receptors are located in the caudate, putamen, and nucleus accumbens, which are the main input nuclei of the basal ganglia. Each dopamine receptor subtype has been found at presynaptic and postsynaptic sites. The D1-like receptors (i.e., D1 and D5) activate adenylate cyclase and increase production of cyclic AMP, whereas the D2-like receptors (i.e., D2, D3, and D4) inhibit adenylate cyclase. Despite having opposite effects on adenylate cyclase, the functional effect produced by each receptor subclass has been elusive. Imbalances in dopamine transmission have been implicated in schizophrenia and other neuropsychiatric disorders, and this has led to the development of several antipsychotic drugs that act on dopamine receptors.

RESOLUTION OF CLINICAL CASE

The case in this chapter describes the classic symptoms of myasthenia gravis, an autoimmune disorder caused by the formation of antibodies directed against nicotinic ACh receptors in skeletal muscle. Following the loss of cholinergic receptors, muscles are less responsive to ACh released from peripheral motor neurons. Most patients with this disease initially experience weakness in the extraocular muscles and the muscles controlling facial expression, swallowing, and chewing. Hence, patients with myasthenia gravis usually present with dysarthria (inarticulate speech), dysphagia (difficulty swallowing), ptosis (drooping eyelids), and diplopia (double vision). These symptoms are intermittent and may disappear for weeks before reappearing. It is important to note that muscle weakness, not fatigue, is an essential element in the diagnosis of myasthenia gravis. If untreated, myasthenia gravis usually affects the respiratory muscles, especially during periods of emotional stress or respiratory infection. In fact, most deaths are attributed to respiratory failure. Consistent with its autoimmune mechanism, the primary relatives of these patients exhibit a significant incidence of other autoimmune disorders such as rheumatoid arthritis or lupus.

Myasthenia gravis is diagnosed by injecting Tensilon (edrophonium chloride), a drug that inhibits acetylcholinesterase, the enzyme at the neuromuscular junction that degrades ACh. Following a Tensilon injection, patients with myasthenia gravis regain muscle strength immediately because the drug increases the concentration of synaptic ACh, which activates the remaining nicotinic receptors that have not been destroyed by the disease. When myasthenia gravis is confirmed, patients often undergo plasmapheresis, a procedure that removes the antibodies circulating in the blood. For long-term management of the disease, patients are maintained on immunosuppressive drugs that reduce the production of antibodies that attack the nicotinic receptors.

REVIEW QUESTIONS

Directions: For each of the following questions, choose the **one best** answer.

1. Which of the following pairs of items are **unlikely** to be located in the same synaptic terminal?
   A. Dense-core vesicles and clear synaptic vesicles
   B. Substance P and glutamate
   C. Acetylcholine (ACh) and glutamate
   D. Tyrosine hydroxylase and dopamine
   E. Mitochondria and clear synaptic vesicles

2. What ion plays a critical role in protein synthesis and muscle contraction?
   A. Ca^{2+}
   B. Cl^-
   C. K^+
   D. Mg^{2+}
   E. Na^+

3. The repetitive seizures in epilepsy are caused by excessive release of which neurotransmitter?
   A. Glutamate
   B. γ-aminobutyric acid (GABA)
   C. Acetylcholine (ACh)
   D. Norepinephrine
   E. Substance P

4. L-dopa ameliorates the symptoms of Parkinson's disease because it does what?
   A. Blocks dopamine autoreceptors
   B. Activates postsynaptic dopamine receptors
   C. Is converted to dopamine by all neurons that contain amino acid decarboxylase
   D. Is converted to dopamine by dopaminergic terminals
   E. Interferes with the hydrolysis of dopamine

5. What causes the motor symptoms associated with myasthenia gravis?
   A. A viral infection that destroys the motor neurons in the spinal cord
   B. A genetic mutation that results in decreased production of acetylcholine
   C. A viral infection that destroys the myelin surrounding peripheral motor neurons
   D. A dietary deficiency in choline intake
   E. An autoimmune disorder that destroys nicotinic receptors

6. What neurotransmitter interacts only with metabotropic receptors?
   A. Glutamate
   B. Dopamine
   C. Acetylcholine
   D. GABA
   E. *N*-methyl-D-aspartate

7. Curare, mustard gas, and α-bungarotoxin produce their lethal effects by doing what?
   A. Altering transmission at the neuromuscular junction
   B. Blocking the synthesis of dopamine
   C. Stimulating mucarinic receptors
   D. Releasing acetylcholine in the CNS
   E. Blocking calcium channels

ADDITIONAL READING

Classic Literature

Curtis DR, Phillis JW, Watkins JC: Chemical excitation of spinal neurons. *Nature* 183:611–612, 1959.

Dale HH, Feldberg W, Vogt M: Release of acetylcholine at voluntary motor nerve endings. *J Physiol* 86:353–380, 1936.

Furshpan EJ, Potter DD: Transmission at the giant motor synapses of the crayfish. *J Physiol (Lond)* 145:289–325, 1959.

Reviews and Landmark Research Articles

Adams ME, Olivera BM: Neurotoxins: overview of an emerging research technology. *Trends in Neurosci* 17:151–155, 1994.

Augustine GJ: How does calcium trigger neurotransmitter release? *Curr Opin Neurobiol* 11:320–326, 2001.

Carlsson A: Perspectives on the discovery of central monoaminergic neurotransmission. *Ann Rev Neurosci* 10:19–40, 1987.

Cooper JR, Bloom FE, Roth RH: *The Biochemical Basis of Neuropharmacology*. New York, NY: Oxford Press, 2003.

Gilman AG: G proteins and dual control of adenylate cyclase. *Cell* 36:577–579, 1984.

Hokfelt T, Millhorn D, Seroogy K, Tsuruo Y, Ceccatelli S, Lindh B, Meister B, Melander T, Schalling M, Bartfai T: Coexistence of peptides with classical neurotransmitters. *Experientia,* 43:768–780, 1987.

Hughes J, Smith HW, Kosterlitz LA, Fothergill, Morgan BA, Morris HR: Identification of two related pentapeptides from the brain with potent opiate agonist activity. *Nature* 258:577–580, 1975.

Miledi R: Transmitter release induced by injection of calcium ions into nerve terminals. *Proc R Soc Lond B* 183:421–425, 1973.

Mody I, Pearce RA: Diversity of inhibitory neurotransmission through GABA(A) receptors. *Trends Neurosci* 27:569–575, 2004.

Murthy VN, De Camilli P: Cell biology of the presynaptic terminal. *Ann Rev Neurosci* 26:701–728, 2003.

Nakanishi S: Molecular diversity of glutamate receptors and implications for brain function. *Science* 258:597–603, 1992.

Rothman SM: Synaptic activity mediates death of hypoxic neurons. *Science* 220:536–537, 1983.

Sealfon SC, Olanow CW: Dopamine receptors: from structure to behavior. *Trends Neurosci* 10:S34–40, 2000.

Sheng M, Kim MJ: Postsynaptic signaling and plasticity mechanisms. *Science* 298:776–780, 2002.

Sieb JP: Myasthenia gravis: emerging new therapy options. *Curr Opin Pharmacol* 5:303–307, 2005.

Sudhof TC: The synaptic vesicle cycle: a cascade of protein-protein interactions. *Nature* 375:645–653, 1995.

Vincent A: Unraveling the pathogenesis of myasthenia gravis. *Nature Rev Immunol* 2:797–804, 2002.

INTERNET RESOURCES

American Parkinson Disease Association
http://www.apdaparkinson.org/

Center for Synaptic Plasticity
http://www.bris.ac.uk/Depts/Synaptic/Welcome.html

Multimedia Neuroscience Education Project of Williams College
http://www.williams.edu/imput/

Muscular Dystrophy Association
http://www.mda.org.au/specific/mdamg.html

Myasthenia Gravis Foundation of America
http://www.myasthenia.org/

National Institute of Neurological Disorders and Stroke
Epilepsy
http://www.ninds.nih.gov/disorders/epilepsy/epilepsy.htm

National Institute of Neurological Disorders and Stroke
Myasthenia Gravis
http://www.ninds.nih.gov/disorders/myasthenia_gravis/myasthenia_gravis.htm

National Parkinson Foundation
http://www.parkinson.org/

National Society for Epilepsy
http://www.e-epilepsy.org.uk/

Neuromuscular Disease Center of Washington University
http://www.neuro.wustl.edu/neuromuscular/

Neurosciences on the Internet
http://www.neuroguide.com/

NIH—The Brain: Understanding Neurobiology (see Student Activities)
http://science.education.nih.gov/supplements/nih2/addiction/default.htm

The Medical Biochemistry Page
http://web.indstate.edu/thcme/mwking/home.html

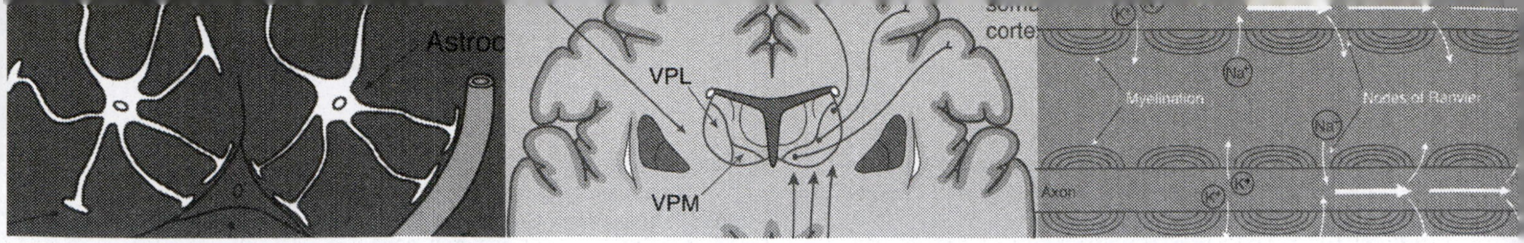

CHAPTER 3

General Organization of the Nervous System

INTRODUCTION OF CLINICAL CASE

When a 67-year-old retired plumber was brought to the emergency department by his wife, he had a flushed complexion and was experiencing shortness of breath and nausea. The patient reported having the worst headache of his life. Onset of the headache several hours earlier was sudden, but poorly localized. The patient reported having few headaches over the last year, but several over the past 2 weeks; none responded to self-medication with aspirin. This headache, unlike the others, was accompanied by a stiff neck. The patient's blood pressure (170/100 mm Hg) and heart rate (90 beats/min) were elevated; his respiration rate was 20 breaths/min and labored. As the physical examination continued, the patient became disoriented, incoherent, stuporous, and finally lost consciousness. The physician ordered a full series of computed tomography (CT) scans of the head and, pending the outcome of the scans, a lumbar puncture.

TERMINOLOGY AND NOMENCLATURE

Neuroscientists use a specialized lexicon to describe the complex three-dimensional organization of the nervous system. To students beginning their study of neuroanatomy, this terminology may seem daunting, but given time, it will prove its worth.

Orientation

The longitudinal orientation of the mammalian nervous system is best appreciated in a quadruped species such as the rat. As Figure 3.1 illustrates, the nervous system of the rat has clear rostral and caudal ends that correspond to its nose and tail. The rat's ventral (or anterior) surface points to the substrate, and its dorsal (or posterior) surface forms the back. In humans, the brain has a pronounced flexure that orients the forebrain almost perpendicular to that of the spinal cord (see Figure 3.1). At spinal and lower brainstem levels, the terms "dorsal" and "ventral" have the same meaning in bipeds and quadrupeds. Further rostrally, however, this flexure affects the meaning of some terms. For example, the terms "dorsal" and "ventral" continue to describe structures that lie above or below the long axis of the brain, but the terms "anterior" and "posterior" relate to the rostrocaudal axis—that is, toward or away from the front of the head.

Three other terms use the midline as their reference point. "Median" means on the midline, and "medial" means toward the midline. Note that a structure may be medial to another yet may not lie on the midline. "Lateral" means away from the midline. Hence, the words "lateral" and "medial" are used with respect to a reference; for example, "A lies lateral to B."

Planes of Section

Sections of the nervous system are typically shown in one of the three major planes: sagittal, coronal (transverse), or horizontal (Figure 3.2). A sagittal section divides the specimen into left and right portions. When a specimen is cut on the midline, it is called a midsagittal section; sections parallel to, but offset from the midline, are in parasagittal planes. A view of the brainstem or spinal cord that is perpendicular to its long axis is a transverse section. A similar section in the forebrain, i.e., that is rostral to the flexure of the neuraxis, is in the

Three major planes of section:
- Sagittal
- Coronal
- Horizontal

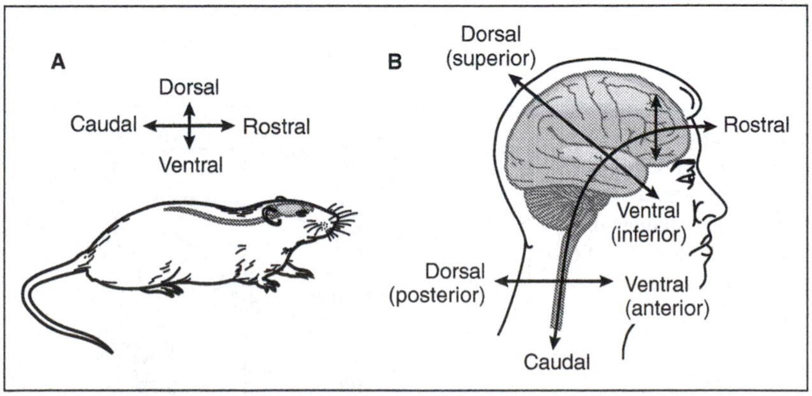

FIG. 3.1. Axes of the Central Nervous System. The directions of orientation used to describe the brain of the rat (A), whose brain is linear, and the human (B), whose brain has a pronounced flexure.

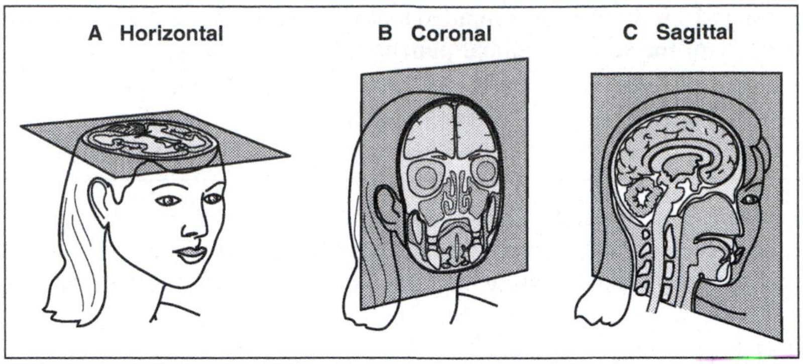

FIG. 3.2. Planes of Section. Panels A, B, and C illustrate the horizontal, coronal, and sagittal planes of section that are used to describe the human brain.

coronal plane. Sections made in the horizontal plane divide the specimen into dorsal and ventral segments. It is common for neuroradiographic studies of the forebrain to be done in the horizontal plane; in the brainstem, it is rare. Oblique sections do not conform to any of these planes.

Pathways

Interhemispheric pathways:
- Corpus callosum
- Anterior commissure
- Posterior commissure
- Hippocampal commissure

Mastery of the organization of the central nervous system (CNS) requires a detailed understanding of its circuitry. A variety of terms are used to distinguish the different types of CNS pathways (Figure 3.3). A collection of axons is called a tract, fasciculus, lemniscus, or pathway. The term funiculus refers to one of the longitudinal bulges in the spinal cord formed by an underlying tract. Pathways whose origin, course, and destination remain on the same side of the nervous system constitute ipsilateral projections; those that cross the midline project contralaterally. Crossing or decussating pathways are common in the nervous system and account for a number of observations including control of the body's musculature by the contralateral side of the brain. Another type of crossing pathway, the commissure, interconnects corresponding regions of the brain or spinal cord. The brain's largest commissure, the corpus callosum, interconnects most parts of the cerebral hemispheres.

Fugit, from Latin, means "to flee" (e.g., *tempus fugit*).

Afferent pathways, which bring information to a nucleus, are often distinguished from efferent pathways that leave a nucleus (*pl.* nuclei). These terms also may be used without reference to a particular nucleus. For example, an afferent projection carries sensory information (e.g., a sour taste), whereas an efferent projection has a motor function

FIG. 3.3. Pathways. Diagram showing the assembly of axons into progressively larger fiber bundles and the names used to distinguish between bundles that cross the midline and those that do not.

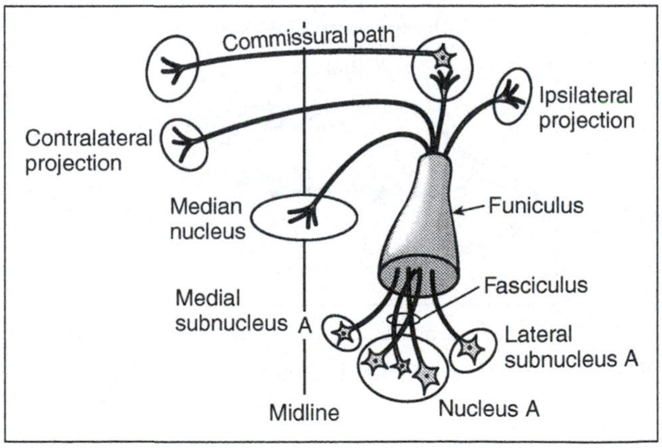

(e.g., innervation of the biceps muscle). Another way to distinguish afferent and efferent pathways is to add the suffix "-fugal" or "-petal" to the nuclear root. For example, efferent projections of the cerebral cortex are corticofugal, and its afferent pathways are corticopetal. In both instances there may be multiple cortical connections, but none are identified with this nomenclature. Another way to specify a pathway is to combine the source and destination nuclei into a new word. For example, a cerebellothalamic projection goes from the cerebellum to the thalamus. This nomenclature designates both the source and destination of the pathway without designating either as sensory or motor or whether the pathway crosses the midline or remains on the ipsilateral side.

NERVOUS SYSTEM

The nervous system has a hierarchical structure that resembles the organization chart of a large corporation. Information gathered by receptors located throughout the body is transmitted to subcortical nuclei, the neural equivalent of corporate departments. This information is transferred to the cerebral cortex where it undergoes further analysis before a plan of action is determined. The action plan is transferred to subordinate systems in the brainstem and spinal cord where implementation takes place. This neural hierarchy, like its corporate counterpart, also enables routine tasks such as reflexes and autonomic regulation to proceed with limited supervision by the cerebral cortex. Complex tasks or those that require cognitive intervention require cortical participation.

Central Nervous System

There are two divisions of the nervous system: the CNS, which consists of the brain and spinal cord, and the peripheral nervous system. The CNS has five parts: (1) telencephalon, (2) diencephalon, (3) mesencephalon, (4) metencephalon, and (5) myelencephalon. The peripheral nervous system is composed of the 12 cranial nerves and the 31 pairs of spinal nerves.

The telencephalon, the most rostral part of the brain, consists of the cerebral cortex and several buried nuclei, the basal ganglia. The diencephalon lies beneath the telencephalon and, consequently, is hidden except for the small portion at the base of the brain that is encircled by the optic tracts and the temporal lobe. The mesencephalon (midbrain), metencephalon (pons and cerebellum), and myelencephalon (medulla) constitute the brainstem, which lies along the ventral surface of the brain. The spinal cord, the most caudal part of the CNS, is continuous with the myelencephalon and extends deep into the vertebral column.

The peripheral nervous system:
- 12 cranial nerves
- 31 spinal nerves

Telencephalon

Cerebral Cortex. The cerebral cortex is a highly convoluted, laminated structure whose appearance is consistent but not identical among individuals. Each convolution, or gyrus (*pl.* gyri), is separated from neighboring gyri by a deep groove called a sulcus (*pl.* sulci). The largest sulcus, the longitudinal fissure, divides the brain into left and right hemispheres. Each hemisphere consists of six lobes whose boundaries are determined by other prominent gyri and sulci. Four of these six lobes are named after the overlying bones of the skull: frontal, parietal, temporal, and occipital. The two remaining lobes, which are not visible externally, are the insular and the limbic lobes.

The two most prominent landmarks on the lateral cortical surface are the central sulcus (fissure of Rolando) and the lateral sulcus (Sylvian fissure; Figure 3.4). The central sulcus separates the frontal and parietal lobes. The lateral sulcus separates the frontal and parietal lobes from the temporal lobe.

The frontal lobe, the largest of the six lobes, includes all of the cortex dorsal to the lateral and cingulate sulci, and rostral to the central sulcus. The precentral gyrus, which forms the anterior bank of the central sulcus, contains the primary motor cortex. Immediately rostral to the precentral gyrus lies the premotor cortex, which has important connections with

The brain has four true lobes:
- Frontal
- Parietal
- Temporal
- Occipital

The brain has two synthetic lobes:
- Insula
- Limbic

Precentral gyrus: primary motor cortex

Broca's area: inferior frontal gyrus of the dominant hemisphere

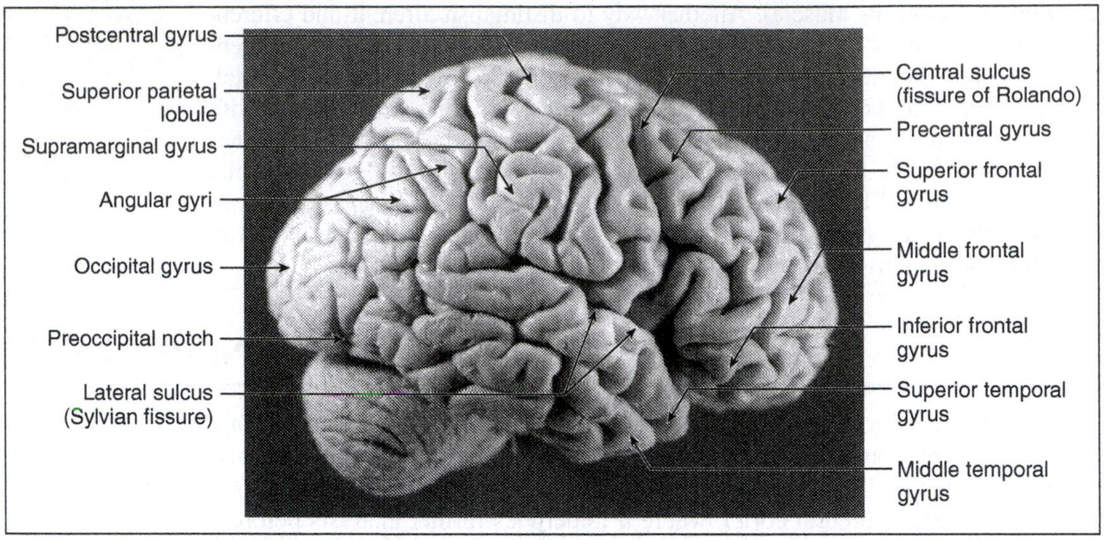

FIG. 3.4. Lateral Surface of the Brain. Anterior is to the right.

the primary motor area. Further rostrally, the frontal lobe consists of the superior, middle, and inferior frontal gyri, which are arranged as three horizontal tiers. The inferior frontal gyrus consists of three parts: the pars orbitalis, the pars triangularis, and the pars opercularis. In the dominant hemisphere, the pars triangularis and opercularis constitute Broca's area, an important region for motor control of language.

Postcentral gyrus: primary somatosensory cortex

The parietal lobe includes all cortex dorsal to the lateral and cingulate sulci between the central sulcus and the anterior border of the occipital lobe. The border between the parietal and occipital lobes is an imaginary line projecting from the parieto-occipital sulcus on the medial surface of the hemisphere to the pre-occipital notch on the lateral aspect of the hemisphere. The postcentral gyrus, which forms the posterior bank of the central sulcus, contains the primary somatosensory cortex and has a topographical representation of the contralateral body. The intraparietal sulcus divides the remainder of the parietal lobe into superior and inferior parietal lobules. A lobule is a group of gyri within one of the six lobes of the brain. The superior and inferior parietal lobules integrate somatosensory, auditory, and visual information from adjacent areas in the temporal, occipital, and parietal lobes.

Heschl's gyrus: primary auditory cortex

One cranial nerve is associated with the telencephalon: Olfactory (I)

- **Occipital lobe:** primary visual cortex

The temporal lobe occupies the ventral bank of the lateral sulcus, fills the entire middle cranial fossa, and shares the same posterior border with the parietal lobe. The surface of the temporal lobe is divided into superior, middle, and inferior gyri, all of which lie parallel to the Sylvian fissure. The superior temporal gyrus, which forms the ventral bank of the Sylvian fissure, contains the transversely oriented gyri of Heschl. This region serves as primary auditory cortex and has important connections with other auditory processing and language comprehension areas in the parietal and frontal lobes. More lateral parts of the temporal lobe, such as the inferior temporal gyrus, mediate pattern recognition and higher-order processing of visual information. The ventral surface of the temporal lobe is formed by the occipitotemporal and parahippocampal gyri (Figure 3.5). The parahippocampal gyrus is an important relay for sensory information bound for the limbic system. Part of the primary olfactory cortex is located at the medial tip of the parahippocampal gyrus, which is called the uncus.

The occipital lobe, lying caudal to the parietal and temporal lobes, comprises the posterior pole of the cerebral cortex. It is the smallest of the four true lobes and is devoted exclusively to vision. Primary visual cortex lies along the banks of the calcarine sulcus, the most prominent groove on the medial surface of the occipital lobe (Figure 3.6). Higher-order visual areas, which begin as a series of bands around the primary visual area, extend rostrally into the caudal parietal and temporal lobes.

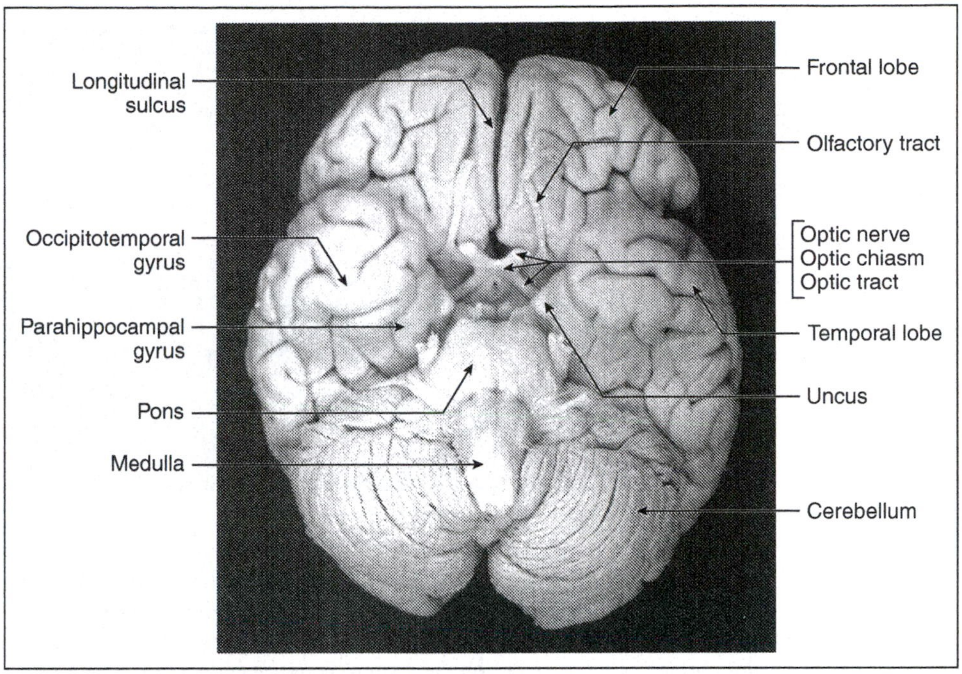

FIG. 3.5. Inferior Surface of the Brain. Anterior is to the top.

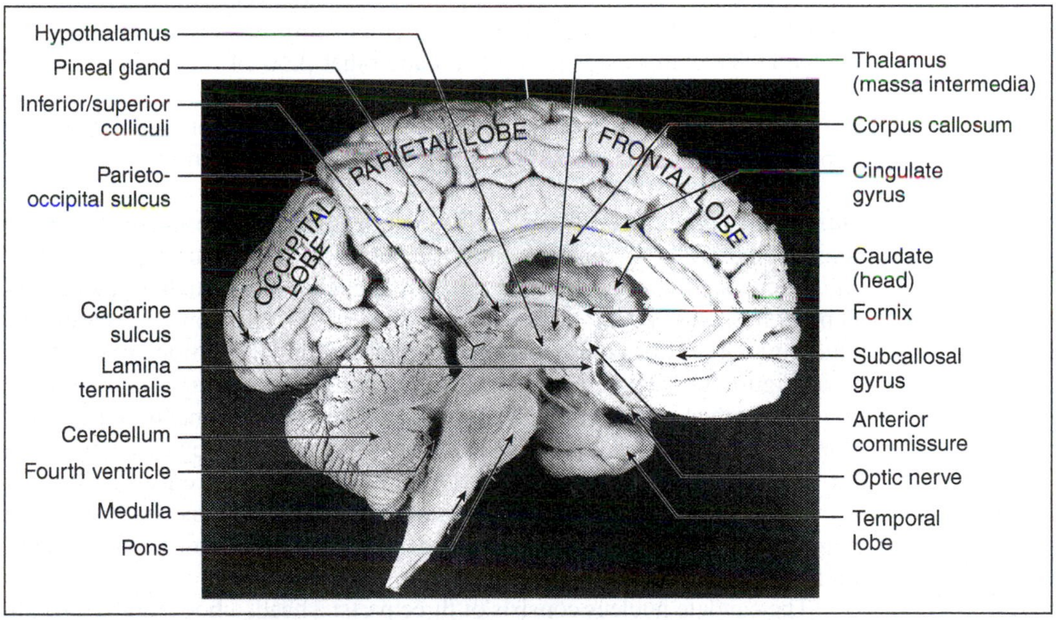

FIG. 3.6. Medial Surface of an Unstained Brain in the Midsagittal Plane. Anterior is to the right.

The insula and the limbic lobe are considered synthetic lobes because their boundaries are less clear. The insula, located deep within the lateral sulcus, can be visualized only after prying the temporal lobe apart from the overlying frontal and parietal lobes (Figure 3.7). The parts of the frontal, parietal, and temporal lobes that cover the insula are called the opercular cortex. In addition to serving as the primary gustatory cortex, the rostral insula has been implicated in cardiovascular, pulmonary, and gastric function.

- **Operculum,** from Latin, means "cover." The operculum covers the insula.
- **Insula:** primary taste cortex

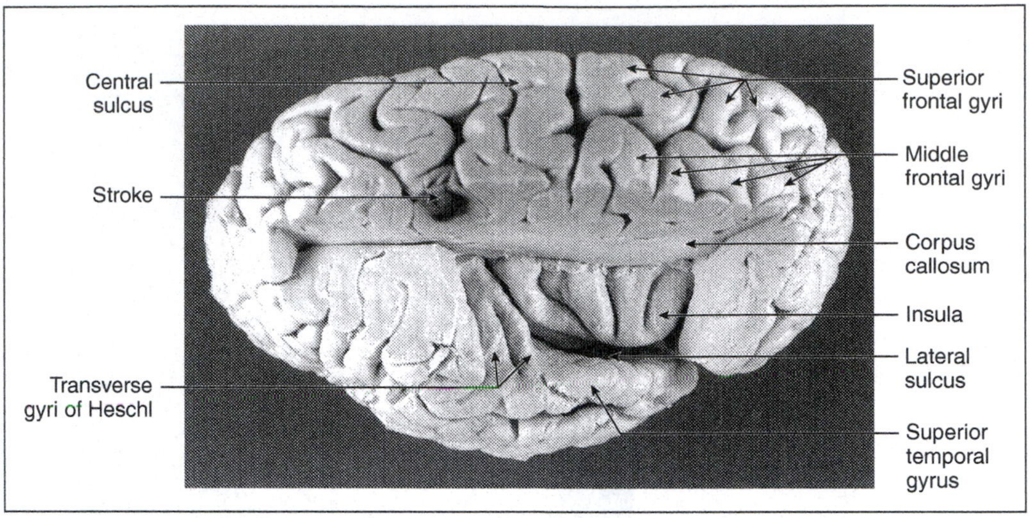

FIG. 3.7. Dorsolateral Aspect of the Brain. (Anterior is to the right.) A wedge of tissue has been removed from the frontoparietal cortex to reveal the underlying insula. The primary auditory cortex is located on the transverse gyri of Heschl along the superior aspect of the temporal lobe. The dark stain on the superior surface of the parietal lobe is a small hemorrhagic stroke, which was large enough to be symptomatic, but not fatal.

Limbic lobe: memory and emotion

The limbic lobe, located on the medial surface of the frontal, parietal, and temporal lobes, includes the subcallosal, cingulate, and parahippocampal gyri as well as the hippocampal formation. Collectively, these regions form a broad arc that surrounds the diencephalon. The hippocampal formation and other parts of the limbic cortex play a critical role in memory formation. Although the functions of the subcallosal and cingulate gyri are not well understood, the available research indicates that both are involved with pain perception, attention, and the visceral aspects of emotional expression.

Basal Ganglia. The basal ganglia include several large nuclei buried in the ventral telencephalon: the caudate nucleus, the putamen, the globus pallidus, and the subthalamic nucleus. Other nuclei located in the telencephalon (nucleus accumbens), the diencephalon (subthalamic nucleus), and the mesencephalon (substantia nigra, ventral tegmental area) have close anatomical and functional relationships with the basal ganglia (Figure 3.8). These nuclei of the basal ganglia are grouped in various ways depending on whether embryologic, anatomic, functional, or connectional criteria are applied. For example, most parts of the caudate and putamen are separated from one another by the anterior limb of the internal capsule, but they often are referred to as the neostriatum because of their functional similarity. The term "corpus striatum" refers to the caudate nucleus, putamen, and globus pallidus, whereas the term "lenticular nucleus" includes only the globus pallidus and the putamen.

The corpus striatum plays a role in movement disorders such as Parkinson's disease, Huntington's disease, and Tourette's syndrome.

The caudate nucleus consists of three parts: a head, a body, and a tail. The head of the caudate is a massive structure that forms the lateral wall of the lateral ventricle's anterior horn. As the body of the caudate nucleus stretches posteriorly, it becomes progressively smaller until it terminates like a tail within the inferior horn of the lateral ventricle. The putamen is the largest nucleus of the basal ganglia, but it can be seen only in sections through the telencephalon. Although the putamen and caudate are continuous rostrally, most of the putamen lies between the lateral margin of the globus pallidus and the external capsule (Figure 3.9). The globus pallidus is an embryologic derivative of the diencephalon but is considered part of the basal ganglia by virtue of its massive input from the neostriatum. The corpus striatum is involved with sensorimotor integration.

The amygdala is an almond-shaped cluster of small nuclei located within the rostral pole of the temporal lobe beneath the uncus (see Figure 3.8). Classically, the amygdaloid

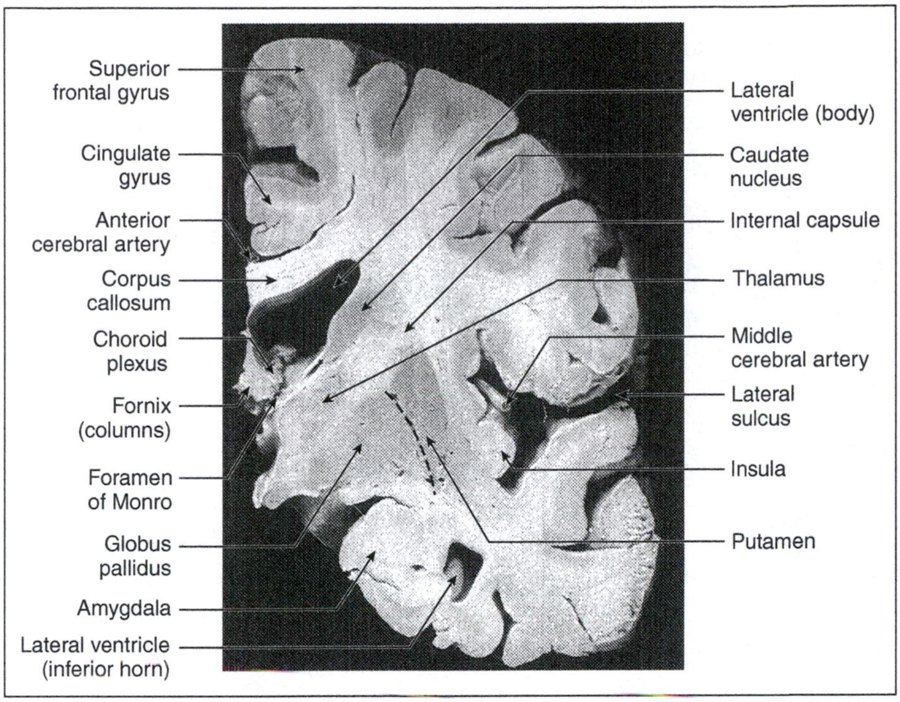

FIG. 3.8. Unstained Coronal Section of the Brain Showing the Basal Ganglia.

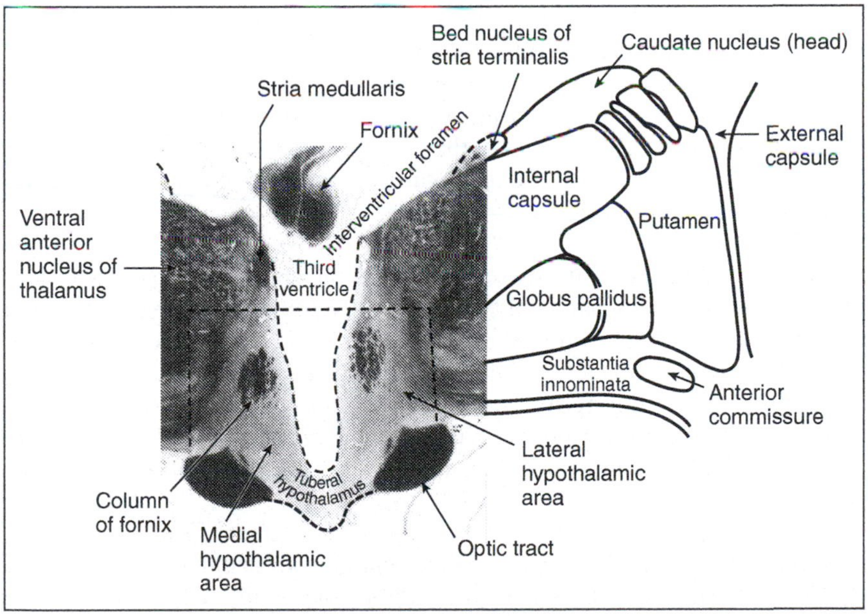

FIG. 3.9. Coronal Section of the Brain at the Level of the Interventricular Foramen.

complex was considered part of the basal ganglia because of its embryologic origin. Its connections with the hypothalamus and its involvement in emotional behavior, however, have led to its inclusion with the limbic system (see Chapter 14).

Diencephalon:
- Thalamus
- Hypothalamus
- Subthalamus
- Epithalamus

Diencephalon. The diencephalon consists of four parts: thalamus, hypothalamus, subthalamus, and epithalamus. The ventral surface of the diencephalon lies exposed at the

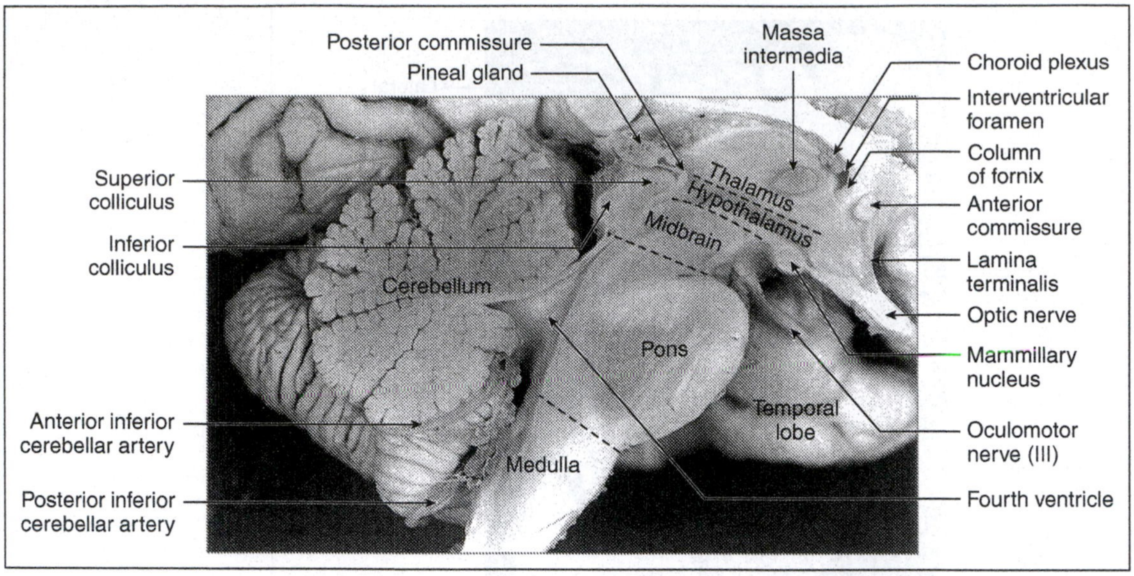

FIG. 3.10. An Enlarged View of Figure 3.6 Showing the Brainstem, Cerebellum, and Diencephalon. Anterior is to the right.

> One cranial nerve is associated with the diencephalon: Optic (II).

base of the brain, but its dorsal surface, which serves as the floor of the lateral ventricle, is hidden by the overlying corpus callosum and cerebral cortex (Figures 3.9 and 3.10). The diencephalon stretches from the lamina terminalis to the posterior commissure, which marks the diencephalic-mesencephalic junction. The lateral boundary of the diencephalon is formed by a large collection of corticofugal and corticopetal fibers called the internal capsule. The slit-like third ventricle located on the midline divides the diencephalon into symmetrical halves. A modest indentation in the wall of the third ventricle, the hypothalamic sulcus, marks the junction between the thalamus and the hypothalamus. The optic nerve is the only cranial nerve that enters the brain through the diencephalon (Figures 3.5 and 3.10).

Thalamus. The thalamus, with its several dozen nuclei, is the largest division of the diencephalon. Both anatomically and physiologically, the thalamus represents an important nexus for many systems of the brain (see Figure 3.10). The structural diversity of the thalamus reflects its functional breadth. The thalamus is a major relay for every sensory system except olfaction during its ascent to neocortex. Several nuclei in the thalamus process information received from the basal ganglia and the cerebellum, and bound for the motor cortices. The remaining thalamic nuclei play vital roles in consciousness, arousal, and sleep.

> The hypothalamus works in concert with the hypophysis.
>
> The hypothalamus is intimately involved with autonomic regulation.

Hypothalamus. The hypothalamus forms the ventral walls and floor of the third ventricle from the lamina terminalis to the caudal border of the mammillary bodies (see Figures 3.9 and 3.10). Laterally, the hypothalamus abuts the internal capsule, the subthalamic nucleus, and the lenticular fasciculus. The hypothalamus, along with the pituitary gland, plays a critical role in the vegetative, regulatory, and cognitive control of core temperature, food and fluid consumption, hormone secretion, sleep, reproduction, and maternal behavior. The intimate relationship between the hypothalamus and the autonomic nervous system has earned it the nickname "chief autonomic ganglion."

Epithalamus. The epithalamus includes the pineal gland and the habenular nuclei, which are located close to the posterior commissure. The pineal gland, which was mistakenly identified by Descartes as the "seat of the soul," is one of the nuclei involved with regulation of the body's diurnal rhythm.

Subthalamus. The subthalamus is a lens-shaped nucleus immediately ventral to the internal capsule and lateral to the hypothalamus. Although derived from the diencephalon, the subthalamus is more closely related to the globus pallidus and usually is discussed with the basal ganglia.

Brainstem. From rostral to caudal, the brainstem includes the midbrain (mesencephalon), the pons (metencephalon), and the medulla (myelencephalon; see Figures 3.6 and 3.10). Each division contains intrinsic nuclei as well as ascending and descending pathways that have sensory, motor, and vegetative functions. Sensory nuclei process somatosensory, auditory, visual, vestibular, gustatory, and visceral information received from the cranial nerves. Motor nuclei control the muscles of the head, face, eyes, and oral cavity, and regulate the thoracic and abdominal viscera. Both sensory and motor nuclei participate in normal reflexes as well as volitional movements initiated by the cerebral cortex.

Brainstem:
- Mesencephalon
- Metencephalon
- Myelencephalon

The midbrain and the pons are divided into dorsal and ventral regions by the cerebral aqueduct and the fourth ventricle, respectively. Cranial nerve nuclei, the reticular formation, and a variety of ascending and descending fiber tracts are located in the ventral region, which is known as the tegmentum. The dorsal part of the midbrain and pons is called the tectum because it serves as their roof plate. Because the dorsal surface of the medulla is formed by the floor of the fourth ventricle, it has no tectum (roof). The fourth ventricle is partially enclosed by the overlying cerebellum and its three massive peduncles that interconnect the cerebellum and the brainstem (Figure 3.11).

Tegmentum: core of the midbrain, pons, and medulla

Tectum, from Latin, means "roof."

Midbrain (Mesencephalon). The junction between the mesencephalon and the diencephalon is marked by the pineal gland, the habenula, the posterior commissure, and the crus cerebri. At the rostral border of the midbrain, the cerebral aqueduct opens into the slit-like third ventricle.

Two paired bumps on the dorsal surface of the mesencephalon, the superior and inferior colliculi, constitute the midbrain tectum (see Figures 3.10 and 3.11). The trochlear nerve (IV), which emerges immediately posterior to the inferior colliculus, is the only cranial nerve that exits from the dorsal surface of the brainstem. Several sensory and motor nuclei, the red nucleus, the reticular formation, and the superior cerebellar peduncle dominate the midbrain tegmentum. The ventral midbrain contains a darkly pigmented nucleus, the substantia nigra, the ventral tegmental area, and the crus cerebri. Degeneration of the nigrostriatal dopaminergic neurons is the anatomical signature of Parkinson's disease (see Chapter 12). The oculomotor nerve emerges from the interpeduncular fossa, the prominent midline cistern formed by the massive pillars of the crus cerebri (Figure 3.12).

Corpora quadrigemina:
- Superior colliculi
- Inferior colliculi

Two cranial nerves are associated with the mesencephalon:
- Oculomotor (III)
- Trochlear (IV)

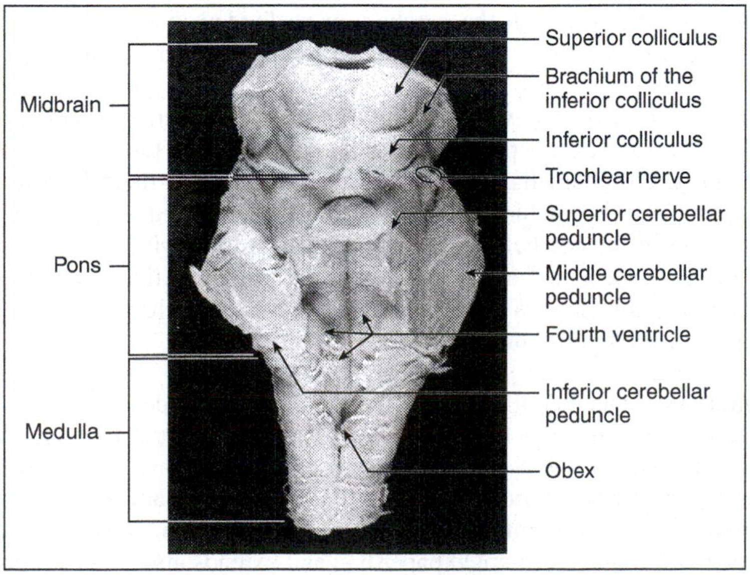

FIG. 3.11. Superior Surface of the Brainstem. Anterior is to the top.

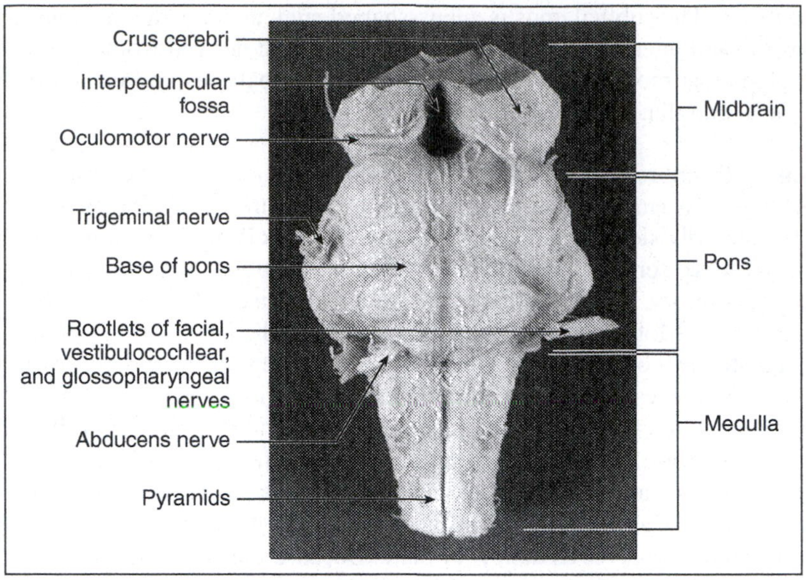

FIG. 3.12. Inferior Surface of the Brainstem. Anterior is to the top.

Four cranial nerves are associated with the pons:

- Trigeminal (V)
- Abducens (VI)
- Facial (VII)
- Vestibulocochlear (VIII)

Cerebellopontine angle: junction of the cerebellum, pons, and medulla

Pons and Cerebellum (Metencephalon). A prominent bulge on the ventral surface of the brainstem marks the location of the pons. This bulge is caused by the underlying pontine nuclei and several large myelinated pathways (see Figure 3.12). The pontine nuclei are a functional bridge between the cerebral cortex and the cerebellum. Efferent projections from the pontine nuclei form the transversely oriented fibers of the middle cerebellar peduncle that wrap around the lateral aspect of the pons and enter the cerebellum.

The dorsal surface of the pons forms the floor of the rostral half of the fourth ventricle. Two bumps in the floor of the fourth ventricle called the facial colliculi mark the locations of the facial nerve where it arches over the abducens nucleus before exiting the brainstem. Four cranial nerves emerge from the pons: the motor and sensory roots of the trigeminal nerve (V), the abducens nerve (VI), the motor and intermediate branches of the facial nerve (VII), and the vestibulocochlear nerve (VIII).

The cerebellum forms the roof of the fourth ventricle above the pons and medulla and is the largest tenant of the posterior cranial fossa (see Figures 3.5, 3.6, and 3.10). Projections from almost every sensory system enable the cerebellum to modulate balance, posture, and fine motor control. Although the cerebellum is divided into cortical and subcortical parts like the neocortex, its internal and external architectures are significantly different.

The cerebellar cortex is divided into two hemispheres by a narrow vermal region on the midline. Hundreds of small and tightly packed gyri called folia obscure the few named sulci of the cerebellar cortex. The cerebellar cortex consists of three lobes: the paleocerebellum, the neocerebellum, and the archicerebellum. Heavily myelinated afferent and efferent axons form the core of the cerebellum, the arbor vitae. Buried within the arbor vitae are four paired nuclei that channel almost all cerebellar output to the rest of the brain. All afferent and efferent connections of the cerebellum traverse the three peduncles that anchor the cerebellum to the brainstem.

Medulla (Myelencephalon). The medulla extends from the caudal border of the pons to the pyramidal decussation, which marks the transition with the spinal cord. The ventral surface of the medulla is marked by the pyramidal tracts (or pyramids) that straddle the midline (see Figure 3.12). An oval bulge located lateral to each pyramid marks the underlying inferior olivary nucleus, which is important for cerebellar function. In transverse sections, the inferior olive resembles a crumpled paper bag and extends almost the entire length of the medulla. Rostrally, the dorsal surface of the medulla serves as the floor of the fourth ventricle (see Figure 3.11). Caudally, the surface of the medulla reveals several pairs of protuberances or tubercles caused by nuclei that are important for somatosensory function. The paired tubercles gracilis, cuneatus, and cinereum are protrusions caused by the underlying nucleus gracilis, nucleus cuneatus, and the spinal trigeminal nucleus, respectively. The inferior cerebellar peduncle forms an elongated bulge on the dorsolateral surface of the rostral medulla.

The medullary tegmentum, like that of the pons and midbrain, contains a dense reticular core surrounded by sensory and motor nuclei. Four cranial nerves emerge from the medulla: the glossopharyngeal nerve (IX), the vagus nerve (X), the spinal accessory nerve (XI), and the hypoglossal nerve (XII).

Four cranial nerves are associated with the medulla:

- Glossopharyngeal (IX)
- Vagus (X)
- Spinal accessory (XI)
- Hypoglossal (XII)

Spinal Cord. The spinal cord retains the elongated shape reminiscent of its early development from the neural tube. Though continuous with the brainstem, the spinal cord is narrower, and its internal and external features are substantially different. Thirty-one pairs of spinal nerves connect the spinal cord with the body. The spinal nerves give the cord a segmented appearance that obscures its functional and anatomic continuity. Although analogous to the cranial nerves of the brainstem, the anatomy of the spinal nerves is significantly different. Each spinal nerve emerges from the cord in two parts: a dorsal root containing only afferent fibers and a ventral root consisting almost exclusively of efferent fibers (see Figure 4.6). To identify specific levels of the spinal cord, the spinal nerves and their corresponding vertebral segments (i.e., cervical, thoracic, lumbar, sacral, and coccygeal) are numbered consecutively from rostral to caudal (e.g., fifth cervical vertebra or C5).

In transverse section, the spinal cord reveals a butterfly-shaped central gray region that is surrounded by an annulus of ascending and descending myelinated tracts (see Figure 4.6). This concentric organization vaguely resembles the brainstem, where the core tegmental region is surrounded by long ascending and descending tracts. The central gray consists of dorsal, ventral, and lateral horns, which are involved with sensory, motor, and autonomic activity, respectively.

Dorsal root: afferent
Ventral root: efferent

The spinal cord is divided into 31 cervical, thoracic, lumbar, sacral, and coccygeal segments.

The spinal cord central gray consists of three horns:

- Dorsal (posterior)
- Ventral (anterior)
- Lateral

Peripheral Nervous System

The peripheral nervous system is composed of all nerve fibers located outside the brain and spinal cord, including the cranial nerves originating in the brain and the paired spinal nerves emerging from the spinal cord. The cranial nerves are listed in Table 3.1 and are described in more detail throughout the book. Functionally, the peripheral nervous system is frequently divided into somatic and autonomic divisions.

Somatic Division. The somatic division of the peripheral nervous system includes both sensory and motor components. The sensory elements include the neurons and axons associated with the dorsal root and cranial nerve ganglia. As the name implies, sensory nerves convey afferent information from skin, joints, muscles, and the thoracic and abdominal organs to the CNS.

The motor elements consist of neurons located in either the brain or the spinal cord whose axons course to their target through the cranial nerves or ventral roots, respectively. Although many of these motor fibers innervate muscles, some project to the autonomic ganglia that supply the viscera.

Autonomic Division. The autonomic division of the peripheral nervous system has components of central and peripheral origin and consists of three separate but intertwined parts: the sympathetic, the parasympathetic, and the enteric nervous systems. In emergency situations, the sympathetic system readies the body for "fight or flight." The parasympathetic system predominates during quiescent periods when it is safe to "rest and digest." The cooperative actions of the sympathetic and parasympathetic systems enable the body to meet varying environmental challenges. Both sympathetic and

Three parts of the autonomic nervous system:

- Sympathetic
- Parasympathetic
- Enteric

Sympathetic function: fight or flight

Parasympathetic function: rest and digest

TABLE 3.1 Cranial Nerves

Cranial Nerves				
Number	**Name**	**Components**	**Function**	**CNS Insertion**
I	Olfactory	Sensory	Smell	Telencephalon
II	Optic	Sensory	Vision	Diencephalon
III	Oculomotor	Mixed	Eye movement	Mesencephalon
IV	Trochlear	Somatomotor	Eye movement	Mesencephalon
V	Trigeminal	Mixed	Sensation from face and mouth Mastication	Metencephalon
VI	Abducens	Somatomotor	Eye movement	Metencephalon
VII	Facial	Mixed	Facial expression Taste	Metencephalon
VIII	Vestibulocochlear	Sensory	Hearing and balance	Metencephalon
IX	Glossopharyngeal	Mixed	Sensation from pharynx, taste buds, and vascular system Gag reflex	Myelencephalon
X	Vagus	Mixed	Autonomic control and sensation	Myelencephalon
XI	Spinal Accessory	Somatomotor	Shoulder and neck movement	Myelencephalon
XII	Hypoglossal	Somatomotor	Tongue movement	Myelencephalon

parasympathetic divisions originate in the CNS and project to peripherally located ganglia prior to reaching their target organs. The enteric nervous system controls the smooth muscles of the gastrointestinal tract, usually independently of the sympathetic and parasympathetic systems.

MENINGES

Layers from the skull to the brain:

- Skull
- Epidural space (caused by hematoma)
- Dura mater
- Subdural space (caused by hematoma)
- Arachnoid
- Pia mater

The human brain, whose consistency resembles that of meringue, requires an extraordinary degree of protection to survive the rigors of everyday life, not to mention rugby, soccer, and skateboarding. The skull provides the first level of protection, but additional mechanisms must prevent the brain from pressing against the inner surface of the skull. This protection is afforded by the meninges, a membranous canopy that suspends the brain within its bony vault. The meninges consist of three layers: the dura mater, the arachnoid, and the pia mater. Additional cushioning and floatation is provided by the cerebrospinal fluid (CSF). The brain's need for chemical stability, though perhaps not as obvious, is just as important. Two complex systems, the blood-brain barrier and the blood-CSF barrier, enable the brain to draw nutrients from the vasculature system while insulating it from the chemical flux in the rest of the body.

Dura Mater

The dura mater, the outermost layer of the meninges, is a thick, parchment-like membrane that serves two functions. First, the dura protects the delicate CNS from trauma. Second, the dura contains specialized cavities or sinuses that link the brain's venous circulation with the systemic circulation.

Dura mater, from Latin, means "tough mother."

Collagen and flattened fibroblasts are arranged into the dura's outer periosteal layer that adheres to the skull, and an inner meningeal layer that is attached to the underlying arachnoid. The periosteal layer is confined to the cranium; the meningeal layer, however, exits the skull through the foramen magnum and lines the entire inner surface of

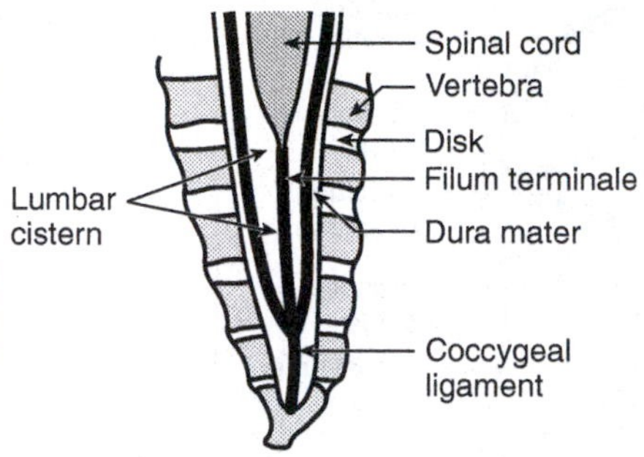

FIG. 3.13. Caudal End of the Dural Sac. The filum terminale secures the spinal cord to the dural sac. The coccygeal ligament anchors the dural sac to the base of the vertebral column. The cauda equina, which fills the lumbar cistern, is not shown.

the vertebral column. A woven cord of the meningeal dura, the coccygeal ligament, anchors the caudal end of the spinal cord to the sacrum of the vertebral column (Figure 3.13). The meninges protect the brain and spinal cord from trauma by suspending them within their bony casings.

Lateral brain stability is provided by the falx cerebri, a sickle-shaped dural reflection located within the midsagittal sulcus (Figure 3.14). The falx cerebri extends from the crista galli of the ethmoid bone to the internal occipital protuberance where it joins the tentorium cerebelli. The tentorium is the broad dural reflection that separates the dorsal surface of the cerebellum from the overlying occipital cortex. In this position, the tentorium partitions the brain into a supratentorial compartment (forebrain and upper brainstem) and an infratentorial compartment (cerebellum and lower brainstem). The midbrain passes through the only opening in the tentorium, which is called the tentorial notch. Unfortunately, increased intracranial pressure may herniate supratentorial structures through the notch and create a life-threatening situation. Gross inspection of the brain reveals two other dural reflections, the falx cerebelli and the diaphragma sellae. The falx cerebelli is the cerebellar analog of the falx cerebri. The diaphragma sellae forms a partition between the base of the brain and the pituitary fossa, the bony receptacle of the pituitary gland.

The middle meningeal artery, a branch of the maxillary artery, supplies the dura.

The tentorium divides the cranial vault into supratentorial and infratentorial compartments.

Cavities between the periosteal and meningeal layers of the dura called dural sinuses link the venous circulation of the brain with the systemic circulation (Figure 3.15). Although most sinuses are located along the edges of dural folds, others line the base of the skull. Together, they provide venous drainage for all cortical and subcortical structures.

Most of the supratentorial dura is innervated by the trigeminal nerve. The dura covering the posterior fossa is innervated primarily by the vagus nerve, with lesser contributions from the glossopharyngeal nerve and the first three cervical nerves. Mechanical traction, irritation, and inflammation of the dura cause headaches.

Sinuses: cavities between the meningeal and periosteal layers of the dura

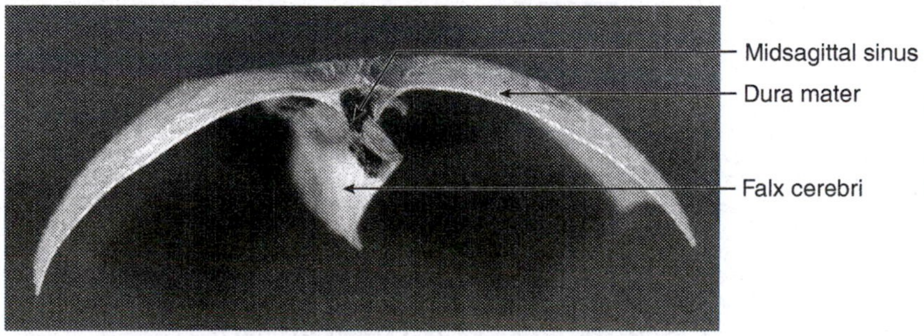

FIG. 3.14. The Dura Mater and the Falx Cerebri Dissected Free from the Skull and Brain. This section of the dura mater was removed from the frontoparietal region and is shown from the front. Occult blood in the midsagittal sinus gives this normally hollow structure its darkened appearance.

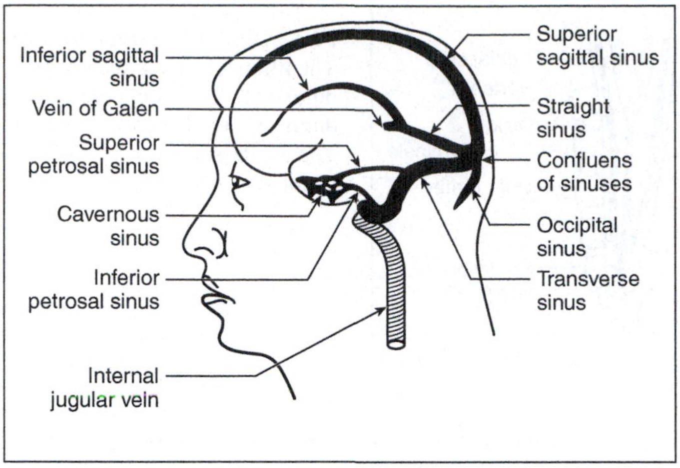

FIG. 3.15. Lateral View of the Head Showing Major Dural Sinuses.

Arachnoid Mater

Hydrocephalus, from Latin, means "water on the brain."

The arachnoid mater consists of fibroblasts arranged into an outer sheet and an underlying web or trabeculae (Figure 3.16). The framework formed by the trabeculae not only secures the meningeal dura to the underlying pia mater, it also creates the subarachnoid space, which contains CSF, arteries, veins, and cranial nerve roots. The subarachnoid space is the conduit for CSF to return to the venous circulation. Passage from the subarachnoid space to the venous circulation takes place through specialized structures called arachnoid granulations or villi (*sing*., villus) located in the walls of the superior sagittal sinus (Figure 3.16). Each villus is formed by an evagination of the outer arachnoid membrane into the dural sinus. Flow of CSF through each villus occurs when fluid pressure in the subarachnoid space exceeds that of the dural sinus. Because reversal of the pressure gradient stops CSF discharge from the subarachnoid space, each villus resembles a one-way valve. If the sinus pressure exceeds the CSF pressure for an extended period (e.g., from a sagittal sinus thrombosis), or if the villi clog following a hemorrhage, hydrocephalus will develop.

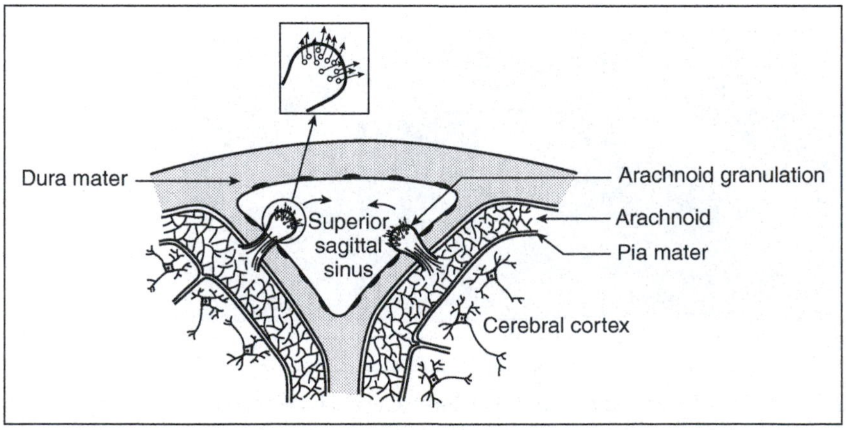

FIG. 3.16. Cross Section of the Midsagittal Sinus Showing Two Arachnoid Granulations.

TABLE 3.2 Ventricular Cisterns

Cistern	Location
Cisterna magna	Post to cerebellum; near foramen magnum
Interpeduncular fossa	Between the cerebral peduncles
Cerebellopontine	Junction of pons, medulla, and cerebellum
Quadrigeminal	Posterior to the colliculi
Prepontine	Ventral to the pons
Ambient	Lateral to the midbrain
Lumbar	Lumbar level of the spinal column

Because the arachnoid follows the contours of the skull more closely than those of the brain, the width of the subarachnoid space increases where the brain's surface does not lie close to the skull. These enlargements or cisterns are normally filled with CSF (Table 3.2). When a hemorrhage is suspected, radiologists check the larger cisterns for signs of occult blood. The largest cistern, the cisterna magna, is located between the base of the cerebellum and the dorsal surface of the medulla. One of the more clinically relevant is the lumbar cistern, which is located in the spinal canal beyond the caudal end of the spinal cord. The lumbar cistern contains CSF as well as the nerve roots that form the cauda equina (see Chapter 4). Percutaneous punctures of the lumbar cistern are used routinely to obtain samples of CSF and to deliver therapeutic agents to the CNS (see Figure 4.2).

Cisterns: CSF-filled enlargements of the subarachnoid space

Pia Mater

The innermost meningeal layer is the pia mater, a delicate membrane that clings to the brain. The pia lacks the strength of the dura and arachnoid, but its tight adhesion to the cortical surface distributes the suspensory forces that secure the brain to the cranium. The pial lining of the spinal cord is secured to the vertebral canal in two ways. A series of pial bands called denticulate ligaments anchor the lateral aspect of the spinal cord to the arachnoid and dural membranes. The denticulate ligaments run the full length of the spinal cord. The caudal end of the spinal pia is secured to the end of the dura sac by the filum terminale (see Figure 3.13).

Hematomas

Hematomas are pools of occult blood formed by either arterial or venous hemorrhage. When intracranial hematomas displace and compress the brain, there may be irreversible brain damage. It is not uncommon for the point of maximum compression to be distant to the site of hematoma formation as in uncal herniations (see Chapter 5). During acute hematoma formation, patients exhibit headaches, lethargy, and mental confusion that may progress to coma and death.

Hemorrhages may form within the parenchyma, but the most common sites are juxtaposed to the dura. Normally, the dura is attached to the inner tablet of the skull and the underlying arachnoid, but trauma may cause hemorrhagic separation of these layers. Arterial bleeding may create a blood-filled space between the periosteal dura and the skull called an epidural hematoma (see Figure 5.32). Subdural hematomas form along the border between the meningeal dura and the underlying arachnoid layer. Subdural hematomas are usually caused by rupture of bridging veins, the short segment of the superficial cerebral veins that cross the arachnoid space (Figure 3.17). Epidural and subdural hematomas represent life-threatening emergencies that require immediate medical care.

Subdural hematomas: venous
Epidural hematomas: arterial

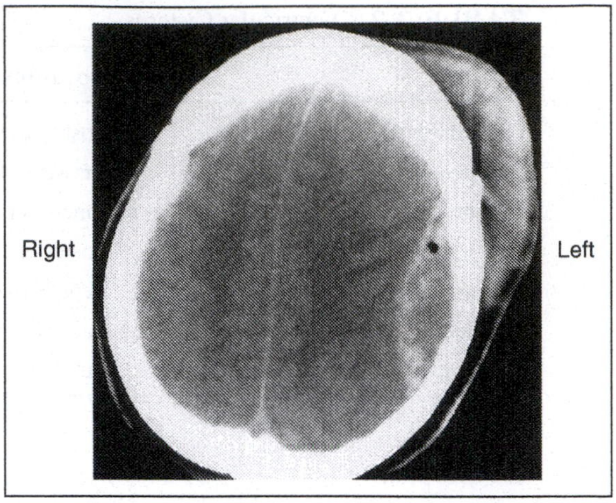

FIG. 3.17. Computerized Axial Tomography Scan of Trauma-Induced Subdural Hematoma over the Left Frontoparietal Area. Note the shift of the midline to the patient's right. (Courtesy of Dr. John Barr, Mid-South Imaging and Therapeutics, Memphis, TN.)

VENTRICULAR SYSTEM

Four parts of the lateral ventricle:
- Anterior horn
- Body
- Posterior horn
- Inferior horn

The ventricular system helps protect, stabilize, and nourish the CNS. Many parts of the ventricular system contain choroid plexus and its plasma-like secretion, CSF. The ventricular system consists of four chambers: the paired lateral ventricles, the third ventricle, and the fourth ventricle.

Lateral Ventricles

The lateral ventricles are paired, C-shaped cavities within the telencephalon. Each lateral ventricle consists of four parts, the anterior horn, the body, and the posterior and inferior horns (Figure 3.18). The anterior horn ends abruptly within the white matter of the frontal

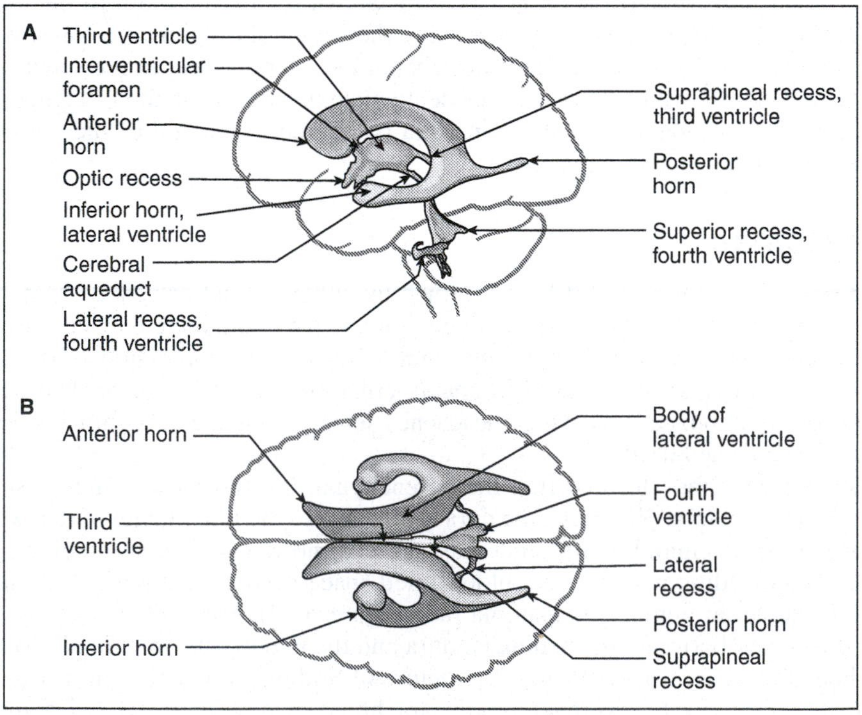

FIG. 3.18. Ventricular System. (A) Lateral view. (B) Dorsal view. Anterior is to the left.

lobe, its medial wall formed by the septum pellucidum and the fornix. The head of the caudate nucleus forms the lateral wall of the anterior horn, and the corpus callosum serves as the roof. The body of the lateral ventricle is located further caudally, its floor formed by the thalamus and the caudate nucleus. As the body of the lateral ventricle sweeps further posteriorly, it joins the inferior and posterior horns at the collateral trigone. The posterior horn terminates within the white matter of the occipital lobe, partially surrounded by fibers of the corpus callosum. The inferior horn descends, enters the temporal lobe, and proceeds rostrally until terminating immediately caudal to the amygdala. The inferior horn is bounded dorsomedially by the tail of the caudate nucleus and ventrally by the hippocampus.

Collateral trigone: atrium

Third Ventricle

The third ventricle is a vertically oriented, slit-like cavity in the diencephalon, bounded anteriorly by the lamina terminalis and laterally by the thalamus and hypothalamus. Rostrally, the third ventricle communicates with the paired lateral ventricles through the interventricular foramen (foramen of Monro). Caudally, the third ventricle tapers to a narrow channel, the cerebral aqueduct (Sylvian aqueduct), that burrows through the mesencephalon and then widens into the fourth ventricle.

Interventricular foramen: connects the lateral and third ventricles

Fourth Ventricle

The fourth ventricle forms a diamond-shaped depression on the roof of the pons and medulla. The walls of the fourth ventricle are formed by the cerebellum and the superior cerebellar peduncles. Two membranes, the anterior and posterior medullary vela (sing., velum), separate the fourth ventricle from the overlying cerebellum. Posteriorly, the fourth ventricle tapers to a point, the obex, and joins the central canal of the spinal cord. Because the central canal of the spinal cord is only open at its rostral end, little CSF enters. Some CSF in the fourth ventricle flows around the perimeter of the spinal cord, but most empties into the subarachnoid space through three perforations in the vela: the foramen of Magendie and the paired foramina of Luschka. The foramen of Magendie is a jagged opening near the midline of the posterior medullary velum, whereas the paired foramina of Luschka are located in the lateral recess of the fourth ventricle at the pontomedullary junction.

Foramen of Magendie: Medial; Foramina of Luschka: Lateral

CHOROID PLEXUS AND CEREBROSPINAL FLUID

Cerebrospinal fluid is a clear, plasma-like liquid that bathes the pial surfaces of the ventricles and the subarachnoid space surrounding the brain and spinal cord. The primary function of CSF is to prevent the brain from striking the skull during quick or violent head movements. The protection afforded by the CSF derives from the brain's natural buoyancy, which distributes the weight of the brain evenly to all of the meningeal surfaces. The brain, spinal cord, ventricles, and subarachnoid spaces contain 120-150 ml of CSF.

Because a 1500 g brain weighs only 50 g when suspended in CSF, it virtually floats.

Cerebrospinal fluid is produced primarily by the choroid plexus, a band of highly vascularized, microvillous tissue within the lateral, third, and fourth ventricles. In the lateral ventricle, the choroid plexus forms a loose trail from the interventricular foramen to the tip of the inferior horn. A dense accumulation of choroid plexus within the collateral trigone, the glomus, calcifies with age and may appear on radiographic films. Some of the choroid plexus in the body of the lateral ventricle enters the third ventricle through the interventricular foramen. Choroid plexus is not found in the anterior or posterior horns of the lateral ventricle or in the cerebral aqueduct. The choroid plexus in the fourth ventricle hangs like moss from the posterior medullary velum and spills through the foramina of Luschka into the subarachnoid space of the cerebellopontine cistern.

Almost 70% of the CSF is derived from the choroid plexus through secretion and filtration of blood plasma; the remaining 30% represents water-soluble metabolic waste discharged by the neuropil surrounding the ventricles. Compared to blood plasma, CSF has lower concentrations of glucose, calcium (Ca^{2+}), protein, and potassium (K^{+}), but

Lumbar punctures must NOT be done in patients with increased intracranial pressure.

higher concentrations of sodium (Na^+), magnesium (Mg^{2+}), and chloride (Cl^-). The concentrations of B and T lymphocytes, monocytes, and neutrophils normally are low.

Changes in the chemical composition of the CSF can be important for diagnosing a variety of disorders. For example, bacterial meningitis and brain abscesses decrease the CSF glucose concentration and increase the neutrophil and protein counts. Viral meningitis, on the other hand, has little effect on the glucose concentration. Multiple sclerosis increases the lymphocyte count as well as the concentration and makeup of immunoglobulin. Increased protein levels may signal a subarachnoid hemorrhage or a CNS tumor. A cautionary note should be added here: Obtaining a CSF sample via a lumbar puncture in patients suspected of having elevated intracranial pressure risks herniation of the cerebellar tonsils through the cisterna magnum. Tonsillar herniation compresses the lower brainstem, causing apnea, circulatory collapse, and coma; prompt treatment is required to avoid death.

Even though 75% of the CSF is produced in the lateral ventricles, all but about 25 ml is found in the subarachnoid space. The flow of CSF begins in the lateral ventricles and proceeds through the interventricular foramina into the third ventricle before squeezing through the cerebral aqueduct into the fourth ventricle. Then the CSF empties into the subarachnoid space through the foramina of Magendie and Luschka. The impetus for CSF flow is provided by pulsation of the choroidal arteries within the ventricles and the coordinated beating of the cilia of the choroidal epithelium. When the hydrostatic force of the CSF exceeds the venous pressure, CSF moves from the subarachnoid space through the arachnoid granulations into the superior sagittal sinus. Most CSF enters the venous circulation through bulk flow; the rest is actively transported. Cerebrospinal fluid in the subarachnoid space around the spinal cord is resorbed by the lymphatic system through the perilymphatic spaces along the spinal veins.

450-500 ml of CSF is produced daily in a system that only holds 120 ml.

Daily secretion of CSF (approximately 450-500 ml) far exceeds the 120-150-ml capacity of the average adult brain. When excess CSF is unable to drain into the dural sinuses, intracranial pressure increases, causing hydrocephalus, which is classified as either non-communicating or communicating. Obstructions within the ventricular system that prevent the normal flow of CSF into the subarachnoid space cause non-communicating hydrocephalus. Non-communicating hydrocephalus is caused by congenital stenosis of the cerebral aqueduct, post-hemorrhagic blood clots, intracranial neoplasms, tuberculosis, and meningitis. Every part of the ventricular system except the lateral ventricle is vulnerable to obstruction, but the most common site is the cerebral aqueduct because of its small diameter. In communicating hydrocephalus, flow of CSF into the subarachnoid space is unimpeded, but flow either within the space or through the villi is blocked or slowed. Although less common than ventricular blockage, extraventricular obstructions may occur almost anywhere in the subarachnoid space. Common causes of communicating hydrocephalus include subarachnoid hemorrhage, excess protein accumulation in patients with CNS infections or tumors, and oversecretion of CSF.

The presenting symptoms of hydrocephalus may include dizziness, headaches, nausea, and vomiting. If intracranial pressure has increased, papilledema may be present (see Chapter 11). Radiographs of the skull may show enlarged ventricular spaces proximal to the occlusion and eventual thinning of the cerebral cortex (Figure 3.19). Hydrocephalus in infants causes skull enlargement with widened fontanelles and, if left untreated, results in severe physical and mental retardation and, ultimately, death.

Less frequently, hydrocephalus develops in the absence of an intraventricular or extraventricular occlusion. In these cases, intracranial pressure is normal and the diagnosis of a communicating hydrocephalus is made. Normal pressure hydrocephalus is indicated by the following triad of symptoms: dementia, urinary incontinence, and gait disturbances. Common causes of communicating hydrocephalus include oversecretion of CSF, impaired CSF absorption, and venous insufficiency. Oversecretion of CSF is rare, but it is found in patients with papillomas (tumors of the choroid plexus). The preferred method of treatment for hydrocephalus (except when caused by metastatic tumors) is surgical implantation of a shunt that either bypasses the obstruction or drains excess CSF from the head into the heart or the peritoneal cavity.

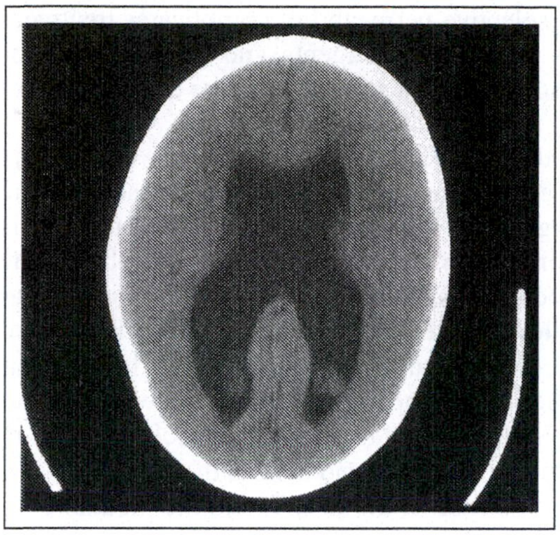

FIG. 3.19. Ventricular Enlargement and Thinning of the Cerebral Cortex Caused by Non-communicating Hydrocephalus. Anterior is to the top. (Courtesy of Dr. John Barr, Mid-South Imaging and Therapeutics, Memphis, TN.)

CHEMICAL ISOLATION OF THE BRAIN

The brain's reliance on the vascular system for its nourishment exposes it to the chemical flux in the rest of the body. The chemical integrity of the CNS is protected by the blood-brain barrier and the blood-CSF barrier. Both barriers are structural partitions that protect the brain and the CSF from potential hazards in the blood.

The blood-brain and blood-CSF barriers are formed by the walls of arterial capillaries within the CNS. Unlike the arterial capillaries in the body, those in the CNS do not allow solutes to pass freely from the blood into the parenchyma or the CSF. In the body, the arterial capillaries have a basal lamina with fenestrated endothelial walls. In the CNS, the endothelial cells of the capillaries are bound to one another with tight junctions. Additional security is provided by the basal lamina, which is reinforced with an outer sheath of astrocytic foot processes that form a barrier around each capillary (Figure 3.20). These barriers allow water, small lipid-soluble solutes, and gases such as oxygen and carbon dioxide to pass freely between the brain or CSF and the blood. Capillary cell walls are slightly permeable to Na^+, K^+, and Cl^-, but they are impermeable to large plasma

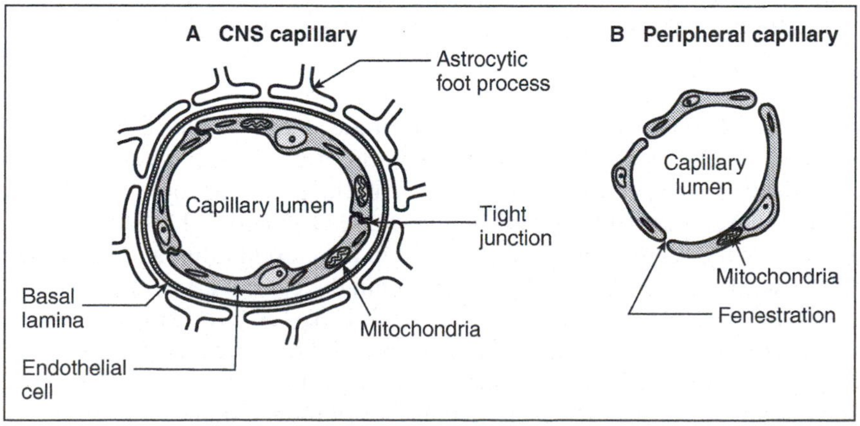

FIG. 3.20. Central and Peripheral Capillaries. (A) The relative impermeability of capillaries in the CNS derives from the tight junctions between the endothelial cells and the continuous lining of astrocytic foot processes. (B) Capillaries in the systemic circulation have a fenestrated lining of epithelial cells that permits most solutes to pass freely between the blood and the interstitial spaces in the tissue. CNS = central nervous system.

proteins and large organic molecules. This selective permeability complicates treatment of intracranial disorders because antibiotics, antineoplastic agents, and many other therapeutic agents cannot enter the brain. Lipid solubility is a common feature of many chemicals that cross the blood-brain barrier.

Circumventricular organs lack a blood-brain barrier.

Area postrema: the brain's emesis center

Despite the widespread distribution of these barriers along the capillaries within the brain and choroid plexus, the barrier is either missing or incomplete in eight areas of the brain: the subfornical organ (SFO), the organum vasculosum of the lamina terminalis (OVLT), the median eminence, the anterior and posterior lobes of the hypophysis, the pineal gland, the area postrema, and the subcommissural organ. These circumventricular organs have fenestrated capillaries that allow solutes to enter and exit the brain. For example, various hormones secreted by the anterior and posterior lobes of the hypophysis pass directly into the systemic circulation. The pineal gland secretes melatonin into the circulation. The area postrema, located in the floor of the fourth ventricle adjacent to the nucleus of the solitary tract, detects circulating toxins and acts as the brain's emesis center. Other circumventricular areas such as the SFO, the OVLT, and the median eminence are chemoreceptor zones that monitor changes in body fluids such as plasma osmolarity and blood glucose levels. The circumventricular organs are discussed further in Chapter 13.

Many brain tumors lack a barrier system, so they readily absorb contrast agents that are detectable by magnetic resonance imaging (MRI) and CT scans. Disruption of the blood-brain barrier accompanies a number of diseases, including multiple sclerosis, AIDS, lead poisoning, and perhaps Alzheimer's disease.

BLOOD SUPPLY OF THE BRAIN AND SPINAL CORD

Humans can survive for several weeks without food and for several days without water. When the brain's supply of oxygen is interrupted for as little as 30 seconds, however, its metabolism is affected. Following 1 minute of anoxia, neural activity begins to falter; by 5 minutes, irreversible cell death begins, followed minutes later by certain death. The brain's vulnerability derives from its high metabolic requirements and severely limited stores of oxygen and glucose.

Arterial Supply

The responsibility for delivering continuous supplies of oxygen and glucose to the brain lies with the elaborate vascular system that derives from the carotid and vertebral arteries.

Carotid Artery Circulation. The common carotid artery ascends the neck, bifurcates, and continues as the external and internal carotid arteries, which supply the face and scalp, and the brain, respectively. The internal carotid artery has four segments: cervical, intrapetrosal, cavernous, and cerebral (Figure 3.21). The cervical branch of the internal carotid artery is the segment in the neck between the carotid bifurcation and the petrous bone of the skull. The intrapetrosal part lies within the carotid canal of the petrous bone. As the internal carotid artery enters the cranium, it passes through the cavernous sinus close to the oculomotor, trochlear, trigeminal, and abducens nerves (Figure 3.22). Arterial bleeding into the cavernous sinus may affect all four cranial nerves. The inferior and middle hypophyseal arteries are the only branches of the internal carotid artery that originate within the intracavernous segment. The cerebral segment begins as the internal carotid artery emerges from the cavernous sinus. The intracavernous and cerebral segments of the internal carotid artery form an S-shaped region called the carotid siphon. The cerebral segment gives rise to three major arteries: the ophthalmic artery, the posterior communicating artery, and the anterior choroidal artery, as well as the superior hypophyseal artery that supplies the hypothalamic-hypophyseal portal system (see Figure 3.23 and

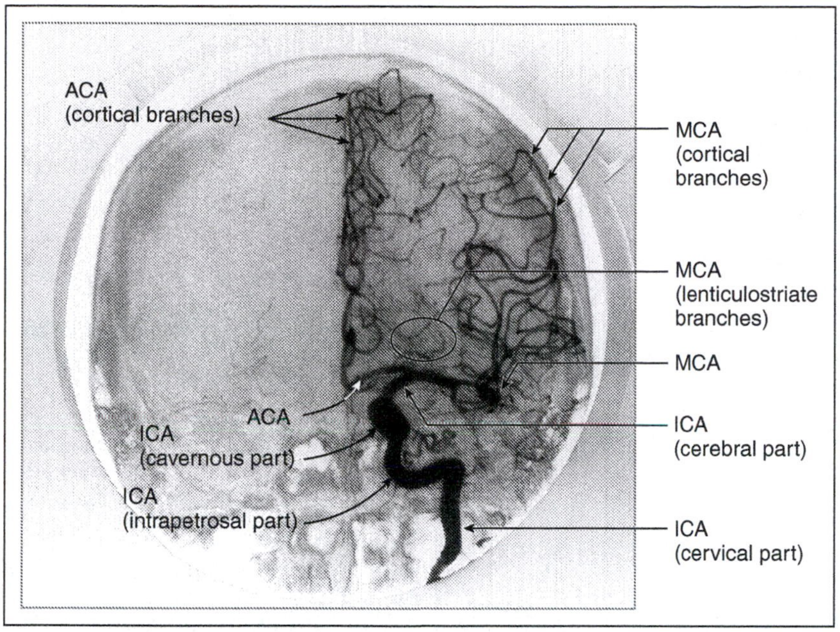

FIG. 3.21. Angiogram. An angiogram in the anterior-posterior plane showing the distributions of the internal carotid artery (ICA), anterior cerebral artery (ACA), and the middle cerebral artery (MCA). (Courtesy of Dr. John Barr, Mid-South Imaging and Therapeutics, Memphis, TN.)

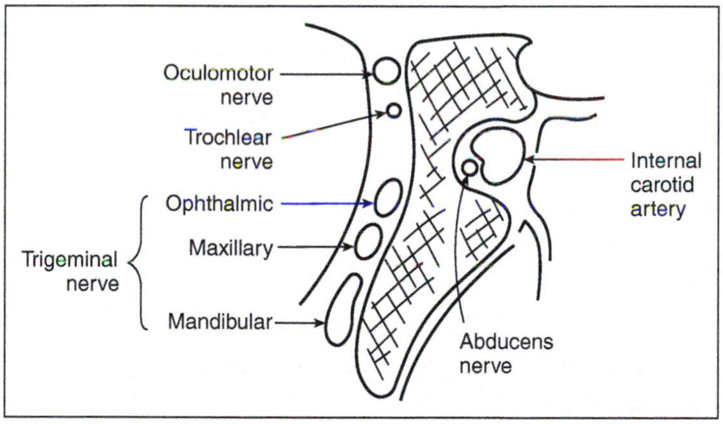

FIG. 3.22. Cavernous Sinus. A coronal section through the cavernous sinus illustrating the proximity of the internal carotid artery to the oculomotor, trochlear, trigeminal, and abducens nerves.

Chapter 13). The ophthalmic artery supplies the optic nerve and retina, as well as the paranasal sinuses and parts of the nose. Small emboli in the systemic circulation may enter the internal carotid artery, lodge in the ophthalmic artery, and trigger monocular visual loss. The anterior choroidal artery passes posterolaterally, enters the inferior horn of the lateral ventricle through the choroidal fissure, and supplies the choroid plexus, the globus pallidus, the hippocampal formation, parts of the internal capsule, the amygdala, and the tail of the caudate. The posterior communicating artery is the link in the circle of Willis between the internal carotid artery and the posterior circulation that arises from the vertebral artery. The internal carotid artery ends at the bifurcation of the anterior and middle cerebral arteries.

> Four segments of the internal carotid artery:
> - Cervical
> - Intrapetrosal
> - Cavernous
> - Cerebral

From its origin at the internal carotid artery, the anterior cerebral artery (ACA) courses rostromedially, crosses the optic nerve, and enters the interhemispheric fissure (see Figure 3.23). Two branches of the ACA, the frontopolar and orbital arteries, supply the frontal pole as well as the orbital and medial surfaces of the frontal cortex. Two larger

FIG. 3.23. Circle of Willis. ACA = anterior cerebral artery; AICA = anterior inferior cerebellar artery; ICA = internal carotid artery; MCA = middle cerebral artery; PCA = posterior cerebral artery; PICA = posterior inferior cerebellar artery; SCA = superior cerebellar artery.

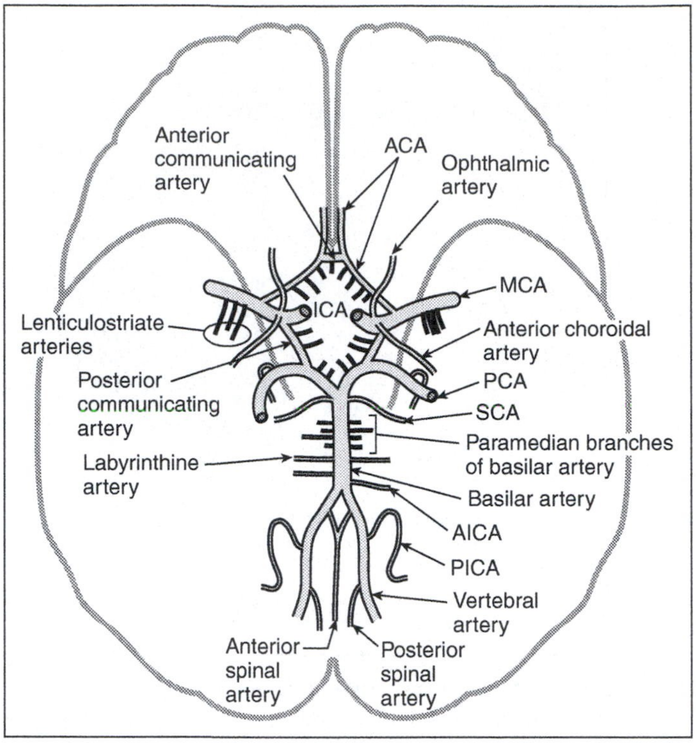

branches, the callosomarginal and the pericallosal arteries, arch around the genu of the corpus callosum and supply the entire medial surface of the frontal and parietal lobes, and part of the adjacent lateral convexity (Figure 3.24). Occlusion of the callosomarginal branch may produce sensory loss, paresis, or both in the contralateral lower limbs.

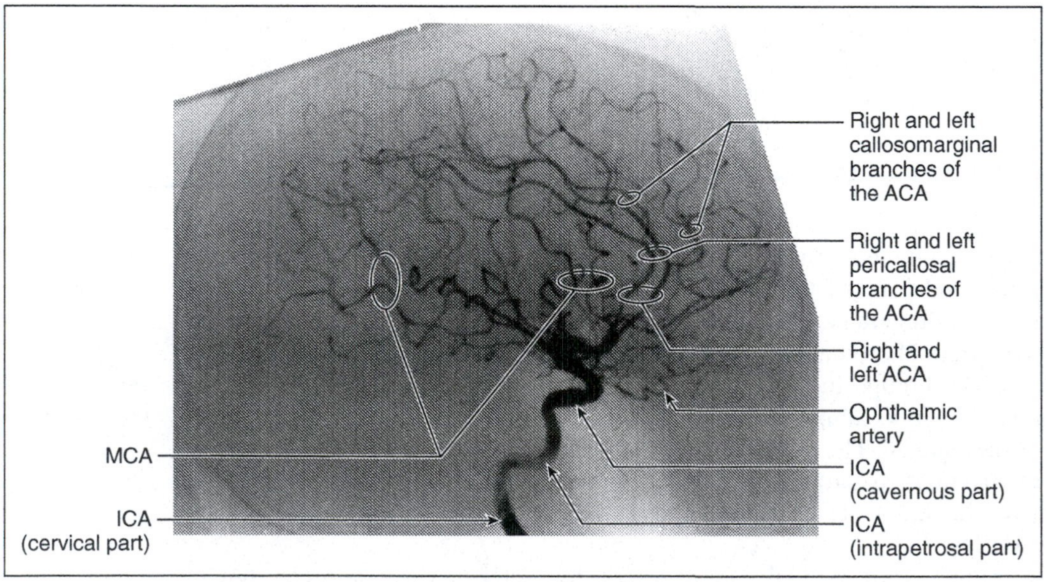

FIG. 3.24. Internal Carotid Artery. A lateral angiogram following injection of the internal carotid artery. Anterior is to the right. ACA = anterior cerebral artery; ICA = internal carotid artery; MCA = middle cerebral artery.

The middle cerebral artery (MCA), which represents the continuation of the internal carotid artery, has the largest and most complex distribution of the major cerebral arteries. From its origin near the circle of Willis, the MCA passes laterally between the frontal lobe and the rostral pole of the temporal lobe. During its course, small penetrating branches called the lenticulostriate arteries enter the brain through the anterior perforated substance and supply blood to the anterior and posterior limbs of the internal capsule and to the corpus striatum (i.e., the globus pallidus, putamen, and caudate nucleus; see Figure 3.23). The first major branches of the MCA are the anterior temporal artery and the orbitofrontal artery, which emerge from the lateral sulcus and blanket the superior and middle temporal gyri and the lateral gyri of the orbitofrontal cortex, respectively. Occlusion of the anterior temporal artery affects the primary auditory cortex and the adjacent auditory association cortices. In the dominant hemisphere, severe language deficits result if this damage includes Wernicke's area, which is located at the posterior terminus of the lateral sulcus.

The middle cerebral artery is the continuation of the internal carotid artery.

The main trunk of the MCA remains within the lateral sulcus and spreads across the insula. Some small arteries penetrate the insula itself, but most emerge from the lateral sulcus and fan out across the frontoparietal cortex. The pre-Rolandic and post-Rolandic arteries supply the primary motor and somatosensory cortices located along the banks of the central sulcus (fissure of Rolando).

Obstruction of the Rolandic branches produces motor and somatosensory deficits of the contralateral torso, upper limbs, or head. Such an occlusion usually spares the lower limbs, because their cortical representations are buried within the longitudinal fissure and are perfused by the ACA.

Vertebral Artery Circulation. The vertebral arteries derive from the subclavian artery and enter the skull through the foramen magnum after threading their way through the foramina of the upper six cervical vertebrae. Inside the cranial vault, the paired vertebral arteries run along the ventrolateral margin of the medulla until they join as the basilar artery at the pontomedullary junction (see Figures 3.23 and 3.25). Three major arteries emerge from the vertebral artery: the posterior inferior cerebellar artery (PICA) and the

Three major arteries emerge from the vertebral artery:
- PICA
- Anterior spinal artery
- Posterior spinal artery

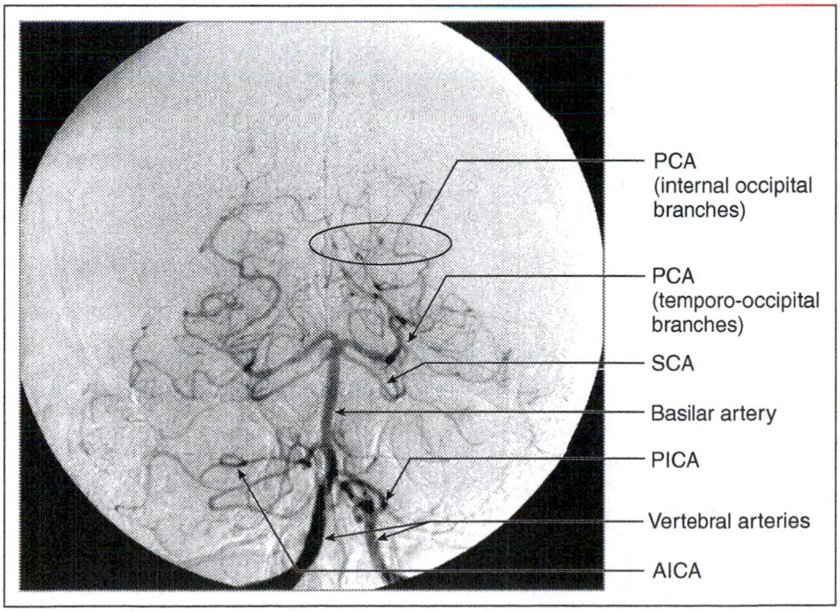

FIG. 3.25. Vertebral Artery. An angiogram in the anterior-posterior plane following injection of the vertebral artery. AICA = anterior inferior cerebellar artery; PICA = posterior inferior cerebellar artery; PCA = posterior cerebral artery; SCA = superior cerebellar artery. (Courtesy of Dr. John Barr, Mid-South Imaging and Therapeutics, Memphis, TN.)

anterior and posterior spinal arteries. The paired vertebral arteries and their tributaries perfuse the brainstem and cerebellum as well as part of the spinal cord, but their territories show considerable variation.

Proximal branches of PICA, the largest branch of the vertebral artery, perfuse the dorsolateral quadrant of the medulla, which contains the nuclei of cranial nerves V, VII, IX, and X (see Figures 3.23, 3.25, and 3.26). More distal branches perfuse the cerebellum. Occlusion of the vertebral artery or PICA produces a constellation of deficits known as the lateral medullary syndrome and Horner's syndrome (see Chapter 5).

Blood supply to the medulla: the spinal and vertebral arteries and their major tributaries

Further caudally, the medulla is supplied by the vertebral arteries and the proximal parts of the anterior and posterior spinal arteries (see Figures 3.23 and 3.26). The anterior spinal artery is formed by the fusion of two small branches that emerge from the vertebral arteries (Figure 3.23). The anterior spinal artery perfuses a U-shaped area along the midline. Medullary structures located further laterally are supplied by the vertebral artery. Occlusion of the anterior spinal artery produces an inferior alternating hemiplegia, characterized by contralateral motor paralysis of the limbs and ipsilateral paralysis of the tongue (see Chapter 5). Proximal branches of the posterior spinal artery perfuse the dorsolateral quadrant of the medulla, and its more distal branches descend to the conus medullaris of the spinal cord.

The anterior and posterior spinal arteries provide the primary vascular supply for the upper cervical segments (see Figure 3.26). Caudal to the cervical level, the continuity of the spinal arteries is maintained by anastomotic connections with radicular arteries,

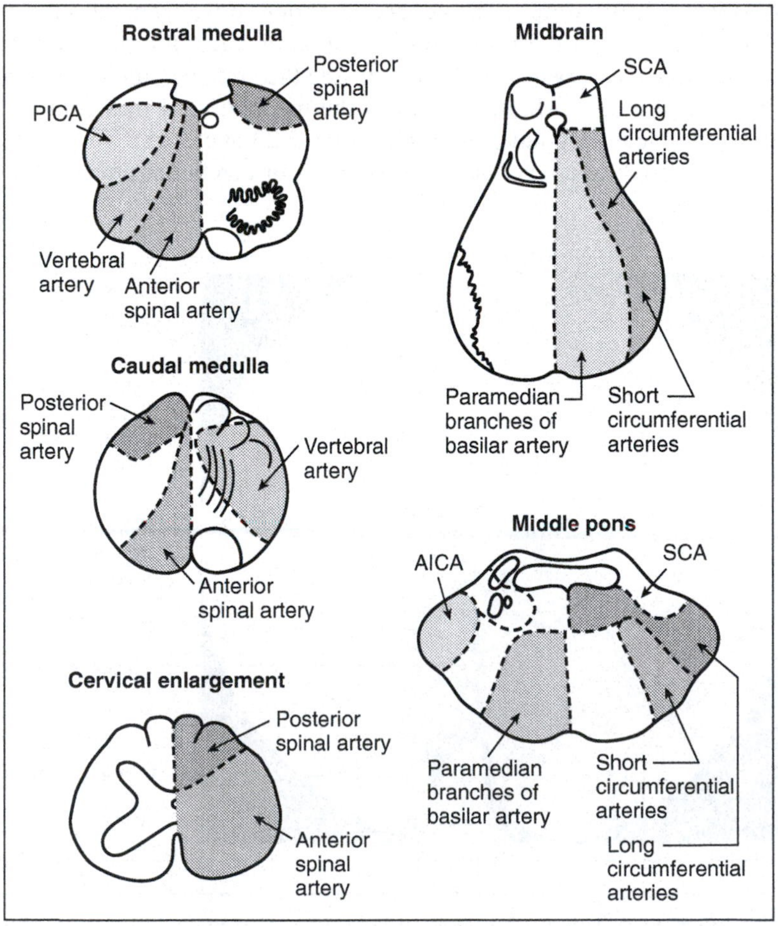

FIG. 3.26. Arterial Supply of the Brainstem and Spinal Cord. AICA = anterior inferior cerebellar artery; PICA = posterior inferior cerebellar artery; SCA = superior cerebellar artery.

which are of segmental origin. Because the radicular arteries are not distributed evenly along the length of the spinal cord, occlusions are more common at spinal levels where the radicular supply is sparse (i.e., T1-T4, L1). From its position within the anterior median fissure, the anterior spinal artery supplies the ventral two-thirds of the spinal cord. The posterior spinal artery supplies a wedge-shaped area of the posterior spinal cord. Ironically, the two posterior spinal arteries perfuse only about one-third of the area that is supplied by the single anterior spinal artery. The perimeter of the lateral funiculus is supplied by a halo of superficial arteries, the arterial vasocorona.

Blood supply to the spinal cord:

- Anterior spinal artery
- Paired posterior spinal arteries
- Radicular arteries

Basilar Artery Circulation. At the pontomedullary junction, the vertebral arteries anastomose to form the basilar artery, which ascends the pons within the basilar sulcus (see Figures 3.23 and 3.25). The basilar artery has many small unnamed branches and three major ones: the labyrinthine artery, the anterior inferior cerebellar artery (AICA), and the superior cerebellar artery (SCA). The labyrinthine artery travels with the eighth cranial nerve through the internal auditory meatus to the inner ear, where it supplies the auditory and vestibular apparati. The distribution of the AICA, like its posterior namesake, varies considerably but usually includes the middle cerebellar peduncle and the choroid plexus of the fourth ventricle, as well as the inferior surface of the anterior cerebellum. The SCA originates from the rostral part of the basilar artery, passes immediately caudal to the root fibers of the oculomotor nerve, and supplies most of the rostral cerebellum. Proximal branches of the SCA perfuse the crus cerebri, portions of the superior and middle cerebellar peduncles, and part of the choroid plexus of the fourth ventricle (see Figure 3.26).

Three major branches of the basilar artery:

- Labyrinthine artery
- AICA
- Superior cerebellar artery

The unnamed branches of the basilar artery are referred to generically as the paramedian and the circumferential arteries. Paramedian branches perfuse the pontine nuclei, the middle cerebellar peduncle, and descending corticofugal fibers (Figures 3.23 and 3.26). Structures located further laterally in the pons are supplied by the short circumferential branches of the basilar artery. Long circumferential branches curve around the pons and supply blood to most of the nuclei and tracts within the dorsolateral pontine tegmentum. In the caudal pons, the long circumferential arteries overlap the proximal branches of the AICA: further rostrally they overlap the area supplied by the SCA.

Posterior Cerebral Artery. As the basilar artery reaches the interpeduncular fossa, it bifurcates and forms the right and left posterior cerebral arteries (see Figure 3.23). An anastomosis between the posterior cerebral artery and the posterior communicating artery provides continuity between the basilar and carotid circulations. The trunk of the posterior cerebral artery passes around the lateral margin of the crus cerebri and climbs to the ventrolateral surface of the cerebral cortex by crossing the tentorium. The two main branches of the posterior cerebral artery are the posterior temporal (temporo-occipital) artery and the internal occipital arteries. The posterior temporal artery supplies the inferior and medial surfaces of the posterior two-thirds of the temporal lobe. The internal occipital artery or its major branches, the parieto-occipital artery and the calcarine artery, supply most of the occipital lobe and a significant portion of the superior parietal lobule. Anastomoses between the posterior and middle cerebral arteries along the calcarine sulcus may preserve visual function following strokes of the occipital lobe (see Chapter 11).

The paired posterior cerebral arteries are the continuation of the basilar artery.

Circle of Willis. The circle of Willis is formed by the posterior communicating arteries, which connect the internal carotid arteries with the proximal portion of the posterior cerebral artery, as well as by the anterior communicating artery, which connects the left and right anterior cerebral arteries (see Figure 3.23). In the event of a stroke, the circle of Willis should allow one side of the brain to be fed by the arteries from the opposite side. Unfortunately, in some individuals there is little collateral circulation because the anterior and posterior communicating arteries are either too small or missing. The circle of Willis is a common site for saccular aneurysms which, if left untreated, may bleed into the subarachnoid space and cause serious neurologic deficits.

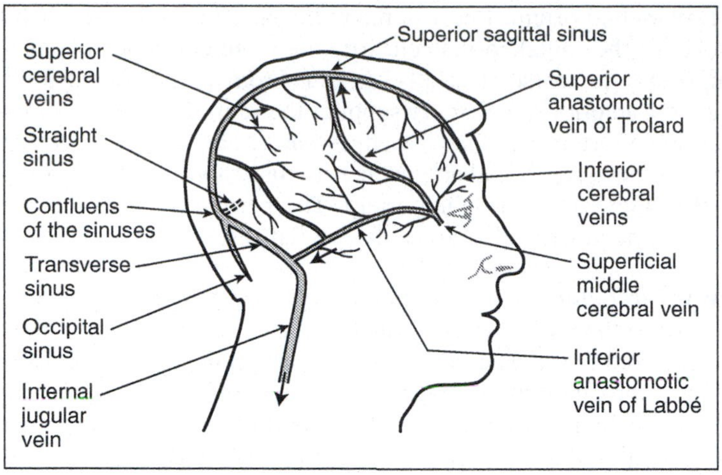

FIG. 3.27. Superficial Veins of the Brain. The arrows indicate the direction of blood flow in the anastomotic veins.

Venous Drainage

Venous drainage of the brain does not run in parallel to its arterial supply. Instead, venous drainage of the brain is accomplished through an elaborate system of veins that shunts blood into the sinuses that eventually drain into the internal jugular vein for return to the systemic circulation. Depending on their location, cerebral veins are classified as superficial or deep. Superficial veins lie on the surface of the cerebral cortex and drain into the large sinuses sandwiched between the meningeal and periosteal layers of the dura (Figure 3.27). Deep veins that serve the internal structures of the brain empty into the great cerebral vein (great vein of Galen) which, in turn, drains into the straight sinus (Figure 3.28).

Deep veins → great cerebral vein → straight sinus → confluens → transverse sinus → internal jugular vein

The venous organization of the spinal cord resembles its arterial supply in that the longitudinal vessels lying on the anterior and posterior surfaces of the cord are supplemented by a series of radicular veins. Although some venous blood ascends and enters the jugular veins, most of it leaves the spinal canal through epidural plexuses that empty into nearby segmental veins.

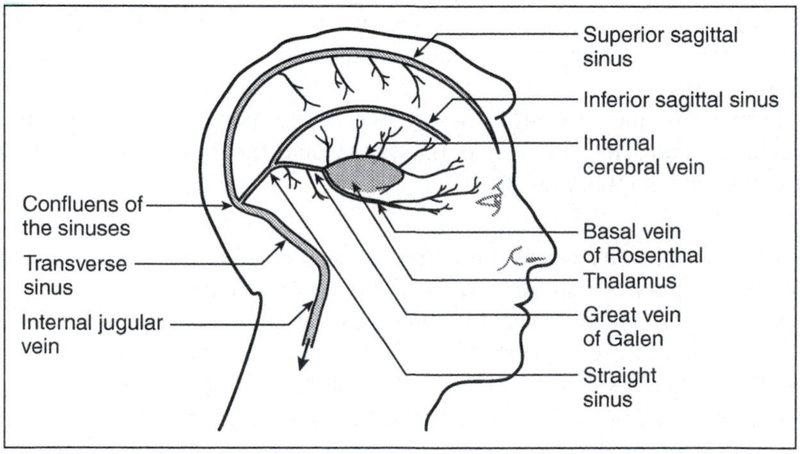

FIG. 3.28. Deep Veins of the Brain.

Superficial Cerebral Veins. The superficial venous circulation differs from the arterial system by being more variable and more reliant on anastomoses. The superficial veins most consistently observed are the superior, middle, and inferior cerebral veins and the large anastomotic veins of Trolard and Labbé (see Figure 3.27).

The medial parts of the frontal and parietal lobes are drained by the superior cerebral veins into the superior sagittal sinus. At the internal occipital protuberance, the superior sagittal sinus joins the occipital sinus and the straight sinus to form the confluens of the sinuses. Venous blood in the confluens of the sinuses flows into the left and right transverse sinuses which curve ventrally and anteriorly around each side of the occipital cortex. These venous curvatures, called the sigmoid sinuses, exit the skull as the internal jugular veins.

The middle cerebral vein lies in the lateral sulcus and drains the adjacent frontal, parietal, and temporal opercular cortices into the anastomotic veins of Trolard and Labbé. The anastomotic vein of Trolard empties into the superior sagittal sinus, while blood in the anastomotic vein of Labbé flows into the transverse sinus.

The inferior cerebral veins drain the ventral surface of the cerebrum into the cavernous, intercavernous, and petrosal sinuses, which line the base of the calvarium. The cavernous sinus surrounds the sella turcica, the bony saddle that partially encapsulates the hypophysis. The proximity of the cavernous sinus to the hypothalamus, the hypophysis, the internal carotid artery, and four cranial nerves makes this a clinically important structure (see Figure 3.22). The intercavernous sinuses form an anastomotic venous grid between the left and right cavernous sinuses. Blood from the cavernous and intercavernous sinuses empties into the superior and inferior petrosal sinuses, which in turn flow into the transverse sinus and internal jugular vein, respectively (see Figure 3.28).

The cavernous sinus encapsulates cranial nerves III, IV, VI, and the ophthalmic and maxillary branches of cranial nerve V.

Deep Cerebral Veins. The two most important deep cerebral veins are the internal cerebral vein and the basal vein (of Rosenthal; Figures 3.28 and 3.29). The internal cerebral vein collects venous blood from the striatum, the thalamus, the hippocampus, and the choroid plexus of the lateral ventricle before running posteriorly along the dorsomedial edge of the thalamus. The basal vein collects venous blood from the medial surface of the temporal pole, the orbital gyri of the frontal lobe, and the insular-opercular cortices. At the posterior border of the thalamus, the left and right cerebral veins fuse into the great cerebral vein, which the basal veins then join. The great cerebral vein courses under the splenium of the corpus callosum and then enters the straight sinus within the midline ridge of the tentorium. The straight sinus enters the confluens of the sinuses (Figure 3.29).

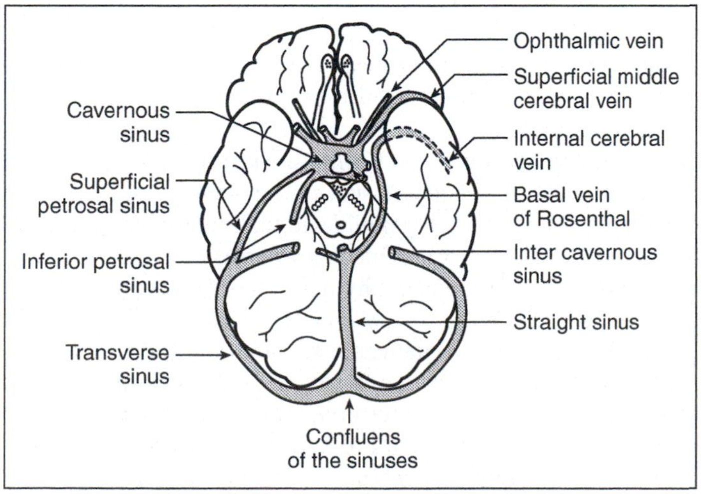

FIG. 3.29. Venous and Sinus Drainage.

Cerebrovascular Accidents

Cerebrovascular accidents are one of the leading causes of mortality and morbidity in the world. The arterial and venous blood supply of the CNS is vulnerable to trauma, disease (e.g., heart disease and diabetes), and normal aging. Other factors such as heredity and lifestyle (e.g., cigarette smoking, diet, and level of exercise) play important roles as well.

> The area of cell death associated with stroke is called an **infarct.**
>
> Strokes are either **hemorrhagic** or **ischemic.**
>
> Stroke is the third leading cause of death in the United States.

Strokes. Strokes are caused by a sudden interruption of the arterial blood supply. Ischemic strokes block blood flow and starve neural tissue located downstream; hemorrhagic strokes bleed into the neuropil. Effective medical care requires the differential diagnosis of ischemic versus hemorrhagic stroke. Anticoagulant therapy, a prudent course of treatment for an ischemic stroke, would be catastrophic for a patient in the midst of a hemorrhagic stroke. The area of cell death caused by a stroke is called an infarct.

Following a stroke, the functions previously performed by the infarcted area are lost. Although loss of motor control is one of the most obvious effects of stroke and the one most people associate with a cerebrovascular accident, sensory, autonomic, and cognitive problems are common as well. The neurons just beyond the infarct form the penumbra, an area of compromised function where the cell function is regained as local edema decreases and the circulation returns to normal.

> **Embolic strokes:** caused by circulating debris called emboli or "floaters"
>
> **Thrombotic strokes:** caused by a blood clot forming on an existing atherosclerotic plaque

Embolic strokes are caused by circulating debris called emboli that occlude the vasculature of the brain or the arteries leading to the brain. Emboli may originate in the heart following a heart attack or during bouts of atrial fibrillation. Others may detach from atherosclerotic plaques or dissections of the carotid or vertebral arteries. Symptom onset is typically abrupt and the clinical signs are usually focal and static. A thrombotic infarct, by comparison, is caused by a local event such as a blood clot forming on an atherosclerotic plaque, and for this reason, symptoms may have a gradual or even stuttering onset. Venous thrombosis may occur in patients with hypercoagulation diseases or disorders, but it is much less common than arterial strokes. The clinical presentation of a venous thrombosis may include headaches (25%) and seizures (10%), typically accompanied by sensory or motor symptoms that do not necessarily indicate the site of the occlusion. For example, contralateral paresis and sensory loss in the arm and face might be caused by occlusion of the middle cerebral artery or the internal cerebral vein.

> Most **TIAs** last about 10 minutes.

In some cases, an embolic stroke is preceded by a transient ischemic attack (TIA), an episode lasting less than 24 hours during which the patient shows all of the neurological signs of a stroke. A TIA is believed to be caused by small emboli that dissolve over the course of the episode. A TIA is time limited and self-resolving, but nevertheless an unmistakable sign that the patient is at high risk for stroke. Anti-coagulant therapy, if instituted within several hours, may dissolve emboli in time to prevent permanent brain damage.

> 13% of all strokes are hemorrhagic.

Hemorrhagic strokes caused by intracranial bleeding may create hematomas within the meninges, as described earlier, or within the parenchyma. Intracranial hemorrhages are common in hypertensive patients because their arterial walls are stiff and brittle. Other causes of hemorrhagic stroke include aneurysms, arteriovenous malformations, trauma, and tumors.

> 40% of all intraparenchymal hemorrhages bleed into the ventricles.
>
> Hemorrhagic strokes have a 30-day mortality rate of 35%–52%.
>
> When a hemorrhagic stroke is suspected, a CT scan should be done, ideally within 24 hours of symptom onset.

Most hemorrhagic strokes are arterial, although trauma may cause bleeding from the bridging veins that cross the subarachnoid space. The majority of hemorrhagic strokes are of supratentorial origin, with the basal ganglia and thalamus being the most common loci. Although some damage is caused by inadequate perfusion, most is caused by physical disruption of the tissue itself. Intraparenchymal hemorrhages that invade the ventricles create an acute noncommunicating hydrocephalus that complicates medical care. The presenting signs and symptoms include headache and vomiting as well as focal deficits related to the size and location of the hemorrhage and hematoma. Symptoms typically progress and the patient's condition deteriorates as long as bleeding continues and intracranial pressure increases. Intracranial pressure is also increased by post-hemorrhagic edema, and for this reason, a lumbar puncture should not be performed until the differential diagnosis between an ischemic and hemorrhagic stroke has been made. The diagnosis

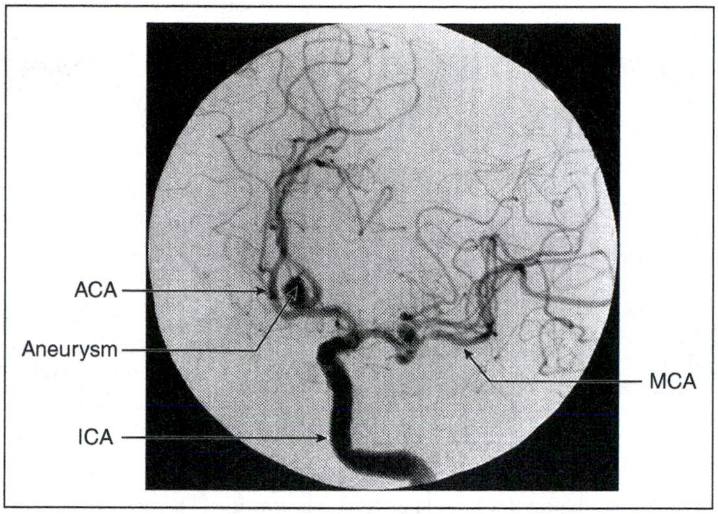

FIG. 3.30. Saccular Aneurysm. Angiogram showing a saccular aneurysm on the anterior communicating artery. ACA = anterior cerebral artery; ICA = internal carotid artery; MCA = middle cerebral artery. (Courtesy of Dr. John Barr, Mid-South Imaging and Therapeutics, Memphis, TN.)

of an intracranial hemorrhage is made after considering the patient's history (e.g., hypertension, smoking, etc.), the onset and progression of the stroke (sudden and progressive), and the results of a CT scan. Despite better control of risk factors and improved medical care over the last few decades, the mortality and morbidity rates for hemorrhagic strokes remain high.

Aneurysms. An aneurysm is a congenital dilatation of an artery caused by weakness in the arterial wall. This weakness is exploited by high blood pressure, smoking, and hypercholesteremia. Saccular or berry aneurysms, the most common type of intracranial aneurysm, are rounded dilatations attached to the main artery by a narrow pedestal (Figure 3.30). Saccular aneurysms are the most common cause of non-traumatic subarachnoid hemorrhages. Approximately 90% of all saccular aneurysms are located on branch points associated with the anterior circulation, (i.e., anterior and middle cerebral arteries, carotid artery, and the anterior rim of the circle of Willis). The first sign of an aneurysm is usually a headache of unprecedented intensity caused by bleeding into the subarachnoid space. Left untreated, an aneurysm may burst or become a source of emboli. The mortality rate following a ruptured aneurysm is approximately 50% at 30 days; a third of these patients die before reaching the hospital. Because the risk of rupture increases as the aneurysm enlarges, surgical intervention is usually reserved for the larger aneurysms. The most effective treatment is isolation of the aneurysm body from the general circulation by placing a small clip on its pedestal.

A patient with a subarachnoid hemorrhage often reports having "the worst headache of my life."

Arteriovenous Malformations. Arteriovenous malformations are congenital shunts between arteries and veins (Figure 3.31A). Although usually focal in nature, arteriovenous malformations may enlarge with age and become symptomatic by hemorrhaging. Patients may present with seizures, headaches, or neurologic deficits, even in the absence of hemorrhage through the abnormally thin walls of these blood vessels. Because arteriovenous anastomoses bypass the normal capillary bed, the adjacent neuropil may linger in a chronic ischemic state. The brain parenchyma within the arteriovenous malformations is typically gliotic, edematous, or necrotic. Large or troublesome arteriovenous malformations require surgical removal, which is best done after the most tortuous vasculature has been embolized (Figure 3.31B).

50%–60% of all arteriovenous malformations present with hemorrhage.

The mortality rate for patients with an arteriovenous malformations is 10%–30%.

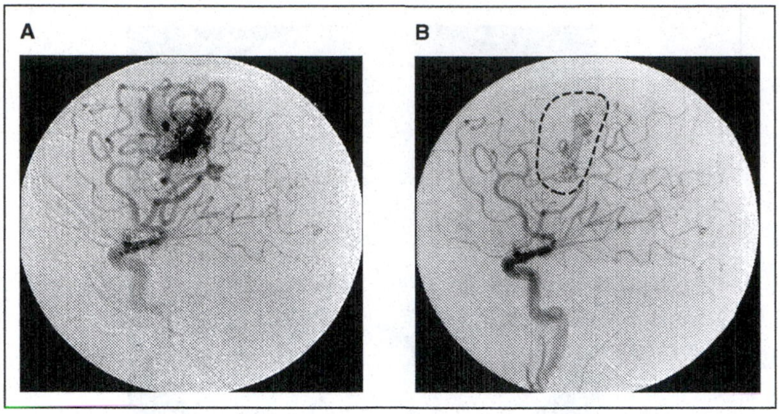

FIG. 3.31. Embolization of an Arteriovenous Malformation. Arteriovenous malformation of the anterior cerebral artery before (A) and after (B) embolization. The dashed line in B show the former distribution of the arteriovenous malformation. Some of the opacities in the post-embolization radiograph are matrix inserted by the surgeon to facilitate embolization. (Courtesy of Dr. John Barr, Mid-South Imaging and Therapeutics, Memphis, TN.)

BRAIN TUMORS

Benign brain tumors, though not metastatic, are still deadly.

The brain, like every other part of the body, is susceptible to tumors. Primary brain tumors originate inside the cranium and constitute 80% of all intracranial neoplasms; the remaining 20% are metastatic derivatives of systemic tumors. Even though most primary brain tumors are benign and indolent, they may cause significant damage or death by infiltrating and displacing healthy neural tissue. Symptoms are caused by pressure exerted by the tumor on local tissue as well as brain herniation at remote sites. Epileptic seizures are the most common manifestation of primary brain tumors.

The World Health Organization has established a histopathological classification system that divides primary brain tumors into nine categories. In adults, almost 50% of all primary tumors are gliomas—that is, tumors that originate from glia. Meningiomas, tumors derived from the meninges, account for another 20%–25% of primary tumors. The third most common type of tumor is the pituitary adenoma. Approximately 70% of all brain tumors in adults are supratentorial.

Gliomas

Gliomas are named according to the type of glial cell from which they originate. Astrocytomas, the most common type of glioma, originate from astrocytes, and for this reason they can be identified by the immunohistochemical marker glial fibrillary acidic protein. Although slow growing, astrocytomas are difficult to remove and may recur in a malignant form. Astrocytomas are commonly found in the cerebral cortex. Radiation and chemotherapy are useful post-surgical adjuvants; unfortunately, not all chemotoxic agents cross the blood-brain barrier. Oligodendrogliomas are derived from oligodendrocytes and are found in the cortical grey matter, the corpus callosum, and the basal ganglia. Ependymonas form in association with the ependymal cells that line the ventricles and are most often seen in young children. Because most ependymonas form in the fourth ventricle, they often press upon the autonomic areas around the area postrema and cause nausea, vomiting, headache, and papilledema. When ependymonas form in the third ventricle, hydrocephalus may develop if CSF flow through the cerebral aqueduct is obstructed.

Meningiomas

Meningiomas are a class of slow-growing tumors that originate in the meninges, usually where the arachnoid villa, cranial nerves, or blood vessels pierce the dura. The most common site of meningioma formation is along the falx cerebri. Meningiomas rarely invade the parenchyma, so their damage is caused primarily through compression and displacement of the brain. These tumors are accompanied by headaches and seizures; more specific symptoms related to brain compression are seen in advanced cases. The slow but inexorable growth of meningiomas requires surgical intervention, but regrowth within 5 years is common.

Meningiomas are tumors of the meninges, which displace rather than invade the brain parenchyma.

Pituitary Adenomas

Pituitary adenomas are slow-growing, benign tumors that arise from the glandular cells of the adenohypophysis (anterior lobe of the pituitary gland). As discussed in Chapter 13, the glandular cells of the adenohypophysis secrete a variety of hormones that regulate growth, metabolism, reproduction, lactation, and the body's reaction to stress. Most pituitary adenomas secrete one of more of these hormones, which predictably increase to abnormally high levels. Secretory pituitary adenomas are usually symptomatic and thus can be detected when they are only 1 mm in diameter. Nonsecreting adenomas produce no symptoms until they grow large enough to irritate the local dura, cause headaches, or in extreme cases, disturb vision by pressing against the underside of the optic chiasm (see Clinical Cases in Chapters 11 and 13). The most common treatment is surgical removal, although some adenomas respond to medications that inhibit secretion of the affected hormone.

Approximately half of all secreting pituitary adenomas release prolactin.

BRAIN INFECTIONS

Brain infections are caused by viruses, bacteria, fungi, parasites, and prions that enter the CNS through the blood, CSF, the gastrointestinal and respiratory tracts, surgical and traumatic wounds, bites, and even the nasal passages. Signs and symptoms vary with the type of infection, but usually include fever, headache, lethargy, photophobia, phonophobia, and nuchal rigidity.

Nuchal rigidity, a stiff neck that resists both active and passive flexion, is the hallmark of meningitis.

One of the more common and most serious infections seen in the clinic is meningitis. Meningitis, an infection of the CSF in the subarachnoid space, may be of bacterial or viral origin. The time course of bacterial meningitis is very rapid, making it more serious than its viral counterpart. Indeed, the time course of bacterial meningitis is so quick that in some cases it may be prudent to begin antibiotic treatment before the diagnosis (by lumbar tap) has been completed. Bacterial meningitis, if left untreated, is usually fatal. Cerebrovascular complications such as stroke and cerebral edema are the two leading causes of death. The ability of bacterial meningitis to spread rapidly through groups living in close quarters makes any outbreak a public health concern. Viral meningitis produces many of the same symptoms as its bacterial namesake, but is less virulent and often resolves spontaneously in 1–2 weeks. Viral infections of the brain parenchyma (viral encephalitis), sometimes in combination with the meninges (meningoencephalitis), are more serious and require quick treatment to prevent permanent disability or death. The most common cause of viral encephalitis is herpes simplex virus type I (HSVI), which attacks limbic structures of the temporal and frontal lobes, often bilaterally. Patients with viral encephalitis exhibit most of the symptoms previously listed for meningitis, as well as anosmia, memory loss, and aphasia due to destruction of limbic tissue. The CNS is also vulnerable to attacks from human immunodeficiency virus (HIV), which opens the door to many opportunistic neurologic infections.

Viral encephalitis (HSVI) attacks limbic areas of the temporal and frontal lobes.

Brain and epidural abscesses are also caused by bacterial infections that originate outside the CNS. Brain abscesses of all sizes produce meningitis-like symptoms; larger abscesses may produce focal signs and symptoms as well as mass effects. Treatment options include antibiotics and drainage (needle aspiration).

Neurosyphillis, which is caused by spirochetes contracted through sexual transmission, produces a host of neurologic problems if left untreated. In the advanced stages of the disease, patients may exhibit paresis, psychosis, and degeneration of spinal cord tracts (tabes dorsalis; see Chapter 4). Lyme disease is caused by a different spirochete carried by deer ticks. In advanced cases, Lyme disease may cause mild menigoencephalitis, marked by the typical symptoms of a meningitis as well as impairments in memory and concentration. Other neurologic symptoms may include cranial and peripheral neuropathies.

MASS EFFECTS AND BRAIN HERNIATION

Tumors, abscesses, edema, hydrocephalus, hematomas, and other mass lesions that form inside the calvarium increase intracranial pressure. Ventricular compression, decreased vascular and CSF volumes, and a shift in fluid from the intracellular to the extracellular compartment can compensate for small increases in pressure. Further increases have many serious and potentially life-threatening consequences.

A midline shift of the ventricles or the calcified pineal gland is a sign of a mass lesion.

Engorgement and elevation of the optic disc is called **papilledema.**

Mass lesions affect the brain both locally and at a distance. Local effects include neurologic deficits related to compression at the lesion site as well as ischemia and headaches due to pressure on blood vessels. Mass lesions produce effacement (flattening) of the sulci, which can be seen on MRI and CT films. Pressure transmitted through the subarachnoid space surrounding the optic nerve compromises venous return from the eye and increases intraocular pressure. Fundoscopic examination of the eye shows engorgement and elevation of the optic disc (see Chapter 11, Figure 11.7). Further pressure increases may cause the brain to herniate from one compartment to another. These herniations are usually visible on CT and MRI films as midline shifts. As a rule, higher pressure causes more pronounced distortion and a less favorable clinical outcome.

A falcine herniation may pinch the anterior cerebral artery and infarct the medial frontoparietal cortex.

Uncal herniations are characterized by a triad of signs: a "blown" pupil, hemiplegia, and diplopia.

Lateral displacement of the cerebral cortex in the anterior cranial fossa may push the cingulate gyrus under the falx cerebri. These falcine herniations are usually asymptomatic unless the falx pinches the anterior cerebral artery. Increases in intracranial pressure are also capable of pushing the uncus, the medial tip of the temporal lobe, through the tentorial notch. Uncal herniation compresses the oculomotor nerve, which initially causes a dilated and unresponsive pupil and may progress to oculomotor impairment and diplopia (see Chapter 5). Progression of an uncal herniation may compress the descending motor fibers of the ipsilateral crus cerebri and produce a contralateral hemiplegia (see Figure 5.32). Compression of the brainstem impairs consciousness, and unless corrective action is begun quickly, it proceeds to coma and ultimately death. Mass lesions of the posterior cranial fossa may herniate the cerebellar tonsils through the foremen magnum. Because brainstem compression caused by a tonsillar herniation jeopardizes respiratory and cardiac function, it represents a dire medical emergency. For this reason, a lumbar puncture should never be performed on a patient with increased intracranial pressure.

RESOLUTION OF CLINICAL CASE

The patient was in the acute phase of a subarachnoid hemorrhage when he arrived at the emergency department. The headache was caused by a saccular aneurysm bleeding into the subarachnoid space. Saccular aneurysms may leak sporadically before more serious bleeding forces the patient to seek emergency care. In this case, the patient experienced intermittent headaches during the preceding few weeks, which in retrospect may have been a symptom of seepage from the aneurysm. Aspirin did little to relieve the pain and, indeed, may have exacerbated the bleeding. During the current episode, the bleeding was worse and the symptoms more serious. Progression of the patient's symptoms to the point of unconsciousness makes this a life-threatening situation. The physician, suspecting a subarachnoid hemorrhage, ordered a CT scan, the technique of choice for visualizing occult blood. If bleeding had been confirmed, pharmacologic intervention would have been instituted to prevent vasospasm and the order for a lumbar puncture would have been canceled. The decision about clipping the aneurysm would have been made after the location of the aneurysm was determined with a series of angiograms.

REVIEW QUESTIONS

Directions: For each question, choose the **one best** answer.

1. Aneurysms typically bleed into
   A. Ventricles
   B. Sinuses
   C. Parenchyma
   D. Subarachnoid space
   E. Epidural space

2. Which of the following conditions is most likely to involve venous blood?
   A. Hemorrhage
   B. Stroke
   C. Epidural hematoma
   D. Subdural hematoma
   E. Aneurysm

3. Which of the following sites is most commonly used to obtain a sample of the cerebrospinal fluid (CSF)?
   A. Lateral ventricle
   B. Lumbar cistern
   C. Subarachnoid space
   D. Cerebellopontine cistern
   E. Superior sagittal sinus

4. What is the major difference between arteriovenous malformations and aneurysms?
   A. Whether they must be treated surgically
   B. Whether they are life threatening
   C. Whether they are prone to hemorrhage
   D. Their location
   E. Whether they cause headaches

5. Which of the following blood vessels forms part of the circle of Willis?
   A. Internal carotid artery
   B. Middle cerebral artery
   C. Superior cerebellar artery
   D. Ophthalmic artery
   E. Cavernous sinus

6. If blue dye were injected into the femoral artery, which area would retain its normal color?
   A. Choroid plexus
   B. Pineal gland
   C. Nucleus of the solitary tract
   D. Area postrema
   E. Liver

7. Which of the following cardiovascular events has the greatest survivability?
   A. Ischemic stroke
   B. Hemorrhagic stroke
   C. TIA
   D. Ruptured aneurysm
   E. Subdural hematoma

8. Where would damage be expected following an occlusive stroke of the middle cerebral artery near the junction with the internal carotid artery?
   A. Thalamus
   B. Primary visual cortex
   C. Inferior temporal gyrus
   D. Basal ganglia
   E. Superior and inferior colliculus

9. Venous return involves deep and superficial veins, which begin as separate drainage systems but eventually unite. Use the letter "S" to indicate which veins and sinuses are part of the superficial system, a "D" for those in the deep system, and a "B" for those that receive flow from both.
   A. Transverse sinus
   B. Great vein of Galen
   C. Internal cerebral vein
   D. Superior sagittal sinus
   E. Vein of Trolard
   F. Basal vein of Rosenthal

10. Which of the following events is most likely to cause a communicating hydrocephalus?
   A. Meningioma
   B. Papilloma
   C. Glioma
   D. Pituitary adenoma
   E. Ependymona

ADDITIONAL READING

Classic Literature

Brightman MW: The intracerebral movement of proteins injected into blood and cerebrospinal fluid of mice. *Prog Brain Res* 29:19–40, 1968.

Gillilan L: The arterial and venous blood supplies to the forebrain (including the internal capsule) of primates. *Neurol* 18:653–670, 1968.

Gillilan L: The correlation of the blood supply to the human brain stem with clinical brain stem lesions. *J Neuropath Exp Neurol* 23:78–108, 1964.

Riggs HE, Rupp C: Variation in form of circle of Willis. The relation of the variations to collateral circulation: anatomic analysis. *Arch Neurol* 8:8–14, 1963.

Roy CS, Sherrington CS: On the regulation of the blood supply of the brain. *J Physiol* 11:85–108, 1890.

Reviews and Landmark Research Articles

Abbott NJ: Dynamics of CNS barriers: evolution, differentiation, and modulation. *Cell Mol Neurobiol* 25:5–23, 2005.

Broderick JP, Brott TG, Duldner JE, Tonsick T, Huster G: Volume of intracerebral hemorrhage: a powerful and easy-to-use predictor of 30-day mortality. *Stroke* 24:987–993, 1993.

Burger PC, Scheithauer BW: *Tumors of the Central Nervous System.* Washington, DC: Armed Forces Institute of Pathology, 1994.

Chae J, Zorowitz RD, Johnston MV: Functional outcome of hemorrhagic and nonhemorrhagic stroke patients after in-patient rehabilitation. *Am J Phys Med Rehabil* 75:177–182, 1996.

Coyle PK: Overview of acute and chronic meningitis. *Neurol Clin* 17:691–710, 1999.

Davson H, Hollingsworth G, Segal MB: The mechanism of drainage of the cerebrospinal fluid. *Brain* 93:665–678, 1970.

DeAngelis LM: Brain tumors. *N Engl J Med* 344:114–123, 2001.

Edwards RJ, Dombrowski SM, Luciano MG, Pople IK: Chronic hydrocephalus in adults. *Brain Pathol* 14:325–336, 2004.

Engelhardt B, Risau W: The development of the blood-brain barrier. In: Greenwood J, Begley D, Segal M. London. *The Development of the Blood-Brain Barrier*. Plenum, 1995.

Goldstein LB, Simel DL: Is this patient having a stroke? *JAMA* 293:2391–2402, 2005.

Grand W, Hopkins LN: *Vasculature of the Brain and Cranial Base: Variations in Clinical Anatomy*. New York, NY: Thieme Medical Publishers, 1999.

Hossmann KA: Viability thresholds and the penumbra of focal ischemia. *Ann Neurol* 36:557–565, 1994.

Laine FJ, Shedden AI, Dunn MM, Ghatak NR: Acquired intracranial herniations: MR imaging findings. *AJR Am J Roentgenol* 165:967–973, 1995.

Laterra J, Brem H: Primary brain tumors in adults. In: Asbury AK, McKhann GM, McDonald WI, Goadsby PJ, McArthur JC. *Diseases of the Nervous System. Clinical Neuroscience and Therapeutic Principles.* Cambridge, UK: University Press, Vol 2:1431–1447, 2002.

Maramattom BV, Wijdicks EFM: Uncal Herniation. *Arch Neurol* 62:1932–1935, 2005.

McKinley MJ, Clarke IJ, Oldfield BJ: Circumventricular organs. In: Paxinos G, Mai J. *The Human Nervous System.* New York, NY: Elsevier, 2nd ed., 2004:563–591.

Mollgard K, Saunders NR: The development of the human blood-brain and blood-CSF barriers. *Neuropath Appl Neurobiol* 12:337–358, 1986.

Porter DG, Bandman O, Thomas DG: Primary intracranial and spinal tumors in adulthood. In: Brandt T, Caplan LR, Dichgans J, Diener HC, Kennard C. *Neurological Disorders. Course and Treatment.* New York, NY: Academic Press, 1996:569–593.

Relkin N, Marmarou A, Klinge P, Bergsneider M, Black PM: Diagnosing idiopathic normal-pressure hydrocephalus. *Neurosurg* 57(suppl 3):S4–16, 2005.

Ribatti D, Nico B, Crivellato E, Artico M: Development of the blood-brain barrier: a historical point of view. *Anat Rec B New Anat* 289:3–8, 2006.

Rizvi R, Anjum Q: Hydrocephalus in children. *J Pak Med Assoc* 55:502–507, 2005.

Rothwell PM, Johnston SC: Transient ischemic attacks: stratifying risk. *Stroke* 37:320–322, 2006.

Salman M: Why does tonsillar herniation not occur in idiopathic intracranial hypertension? *Med Hypotheses* 53:270–271, 1999.

Scott TF: Cerebral herniation after lumbar puncture in sarcoid meningitis. *Clin Neurol Neurosurg* 102:26–28, 2000.

Scremin OU: Cerebral vascular system. In: Paxinos G, Mai J. *The Human Nervous System.* New York, NY: Elsevier, 2nd ed., 2004:1325–1348.

Sullivan HC: Fatal tonsillar herniation in pseudotumor cerebri. *Neurol* 41:1142–1144, 1991.

Tatu L, Moulin T, Bogousslavsky J, Duvernoy H: Arterial territories of human brain: brainstem and cerebellum. *Neurol* 47:1125–1135, 1996.

Tatu L, Moulin T, Bogousslavsky J, Duvernoy H: Arterial territories of human brain: cerebral hemispheres. *Neurol* 50:1699–1708, 1998.

Vanneste JA: Diagnosis and management of normal-pressure hydrocephalus. *J Neurol* 247:5–14, 2000.

INTERNET RESOURCES

The Brain Aneurysm Foundation
http://www.bafound.org/info/index.php

California State University, Chico
Neuroanatomy of Speech, Swallowing and Language
http://www.csuchico.edu/~pmccaff/syllabi/CMSD%20320/362%20index.html

Duke University
NeuroAnatomy Web Resources
http://pathology.mc.duke.edu/neuropath/nawr/nawr_index.html

Harvard University
The Whole Brain Atlas
http://www.med.harvard.edu/AANLIB/home.html

The Hydrocephalus Foundation, Inc. (HyFI)
http://www.hydrocephalus.org/

Indiana University
Brain Images
http://users.ipfw.edu/sweazey/grosssections.htm

Loyola University (Chicago)
Medical Neuroscience
http://www.meddean.luc.edu/lumen/MedEd/Neuro/Neuro.html
McGill University
CNS Learning Center
http://sprojects.mmi.mcgill.ca/cns/histo/systems/systems.htm
http://sprojects.mmi.mcgill.ca/brain/contents.htm
Michigan State University
The Human Brain Atlas
http://www.msu.edu/~brains/brains/human/index.html
National Institute of Neurological Disorders and Stroke
Stroke Page
http://www.ninds.nih.gov/disorders/stroke/stroke.htm
Microcephaly Information Page
http://www.ninds.nih.gov/disorders/microcephaly/microcephaly.htm
Hydrocephalus Information Page
http://www.ninds.nih.gov/disorders/hydrocephalus/hydrocephalus.htm
Normal Pressure Hydrocephalus Information Page
http://www.ninds.nih.gov/disorders/normal_pressure_hydrocephalus/normal_pressure_hydrocephalus.htm
Meningitis and Encephalitis Information Page
http://www.ninds.nih.gov/disorders/encephalitis_meningitis/encephalitis_meningitis.htm
Cerebral Aneurysm Information Page
http://www.ninds.nih.gov/disorders/cerebral_aneurysm/cerebral_aneurysm.htm
Texas Tech University
Texas Tech Neuro Atlas
http://www.ttuhsc.edu/som/courses/neuro/wygrt/index.html
Uniformed Services University
Cranial Nerves
http://rad.usuhs.mil/cranial_nerves/timrad.html
Vascular Supply
http://rad.usuhs.mil/rad/stroke/index.html
University of California at Los Angeles
Web-Atlas
http://www.radnet.ucla.edu/sections/DINR/index.htm
University of Debrecen, Hungary
Department of Neurology Link List
http://www.neuropat.dote.hu/anatomy.htm
University of Idaho
Brain Atlases
http://www.sci.uidaho.edu/med532/start.htm
University of Manchester, UK
Cranial Nerves
http://www.teaching-biomed.man.ac.uk/resources/wwwcal/cranial_nerves/
University of Utah
Anatomy-Histology Tutorials
http://www-medlib.med.utah.edu/WebPath/HISTHTML/HISTO.html
University of Washington
Digital Anatomist Project
http://www9.biostr.washington.edu/da.html
University of Wisconsin Medical School
Brain Vasculature
http://www.neuroanatomy.wisc.edu/angiograms/bldsup.html
http://www.neuroanatomy.wisc.edu/angiograms/coronal.html
Washington University School of Medicine
Coronal and Horizontal Sections
http://thalamus.wustl.edu/course/corhor.html
Yale University School of Medicine
Cranial Nerves
http://info.med.yale.edu/caim/cnerves/contents.html

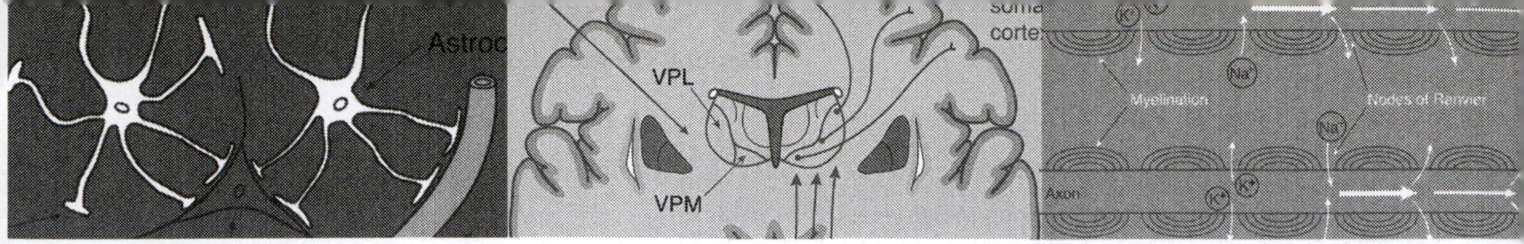

CHAPTER 4

Spinal Cord and Peripheral Nerves

INTRODUCTION OF CLINICAL CASE

A 30-year-old man was brought to the emergency department of a local hospital after he had been seriously injured in a knife fight. The man was conscious and showed no signs of confusion. An examination revealed multiple bruises and lacerations as well as a piercing knife wound in his back, just to the right of the midline at the first thoracic vertebra (T1). Pupillary, gag, and corneal reflexes were normal, and a full range of eye movements was present. The tongue protruded on the midline, and all facial movements were normal. The man could move both arms and his left leg, but not his right leg. Deep tendon reflexes were absent in the right leg, which exhibited flaccid paralysis. There was no response to pinprick on the left side of the body below T3. The right side was responsive to pinprick, but sensation for light touch and vibration was lost on the right side below T1. The victim's condition was unchanged 2 months later, except the right leg showed hyperactive deep tendon reflexes, and Babinski's sign was present when the plantar surface of the right foot was stroked.

INTRODUCTION TO THE SPINAL CORD

The spinal cord represents the caudal end of the central nervous system (CNS). In conjunction with the peripheral nerves, the spinal cord forms a functional system that is essential for the sensory and motor activities of the body. The peripheral nervous system contains millions of nerve fibers that transmit sensory activity to the spinal cord and motor commands to the skeletal muscles. As part of the CNS, the spinal cord contains neural circuits needed for sensory integration and muscular coordination. In the clinic, the functional integrity of these circuits is evaluated by examining limb reflexes, muscular strength, and cutaneous sensitivity. Damage to the spinal cord or peripheral nerves is indicated by weakness, paralysis, or insensitivity to sensory stimulation.

GROSS ANATOMY OF THE SPINAL CORD

The cauda equina resembles a horse's tail.

The spinal cord is a cylindrical structure that extends through the neural canal of the vertebral column. The rostral end of the spinal cord continues into the medulla through the foramen magnum, and its caudal end terminates in the conus medullaris, as shown in Figure 4.1. The spinal cord develops from the caudal two-thirds of the neural tube, and in early embryologic development it occupies the entire length of the vertebral column. As the embryo develops, however, the caudal end of the spinal cord ascends with respect to the spine so that, at birth, the conus medullaris lies at the third lumbar vertebra (L3). The differential growth of the spinal cord and vertebral column continues until adulthood, at which time the conus medullaris has risen to the first lumbar vertebra (L1). This differential growth creates an elongated space in the caudal end of the spinal canal that is called the lumbar cistern. Nerve roots emerging from the lumbosacral segments descend through the lumbar cistern and are called the "cauda equina" because they resemble a horse's tail. Hypodermic needles can be inserted into the lumbar cistern without damaging the spinal cord (Figure 4.2). This technique is used to withdraw cerebrospinal fluid for its diagnostic value or to inject drugs that block the pain associated with labor and delivery.

The 31 pairs of spinal nerves that emerge from the spinal cord impose a segmental organization that is used to identify different levels of the spinal axis. Each segment is numbered according to the vertebra associated with the departing spinal nerve: 8 cervical (C1-C8), 12 thoracic (T1-T12), 5 lumbar (L1-L5), 5 sacral (S1-S5), and 1 coccygeal. In the cervical segments, nerves C1-C7 emerge rostral to the vertebra with the same number; nerve C8 emerges rostral to the first thoracic vertebra. The remaining spinal nerves emerge caudal to the corresponding vertebra (Figure 4.3).

Vertebral Column

The bony vertebrae and spinal nerves have a spatial configuration that permits flexible support of the vertebral column during normal motor activities. As shown in Figure 4.4, the spinal cord is protected by virtue of its position within the neural canal of the bony vertebrae. Generally, an intervertebral disk is located between each vertebral body; exceptions are the sacrum and coccyx, which are fused vertebrae. The disks act as shock absorbers and are composed of the nucleus pulposus, a soft, pulpy material surrounded by denser connective tissue called the annulus fibrosus. Longitudinal ligaments attached to the vertebral bodies hold the disks in place when the vertebral column bends during movement. Each spinal nerve passes through the intervertebral foramen that lies posterior to the pedicle of the neural arch (Figure 4.4). Among older individuals, disks may rupture and herniate into the neural canal (Figure 4.5). If a herniated disk impinges upon the spinal cord or nerve root, it will cause severe pain, paralysis, or loss of sensation.

FIG. 4.1. Posterior View of the Spinal Cord. Different parts of the spinal cord, including the cervical and lumbar enlargements, are shown with respect to the dorsal roots and dorsal root ganglia. Note the absence of a dorsal nerve root at segment C1.

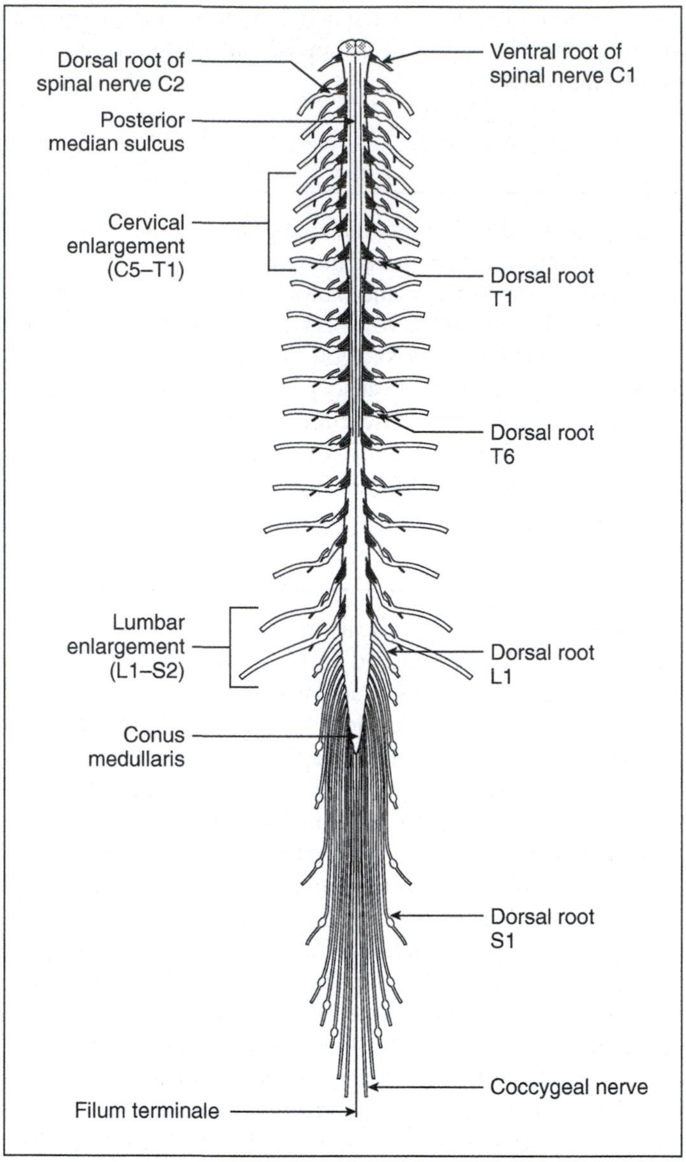

FIG. 4.2. Injection into the Lumbar Cistern. This lateral view shows a lumbar puncture to inject narcotics or local anesthetics into the lumbar cistern, or to take a sample of cerebrospinal fluid.

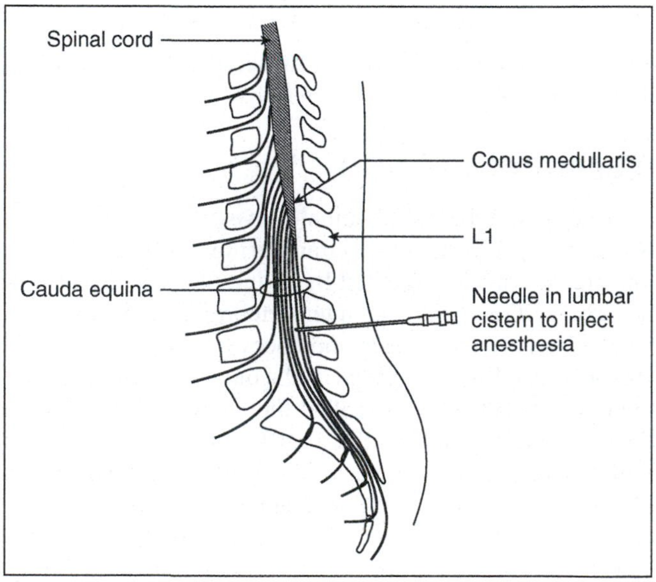

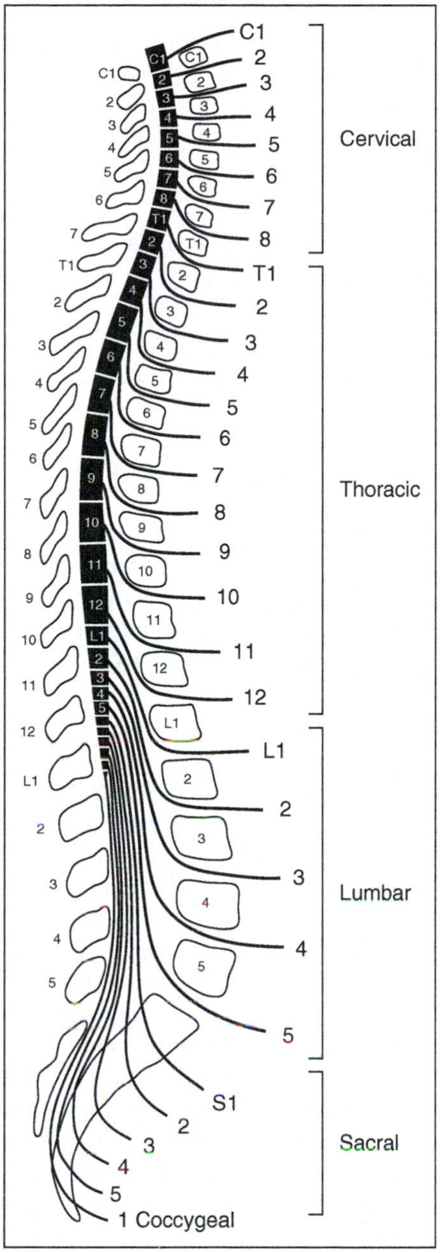

FIG. 4.3. Spinal Cord and Vertebral Segments. This drawing shows the relationship between the bony vertebral bodies and the spinal nerves emerging from each segment of the spinal cord.

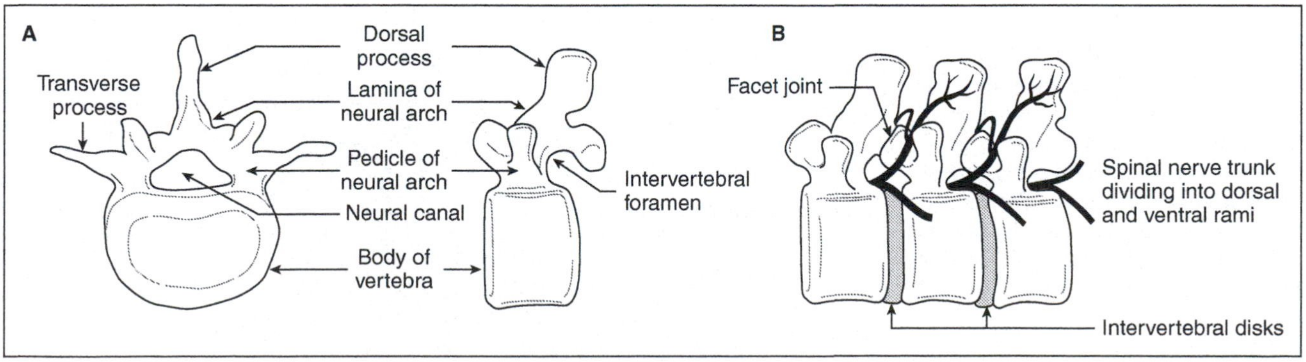

FIG. 4.4. Bony Vertebrae. (A) Superior and lateral views of a typical vertebra. (B) Lateral view showing spinal nerves emerging from the intervertebral foramina of successive vertebrae.

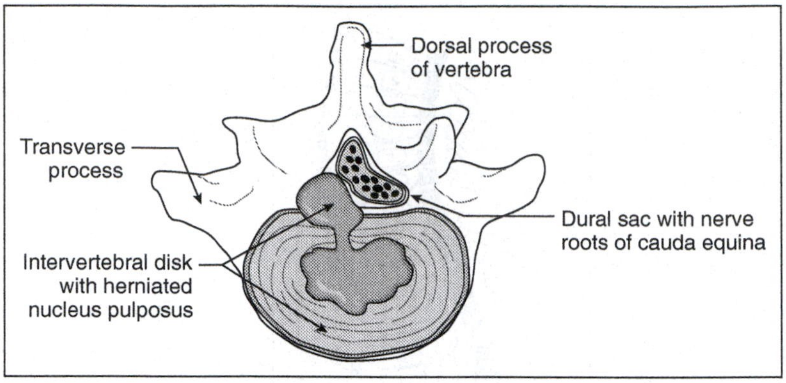

FIG. 4.5. Herniated Disk. Transverse view of a herniated disk at the level of the lumbar cistern. The herniation compresses nerve roots that innervate the lower back and legs.

Longitudinal Organization of the Spinal Cord

The spinal cord varies in diameter throughout its length because of variations in the number of neurons and axons at different spinal levels. The cord has two enlargements, one at the cervical level and another at the lumbar level; these enlargements are caused by the large number of neurons that innervate the skin, joints, and muscles of the limbs. The cervical enlargement, which is 1.5 cm wide, extends from C5 to T1 and gives rise to nerve roots that form the brachial plexus. Nerve roots for the lumbosacral plexus emerge from segments in the lumbar enlargement that extends from L1 to S2. The upper cervical region (C1-C4) is narrower than the cervical and lumbar enlargements, but it is wider than the thoracic region because it contains all ascending and descending fiber tracts passing between the brain and spinal cord. The narrowest part of the spinal cord, the thoracic region, is only 1.0 cm wide and gives rise to the intercostal nerves.

Several fissures extend the length of the spinal cord. On the midline, the deep anterior median fissure and the shallow posterior median septum nearly divide the spinal cord into symmetrical halves (Figure 4.6). On each side, a posterolateral sulcus marks the entry of dorsal nerve roots. Similarly, an anterolateral sulcus is located at the site where the ventral nerve roots emerge from the anterior surface of the cord. The nerve roots and their associated fissures provide gross landmarks that separate the spinal white matter into different sections.

Collections of myelinated axons that transmit sensory or motor information along the length of the spinal cord are located within three pairs of funiculi. Within each funiculus, related groups of axons are bundled into tracts or fasciculi that convey similar types of information. The posterior funiculus, which is located between the dorsal nerve roots and the posterior median sulcus, contains fiber bundles that transmit somatosensory information to the brain. In the cervical and upper thoracic segments (C1-T6), an additional

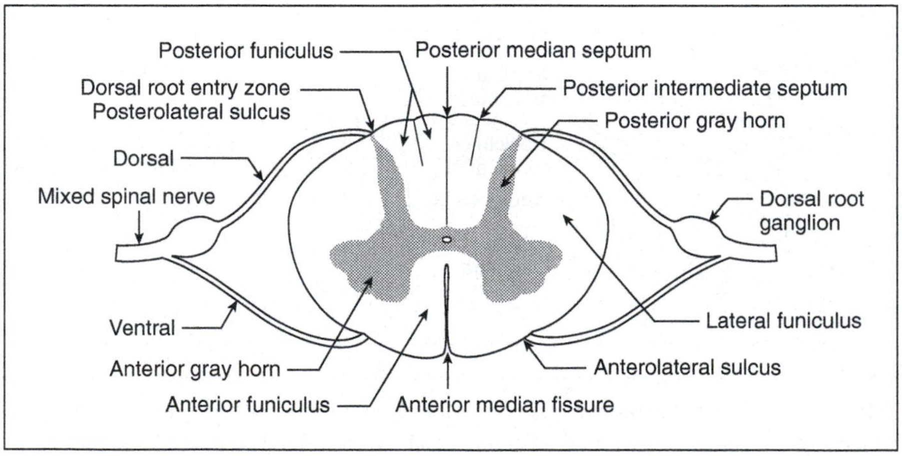

FIG. 4.6. Spinal Cord Landmarks. This drawing identifies the major landmarks of the spinal cord. The central gray region is surrounded by three pairs of funiculi consisting of myelinated fiber tracts. The dorsal and ventral roots are closely associated with the posterior and anterior gray horns, respectively.

fissure, the posterior intermediate septum, subdivides the posterior funiculus into the fasciculus gracilis and the fasciculus cuneatus. The lateral funiculus, located between the dorsal and ventral nerve roots, has both ascending (sensory) and descending (motor) nerve tracts. The anterior funiculus, located between the ventral nerve roots and the anterior median fissure, also contains a mixture of ascending and descending tracts.

Transverse Organization of the Spinal Cord

A transverse section through an unstained spinal cord reveals a central gray region surrounded by the posterior, lateral, and anterior funiculi (Figure 4.6). This central gray region contains symmetrical pairs of posterior and anterior horns that resemble the wings of a butterfly. Because transverse sections of the human spinal cord are usually shown with the posterior horns on top, the horns are often identified as being dorsal (i.e., posterior) or ventral (i.e., anterior). The gray appearance of the central region is due to the presence of neuronal cell bodies and their dendritic processes. By comparison, the surrounding funiculi have a pale appearance because they contain myelinated axons. Both the gray and white matter regions in the spinal cord are infiltrated by small blood vessels and glial cells.

Different levels of the spinal cord can be distinguished on the basis of size, shape, and the relative proportions of white and gray matter. Some nuclei and fiber tracts are found only at certain levels of the spinal cord, and this contributes to the distinct appearance of transverse sections at different levels of the spinal cord. Figure 4.7 shows a flowchart that uses the size, shape, and topography of white and gray matter to determine the level of the spinal cord.

Cervical Levels. Transverse sections through the cervical cord have an oval shape dominated by large funiculi. The funiculi are largest in the cervical segments because (1) the ascending sensory tracts become larger with the addition of more axonal fibers as the tracts proceed toward the brainstem, and (2) the descending motor tracts gradually taper in diameter at successive lower levels as motor fibers leave the tract to innervate groups of

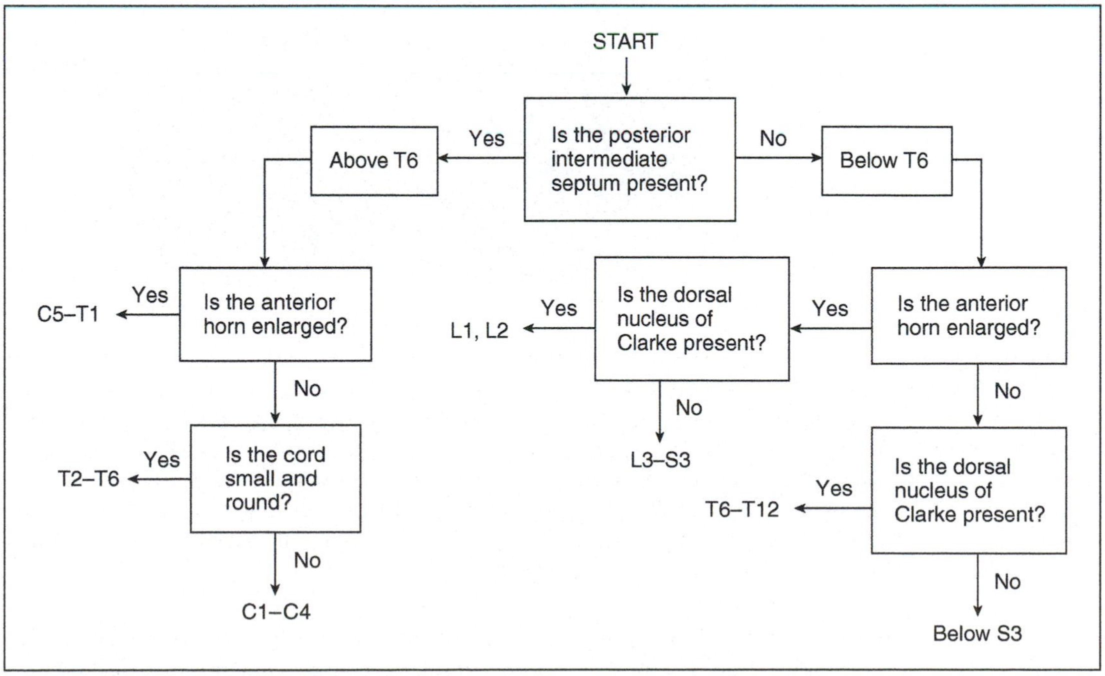

FIG. 4.7. Determination of Spinal Level. This flowchart can be used to determine the approximate level of a transverse section of spinal cord.

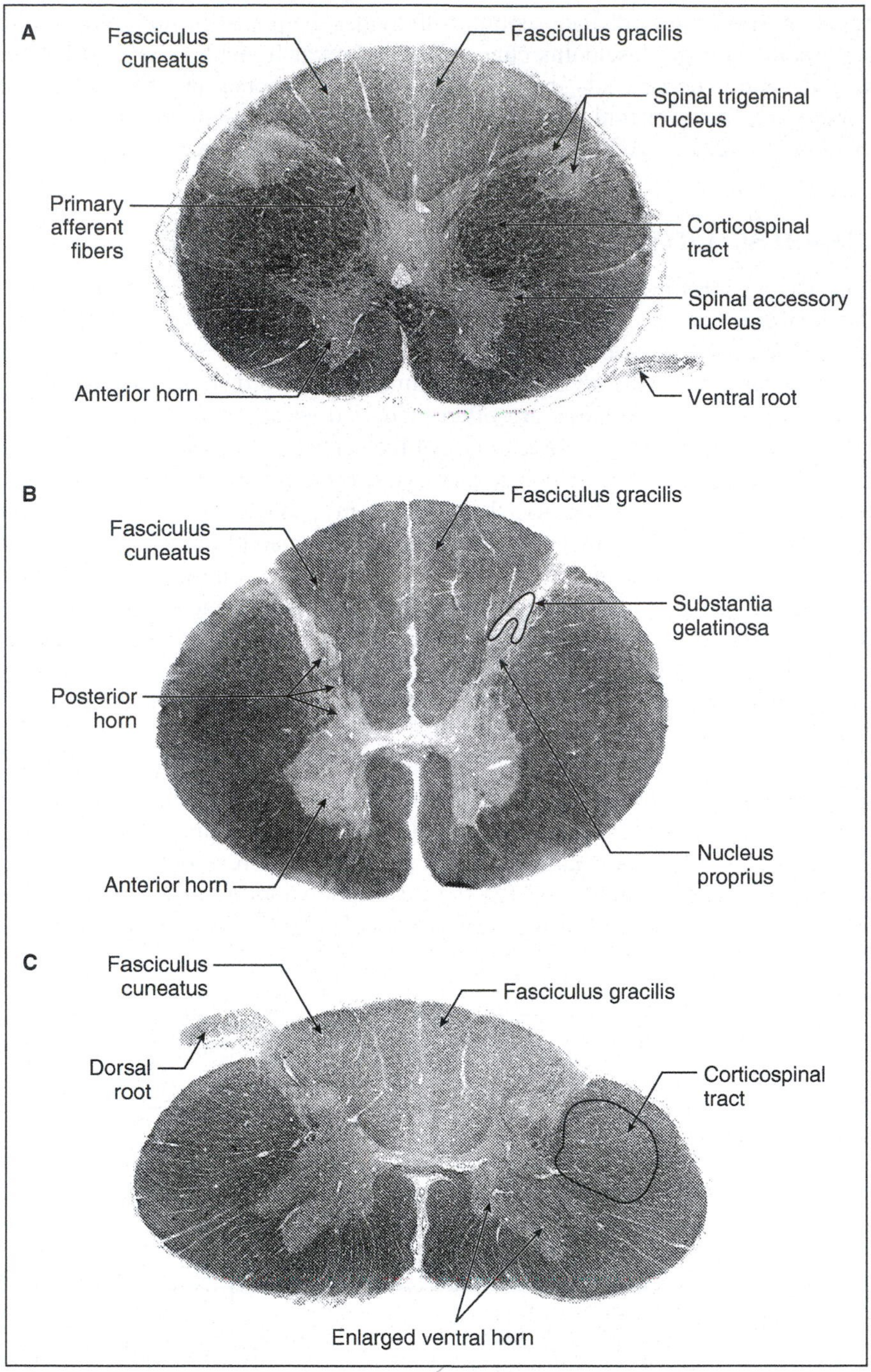

FIG. 4.8. Transverse Sections of the Spinal Cord. Selected levels of the spinal cord reveal characteristic differences in the size, shape, and topography of the central gray and surrounding white matter regions. (A) Section through C1, just caudal to the pyramidal decussation. (B) Section through C4, just rostral to the cervical enlargement. (C) Section of the cervical enlargement at C7. (D) Section through the thoracic level at T10. (E) Section through the lumbar enlargement at L3. (F) Section through the sacral spinal cord.

motor neurons. In the posterior funiculus, the posterior intermediate sulcus separates the fasciculus gracilis from the more lateral fasciculus cuneatus. In the lower half of the cervical cord, C5-C8, the posterior and anterior horns are enlarged because they contain additional neurons to innervate the upper limbs. Figure 4.8 compares transverse views of cervical segments with other levels of the spinal cord.

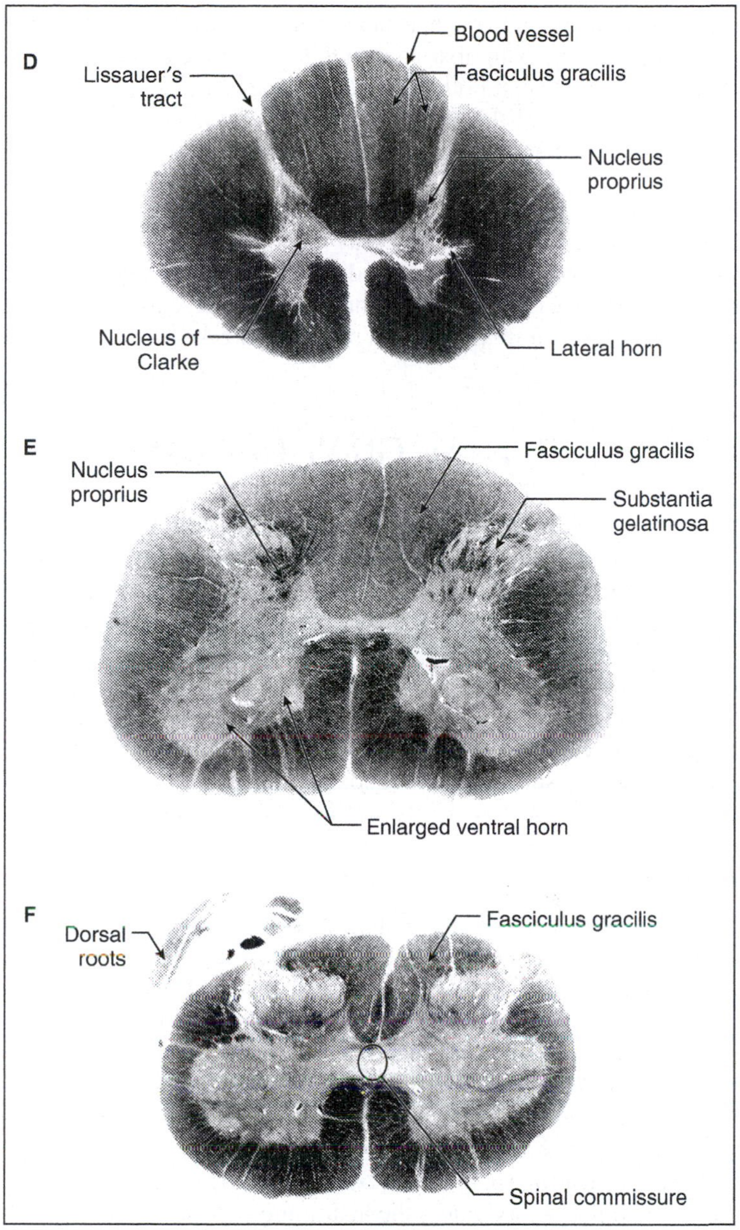

FIG. 4.8. *(Continued)*

Thoracic Levels. With the exception of thoracic segment T1, transverse sections through the thoracic cord are smaller because the central gray region requires few neurons to innervate the intercostal muscles of the trunk. Thoracic segments have a small lateral horn that protrudes into the lateral funiculus, halfway between its slender posterior and anterior horns. The lateral horn is comprised of an intermediolateral cell column that contains preganglionic sympathetic neurons of the autonomic nervous system. All thoracic segments contain the dorsal nucleus of Clarke, a group of large neurons at the base of the posterior horn that is most prominent in segments T10-T12 (Figure 4.8). Upper thoracic segments T1-T6 are distinguished from lower thoracic segments by the presence of the fasciculus cuneatus.

Lumbar Levels. Transverse sections through the lumbar cord have large posterior and anterior horns with a relatively small proportion of white matter. In lumbar segments, the fasciculus gracilis has a boomerang shape and is relatively narrow compared to sections of the thoracic spinal cord. Upper lumbar segments L1-L2 have a lateral horn and a prominent dorsal nucleus of Clarke, but both of these landmarks are absent in lower lumbar segments L3-L5. The large size of the anterior horn in the lumbar enlargement is due to the addition of motor neurons that innervate the muscles of the lower limbs (Figure 4.8).

Sacral Levels. Sections through the sacral cord are characterized by small amounts of white matter, a relatively large proportion of gray matter, and a thick gray commissure in the center of the cord. With successively more caudal sections, sacral segments diminish in size, and the three funiculi become progressively thinner. Coccygeal segments resemble sacral segments in appearance but have a smaller diameter (see Figure 4.8).

CYTOARCHITECTURE OF THE CENTRAL GRAY REGION

The central gray region of the spinal cord is composed of a network of neurons with different sizes, shapes, and connections. Neurons in the central gray region receive afferent projections from the dorsal root ganglia, from other parts of the central gray region (intersegmental connections), and from the brainstem or cerebral cortex (suprasegmental connections). Many neurons in the central gray region innervate peripheral targets, such as muscles and autonomic ganglia, or project to other parts of the CNS. Spinal cord neurons whose processes remain entirely in the CNS can project locally (interneurons), to neighboring segments of the central gray region (intersegmental connections), or to nuclei in the brainstem or thalamus (suprasegmental connections).

Rexed Laminae

In the early anatomical studies of the spinal cord, the terminology for describing its cytoarchitecture was inconsistent and only a few nuclear groups were widely recognized. In 1952, Bror Rexed made much thicker transverse sections of the spinal cord and discovered a laminar pattern composed of distinct cell columns that extended throughout the longitudinal axis of the cord. The classification system of Rexed uses Roman numerals to identify nine laminae progressing ventrally from the superficial aspect of the dorsal horn (lamina I) to the motor neurons of the ventral horn (lamina IX). The region surrounding the central canal is classified as lamina X.

The laminar classification system of Rexed is used by most anatomists, but it is difficult to detect the cellular layers unless the histologic sections are at least 100 μm thick. Some nuclei are confined to a single Rexed lamina; in such cases, the name of the nucleus may be used interchangeably with the laminar designation. In other cases, spinal cord nuclei extend across Rexed laminae or are located in one part of a specific lamina. Table 4.1 indicates the anatomic relationships and identified functions of several nuclei located at different levels of the spinal cord.

Connections of the Spinal Nerve Roots

Posterior horn: sensory functions

The functional anatomy of the central gray region can be understood by considering the connections of the dorsal and ventral nerve roots. All dorsal nerve root fibers convey sensory impulses, and virtually all of them have collateral axons that terminate in the posterior horn. Hence, neurons in the posterior horn receive synaptic inputs from fibers conveying sensory information from the skin, joints, and muscles. Nerve fibers entering the posterior horn are classified as general somatic afferents (GSA) or general visceral afferents (GVA), and their cell bodies are located in the dorsal root ganglia.

TABLE 4.1 Subdivisions of the Central Gray Region

Spinal Nucleus	Rexed Lamina	Spinal Levels	Functions
Dorsomarginal nucleus	I	All	Anterolateral system
Substantia gelatinosa	II	All	Modulates pain and temperature inputs
Nucleus proprius	III and IV	All	Cutaneous and nociceptive processing
Not named	V	All	Anterolateral system
Not named	VI	Enlargements	Proprioceptive processing
Dorsal nucleus of Clarke	VII	T1-L3	Posterior spinocerebellar tract
Intermediomedial nucleus	VII	All	Visceral processing
Intermediolateral nucleus	VII	T1-L3	Preganglionic sympathetic neurons
Sacral parasympathetic nucleus	VII	S2-S4	Preganglionic parasympathetic neurons
Not named	VIII	All	Receives descending brain projections
Medial motor neurons	IX	All	Innervates axial muscles
Lateral motor neurons	IX	Enlargements	Innervates limb muscles
Phrenic nucleus	IX	C3-C5	Innervates diaphragm
Spinal accessory nucleus	IX	Medulla-C5	Innervates strenocleidomastoid, trapezius

By comparison, at least 80% of the ventral nerve root fibers have efferent functions. These efferent fibers originate from cell bodies located in the anterior or lateral horns. Ventral root fibers originating from the lateral horn represent preganglionic, general visceral efferent (GVE) fibers of the sympathetic nervous system. Ventral nerve roots that originate from cell bodies in the anterior horn are classified as general somatic efferent (GSE) fibers because they innervate skeletal muscles. A small portion (about 15%) of fibers in the ventral nerve root do not follow this functional convention; these are nociceptive afferent fibers that enter the cord through the ventral rather than through the dorsal root entry zone.

Anterior horn: motor functions

Posterior Horn

The posterior horn is primarily sensory in function. Located between the lateral and posterior funiculi, the posterior horn receives most of its inputs from afferent fibers that enter the cord at the dorsal root entry zone. Many of these incoming fibers send bifurcating axons rostrally and caudally in Lissauer's tract for a few segments before entering the posterior horn. After leaving Lissauer's tract, the small-diameter nociceptive fibers enter the lateral aspect of the posterior horn, whereas the wider cutaneous fibers proceed more medially as shown in Figure 4.9. Both sets of fibers use excitatory neurotransmitters; glutamate is found in the terminals of cutaneous fibers, whereas glutamate and substance P are co-localized in the terminals of the nociceptive fibers.

Depending upon the level of the cord, the posterior horn is composed of five or six cell layers (Rexed laminae) that vary in thickness, neuronal composition, and anatomic connections. The superficial rim of the posterior horn contains a thin layer of neurons known as Rexed lamina I or the posteromarginal nucleus (Figure 4.9). The posteromarginal nucleus receives inputs primarily from thin fibers conveying nociceptive information. Lamina II, located below the posteromarginal nucleus, has a pale appearance resembling gelatin and, for this reason, is known as the substantia gelatinosa. The substantia gelatinosa has small neurons with high concentrations of enkephalin, and it receives synaptic inputs from both cutaneous and nociceptive nerve fibers. Rexed laminae III and IV, which

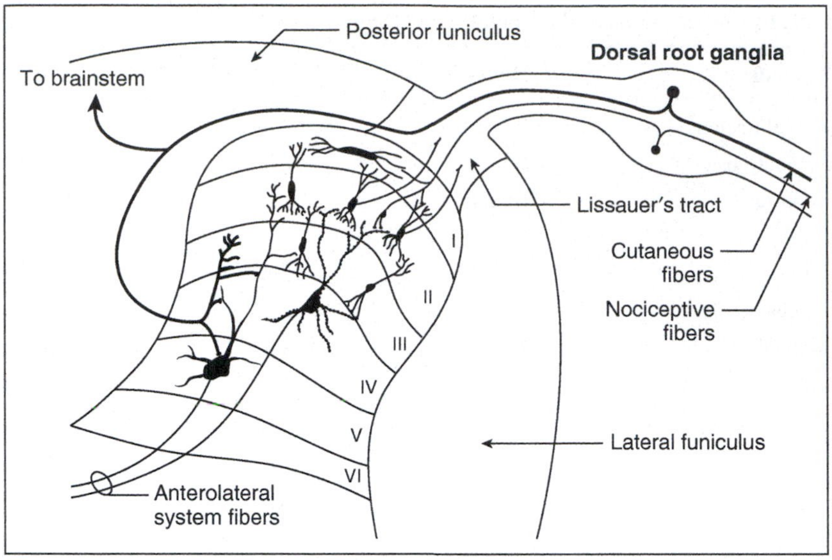

FIG. 4.9. Cytoarchitecture of the Posterior Horn. In the cervical and lumbar enlargements, the posterior horn is composed of Rexed laminae I-VI. Note that each layer in the posterior horn is characterized by different types of neurons. Large-diameter and small-diameter afferent fibers enter the cord through Lissauer's tract before diverging into medial (large fibers) and lateral (small fibers) groups. After entering the spinal cord, the larger fibers proceed medially and ascend the posterior columns. Collaterals of these large fibers enter the medial side of the posterior horn and terminate in its deeper layers, especially in laminae III, IV, and V. By comparison, the thin fibers proceed to the lateral side of the posterior horn and terminate in laminae I, II, IV, and V. Laminae I, IV, and V contain projection neurons whose axons cross the midline before ascending in the lateral funiculus to convey nociceptive information to the brain.

comprise the nucleus proprius (or proper sensory nucleus), receive inputs mainly from cutaneous fibers and, to a lesser extent, from nociceptive fibers. Rexed lamina IV is the thickest layer of the dorsal horn and contains many large multipolar neurons. Neurons in Rexed lamina V, which extends across the neck of the dorsal horn, receives inputs from both cutaneous and nociceptive fibers. The neurons forming Rexed lamina VI are located along the base of the dorsal horn, but these are present only in the cervical and lumbar enlargements. The medial part of lamina VI receives input from Golgi tendon organs, muscle spindles, and nociceptive free nerve endings. The lateral part of lamina VI receives descending projections from the motor cerebral cortex.

Local Pain Circuits. The posterior horn plays a significant role in coding the intensity and quality of somatosensory sensations, including those related to pain. Neurons located in laminae I, IV, and V, and some in laminae VI and VII, respond to intense thermal or tissue-damaging stimulation and send long ascending projections to specific parts of the brainstem and thalamus. These pain-related projections are called the anterolateral system because they are located in the anterior part of the lateral funiculus. The anterolateral system responds to noxious thermal or intense mechanical stimulation, as well as to cutaneous inputs that signal light touch or pressure. The convergence of these different submodalities causes the anterolateral system to discharge at low rates during cutaneous (non-noxious) stimulation and at higher rates during more intense stimulation (Figure 4.10). Given these response properties, neurons in the anterolateral system are said to respond over a wide dynamic range. This suggests that pain intensity is coded, in part, by the rate of activity among the fibers in the anterolateral system.

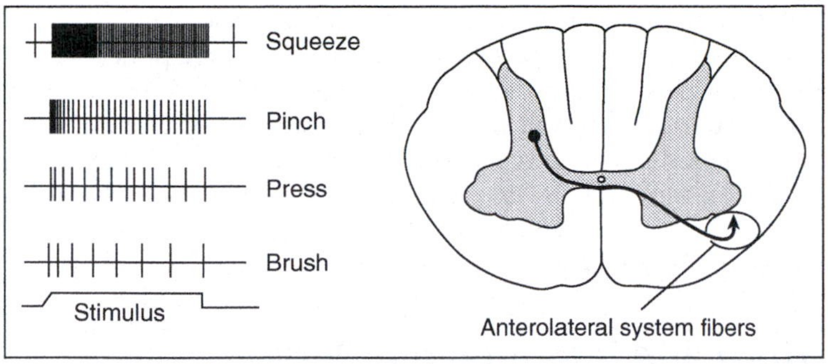

FIG. 4.10. Responses to Convergent Inputs in the Posterior Horn. Many neurons in the posterior horn receive both cutaneous and nociceptive inputs from the periphery. Located mainly in lamina IV and V, the discharge rates of these neurons encode the intensity of the peripheral stimulus. Known as wide dynamic range neurons, their axons project to the brainstem and thalamus as part of the anterolateral system.

Substantia gelatinosa is a neural gate for blocking pain.

Physiologic studies indicate that enkephalin is a neurotransmitter that inhibits the transmission of pain information through the anterolateral system (Figure 4.11). Enkephalinergic neurons in the substantia gelatinosa (lamina II) send their axons dorsally into lamina I and into the overlying Lissauer's tract where they ascend or descend a few segments before reentering laminae I and II. Although the substantia gelatinosa does not send axons ventrally into laminae III, IV, and V, neurons in these underlying layers have dendrites that branch into the substantia gelatinosa where they receive enkephalinergic innervation. In addition, descending projections from the brainstem activate the substantia gelatinosa, causing it to release enkephalin and inhibit the projection neurons

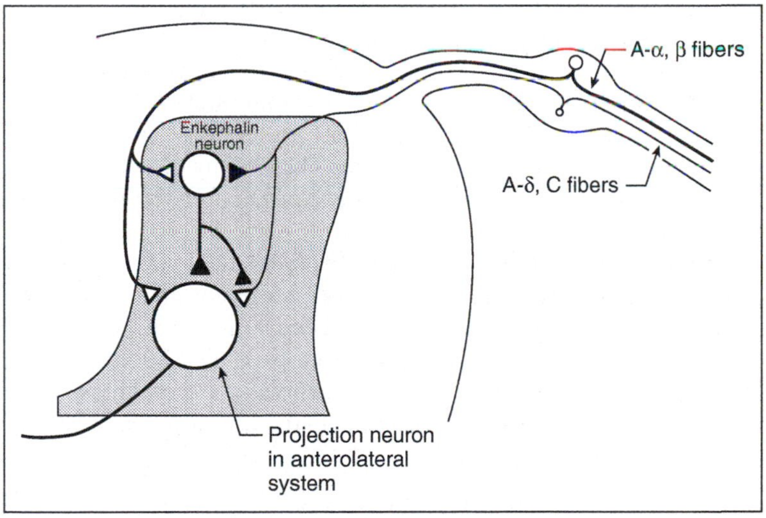

FIG. 4.11. Pain Control Circuits in the Posterior Horn. A schematic illustration of the gate-control mechanism for modulating nociception in the posterior horn. Inhibitory synapses are indicated by filled terminals; excitatory synapses are indicated by open terminals. Enkephalinergic neurons in the substantia gelatinosa inhibit projection neurons directly and can inhibit the release of excitatory transmitters from the C fibers. Enkephalinergic neurons can be activated either by cutaneous stimulation (A-α fibers) or by descending projections from the brainstem (not shown). Note that collaterals of the incoming nociceptive fibers inhibit the enkephalinergic neurons in the substantia nigra but excite the projection neurons of the anterolateral system. The neurons that give rise to the anterolateral system exhibit wide dynamic responses because they receive inputs from both cutaneous and nociceptive afferents.

of the anterolateral system. Hence, the substantia gelatinosa controls or "gates" the efficacy of transmission between peripheral pain fibers and the projection neurons of the anterolateral system. This view, known as the gate-control theory of pain transmission, was first proposed by Melzack and Wall in 1967 (Figure 4.11). Because the substantia gelatinosa receives cutaneous inputs, it is possible to activate this inhibitory system by gently stimulating the skin; this explains why we derive some pain relief by rubbing the skin around an injury. Opiates and other narcotic drugs relieve pain because they act as agonists at presynaptic and postsynaptic enkephalin binding sites in the posterior horn.

Lateral Horn and Intermediate Region

The region between the posterior and anterior horns contains several nuclei that lie in different parts of Rexed lamina VII. These nuclei receive a variety of afferent connections, including inputs from primary sensory fibers, intersegmental connections from other parts of the spinal cord, and descending suprasegmental inputs from the cerebral cortex and other brain regions. The functional diversity of lamina VII reflects the significant differences in their afferent and efferent connections (Table 4.1).

The dorsal nucleus of Clarke, which lies in the medial part of lamina VII from C8 to L2, contains large neurons that receive inputs from several types of muscle receptors, including annulospiral endings, flower spray endings, and Golgi tendon organs. When viewed in transverse sections, the dorsal nucleus of Clarke is most prominent in the lower segments of the thoracic cord because this region receives the bulk of inputs from the muscles of the leg. Axonal projections from the dorsal nucleus of Clarke form the posterior spinocerebellar tract, which is located in the lateral funiculus. This uncrossed pathway conveys sensory information about the position, length, and dynamic activity of the muscles to the cerebellum.

The intermediolateral nucleus is a cholinergic cell column located in the lateral horn from T1 to L2. It contains large preganglionic sympathetic neurons whose axons emerge from the ventral root. The lateral horn does not extend into sacral levels, but a group of cholinergic neurons occupies a similar position in the lateral part of lamina VII from S2 to S4. These sacral neurons give rise to the preganglionic parasympathetic fibers of the pelvic nerves. An intermediomedial nucleus lies ventral to the dorsal nucleus of Clarke and receives afferent projections from peripheral fibers innervating the thoracic and abdominal viscera. The intermediomedial nucleus is present at all levels of the cord, and it sends local projections to the intermediolateral nucleus of the lateral horn.

Some neurons in the region between the intermediolateral nucleus and posterior horn receive convergent inputs from visceral and somatic afferent fibers. These neurons send their axons into the anterolateral system and, because they can be activated by either visceral or cutaneous inputs, they mediate "referred pain" sensations. For example, pain associated with myocardial infarction, kidney infection, or visceral muscle sensations are often perceived as cutaneous sensations that radiate into the arm, upper chest, lower back, or other areas of the body.

Anterior Horn

The anterior horn lies between the lateral and anterior funiculi and contains large and small neurons concerned with voluntary and reflexive movements. Consistent with this role, the ventral horn receives descending inputs from brain regions concerned with motor functions, including the cerebral cortex, the red nucleus, and the reticular formation. To execute reflexes, neurons in the anterior horn receive sensory information from peripheral receptors either directly from the dorsal nerve roots or indirectly via intersegmental pathways that originate from neurons in the posterior horn (Figure 4.12).

The anterior horn consists of Rexed laminae VIII and IX, and the ventral parts of lamina VII. Lamina VIII varies in size and is located mainly in the medial part of the ventral horn, especially at levels associated with the spinal enlargements. Lamina VIII

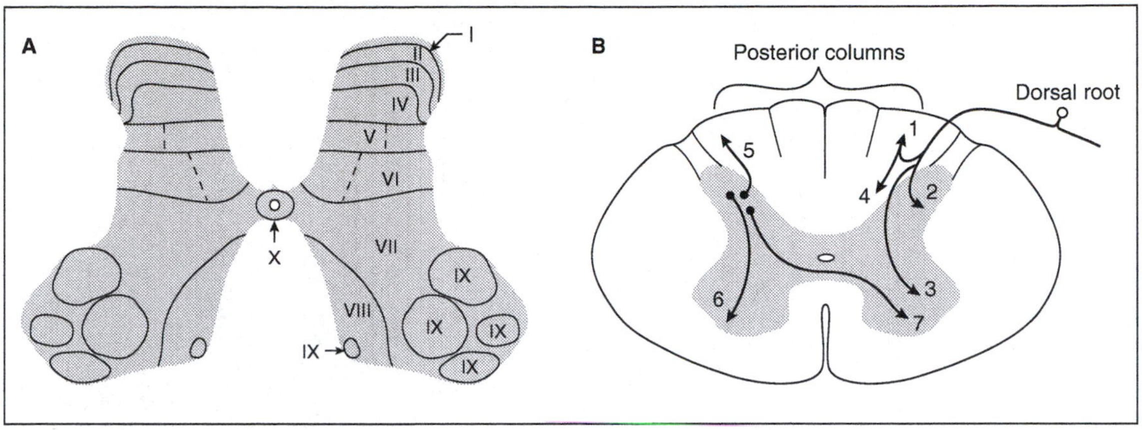

FIG. 4.12. Afferent Connections in the Central Gray Region. (A) Relative location of Rexed laminae in the central gray region of the spinal cord. (B) Major routes for transmission of afferent information in the spinal cord. Primary afferent fibers project to several areas including: (1) the posterior columns, (2) the posterior horn, and (3) the anterior horn. Some collateral fibers may descend several segments before terminating in the central gray region (route 4). Some posterior horn neurons send ascending projections to the brain via the posterior columns (route 5), whereas others project either ipsilaterally (route 6) or contralaterally (route 7) to the anterior horn of neighboring levels of the spinal cord. Routes 2, 3, 4, 6, and 7 are needed to mediate spinal reflexes.

receives descending inputs from the brainstem that are important for modulating motor tone. Finally, the motor neurons that innervate the skeletal muscles reside in clusters that form lamina IX.

Alpha-motor neurons provide the final common pathway to skeletal muscles.

Alpha-Motor Neurons. The anterior horn is a critical component of the motor system because it contains the alpha (α) motor neurons whose emerging axons form the ventral root. Alpha-motor neurons are large, multipolar neurons in lamina IX that innervate the long, extrafusal fibers of the peripheral muscles. Consistent with this function, α-motor neurons release acetylcholine (ACh) from their synaptic terminals in the neuromuscular junction. Because all descending motor commands must converge onto α-motor neurons, the axons of the α-motor neurons are often called the "final common pathway."

Gamma-Motor Neurons. Lamina IX also contains smaller gamma (γ) motor neurons that innervate specialized receptors in the muscles known as muscle spindles. Gamma-motor neurons also release ACh at their synapses to cause contraction of the short intrafusal fibers within the muscle spindles.

Motor Neuron Nuclei. Small collections of α-motor and γ-motor neurons are topographically organized to innervate specific groups of muscles. Medial groups of motor neurons innervate the axial musculature (e.g., the intercostal muscles). The lateral groups are relatively small in thoracic levels but are substantially larger in the cervical and lumbar enlargements because they innervate a large number of muscles in the upper and lower limbs. In the cervical enlargement, for example, the motor neurons located most laterally innervate the most distal muscles of the hand, whereas those located more medially innervate more proximal muscles controlling the shoulder and upper arm (Figure 4.13). In addition, motor neurons innervating the extensors are located ventral to those innervating the flexors.

Phrenic nucleus: "Cut C4, breathe no more."

One of the most important motor nuclei in the spinal cord is the phrenic nucleus. Located in lamina IX from C3 to C5, the phrenic nucleus innervates the diaphragm. Together with motor neurons controlling the intercostal muscles, the phrenic nucleus regulates inspiration by integrating descending projections from the motor cortex (voluntary control) and caudal brainstem (involuntary autonomic control). This interconnected

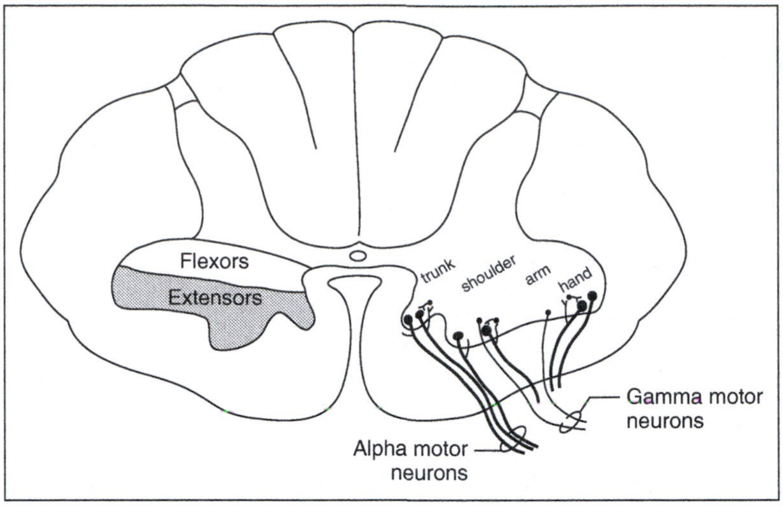

FIG. 4.13. Topography of the Motor Neurons in the Ventral Horn. The left side indicates the general position of motor neurons innervating the flexors or extensors of the upper limb. The right side indicates the medial to lateral organization of motor neurons that innervate proximal and distal muscles, respectively. Each cluster contains α- and γ-motor neurons as well as local inhibitory neurons known as Renshaw cells. Axon collaterals from the motor neurons activate the Renshaw cells to provide recurrent inhibition.

suprasegmental system determines the rhythm, rate, and depth of respiratory movements during the different stages of sleep. Damage to the phrenic nucleus or nerve produces respiratory paralysis and leads to death unless there is immediate intervention.

Poliomyelitis. Poliomyelitis (polio) is an acute viral disease that causes degeneration of α-motor neurons in the anterior horns. Although the severity and spatial extent of the infected sites may vary, the disease invariably produces muscular paralysis and atrophy. In addition to attacking the spinal cord, poliomyelitis may destroy the motor nuclei in the brainstem that control swallowing and respiration. Fortunately, polio is easily prevented by childhood vaccination.

SPINAL NERVES

Peripheral nerves are responsible for afferent and efferent communication between the body and the central nervous system. The cell bodies of afferent nerve fibers are located in the dorsal root ganglia, near the dorsal root entry site. Peripheral afferent neurons are classified as pseudounipolar neurons because only a single axonal process emanates from the soma before bifurcating into a distal branch that innervates the periphery and a proximal branch that enters the spinal cord. The peripheral area innervated by a single dorsal nerve root is called a dermatome. The collection of dermatomes innervated by all of the dorsal nerve roots forms a standard dermatomal map that is used clinically to determine the spinal segments associated with impaired sensitivity (Figure 4.14).

The efferent fibers of the ventral nerve root originate from cell bodies located in the lateral or ventral horns of the spinal cord. After leaving the spinal cord, these efferent fibers merge with the distal processes of the afferent fibers to form a mixed spinal nerve. Efferent fibers originating from motor neurons in lamina IX proceed to the skeletal muscles and terminate in neuromuscular junctions. The topographic sequence of muscles innervated by neighboring ventral nerve roots is similar but not identical to the dermatomal map; nonetheless, the dermatomal map is often used to state clinical findings regarding the level of muscle impairment.

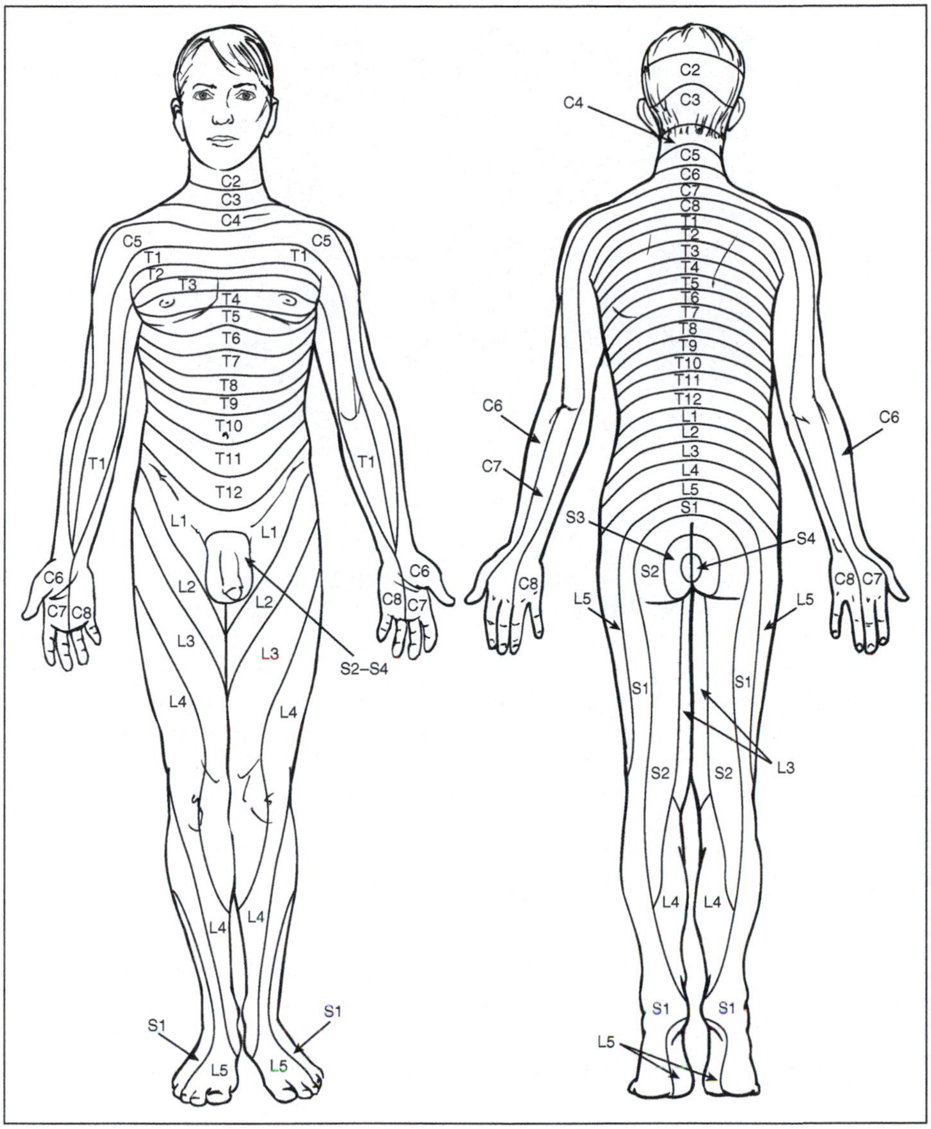

FIG. 4.14. Dermatome Map. Each dermatome represents the body region that receives afferent innervation from a specific dorsal nerve root. The dermatomal map shows the pattern of innervation for all segments of the spinal cord and is divided into cervical, thoracic, lumbar, and sacral regions.

Spinal nerves contain axons, Schwann cells, connective tissue coverings, and blood vessels (Figure 4.15). The entire nerve is wrapped by an outer layer of epineurium that forms a loose connective sheath. Composed of collagen and fibroblasts, the highly elastic epineurium is continuous with the dura and usually ends near the distal termination of small nerve branches. Inside the epineurium is another connective covering, the perineurium, which wraps around bundles of myelinated and unmyelinated axons. The perineurial cells continue to the distal ends of some nerves to form encapsulated endings such as Pacinian corpuscles or muscle spindles. The innermost layer of connective tissue, the endoneurium, ensheathes individual nerve fibers and provides an important substrate for the regrowth of peripheral nerve fibers after injury.

Compound Action Potentials

A cross section of a peripheral nerve shows that the diameter of individual axons can vary substantially (Figure 4.15). The largest axons are approximately 20 μm in diameter and

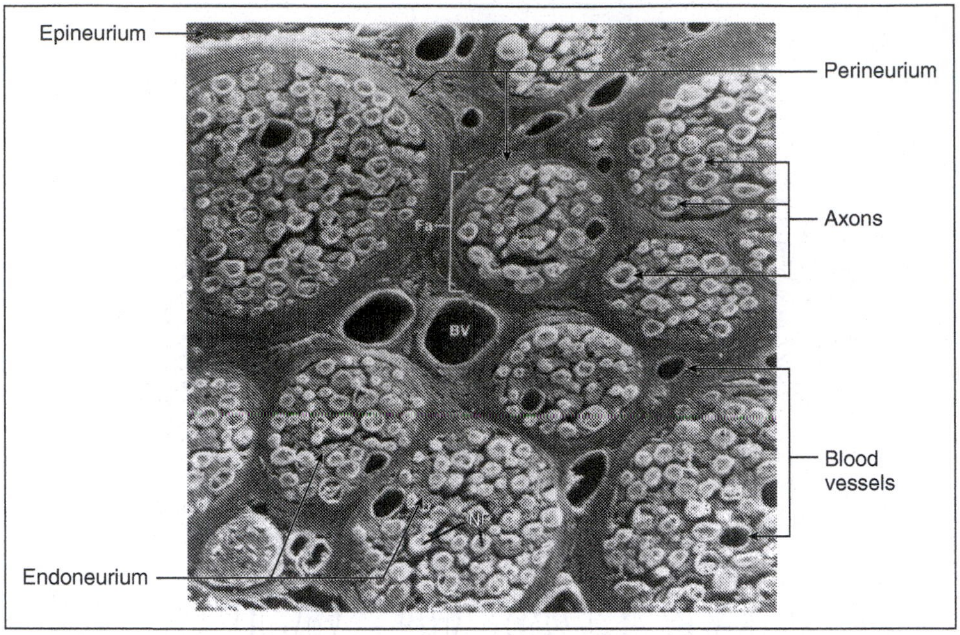

FIG. 4.15. Transverse View of a Peripheral Nerve. This scanning electron micrograph shows a freeze-fractured preparation of peripheral nerve. A band of loose connective tissue, the epineurium, encircles groups of fibers called fascicles (Fa). Each fascicle is covered by perineurium, and individual nerve fibers (NF) within the fascicle are wrapped by a thin layer of endoneurium. Blood vessels (BV) located within the endoneurium or perineurium supply nutrients to the nerve. (Electron micrograph reprinted with permission from Kessel RG, Kardon RH: *Tissues and Organs*. San Francisco, CA: W. H. Freeman, 1979:79.)

heavily myelinated, whereas the smallest axons are less than 1 μm in diameter and unmyelinated. In the 1930s, a series of physiology experiments by Erlanger and Gasser demonstrated the functional importance of the variance in fiber diameter. As shown in Figure 4.16, when the distal part of a peripheral nerve is electrically stimulated, a compound

FIG. 4.16. Compound Action Potentials. (A) The distal portion of a peripheral nerve is electrically stimulated while a more proximal electrode monitors changes in membrane potentials. (B) Compound action potentials are recorded as a series of waves that correspond to the summed activity that is transmitted by populations of fibers with different diameters and conduction velocities.

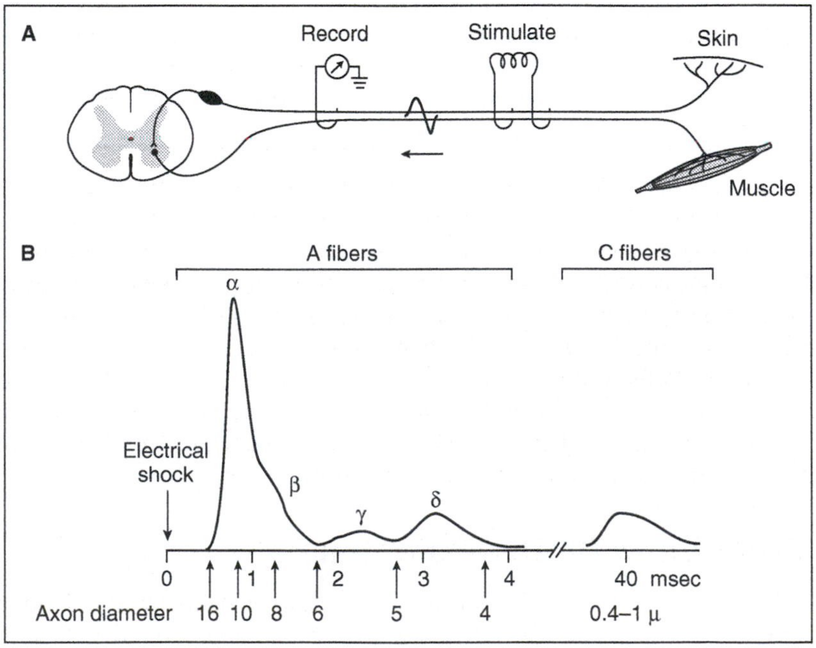

TABLE 4.2 Peripheral Nerve Fiber Classifications

Location	Classification	Function	Axon diameter (μm)	Conduction velocity (m/sec)
Dorsal roots				
	Ia (A-α) GSA	Muscle spindles	12–20	70–120
	Ib (A-α) GSA	Golgi tendon organs	10–18	60–100
	II (A-β) GSA	Flower spray endings	6–12	35–70
	II (A-β) GSA	Tactile receptors	6–12	35–70
	III (A-δ) GSA	Pain, temperature	1–6	10–40
	IV (C) GSA	Pain, temperature	< 1	0.5–2
Ventral roots				
	α—GSE	Extrafusal muscle fibers	12–20	70–120
	γ—GSE	Intrafusal muscle fibers	3–6	15–40

Note: GSA = general somatic afferent; GSE = general somatic efferent.

action potential is recorded by an electrode located proximally. A compound action potential contains several peaks or waves of neural activity that represent the summated response of multiple fibers. By comparing the peaks in the compound action potential with the distribution of fiber diameters in a peripheral nerve, Erlanger and Gasser deduced that conduction velocity is related to fiber diameter. The conduction velocity (in m/sec) of a large-diameter axon can be estimated by multiplying the diameter (in μm) by a factor of 5 or 6. For smaller fibers, multiplying the diameter by 4 provides an accurate estimate of conduction velocity.

The waves in a compound action potential represent different functional categories of nerve fibers (Table 4.2). The first wave of activity, the "A" wave, corresponds to fast-conducting impulses transmitted along large-diameter, heavily myelinated fibers. This wave contains several smaller peaks identified by the Greek letters α, β, γ, and δ. A second Roman numeral system was developed to categorize dorsal nerve fibers according to their diameter, and the two systems are used interchangeably. The fastest axons, A-α fibers, conduct action potentials at 60-120 m/sec. These axons include nerve fibers related to muscle performance, such as α-motor neurons and the afferent fibers that innervate the muscle spindles and Golgi tendon organs. The next fastest (35-70 m/sec) peripheral axons, the A-β fibers, innervate mechanoreceptors responsible for cutaneous sensations. The γ-motor neurons have conduction velocities (15-40 m/sec) that are substantially slower, but not as slow as the thinly myelinated A-δ fibers that convey sensations of sharp pain, cold, or heat. The second wave, composed of "B" fibers, reflects activity in preganglionic sympathetic fibers that originate from cell bodies in the lateral horn. These nerve fibers are lightly myelinated, but only conduct at 3-15 m/sec. Preganglionic sympathetic fibers leave the ventral root soon after emerging from the anterior horn and proceed toward the sympathetic chain ganglia. Consequently, the summated potentials generated by the B fibers are not seen in the compound action potential when the stimulating and recording electrodes are located more distally (Figure 4.16). Finally, the slowest peripheral axons are "C" fibers. These small-diameter, unmyelinated axons innervate free nerve endings and convey sensations of dull, aching pain.

SPINAL REFLEXES

Reflexes are involuntary, stereotypical movements that are mediated by a small number of neural elements. At a minimum, all reflexes involve sequential activation of the following components: (1) peripheral sensory receptors, (2) afferent nerve fibers, (3) efferent nerve fibers, and (4) effectors such as smooth or skeletal muscles. Most spinal reflexes also

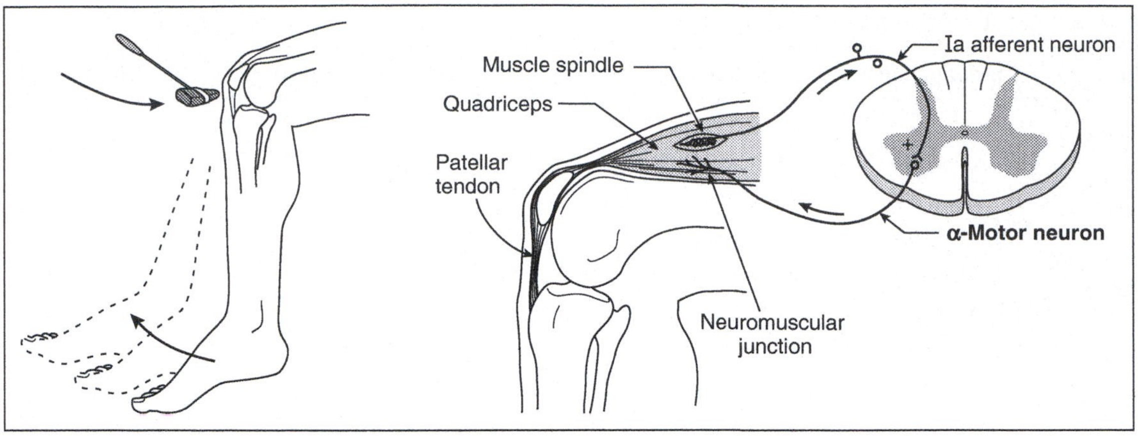

FIG. 4.17. Myotactic Reflex Circuit. Tapping the patellar tendon stretches the quadriceps muscle. This activates the primary afferent fibers that innervate the muscle spindles; the incoming impulses cause monosynaptic excitation of α-motor neurons that project back to the stretched muscle. This motor feedback causes abrupt leg extension or a "knee jerk."

involve one or more central gray interneurons that relay sensory information from the afferent nerve fibers to several populations of motor neurons located across different spinal segments. Hence, reflexes vary in complexity according to the number of neuronal connections that are needed to coordinate different sets of muscles.

Spinal reflexes may occur independently of descending inputs from the brain. In most instances, however, supraspinal influences modulate muscle tone and may either reduce or enhance the execution of a spinal reflex. Regardless of the involvement of supraspinal influences, spinal reflexes are tested in the clinic to assess the functional integrity of the spinal cord and its connections with the peripheral nerves.

Stretch Reflexes

The simplest spinal reflex is called the stretch or myotactic reflex because it occurs in response to stretching a skeletal muscle. When a skeletal muscle is abruptly stretched, the muscle contracts to prevent its fibers from being damaged. Tapping the patellar tendon, for example, causes a sudden stretch of the quadriceps muscle, which then contracts to move the lower leg in a quick jerk (Figure 4.17). To understand myotactic reflexes and their clinical importance, it is necessary to understand the structure of muscle spindles and the function of the γ-motor system.

Muscle spindles detect muscle stretch.

Muscle Spindles. Striated muscles are composed mainly of elongated extrafusal fibers that perform the "work" of the muscle by contracting when ACh stimulates them. Muscles also contain specialized sensory receptors, known as muscle spindles, that signal when the muscle is stretched. Each muscle spindle consists of a few short, intrafusal fibers whose ends are attached to the longer extrafusal fibers. In contrast to the extrafusal fibers, however, intrafusal fibers do not contribute to the overall force of the muscle when it contracts. Two types of intrafusal fibers exist, and both have a multinucleated central region that extends into contractile endings (Figure 4.18). One type, the nuclear bag fiber, has a broad nuclear area in which the nuclei are clustered in a central "bag" region. Nuclear chain fibers, on the other hand, are slender because the nuclei are aligned in single file. Muscle spindles contain a variable number of intrafusal fibers, but usually have two or three nuclear bag fibers and between four and eight nuclear chain fibers.

Muscle spindles are innervated by two types of afferent fibers that signal when the muscle is stretched. The primary afferent fiber is a large-diameter axon (Group Ia) that enters the encapsulated receptor and branches into collaterals that wrap around the central

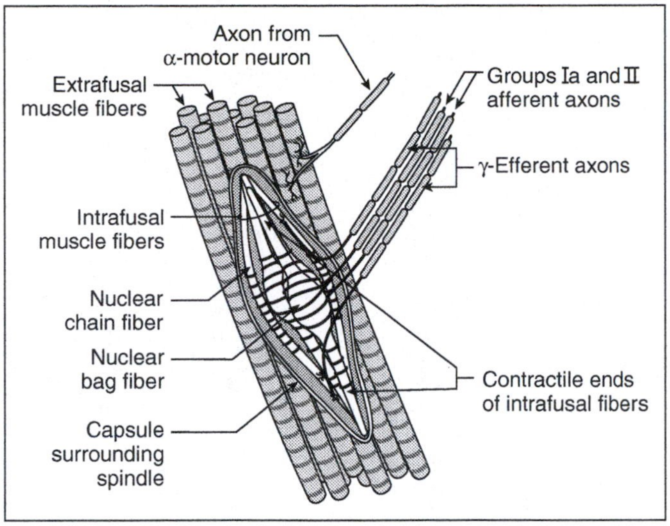

FIG. 4.18. Anatomy of a Muscle Spindle. Nuclear bag and nuclear chain fibers are innervated by a single group Ia annulospiral ending that wraps around the central portion of both sets of intrafusal fibers. Group II flower spray endings also innervate the nuclear chain fibers. The contractile ends of both types of intrafusal fibers receive efferent projections from γ-motor neurons.

nuclear region of each intrafusal fiber in the muscle spindle. These afferent fibers are called annulospiral endings because they make a spiral as they encircle the intrafusal fiber. Secondary innervation is provided by thin axons (Group II) that innervate the nuclear chain fiber on each side of the annulospiral ending. These endings are also called flower spray endings because they form a "spray" of contacts that resemble a flower. Both sets of afferent fibers are inactive in the absence of tension along the middle region of the intrafusal fiber; they discharge only when the central part of the intrafusal fiber is stretched. Because intrafusal fibers are connected in parallel to the extrafusal fibers, they are stretched whenever the extrafusal muscle is stretched.

The myotactic reflex is mediated by a simple neural circuit that contains two neurons and one intervening synapse (see Figure 4.17). Afferent fibers from muscle spindles (Ia, II) enter the posterior horn and proceed to lamina IX, where they synapse with α-motor neurons. Consequently, stretching a muscle and its muscle spindles triggers a series of afferent impulses that activate the α-motor neurons to produce an immediate contraction of the stretched muscle. Hence, the myotactic reflex protects the muscle from excessive stretch because it is mediated quickly by monosynaptic connections between fast-conducting nerve fibers.

Gamma-motor neurons regulate muscle spindles.

Gamma-Motor System. Intrafusal and extrafusal muscle fibers usually contract simultaneously during voluntary movements. This process, called alpha-gamma coactivation, allows the intrafusal muscle fibers to maintain the sensitivity of the muscle spindles to any unexpected or abrupt stretch over a wide range of muscle lengths. To perform this function, the contractile ends of the intrafusal fibers are innervated by γ-motor neurons originating in the anterior horn. In response to ACh released by the γ-motor neurons, the ends of the nuclear bag and chain fibers contract, thereby stretching the central region. This maintains tension in the central part of the muscle spindle when the muscle shortens during contraction (Figure 4.19). Hence, muscle spindles are in a constant state of readiness and are able to detect unexpected muscle stretches across a wide range of muscle lengths. In general, the γ-motor system acts as a feedback loop that enables the nervous system to acquire information continuously about the status of the muscles even as their length changes continuously during the course of multiple, rapid movements.

The pathways mediating the myotactic reflexes are also involved in maintaining muscle tone. Muscle tone is not an inherent property of muscle tissue but involves a minimal degree of contraction that is imposed by the nervous system without conscious effort.

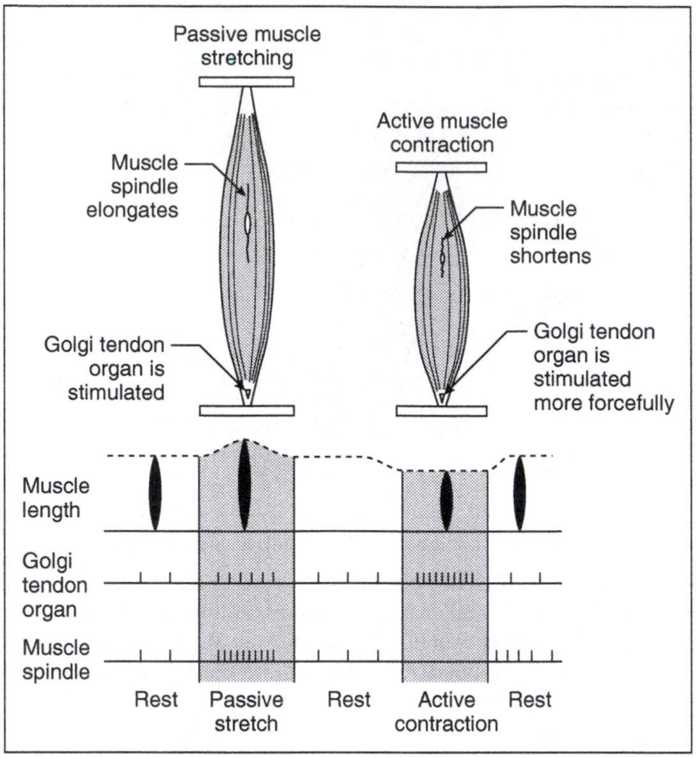

FIG. 4.19. Muscle Receptor Mechanisms. This drawing compares the activity of afferent fibers from the Golgi tendon organs and muscle spindles during different states of muscle contraction. Muscle spindles lie parallel to the extrafusal fibers of a muscle and are activated when the muscle is passively stretched. If the muscle contracts, however, the shortening of the muscle causes a decrease in tension along the length of the muscle spindle, and the annulospiral fibers (group Ia) are silenced. Golgi tendon organs lie in series with the muscles and are moderately active when the muscle is passively stretched; they become more active when the muscle actively contracts.

Descending supraspinal tracts regulate muscle tone by activating the γ-motor neurons on each side of the muscle spindle so that tension is increased in the nuclear bag region (see Figure 4.18). Activation of the annulospiral endings and the consequent increase in activity of the Ia fibers leads to activation of the α-motor neurons. Hence, this multisynaptic circuit maintains a minimum degree of muscle contraction or tone. Muscles normally show muscle tone, and the lack of muscle tone is considered a pathologic sign of ventral root damage.

Tendon Reflexes

Golgi tendon organs detect increases in tendon tension.

Golgi tendon organs signal the degree of tension that develops along a tendon during intense muscle contraction. Located in the myotendinous junction, each Golgi tendon organ consists of a network of collagenous fibers surrounded by a membranous capsule (Figure 4.20). A large sensory fiber (group Ib) enters the receptor and splits into several processes to infiltrate the collagen bundles. In contrast to muscle spindles, Golgi tendon organs are not activated by abrupt stretching of the muscle because most of the resulting tension is distributed uniformly across the length of the passively stretched muscle fibers. Instead, Golgi tendon organs increase their activity most when tension in the tendon is increased during active muscle contraction. Because Golgi tendon organs are connected "in series" with the extrafusal muscle fibers, the contraction produces a large increase in tendon tension that, in turn, activates the Ib fibers. The influence of muscle contraction on the activity of fibers coming from the muscle spindles and Golgi tendon organs is illustrated in Figure 4.19.

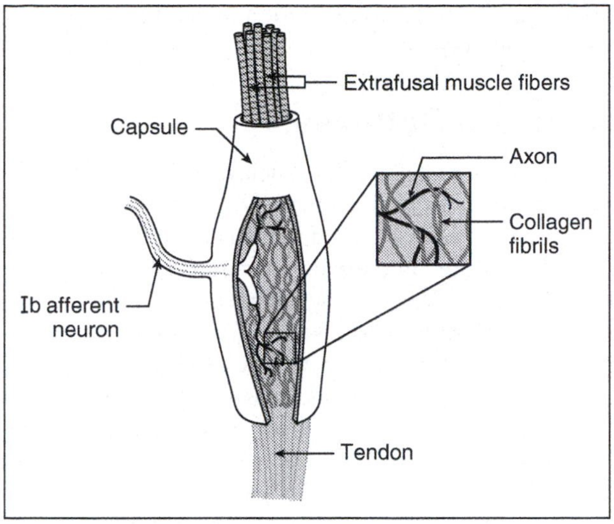

FIG. 4.20. Anatomy of a Golgi Tendon Organ. Encapsulated receptors located in the myotendinous junctions are innervated by a large Ib fiber that arborizes into a plexus of endings scattered throughout a mass of collagen fibrils.

Clasp-Knife Reflex

The exact role of the Golgi tendon organs during normal motor activity is not completely clear. Experiments have shown, however, that electrical stimulation of Ib fibers during muscle contraction produces immediate relaxation of the contracted muscle. This phenomenon, called autogenic inhibition, is a form of feedback inhibition mediated by a disynaptic circuit in the central gray region. As shown in Figure 4.21, afferent Ib fibers from Golgi tendon organs activate inhibitory neurons in the central gray that, in turn, suppress the α-motor neurons that supply the same muscle.

Spasticity is characterized by stiff, hypertonic muscles.

The influence of autogenic inhibition can be observed in patients sustaining certain spinal cord injuries. When the corticospinal tract is severed, patients are unable to control their limbs voluntarily because the descending signals from the motor cortex never reach the motor neurons in the anterior horn of the spinal cord. If the dorsal and ventral roots remain intact, spinal reflexes persist but are greatly modified by the loss of supraspinal inputs from motor cortex. In such cases, the limbs show spasticity as indicated by an increase in muscle tone and resistance to any passive movements. If the physician applies sufficient force to the limb, it gradually moves until a point is reached where all resistance disappears and the limb folds suddenly like the blade of a pocket knife. This "clasp-knife"

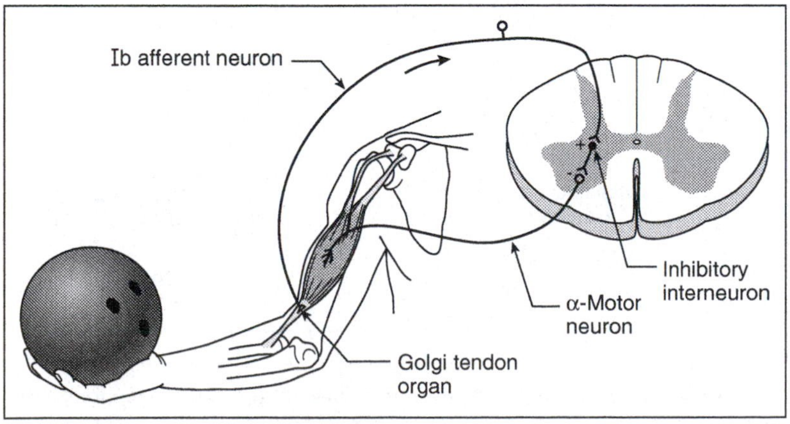

FIG. 4.21. Autogenic Inhibition. When a muscle is strongly contracted, impulses from the Golgi tendon organs excite spinal interneurons that, in turn, inhibit the α-motor neurons supplying the contracted muscle. This circuit mediates the clasp-knife reflex.

response is due to autogenic inhibition that develops when tendon tension surpasses the threshold level for activating the Golgi tendon organs.

Flexor and Crossed Extension Reflexes

The central gray region of the spinal cord contains a network of neuronal connections that coordinate the output of multiple sets of motor neurons that innervate antagonistic muscles on both sides of the body. This spinal circuitry was discovered in the late 1800s by Charles Sherrington and others who studied spinal reflexes in animals after transecting the upper cervical cord. In addition to mediating spinal reflexes, these intersegmental circuits are activated by descending signals from the brain so that both sides of the body are coordinated during walking and other complex activities that involve bilateral movements.

The simultaneous movements that comprise the flexor and crossed extension reflexes demonstrate the function of intersegmental connections. A flexor reflex is a rapid withdrawal of a limb that is triggered by a noxious stimulus such as stepping on a tack. This stimulates free nerve endings in the foot, which then transmits pain signals to different groups of spinal neurons (Figure 4.22). In response to this nociceptive input, intersegmental circuits are activated that lift the ipsilateral foot (flexor or withdrawal reflex) and extend the contralateral leg (crossed extension reflex). The circuits that mediate these movements extend across multiple segments of the spinal cord because the agonist and antagonist muscles that move the two legs are innervated by ventral roots that emerge from different levels of the lumbosacral enlargement.

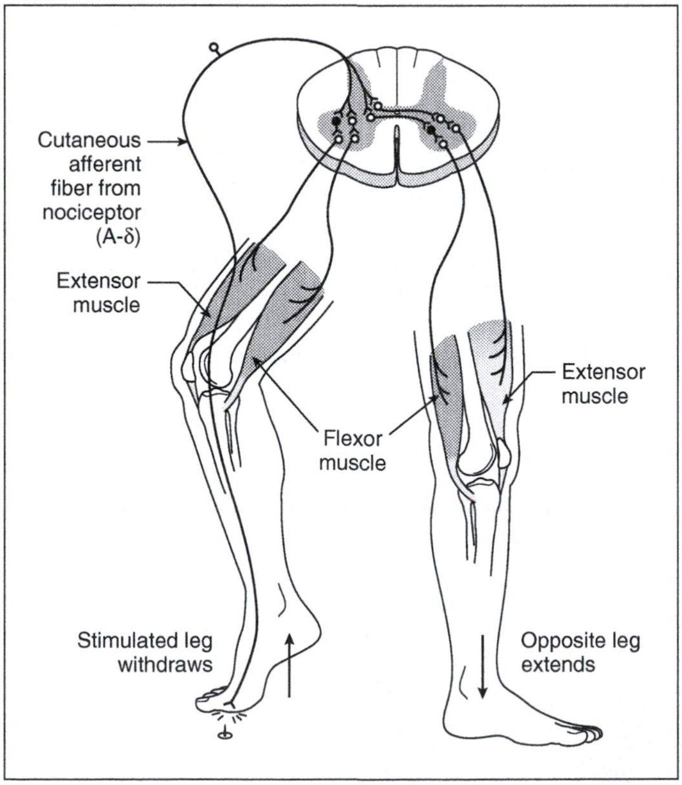

FIG. 4.22. Flexor and Crossed Extension Reflexes. In response to noxious inputs, intersegmental circuits in the spinal cord mediate limb withdrawal while simultaneously causing extension of the opposite limb. Flexor and extensor movements of each limb are mediated by parallel sets of neural connections that activate one set of muscles while inhibiting the antagonist muscles. These hard-wired connections illustrate the principle of reciprocal innervation. Filled neurons are inhibitory; unfilled neurons are excitatory.

Principle of Reciprocal Innervation. The withdrawal and crossed extension reflexes involve activation of several multisynaptic circuits connecting neighboring segments of the spinal cord. An essential feature of these intersegmental circuits is the reciprocal innervation of agonist and antagonist muscle groups (Figure 4.22). Inside the central gray region, primary afferent fibers diverge to control different muscle groups in each limb. Thus, the flexor response is controlled by neurons projecting to two populations of interneurons in the ipsilateral anterior horn: (1) one set that excites α-motor neurons innervating the flexors and (2) another set that inhibits α-motor neurons innervating the extensors. Without reciprocal innervation, a limb would not move smoothly because the antagonist muscles would not be coordinated.

Reciprocal innervation mediates activation of one muscle and simultaneous inhibition of its antagonist.

Intersegmental projections that connect the two sides of the spinal cord are an elaboration of the principle of reciprocal innervation. When nociceptive stimulation triggers flexion of one leg, extension of the contralateral leg is mediated by posterior horn neurons that project across the midline to the contralateral anterior horn. These crossed projections activate two populations of interneurons: (1) one set that excites the extensor α-motor neurons and (2) another set that inhibits the flexor α-motor neurons.

SPINAL CORD TRACTS

Three pairs of funiculi surround the central gray region and contain myelinated fibers that convey information to and from the spinal cord. Bundles of fibers having the same origin, course, and terminations are organized into tracts or fasciculi in specific regions of the spinal cord (Figure 4.23). Essentially, three types of fiber tracts are present in the spinal cord: (1) intersegmental, (2) ascending, and (3) descending. Intersegmental fibers project rostrally or caudally in the propriospinal tract that surrounds the outer edge of the central gray region, and these projections coordinate the different muscle groups that mediate spinal reflexes. Ascending fiber tracts convey sensory information to the thalamus, cerebellum, or brainstem. Descending projections enable the cerebral cortex and brainstem to communicate with the spinal cord so that the brain can execute motor commands or modulate incoming sensory transmission.

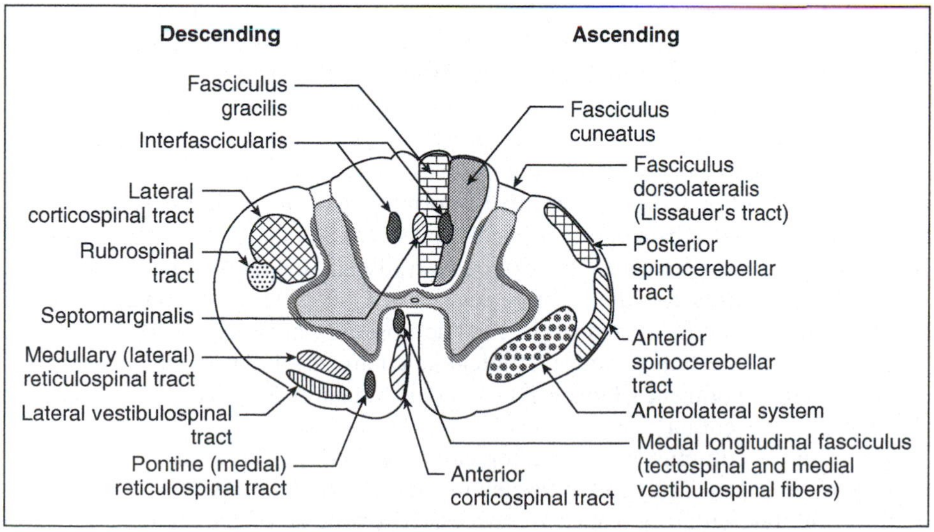

FIG. 4.23. Ascending and Descending Spinal Tracts. This diagram indicates the size and position of the spinal tracts in the paired funiculi. Ascending tracts are shown on the right side, and descending tracts are shown on the left side.

Ascending Tracts

A variety of encapsulated mechanoreceptors and free nerve endings are distributed throughout the skin, joints, and muscles. By converting physical energy into neural activity, these receptors transduce cutaneous, noxious, thermal, and kinesthetic stimulation into a series of action potentials or sensory signals that represent specific sensations. Conscious awareness of these sensations occurs only when these signals are transmitted to the cerebral cortex. All somatosensory sensations that reach consciousness ascend the spinal cord through either the posterior column-medial lemniscal system or through the anterolateral system. A third ascending system, the spinocerebellar pathway, conveys information from the muscle spindles and Golgi tendon organs to the cerebellum, but these signals are not consciously perceived.

Ascending spinal tracts have traditionally been described as having specific sensory functions. This view has arisen largely because many afferent fibers represent specific submodalities and project primarily into one of the ascending spinal tracts. In fact, most afferent fibers entering the spinal cord have collaterals that distribute sensory information for a given modality to several spinal tracts. Thus, most ascending spinal tracts convey sensory information from more than one modality, and most modalities ascend through multiple routes. Consistent with this view, patients who sustain complete damage to one ascending pathway usually have some remaining sensitivity to the affected modality. Nonetheless, these individuals generally exhibit some behavioral impairment, especially in tasks that require integration of multiple sensory channels. In other instances, however, damage to a sensory tract may produce only a temporary sensory loss. Recovery of the affected sensations may occur if other pathways are able to compensate for the damaged tract. Although these mechanisms are poorly understood, such recovery indicates that some functional redundancy exists across the ascending spinal projections.

Posterior Columns

The posterior columns are located in the posterior funiculus and consist of a pair of myelinated fiber tracts, the fasciculus gracilis and the fasciculus cuneatus, that lie on both sides of the midline. The fasciculus gracilis lies adjacent to the midline, ascends the entire length of the spinal cord, and terminates in the nucleus gracilis at the caudal end of the medulla. The fasciculus cuneatus, which is present only in segments rostral to T6, lies lateral to the fasciculus gracilis. The fasciculus cuneatus ascends to the rostral end of the spinal cord and terminates in the nucleus cuneatus, which lies lateral to the nucleus gracilis. All fibers in the posterior columns remain ipsilateral to their site of origin (Figure 4.24).

Approximately 75% of the fibers in the posterior columns are derived from primary afferent neurons whose cell bodies are located in the dorsal root ganglia. These fibers are mainly large-diameter axons (A-β) that innervate a variety of encapsulated receptors in the skin, joints, and deep tissues such as the muscles. Hence, the posterior columns transmit cutaneous, kinesthetic, and proprioceptive information from the limbs and trunk to the brain. Most A-β nerve fibers enter the medial part of the dorsal root entry zone and then bifurcate into two main branches that extend rostrally and caudally along the lateral edge of the posterior column for one or more segments. Collateral axons emerge from these branches at regular intervals and project to the posterior horn, either to mediate spinal reflexes or to convey inputs to sites that integrate cutaneous and nociceptive information. The main ascending branches, however, proceed up the entire length of the cord and terminate in the caudal medulla.

The posterior columns are somatotopically organized so that the lower part of the body is represented medially in the fasciculus gracilis and the upper body is represented laterally in the fasciculus cuneatus. At successive segments of the spinal cord, primary afferent fibers are added laterally to the fibers ascending from lower levels. Thus, fibers coming in from the foot, leg, and lower trunk lie closest to the midline in the fasciculus gracilis. Rostral to T6, fibers innervating the upper trunk, arm, shoulder, neck, and posterior head lie progressively more lateral in the fasciculus cuneatus.

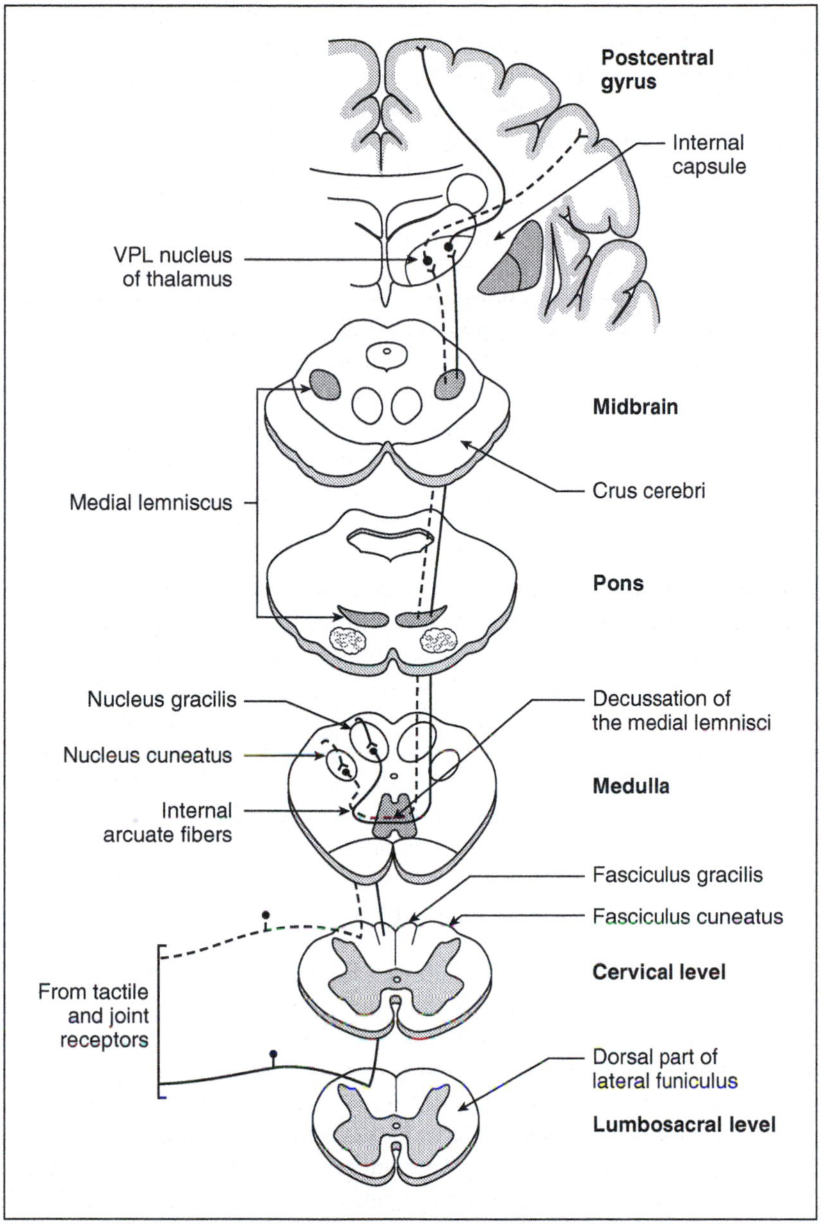

FIG. 4.24. Posterior Column-Medial Lemniscal System. Primary afferent fibers conveying tactile and kinesthetic information bifurcate at the dorsal root entry zone. The main axon ascends ipsilaterally in the posterior column and terminates in the caudal medulla. Fibers representing the lower trunk or leg ascend in the fasciculus gracilis and terminate in the nucleus gracilis. Fibers representing the upper trunk or arm ascend in the fasciculus cuneatus and terminate in the nucleus cuneatus. Second-order neurons in these nuclei send projections across the midline to ascend in the medial lemniscus and terminate in the ventroposterolateral (VPL) nucleus of the thalamus. Third-order neurons in the VPL nucleus project to the primary somatosensory cortex in the postcentral gyrus. The posterior columns and medial lemniscal pathways maintain a somatotopic organization throughout their ascent.

The increased number of afferent fibers coming from the legs and arms causes considerable widening of the fasciculus gracilis and fasciculus cuneatus at the lumbar and cervical enlargements, respectively. In addition, the posterior columns contain two smaller tracts, which enable sensory information to descend short distances within the cord. The fasciculus interfascicularis and the septomarginal fasciculus perform these tasks for the cervical and lumbar regions of the cord, respectively (see Figure 4.23).

Posterior columns:
- Cutaneous or kinesthetic sensations
- Spatial integration
- Complex tactile discriminations

According to classical teaching, the posterior columns are composed exclusively of first-order neurons (i.e., primary afferent neurons). More recent studies, however, indicate that 25% of the fibers in the posterior columns originate from second-order neurons whose cell bodies are located in the posterior horn. The posterior horn receives inputs from several different submodalities, and many neurons in this region may exhibit multimodal response properties. Furthermore, each segment of the posterior horn receives inputs from afferent neurons that innervate neighboring dermatomes. The convergence of information across adjacent dermatomes indicates that neurons in the posterior horn integrate information across a wide region of skin. This view is consistent with evidence showing that focal damage to the posterior columns does not prevent sensory detection but can impair a patient's ability to perform more complex discriminations. For example, patients with a lesion in the posterior columns are unable to distinguish separate skin sites in the affected dermatomes (i.e., impaired two-point discrimination). Moreover, they cannot determine the direction of stimulus motion or identify letters traced on the skin. In addition, because the fasciculus cuneatus contains fibers from encapsulated joint endings, damage to this fasciculus interferes with the ability to judge the shape or size of an object placed in the palm.

The lemniscus is a ribbon-like tract.

Medial Lemniscal System. Neurons contributing to the posterior columns comprise the first part of a multisynaptic route for transmitting somatosensory information to the cerebral cortex. Because neurons in the nucleus gracilis and nucleus cuneatus comprise the second link of this multisynaptic route to the cortex, they are called second-order neurons. These neurons project across the midline and ascend contralaterally through a narrow tract called the medial lemniscus. The medial lemniscus terminates on third-order neurons located in the ventroposterolateral (VPL) nucleus of the thalamus. Neurons in the nucleus VPL project ipsilaterally to the postcentral gyrus of the cerebral cortex, which is also known as the primary somatosensory area. The posterior column-medial lemniscal system is composed exclusively of neurons with wide, heavily myelinated axons that transmit cutaneous information from the periphery to consciousness with minimal delay.

Tabes dorsalis:
- Posterior columns destroyed
- Impairment of kinesthesia
- Broad-based, ataxic gait

Tabes Dorsalis. Tabes dorsalis is a manifestation of tertiary neurosyphilis that results in the destruction of the dorsal root ganglia and their central processes, especially the myelinated fibers in the fasciculus gracilis. Initially, this disease is characterized by intermittent pain and paresthesia (i.e., an abnormal burning or prickly sensation) caused by irritation of the dorsal roots. In time, progressive degeneration of the posterior columns produces a loss of cutaneous sensation, diminished tendon reflexes, reduced muscle tone, and marked impairment of the sense of limb position. To compensate for the loss of kinesthetic sense, such patients usually walk with a broad-based, ataxic gait with eyes directed to the floor.

Anterolateral System

The anterolateral system is a collection of fibers ascending through the anterior part of the lateral funiculus. It is a crossed, multisynaptic pathway whose fibers originate mainly from neurons in Rexed laminae I, IV, and V of the posterior horn. Axons in the anterolateral system project across the midline via the anterior white commissure and proceed toward the lateral funiculus where they ascend the spinal cord and terminate in a variety of brainstem targets (Figure 4.25). Four groups of fibers have been distinguished in the anterolateral system on the basis of their anatomic projections: (1) spinothalamic, (2) spinoreticular, (3) spinomesencephalic, and (4) spinotectal tracts.

The spinothalamic tract is the best known tract in the anterolateral system because of its clinical importance for conveying sensations of pain and temperature. Neurons contributing to the spinothalamic tract, however, do not respond only to noxious stimulation. Because spinothalamic neurons have extensive dendritic arborizations throughout the posterior horn, they receive convergent inputs from both cutaneous and nociceptive modalities. Consequently, spinothalamic neurons exhibit moderate discharge rates during cutaneous stimulation and higher discharge rates during more intense, noxious stimulation. As indicated

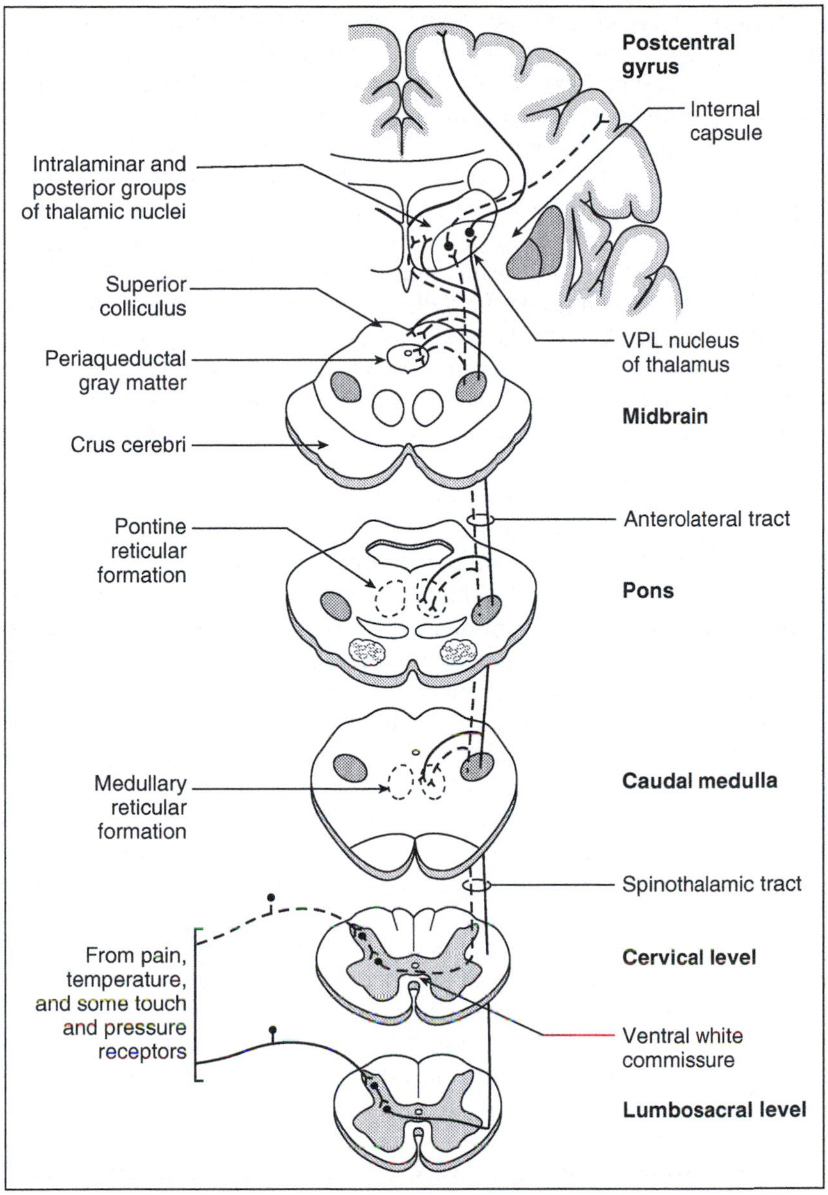

FIG. 4.25. Anterolateral System. Primary nociceptive fibers enter the spinal cord and terminate on neurons in the posterior horn. Second-order neurons, originating in laminae I, IV, and V, send projections across the midline and ascend the spinal cord through the anterior part of the lateral funiculus. While traversing the brainstem, different fibers terminate in the reticular formation (spinoreticular), the periaqueductal gray region (spinomesencephalic), the superior colliculus (spinotectal), or the thalamus (spinothalamic). Spinothalamic fibers terminate in the ventroposterolateral (VPL) nucleus and the intralaminar nuclei. The intralaminar nuclei also receive multisynaptic projections from the reticular formation; this is an additional route by which nociceptive information reaches the thalamus. The thalamic nuclei project to cerebral cortex, where the conscious perception of pain takes place.

earlier (see Figure 4.10), spinothalamic neurons have a wide dynamic range of responsiveness that encodes stimulus intensity. A few neurons in the spinothalamic tract, however, may respond more strongly to cutaneous inputs than to noxious stimulation. Thus, fibers responding primarily to cutaneous or nociceptive inputs are intermingled in the anterolateral system, and this explains why loss of the posterior columns does not completely abolish the ability to detect cutaneous stimulation.

Neospinothalamic tract:
Conveys sharp, well-localized pain
Receives input from a-δ fibers

Paleospinothalamic and spinoreticular tracts:
Convey dull, aching, slow pain
Receive inputs mainly from C fibers

Pain Perception. Different perceptual qualities of pain are mediated by different groups of fibers in the spinothalamic tract. One group of fibers, the neospinothalamic tract, originates mainly from laminae I and V and terminates in the VPL nucleus of the thalamus. These neurons receive inputs primarily from A-δ fibers and are responsible for fast conduction of well-localized sensations and other discriminative aspects of sharp, prickly pain. The paleospinothalamic tract, on the other hand, originates from neurons located more deeply in the posterior horn and projects to the intralaminar thalamic nuclei (e.g., central lateral nucleus). Additional neurons in the anterolateral system terminate in the reticular formation, which transmits pain information multisynaptically to the intralaminar nuclei of the thalamus. In contrast to the VPL nucleus, the intralaminar thalamus is not somatotopically organized. Consistent with this evidence, paleospinothalamic and spinoreticular fibers probably mediate sensations of dull, aching pain that are conveyed more slowly to the anterolateral system by the unmyelinated C fibers. These central projections to the intralaminar thalamus are thought to have a role in the affective components of pain.

Chronic Pain. In the past, neurosurgeons transected the anterolateral pathways to relieve suffering in patients with intractable pain. These surgeries, called cordotomies, produced immediate analgesia if the transection occurred two segments above the highest dermatome exhibiting pain. Cuts at a higher level were necessary because nociceptive fibers ascend in Lissauer's tract before entering the posterior horn, and the fibers in the anterolateral system ascend one or two more segments as they decussate through the spinal commissure. Furthermore, the transection must affect the deepest fibers that lie adjacent to the ventral horn because superficial cuts would only affect the spinothalamic fibers representing the most caudal dermatomes of the body. At each level of the spinal cord, spinothalamic fibers are added medially to those fibers ascending from more caudal segments. Hence, the anterolateral system has a mediolateral somatotopic organization that is opposite to that of the posterior columns.

Anterolateral cordotomies produce immediate contralateral analgesia, but the effect usually lasts only a few months. Although the reason for this is not entirely understood, recent studies indicate that some nociceptive fibers ascend the spinal cord via the posterior columns. Presumably, the terminal synapses of the intact nociceptive fibers in the posterior columns become more efficacious in transmitting pain information to the thalamus following degeneration of the lesioned fibers in the spinothalamic tract. Whatever the explanation, this phenomenon illustrates the functional plasticity of the spinal cord pathways.

Syringomyelia:
Bilateral sensory loss of pain and temperature
Produced by cavities in central gray region

Syringomyelia. In contrast to the recovery of pain sensations following a lateral cordotomy, functional recovery does not occur if the loss of nociceptive perception is produced by syringomyelia. As the name implies, syringomyelia involves the formation of an elongated cavity or syrinx around the region of the central canal. This chronic condition is usually caused by congenital defects in the neural tube or by gliosis within the central part of the cord following certain types of trauma. In either case, syringomyelia is characterized by a dissociated sensory loss in which the sense of touch is preserved but pain and thermal sensitivity are impaired because the decussating spinothalamic fibers are destroyed by a cavity in the central part of the cord. Although syringomyelia may affect lumbar or sacral segments, syrinx formation is most common in consecutive segments of the cervicothoracic cord, and this produces bilateral loss of pain sensitivity in the shoulders and arms. If the syrinx enlarges laterally and invades the ventral horns, the patient experiences weakness and atrophy of the upper limbs.

Spinomesencephalic and Spinotectal Tracts

Additional fibers in the anterolateral system proceed to rostral levels of the brainstem, where they terminate either in the periaqueductal gray (spinomesencephalic) or in deep layers of the superior colliculus (spinotectal). The spinomesencephalic tract projects to parts of the periaqueductal gray that contain high concentrations of endorphin, a neuropeptide important for controlling pain. The periaqueductal gray sends descending projections to both the pons and the medulla. In turn, separate nuclei in these brainstem regions project to the posterior horn of the spinal cord and activate the enkephalinergic neurons in the substantia gelatinosa. Thus, the spinomesencephalic tract represents the afferent limb of a feedback loop that is critical for supraspinal regulation of pain sensitivity.

The superior colliculus is involved in controlling eye and head movements during changes in visual attention. Hence, the spinotectal tract directs visual attention to body regions that experience intense somatosensory stimulation.

Spinocerebellar Tracts

Proprioception is the sensory modality concerned with limb position and includes the sense of stationary position as well as the sense of limb movement known as kinesthesia. The spinocerebellar pathways transmit proprioceptive information from the limb muscles and their joints to the cerebellum, which controls posture and coordinates fine movements. Thus, the spinocerebellar tracts convey information about the length, tension, and position of the limb muscles. The posterior and anterior spinocerebellar tracts convey proprioceptive information from the lower body, whereas the cuneocerebellar tract has the equivalent role for the upper body. All of these tracts originate from second-order neurons that receive primary inputs from deep receptors located in the muscles and joints (Figure 4.26). Although some proprioceptive and kinesthetic information is transmitted by the posterior column-medial lemniscal system to the cerebral cortex, we are not conscious of the proprioceptive information that is sent to the cerebellum.

Posterior Spinocerebellar Tract. The posterior spinocerebellar tract originates from neurons in the dorsal nucleus of Clarke, which is located in Rexed lamina VII and extends from segments C8 to L2. Clarke's nucleus receives inputs mainly from deep receptors such as muscle spindles, Golgi tendon organs, encapsulated joint endings and, to a lesser extent, cutaneous mechanoreceptors in the leg and lower trunk. Because the dorsal nucleus of Clarke does not extend below L3, deep afferent fibers that enter the cord at more caudal levels must ascend through the fasciculus gracilis before terminating in Clarke's nucleus. This explains why Clarke's nucleus is more prominent in segments T10-T12 than in more rostral sections of the thoracic cord. Second-order axons emerge from the dorsal nucleus of Clarke and proceed to the extreme edge of the lateral funiculus to form the posterior spinocerebellar tract, a superficial layer of fibers lying ventral to the dorsal root entry zone. In the brainstem, the posterior spinocerebellar tract merges with other fiber tracts to form the inferior cerebellar peduncle before terminating in the ipsilateral vermis of the cerebellum.

Anterior Spinocerebellar Tract. The anterior spinocerebellar tract differs from the posterior spinocerebellar tract in several ways. First, it originates from cells scattered throughout Rexed laminae V, VI, and VII in spinal segments caudal to L1. Second, the neurons of the anterior spinocerebellar tract receive inputs from a more diverse group of sources including Golgi tendon organ fibers, several types of mechanoreceptor fibers, and descending spinal tracts. Finally, the anterior spinocerebellar tract crosses the midline twice. Thus, second-order neurons contributing to this tract project across the spinal midline and ascend the cord as a superficial layer of fibers just lateral to the anterolateral system. However, instead of entering the cerebellum through the inferior cerebellar peduncle, these fibers continue further rostrally and enter the cerebellum through the superior cerebellar peduncle before crossing the midline again to innervate the ipsilateral vermis of the cerebellum.

Cuneocerebellar Tract. Proprioceptive information coming from the arm does not ascend the spinal cord in two separate fiber bundles like the posterior or anterior spinocerebellar tracts that convey information from the leg. Instead, type la and lb fibers from the arm enter the ipsilateral fasciculus cuneatus, ascend to the medulla, and terminate on

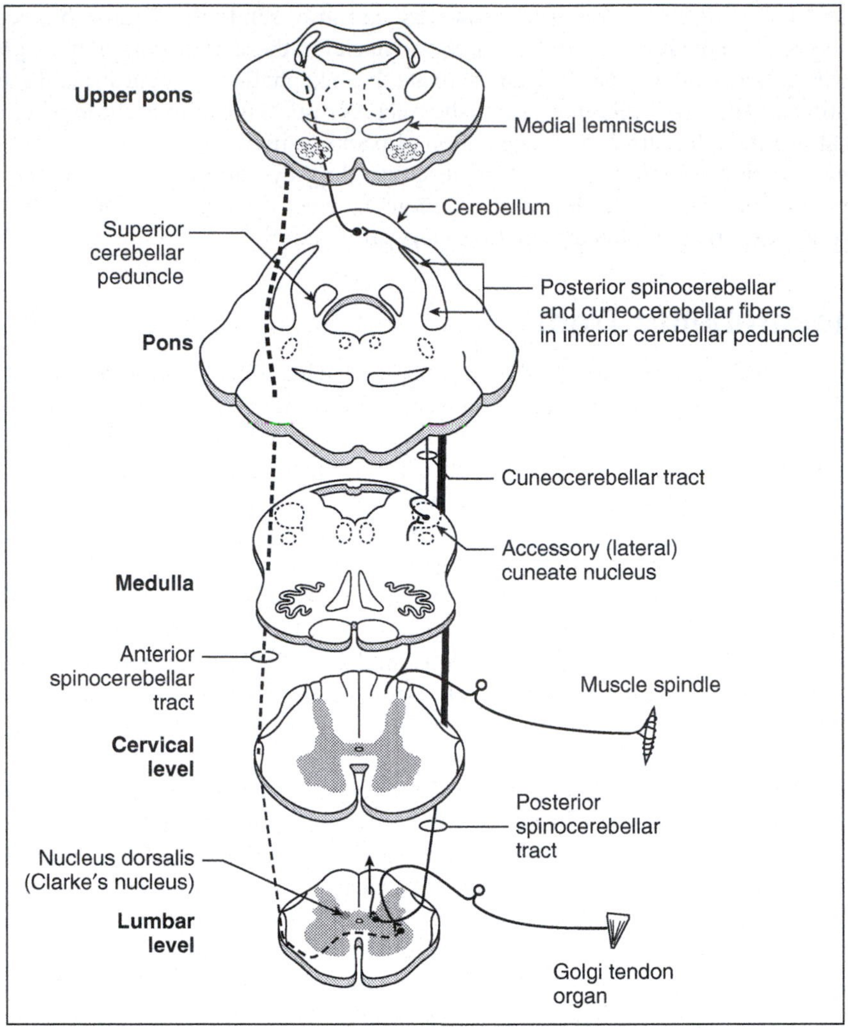

FIG. 4.26. Spinocerebellar Pathways. Primary afferent fibers from muscle spindles and Golgi tendon organs in the leg muscles enter the spinal cord and terminate in the dorsal nucleus of Clarke and surrounding parts of the posterior horn. The posterior spinocerebellar tract is an uncrossed tract that originates in the dorsal nucleus of Clarke. The anterior spinocerebellar tract is a crossed tract that originates in second-order neurons in laminae V, VI, and VIII. Primary afferent fibers from receptors in the hand and arm muscles ascend through the ipsilateral fasciculus cuneatus before terminating in the external cuneate nucleus. The cuneocerebellar tract originates in the external cuneate nucleus. The posterior spinocerebellar and cuneocerebellar tracts enter the inferior cerebellar peduncle and terminate in the ipsilateral cerebellar cortex. The anterior spinocerebellar tract enters the superior cerebellar peduncle and crosses the midline a second time before terminating in cerebellar cortex.

second-order neurons in the lateral cuneate nucleus (also called the accessory or external cuneate nucleus). The lateral cuneate nucleus lies lateral to the nucleus cuneatus and is considered the upper limb equivalent of the dorsal nucleus of Clarke. Efferent fibers from the lateral cuneate nucleus form the cuneocerebellar tract and merge with other fibers of the inferior cerebellar peduncle before terminating in the ipsilateral vermis of the cerebellum.

Descending Tracts

Many regions of the brain send descending projections to the spinal cord to execute skeletal movements, regulate autonomic functions, or modulate the transmission of incoming sensory inputs. All of these descending systems terminate on neurons located in the central gray of the spinal cord. The corticospinal tract is the major pathway for controlling voluntary movements, and it is the only tract that transmits impulses from the cerebral cortex directly to the spinal cord. The actions of the corticospinal system are supplemented by other descending fiber systems that originate in the brainstem and play a role in modulating muscle tone and spinal reflexes. These descending pathways include the rubrospinal, reticulospinal, vestibulospinal, and tectospinal tracts.

Corticospinal Tracts

Voluntary, highly skilled movements are dependent on neural impulses transmitted through the corticospinal tract. Corticospinal fibers originate from neurons in the cerebral cortex, and they descend ipsilaterally through the internal capsule and crus cerebri before passing through the pyramidal tract on the anterior surface of the medulla (Figure 4.27). At the spinomedullary junction, approximately 90% of the corticospinal fibers cross the midline through the pyramidal decussation and continue their descent as the lateral corticospinal tract (Figure 4.28). The lateral corticospinal tract resides in the posterior part of the lateral funiculus, just lateral to the posterior horn. Lateral corticospinal fibers are somatotopically organized so that fibers destined to reach the lumbosacral cord are located lateral to those terminating in the cervicothoracic cord. About 8% of the corticospinal fibers remain uncrossed on the anterior surface of the spinal cord to form the anterior corticospinal tract. Fibers of the anterior corticospinal tract eventually cross the midline at

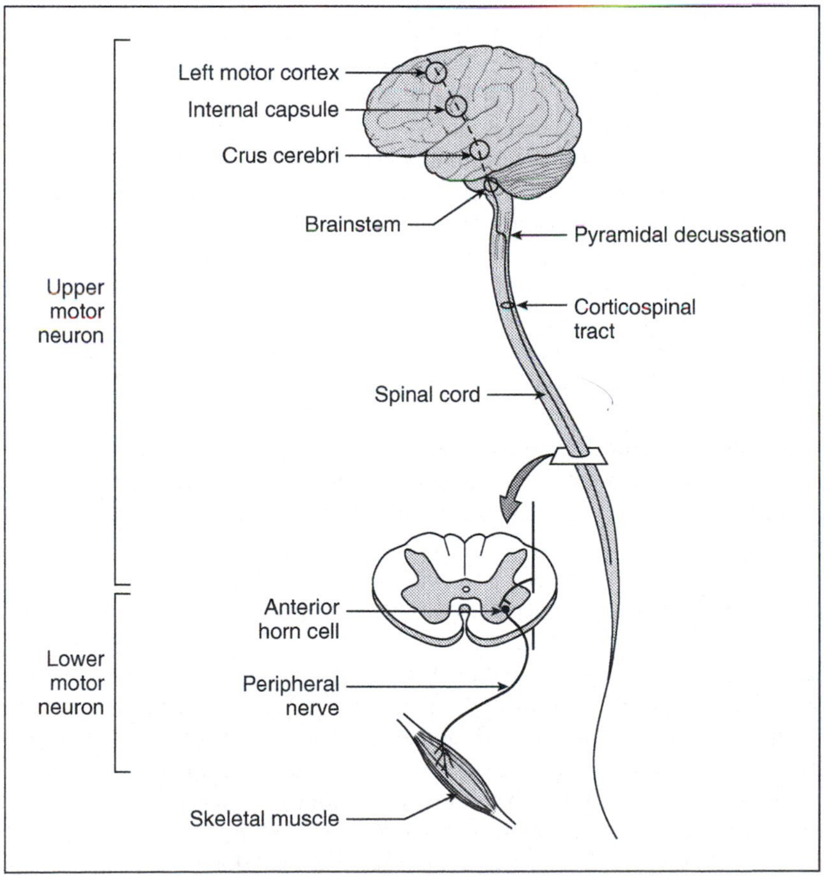

FIG. 4.27. Upper and Lower Motor Neurons. The corticospinal tract originates in the cerebral cortex, and descends through the internal capsule and brainstem before terminating at every level of the spinal cord. Corticospinal neurons are upper motor neurons that terminate in the anterior horn to innervate lower motor neurons. Lower motor neurons comprise the final common pathway to the peripheral muscles.

FIG. 4.28. Pyramidal Decussation. The pyramidal tract lies along the anterior surface of the medulla and contains corticospinal fibers exclusively. At the spinomedullary junction, approximately 90% of the corticospinal fibers cross the midline through the pyramidal decussation and descend through the lateral funiculus as the lateral corticospinal tract. The remaining fibers descend ipsilaterally as the anterior corticospinal tract and most of these fibers eventually cross the midline at the level of termination.

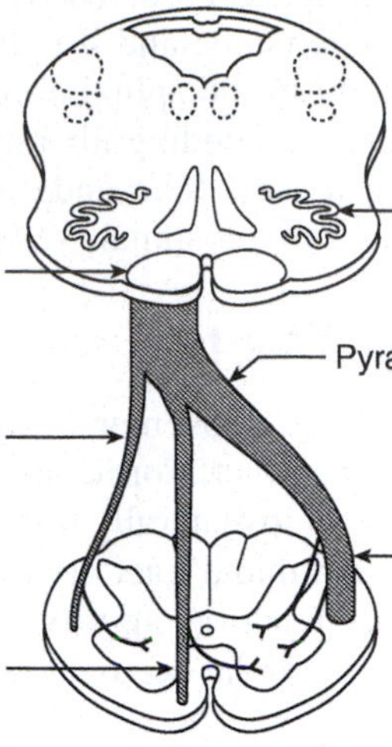

the spinal cord segment in which they terminate. Only 2% of the corticospinal fibers descend uncrossed within the lateral funiculus.

Consistent with its role in motor control, most fibers in the corticospinal tract originate from motor regions in the frontal lobe. Slightly more than 30% of the fibers originate from primary motor cortex (Brodmann area 4), and another 30% come from premotor cortex (Brodmann area 6). Surprisingly, nearly 40% of corticospinal fibers originate from somatosensory areas in the parietal lobe. These sensory-related fibers terminate in the posterior horn to modulate the transmission of afferent inputs.

The lateral corticospinal tract descends the entire length of the spinal cord, but more than half (about 55%) of its axons terminate in cervical regions representing the neck and upper limbs. Approximately 25% of corticospinal fibers terminate in the lumbosacral enlargement to control the lower limbs; the remaining fibers terminate throughout the thoracic cord. Although some (about 10%) corticospinal fibers terminate directly on α-motor neurons in the anterior horn, most fibers terminate on nearby interneurons that, in turn, control the output of the α-motor neurons. The corticospinal tract is concerned primarily with controlling the flexor muscles, which are responsible for the fine, dextrous movements used by the arm and hand to manipulate objects.

Upper and Lower Motor Neurons. Neurons in the anterior horn that give rise to the ventral spinal roots are called "lower motor neurons." These neurons constitute the final common pathway because they provide the final link between the nervous system and the peripheral muscles (see Figure 4.27). Neurons that project to the final common pathway are called "upper motor neurons." The corticospinal tract is composed of upper motor neurons; indeed, the phrase "upper motor neuron" is often considered synonymous with the lateral corticospinal tract.

Lower motor neuron lesions:
- Hypotonia
- Areflexia
- Muscle atrophy
- Fasciculations

Upper motor neuron lesions:
- Spasticity
- Clonus
- Hyperactive tendon reflexes
- Clasp-knife phenomenon
- Babinski's sign

When lower motor neurons are damaged by disease or trauma, the muscles atrophy and exhibit flaccid paralysis. Neurologic signs of a lower motor neuron lesion include: (1) loss of muscle tone (hypotonia), (2) absence of spinal reflexes (areflexia), (3) muscular atrophy, and (4) muscular fasciculations. Fasciculations are probably caused by ACh release at the neuromuscular junction during the course of motor neuron degeneration. Thereafter, the muscles are completely paralyzed and exhibit no motor tone.

Symptoms of an upper motor lesion are produced by damaging the corticospinal tract at any level of the neuraxis. Lesions of the corticospinal tract cause distinct neurologic symptoms that differ from those produced by lower motor neuron pathology. A lesion of the corticospinal tract is usually indicated if muscles participate in spinal reflexes but are not under voluntary control. Transection of the lateral corticospinal tract causes spasticity, which is a state of heightened muscular tone (hypertonia) and rigidity. Spastic paralysis is characterized by hyperactive deep tendon (myotatic) reflexes and increased resistance to passive movement of the limb. Corticospinal lesions cause spinal reflexes to exhibit rapid reverberations or clonus because the reflexive movements are no longer modulated by descending inputs. Pathologic reflexes such as the clasp-knife phenomenon and Babinski's sign are also observed with upper motor neuron lesions. Babinski's sign is a dorsiflexion of the toes in response to lightly stroking the sole of the foot; although it generally indicates loss of corticospinal function, it is also seen in intoxicated adults and in infants before the corticospinal tract has fully developed.

Amyotrophic Lateral Sclerosis. Amyotrophic lateral sclerosis is a progressive disease of unknown etiology that affects upper and lower motor neurons without altering the sensory systems. This disease causes degeneration of the corticospinal tracts and anterior horn neurons; consequently, signs of both upper and lower motor neuron paralysis are present. The muscles of the arm and hand gradually show signs of lower motor neuron lesions, including weakness, atrophy, and fasciculations. Until the anterior horn cells are affected, the patient exhibits upper motor neuron signs, including hyperreflexia, clonus, and Babinski's sign. Motor neurons in the brainstem are also affected, and much later, the disease impairs bladder and bowel function as the descending autonomic fibers degenerate.

Amyotrophic lateral sclerosis:
- Progressive, diffuse degeneration
- Destroys lower and upper motor neurons
- Leads to muscular paralysis

Spinal Shock. When the descending tracts of the spinal cord are severely injured, a period of spinal shock ensues that is characterized by flaccid paralysis and areflexia. Spinal shock occurs even if the ventral roots are intact, and it usually lasts for several weeks or months. Eventually, the limbs become spastic and exhibit hyperactive deep tendon reflexes. The reason for the temporary loss of reflex activity is not understood, but it appears to involve the loss of facilitating influences exerted by descending fiber systems on the reflex circuits of the spinal cord. As the descending fibers degenerate, connections in the reflex circuits become stronger and their functions are re-established to a greater degree than prior to the injury. Patients with spinal shock lose bladder function temporarily and must be catheterized to reduce distention until reflex voiding develops.

Spinal shock:
- Temporary loss of reflexes, muscle tone
- Produced by spinal cord trauma

Rubrospinal Tract

The red nucleus is a large structure in the midbrain that receives direct ipsilateral projections from motor and premotor cortical regions (Brodmann areas 4 and 6) via corticorubral pathways that descend through the internal capsule. The rubrospinal tract originates from magnocellular neurons in the red nucleus and crosses the midline in the ventral tegmental decussation. After descending through the brainstem, the rubrospinal tract enters the lateral funiculus and is partially intermingled with fibers of the lateral corticospinal tract. Rubrospinal fibers descend the entire length of the cord and terminate in laminae V, VI, and VII (Figure 4.29). Together, the corticorubral and rubrospinal pathways augment the functions of the corticospinal tract by facilitating flexor movements. In animals, for example, electrical stimulation of the red nucleus causes contraction of the contralateral flexors while inhibiting the motor neurons that innervate the extensors.

Tectospinal Tract

The tectospinal tract originates from the deep layers of the superior colliculus and crosses the midline in the dorsal tegmental decussation (Figure 4.29). Tectospinal fibers descend in the anterior funiculus and project to neurons located in laminae VI, VII, and VIII of spinal segments C1 to C4. The superior colliculus receives projections from the visual, auditory, and somatosensory systems, and integrates these sensory modalities to construct a representation of body movements relative to extrapersonal space. Thus, the superior colliculus determines the eye and head movements that are needed to redirect visual attention. To mediate these functions, it projects to the motor nuclei that orient the head and eyes to novel stimuli in the visual field or to different parts of the body. By projecting to neurons in the upper four segments of the spinal cord, the tectospinal tract provides a route for activating the motor neurons that control the position of the head and neck.

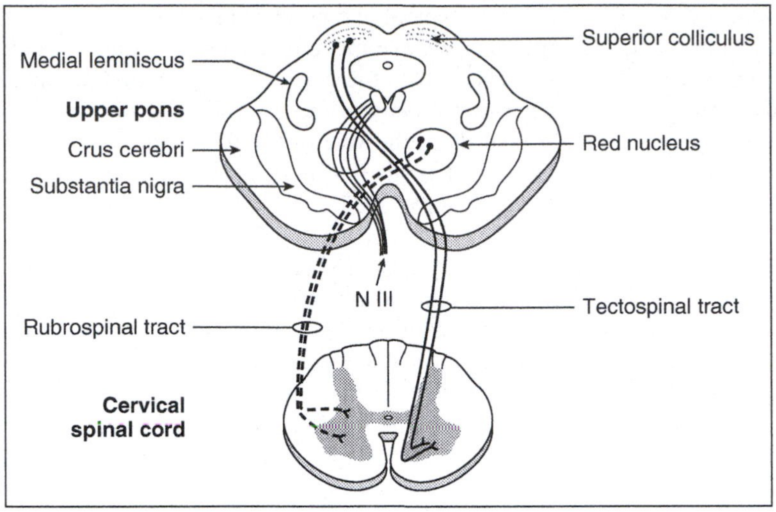

FIG. 4.29. Tectospinal and Rubrospinal Pathways. The rubrospinal tract originates in the red nucleus and crosses through the ventral tegmental decussation before descending through the brainstem and spinal cord. Rubrospinal fibers terminate in laminae V, VI, and VII, and are involved in controlling flexor movements. The tectospinal tract originates in the deep layers of the superior colliculus and crosses the midline through the dorsal tegmental decussation. The tectospinal tract descends through the anterior funiculus of the spinal cord and terminates on neurons in laminae VI, VII, and VIII of the upper cervical segments.

Reticulospinal Tracts

The reticular formation is able to exert widespread influences throughout the neuraxis because it consists of a large number of nuclei that project extensively throughout the brain and spinal cord. Many actions of the reticular formation are undoubtedly directed by corticoreticular fibers that originate from premotor cortex (Brodmann area 6) and terminate bilaterally in the pontine and medullary reticular nuclei. These nuclei, in turn, send descending projections to the ipsilateral spinal cord. The lateral reticulospinal tract originates from large neurons in the medullary reticular formation (nucleus gigantocellularis), whereas the medial reticulospinal tract originates from the pontine reticular formation (nucleus oralis and caudalis). Although these tracts are segregated, both sets of fibers terminate mainly in the medial and ventral regions of laminae VII, VIII, and IX through all levels of the spinal cord (Figure 4.30). The reticulospinal tracts can facilitate or inhibit spinal circuits involved in reflexive or voluntary movements. Because of widespread influences from the motor and somatosensory cortices, the multisynaptic corticoreticulospinal pathways are a major alternative to the corticospinal tract for controlling spinal motor neurons.

The reticular formation is essential for controlling the autonomic activities of the spinal cord. Visceral regions of the reticular formation contain neurons that receive inputs from the hypothalamus and from parasympathetic nuclei associated with the cranial nerves (see Chapter 5). Descending fibers in the lateral reticulospinal tract project to sympathetic and parasympathetic centers of the spinal cord that are concerned with the cardiovascular, respiratory, gastrointestinal, and urinary systems. As such, these fibers can modulate heart rate, respiratory rate, blood pressure, perspiration, and pupillary dilation, as well as other autonomic functions.

Vestibulospinal Tracts

The lateral and medial vestibular nuclei send separate descending projections to the spinal cord through the lateral and anterior funiculi, respectively. These are mainly uncrossed fiber projections that terminate in laminae VII and VIII, which, in turn, interact with the

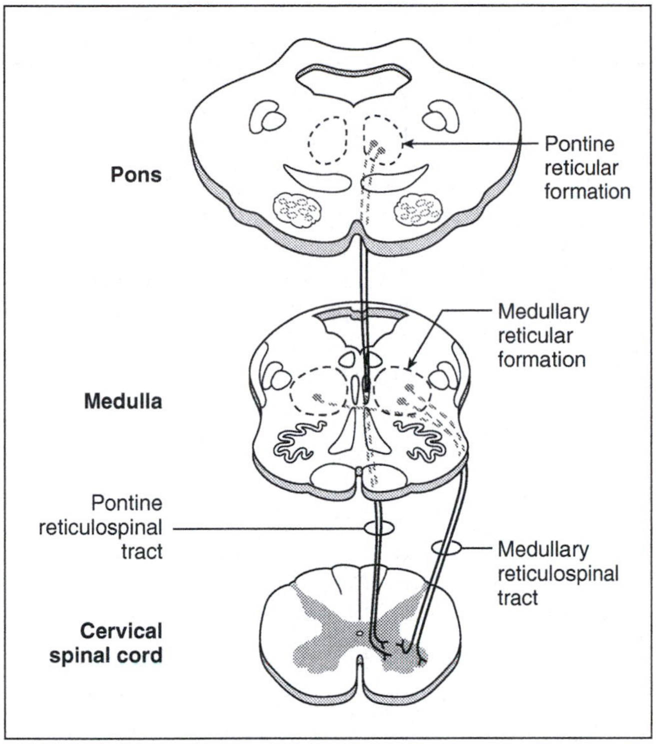

FIG. 4.30. Reticulospinal Pathways. The pontine reticulospinal pathways are uncrossed fiber tracts that descend in the anterior funiculus to all levels of the spinal cord and terminate on neurons in lamina VIII. The medullary reticulospinal fibers descend bilaterally in the anterior part of the lateral funiculus and terminate in laminae VII and IX.

α-motor and γ-motor neurons of lamina IX. Both the medial and lateral vestibulospinal tracts facilitate muscle stretch reflexes and enhance contraction of extensor muscles, especially during reflexive movements that occur in response to falling. The vestibulospinal pathways coordinate the movements of the eyes, head, and limbs in response to angular or linear acceleration. The functions of these pathways are discussed in Chapter 9.

RESOLUTION OF CLINICAL CASE

The clinical case at the beginning of this chapter presents symptoms that characterize the Brown-Séquard syndrome. Although rare, this syndrome is a classic demonstration of the clinical signs that illustrate the differential course of the ascending and descending spinal tracts. After recovery from spinal shock, the limbs caudal to the hemisection develop spastic paralysis on the ipsilateral side. Voluntary movements of the affected limb are absent because the lateral corticospinal tract has been transected ipsilaterally. Deep tendon reflexes are hyperactive, and resting muscle tone is elevated because the muscles are still innervated by α-motor neurons originating from the anterior horn. There is complete loss of touch, proprioception, and kinesthetic sense because the ipsilateral posterior columns and spinocerebellar tracts are damaged. The perception of pain and temperature is lost contralaterally two segments below the wound because the transection interrupts the anterolateral system whose fibers decussate over the course of one to two segments from their site of origin. In many instances, a focal lesion in the spinal cord or brainstem produces a constellation of symptoms affecting opposite sides of the body because the decussating fibers of one tract are near other structures that present ipsilateral symptoms when damaged. Hence, it is important for the clinician to recognize that crossed findings may indicate focal neuropathology.

REVIEW QUESTIONS

Directions: For each of the following questions, choose the **one best** answer.

1. During a traffic accident, an individual suffered a complete dislocation of the spinal cord at C4-C5. What would you expect to see a year after the accident?
   A. Sensitivity to pinpricks on the limbs
   B. Hypotonia of the limb muscles
   C. Hyperactive deep tendon reflexes
   D. Areflexia
   E. Volitional bladder emptying

2. A woman is insensitive to noxious stimulation of both arms, but all other neurologic functions are normal. Where is the lesion?
   A. Posterior funiculus above C5
   B. Commissure of the spinal cord at C5-C8
   C. Dorsal roots of both cervical enlargements
   D. Ventral horns of both cervical enlargements
   E. Nucleus cuneatus on both sides of the medulla

3. After experiencing burning pain in the legs for several weeks, a patient shows diminished tendon reflexes and loss of kinesthetic sense. What condition is indicated by these symptoms?
   A. Syringomyelia
   B. Tabes dorsalis
   C. Amyotrophic lateral sclerosis
   D. Brown-Séquard syndrome
   E. Complete transection of the cord at C4

4. Weakness, fasciculations, and atrophy of the muscles of the hands and arms without sensory loss suggest a pathologic process involving which of the following neural structures?
   A. Lateral horn
   B. Anterior horn
   C. Lateral corticospinal tract
   D. Posterior horn
   E. Dorsal root ganglia

5. When narcotics are injected into the lumbar cistern to produce analgesia, where do they exert their pharmacologic effects?
   A. Anterior horn
   B. Dorsal nucleus of Clarke
   C. Phrenic nucleus
   D. Intermediolateral cell column
   E. Substantia gelatinosa

6. The clasp-knife reflex indicates which of the following conditions?
   A. Lower motor neuron disease
   B. Upper motor neuron disease
   C. Spinal shock
   D. Poliomyelitis
   E. Normal deep tendon reflexes

7. Muscle spindles are essential for initiating which of the following reflexes?
   A. Babinski's reflex
   B. Crossed extension reflex
   C. Clasp-knife reflex
   D. Myotatic reflex
   E. Flexor reflex

8. Which of the following conditions would be produced by a lesion of the pyramidal tract?
   A. Hypotonia
   B. Fasciculations
   C. Areflexia
   D. Spasticity
   E. Muscular atrophy

9. Following a small puncture wound in the lower back, a patient is insensitive to touching the skin on the left leg, but voluntary movements and sensitivity to pinprick remains normal on both sides of the body. What part of the spinal cord is damaged?
   A. Left fasciculus gracilus at L1
   B. Left spinothalamic tract at T11
   C. Right spinothalamic tract at T11
   D. Left fasciculus cuneatus at L1
   E. Left corticospinal tract at L1

10. Which of the following neural structures are directly interconnected?
   A. Dorsal nucleus of Clarke—nucleus gracilis
   B. Substantia gelatinosa—Rexed lamina VIII
   C. Dorsal root ganglia—cerebral cortex
   D. Rexed lamina II—thalamus
   E. Cerebral cortex—Rexed lamina IX

ADDITIONAL READING

Classic Literature

Erlanger J, Gasser HS: *Electrical Signs of Nervous Activity.* Philadelphia, PA: University of Pennsylvania Press, 1937.

Melzack R, Wall PD: Pain mechanisms: a new theory. *Science.* 150:971–979, 1965.

Rexed B: The cytoarchitectonic organization of the spinal cord in the cat. *J Comp Neurol.* 96:415–496, 1952.

Sherrington CS: *The Integrative Action of the Nervous System.* New Haven, CT: Yale University Press, 1947 (original copyright 1906).

Reviews and Landmark Research Articles

Bortoff GA, Strick PL: Corticospinal terminations in two new-world primates: further evidence that corticomotoneuronal connections provide part of the neural substrate for manual dexterity. *J Neurosci* 13:5105–5118, 1993.

Brodal A: The somatic afferent pathways. In *Neurological Anatomy in Relation to Clinical Medicine*, 3rd ed. New York, NY: Oxford University Press, 1981: 46–147.

Brown AG: *Organization in the Spinal Cord.* New York, NY: Springer, 1981.

Darian-Smith I: Touch in primates. *Ann Rev Psychol* 33:155–194, 1982.

Davidoff RA: The dorsal columns. *Neurol* 39:1377–1385, 1989.

Davidoff RA, Hackman JC: Aspects of spinal cord structure and reflex function. *Neurol Clin* 9:533–550 (1991).

Edgarton VR, Tillakaatne NJ, Bigbe AJ, de Leon RD, Roy RR: Plasticity of the spinal neural circuitry after injury. *Ann Rev Neurosci* 27:145–167, 2004.

He SQ, Dum RP, Strick PL: Topographic organization of corticospinal projections from the frontal lobe: motor areas on the lateral surface of the hemisphere. *J Neurosci* 13:952–980, 1993.

He SQ, Dum RP, Strick PL: Topographic organization of corticospinal projections from the frontal lobe: motor areas on the medial surface of the hemisphere. *J Neurosci* 15:3284–306, 1995.

Koerber HR, Mirnics K, Brown PB, Mendell LM: Central sprouting and functional plasticity of regenerated primary afferents. *J Neurosci* 14:3655–3671, 1994.

Martin JH: The corticospinal system: from development to motor control. *Neuroscientis.* 11:161–173, 2005.

Nathan PW, Smith MC, Cook AW: Sensory effects in man of lesions of the posterior columns and of some other afferent pathways. *Brain* 109:1003–1041, 1986.

Nathan PW, Smith MC, Deacon P: The corticospinal tracts in man: course and location of fibres at different segmental levels. *Brain* 113:303–324, 1990.

Price DD, Hayes RL, Ruda M, Dubner R: Spatial and temporal transformations of input to spinothalamic tract neurons and their relation to somatic sensations. *J Neurophysiol* 41:933–947, 1978.

Smith MC, Deacon P: Topographical anatomy of the posterior columns of the spinal cord in man: the long ascending fibres. *Brain* 107:671–698, 1984.

Snyder R: The organization of the dorsal root entry zone in cats and monkeys. *J Comp Neurol* 174:47–70, 1977.

Wall PD, Noordenbos W: Sensory functions which remain in man after complete transection of the dorsal columns. *Brain* 100:641–653, 1977.

Willis WD, Westlund KN: Neuroanatomy of the pain system and of the pathways that modulate pain. *J Clin Neurophysiol* 14:2–31, 1997.

Woodbury CJ, Ritter AM, Koerber HR: On the problem of lamination in the superficial dorsal horn of mammals: a reappraisal of the substantia gelatinosa in postnatal life. *J Comp Neurol* 417:88–102, 2000.

Zehr EP, Stein RB: What functions do reflexes serve during human locomotion? *Prog Neurobiol* 58:185–205, 1999.

INTERNET RESOURCES

Anaesthesia UK
Acute Pain
http://www.frca.co.uk/SectionContents.aspx?sectionid=148

Digital Anatomist Project
http://www9.biostr.washington.edu/da.html

Miami Project to Cure Paralysis
http://www.miamiproject.miami.edu/

Neuroanatomy and Neuropathology on the Internet
http://www.neuropat.dote.hu/

Spinal Cord Injury Information Network
http://www.spinalcord.uab.edu/

Spinal Cord Injury Resource Center
http://www.spinalinjury.net/index.html

Temple University Course on Neuroanatomy
http://courses.temple.edu/neuroanatomy/lab/index.htm

University of Wisconsin Global Anatomy Home Page
http://www.neuroanatomy.wisc.edu/

Virtual Hospital
http://www.vh.org/adult/provider/anatomy/BrainAnatomy/BrainAnatomy.html

Whole Brain Atlas
http://www.med.harvard.edu/AANLIB/home.html

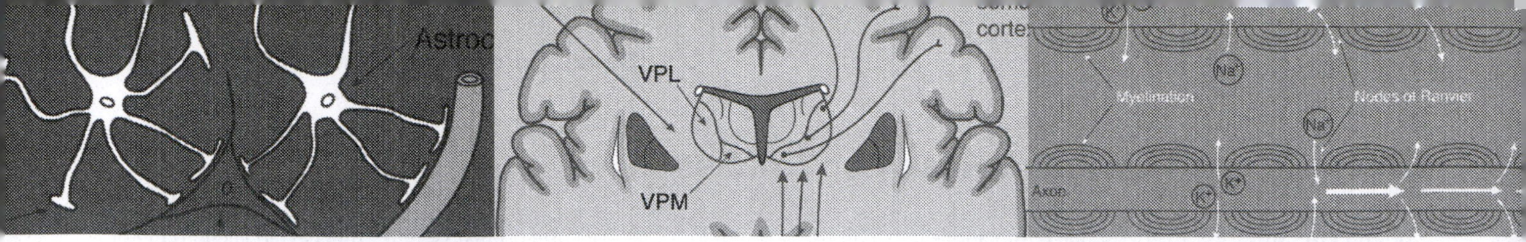

CHAPTER 5

Brainstem and Cranial Nerves

INTRODUCTION OF CLINICAL CASE

A 60-year-old male stockbroker made an appointment with his doctor because he felt dizzy and had experienced other symptoms. This patient had a long history of smoking cigarettes and consuming three or more alcoholic beverages each day, behavior that undoubtedly contributed to the hypertension for which he took medication. On the morning of the appointment, his right eyelid drooped and he had difficulty swallowing food at breakfast. During the physical examination, his blood pressure was elevated, but respiration and heart rate were normal. Ptosis was present in the right eye, and when the doctor gently lifted the eyelid, the right pupil was slightly smaller than the left pupil. Both eyes showed pupillary light reflexes and displayed normal eye movements. Facial expression was normal, but the corneal reflex and pain sensation were depressed on the right side. The skin on the right side of the face was dry and did not perspire. Hearing was normal for a 60-year-old person, but the man was unable to maintain his balance after closing his eyes. Although speech was noticeably hoarse, there was no inflammation of the nose, throat, or ear canals. The tongue protruded on the midline, but the uvula deviated toward the left and the right palate drooped. Both arms and legs had normal strength, and deep tendon reflexes were intact. The response to pinprick was noticeably weaker on the left side of the body even though the patient could detect light touch equally well on both sides.

INTRODUCTION

The brainstem lies rostral to the spinal cord and is subdivided into the medulla, pons, and midbrain. Most cranial nerves are connected to specific brainstem nuclei that control the sensory and motor functions of the head. Extensive interconnections between these nuclei and other parts of the brainstem help mediate simple reflexes and regulate more complex functions such as respiration, sleep, and consciousness. The brainstem also contains large bundles of axons that interconnect the spinal cord and brainstem with more rostral parts of the nervous system. Focal damage in the brainstem usually produces a constellation of neurologic symptoms because it contains many compact and functionally diverse structures that reside in close proximity. Furthermore, damage to brainstem regions that mediate vital autonomic functions may lead to death.

GENERAL ORGANIZATION OF THE BRAINSTEM

The organization of the brainstem follows a pattern similar to that seen in the spinal cord. In both regions, nuclear groups are segregated according to their connections with peripheral nerve fibers. In the spinal cord, afferent nerve fibers project to sensory nuclei in the dorsal horn, whereas the efferent nerve fibers originate from motor nuclei in the ventral horn. A similar pattern is evident in the brainstem, although the relative locations of the sensory and motor nuclei are slightly different because the sensory nuclei in the brainstem are displaced more laterally during the course of embryologic development.

Transverse Organization

As in the spinal cord, the sensory and motor nuclei in the brainstem are derived, respectively, from the alar and basal plates of the neural tube. During development, the dorsal part of the rostral neural tube becomes thinner, and this allows the lateral walls of the neural tube to unfold. This process causes the alar plates to move lateral to the basal plates. With further cellular proliferation, the sensory and motor nuclei of the brainstem undergo further differentiation into somatic and visceral subdivisions (Figure 5.1).

As in the spinal cord, nuclei in the brainstem are classified according to their association with the sensory or motor components of the cranial nerve fibers. Although most cranial nerve nuclei have "general" somatic or visceral functions, some are classified as "special" because they are involved in special functions such as taste, hearing, or speech. All cranial nerve nuclei are classified according to the following categories:

> **Motor brainstem nuclei** are located medially.
> **Sensory brainstem nuclei** are located laterally.

- General somatic efferent (GSE) nuclei give rise to cranial nerve fibers that innervate somatic musculature.
- General visceral efferent (GVE) nuclei give rise to parasympathetic preganglionic fibers that innervate the peripheral parasympathetic ganglia.

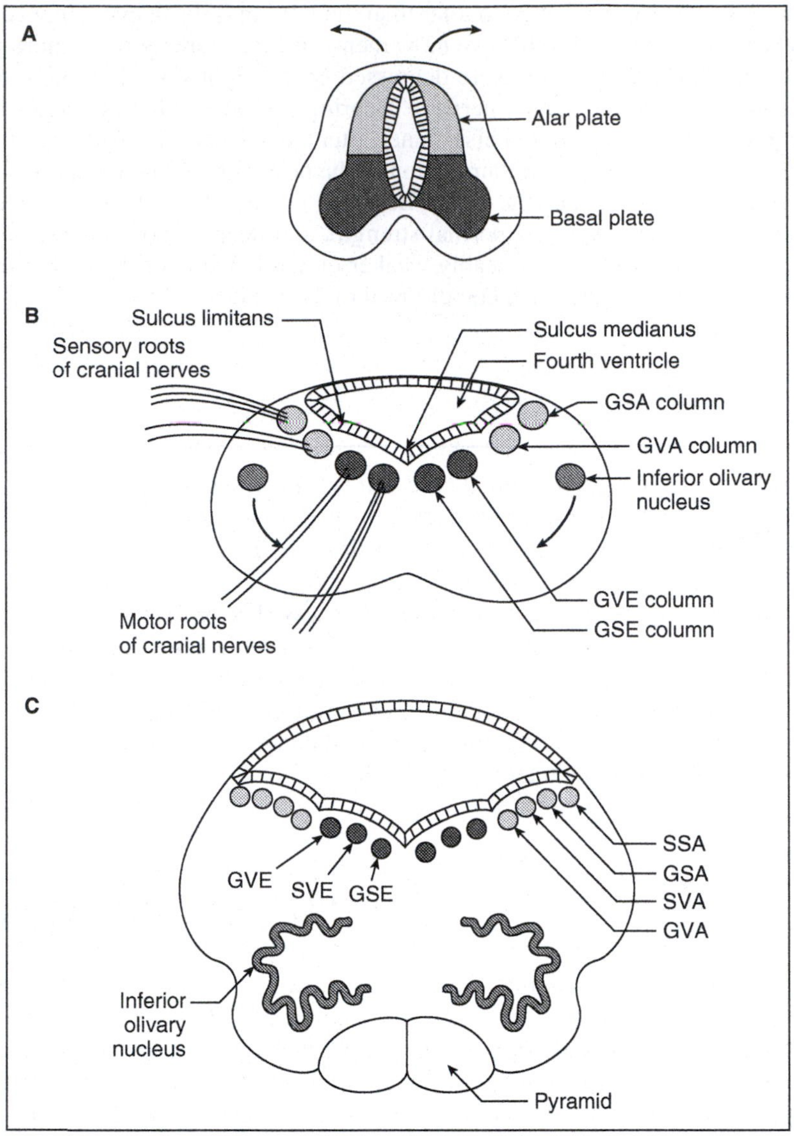

FIG. 5.1. Location and Development of Functional Cell Columns in the Brainstem. (A) Relative position of the alar (sensory) and basal (motor) plates in the embryonic brainstem. (B) During development, the lateral walls of the neural tube unfold to form the medulla and other parts of the brainstem. (C) Neuronal proliferation results in further subdivision of the cell columns into general and special cranial nerve nuclei. GSA = general somatic afferent; GVA = general visceral afferent; GVE = general visceral efferent; GSE = general somatic efferent; SSA = special somatic afferent; SVA = special visceral afferent; SVE = special visceral efferent.

- General visceral afferent (GVA) nuclei receive afferent fibers from receptors located in the thoracic and abdominal viscera.
- General somatic afferent (GSA) nuclei receive afferent fibers from mechanoreceptors in the skin, muscles, and joints.
- Special visceral efferent (SVE) nuclei innervate striated muscles of branchiomeric origin such as the muscles of the larynx, pharynx, and face.
- Special visceral afferent (SVA) nuclei receive projections from taste receptors located in the oral cavity.
- Special somatic afferent (SSA) nuclei receive afferent projections from fibers concerned with hearing or balance.

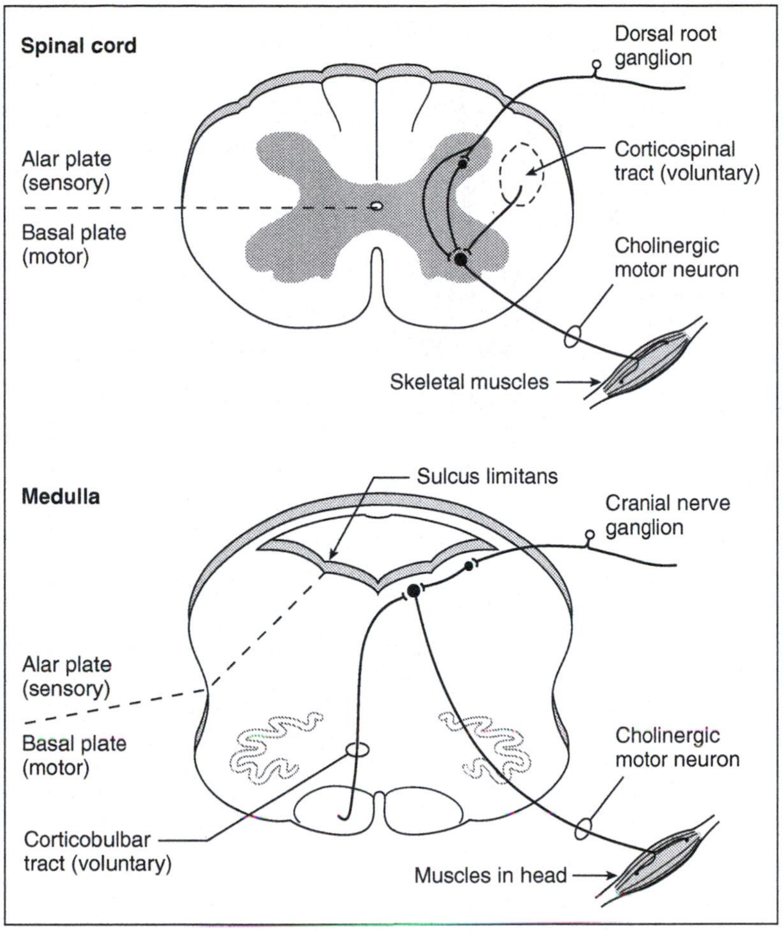

FIG. 5.2. Comparison of Spinal Cord and Medulla. Sensory and motor nuclei in the spinal cord and brainstem are located in separate regions of the spinal cord and medulla. Similar circuits in the spinal cord and brainstem mediate reflexive movements and execute voluntary motor commands issued from the cerebral cortex.

The brainstem contains neural circuits similar to those in the spinal cord that mediate skeletal reflexes. Thus, afferent projections from sensory receptors in the head are conveyed by nerve fibers whose cell bodies are located in various cranial ganglia. The cranial ganglia, which are analogous to the dorsal root ganglia of the spinal cord, contain pseudounipolar neurons whose proximal axons enter the brainstem and terminate in sensory nuclei located lateral to the sulcus limitans. These sensory nuclei project medially to a variety of motor nuclei that innervate the striated muscles in the head, face, and intraoral cavity as well as the autonomic ganglia that control glands or smooth muscles. Hence, cranial nerve reflexes are mediated by sets of neural circuits that resemble the multisynaptic reflex arcs in the spinal cord (Figure 5.2).

> **Cranial nerve reflexes** depend upon connections between sensory and motor nuclei.

> The **corticobulbar tract** consists of cortical projections to the cranial nerve nuclei. Many fibers in this tract are upper motor neurons that mediate motor activity in the head.

The cranial motor nerves originate from visceral and somatic motor nuclei that are reminiscent of the lateral and ventral horns in the spinal cord. As in the spinal cord, brainstem motor neurons use acetylcholine at their synaptic terminals to communicate with peripheral muscles or autonomic ganglia. Hence, the motor nuclei in the brainstem are lower motor neurons, and damage to a motor nucleus or its efferent fibers will cause muscular paralysis.

In addition to receiving sensory inputs to mediate reflexive movements, the motor nuclei in the brainstem receive signals from the motor cortex to execute voluntary movements. Corticobulbar projections descend through the internal capsule and crus cerebri before synapsing on specific sets of cranial nerve nuclei in the midbrain, pons, or medulla (Figure 5.3). In cases in which corticobulbar fibers innervate motor nuclei, these fibers are

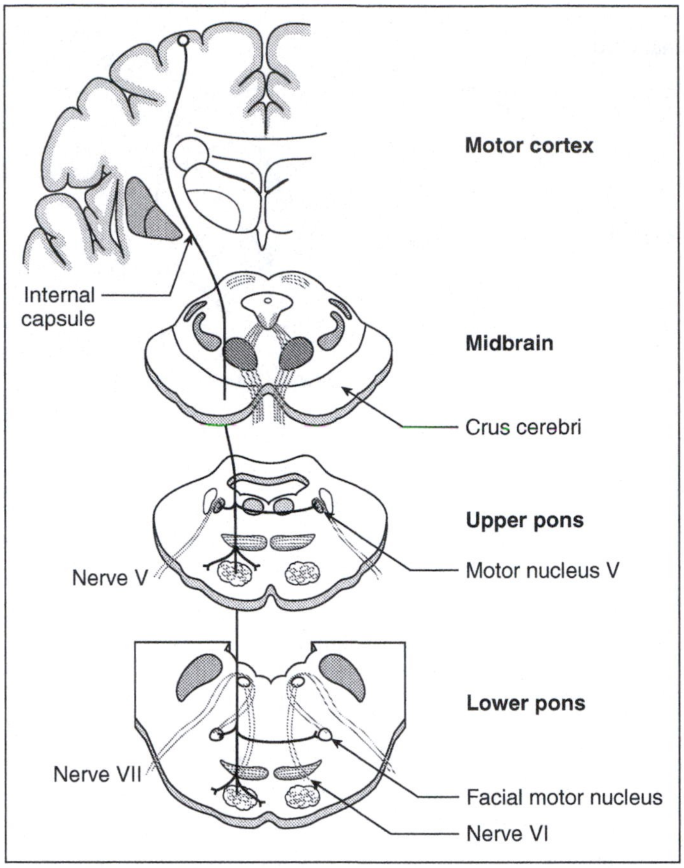

FIG. 5.3. Corticobulbar and Corticopontine Projections. Corticobulbar and corticopontine projections descend through the internal capsule and crus cerebri. Most corticobulbar fibers innervate the motor nuclei in the brainstem directly or indirectly (via the reticular formation) to mediate voluntary control of motor activity in the head. Other corticobulbar fibers project to sensory nuclei in the brainstem to modulate sensory transmission. Corticopontine fibers project ipsilaterally to the pontine nuclei, which in turn project to the contralateral cerebellar cortex (not shown).

analogous to the corticospinal tract because they function as upper motor neurons. In contrast to the corticospinal tract, which projects almost exclusively to the contralateral side, corticobulbar projections are predominately bilateral. Depending on the specific fibers that are affected, corticobulbar lesions impair voluntary movements of the face, eyes, mouth, tongue, or larynx.

Longitudinal Organization

Cranial nerve nuclei are arranged in longitudinal cell columns that extend rostrocaudally as shown in Figure 5.4. In general, sensory nuclei are elongated (up to several millimeters) and contain a huge number of very small neurons. By comparison, neurons in the motor nuclei are larger and are clustered into smaller, more compact groups. A few motor groups in the medulla, however, extend rostrocaudally for several millimeters and give rise to multiple nerve rootlets that emerge at regular intervals as efferent fibers for cranial nerves IX, X, XI, and XII.

Many sensory nuclei in the brainstem receive afferent fibers from more than one cranial nerve. Multiple inputs occur in cases in which afferent fibers of the same modality enter the brainstem through different cranial nerves and project to different rostral-caudal levels of the same sensory nucleus. By comparison, only the nucleus ambiguus contributes efferent fibers to more than one cranial nerve.

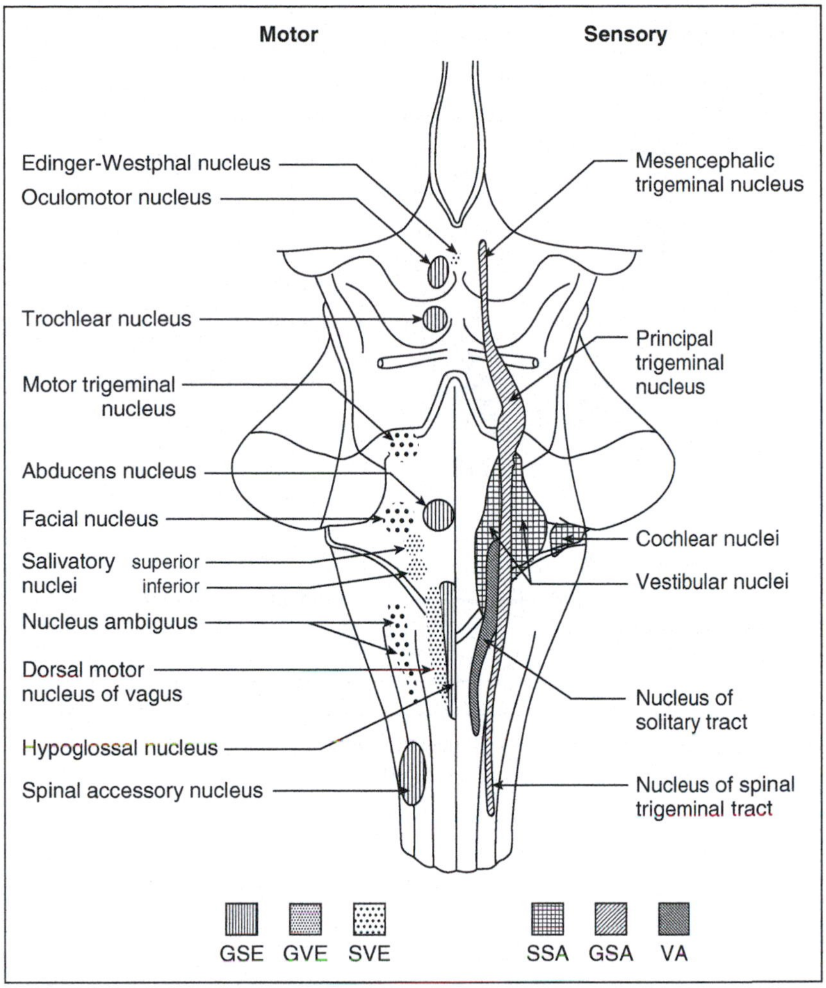

FIG. 5.4. Location of Sensory and Motor Nuclei in the Brainstem. Diagram of the sensory and motor cell columns extending through the brainstem. Each cell column is coded as indicated by the legend. GSE = general somatic efferent; GVE = general visceral efferent; SVE = special visceral efferent; SSA = special somatic afferent; GSA = general somatic afferent; VA = visceral afferent.

MEDULLA

The medulla represents the transition from the spinal cord to the brain. Located in the most caudal part of the brainstem, it contains many structures that are continuous with the upper cervical segments of the spinal cord. At progressively more rostral levels, however, the medulla acquires additional nuclei and fiber tracts that cause an expansion in its diameter.

The spinomedullary junction occurs where the pyramidal decussation interrupts the anterior median fissure on the ventral surface of the spinal cord (Figure 5.5). Rostral to this decussation, the pyramidal tracts lie adjacent to the midline and extend the entire length of the medulla. In the rostral medulla, each pyramidal tract is flanked by a large protruding mass called the inferior olivary nucleus. The olivary nuclei are bounded by the preolivary (or anterolateral) and postolivary sulci. A series of hypoglossal nerve rootlets emerge from the preolivary sulcus, which lies between the pyramidal tract and the inferior olive. The postolivary sulcus contains emerging rootlets from the glossopharyngeal (IX), vagal (X), and spinal accessory (XI) nerves.

On the lateral and dorsal surfaces of the medulla, the longitudinal tracts and sulci of the spinal cord continue without interruption (Figure 5.6). The dorsal (or posterior)

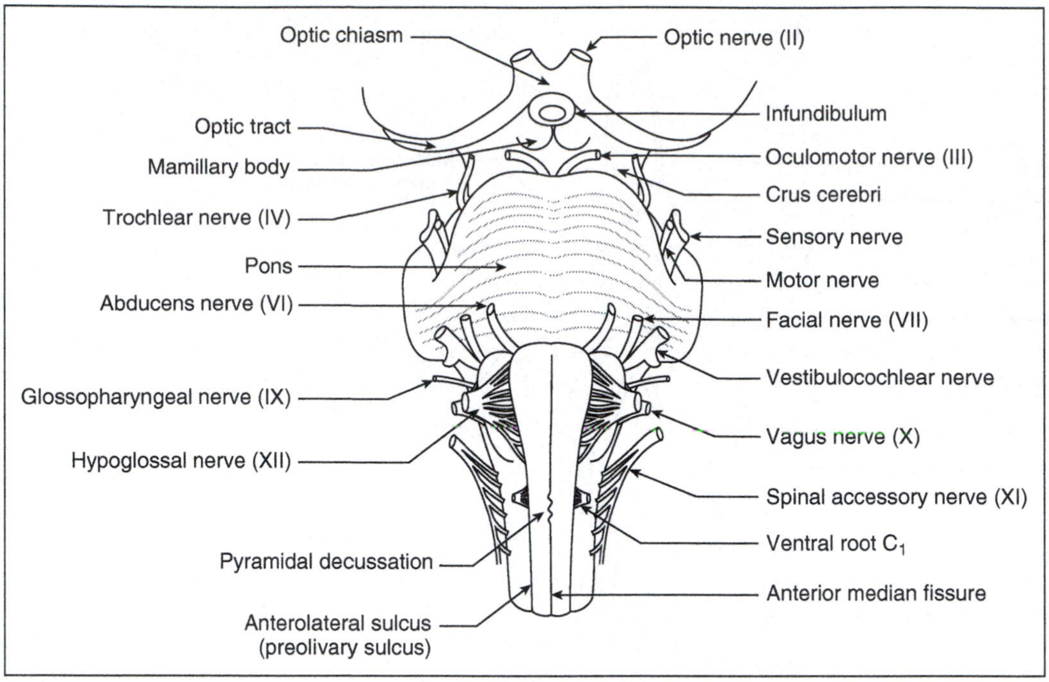

FIG. 5.5. Ventral Surface of the Brainstem. A drawing of the ventral (or anterior) surface of the medulla, pons, and midbrain showing the emergence of cranial nerves II-XII and other major landmarks.

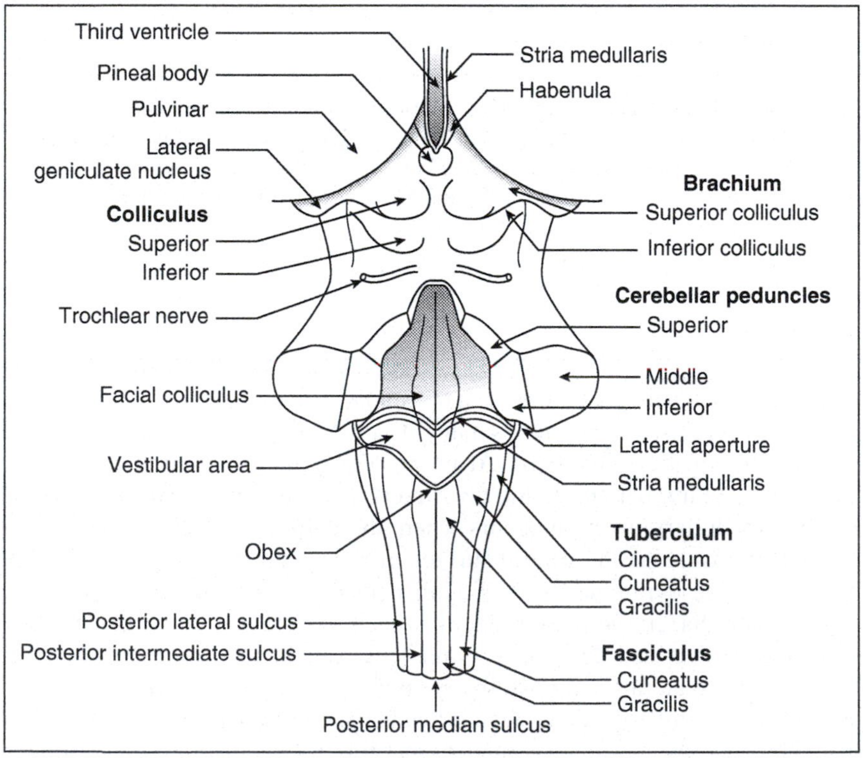

FIG. 5.6. Dorsal Surface of the Brainstem. A drawing of the dorsal (or posterior) surface of the medulla, pons, and midbrain after removal of the cerebellum.

columns lie on both sides of the posterior median sulcus, which terminates at the obex, a midline point that marks the caudal end of the floor of the fourth ventricle. On each side of the obex are small protuberances called the tuberculum gracilis, tuberculum cuneatus, and tuberculum cinereum. These elevations mark the underlying nucleus gracilis, nucleus cuneatus, and spinal trigeminal tract and nucleus, respectively. A shallow groove called the posterior intermediate sulcus separates the nucleus gracilis from the more lateral nucleus cuneatus, whereas the posterolateral sulcus separates the tuberculum cuneatus from the tuberculum cinereum.

Tuberculum, from Latin, means small lump, or elevation.

The dorsal surfaces of the medulla and pons form the floor of the fourth ventricle, which is hidden by the overlying cerebellum. Rostral to the obex are the hypoglossal trigones, a pair of small bumps that mark the underlying hypoglossal nuclei on each side of the midline. More laterally, the vagal trigone overlies the dorsal motor nucleus of the vagus. Lateral to the sulcus limitans are the vestibular area and the cerebellar peduncles, which form the lateral wall of the fourth ventricle. More rostrally, the boundary between the medulla and pons occurs where the thin fibers of the stria medullares traverse the floor of the fourth ventricle.

Internal Structures of the Medulla

The organization of the medulla is best understood by studying its internal structures as they appear in transverse sections. Figure 5.7 illustrates the position of the major structures in the medulla, including cranial nerves X and XII.

Pyramidal Tract and Its Decussation

The most prominent feature in transverse sections of the spinomedullary junction is the decussation of the pyramidal tracts (Figure 5.8). The pyramidal decussation consists of large bundles of corticospinal fibers that cross the midline obliquely as they proceed

The **pyramidal decussation** allows the motor cortex to control the opposite side of the body.

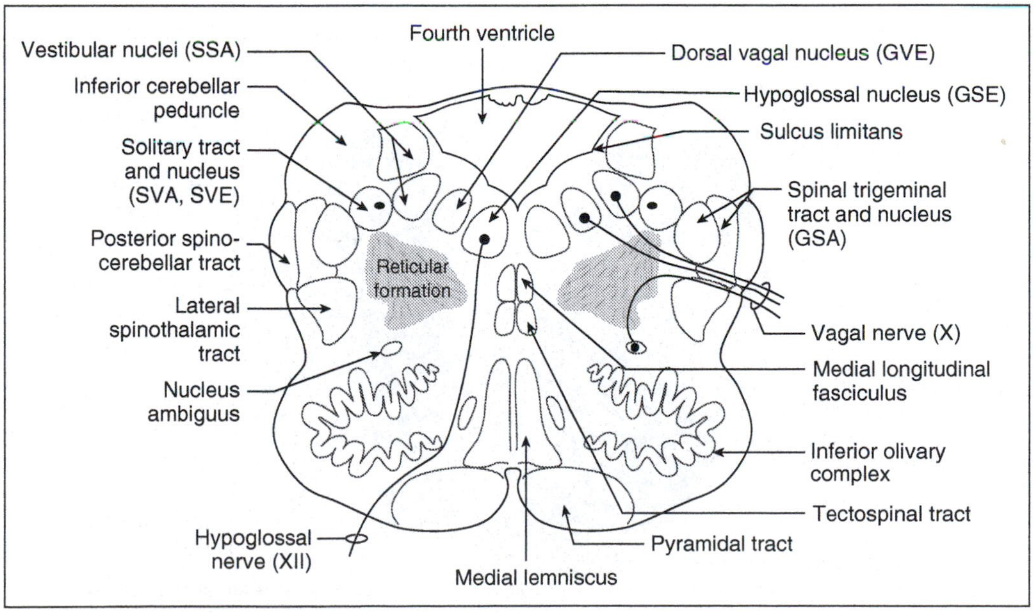

FIG. 5.7. Transverse Organization of the Medulla. This drawing indicates the position of the major nuclei and fiber tracts in the medulla organized according to their functional components. GSE = general somatic efferent; GVE = general visceral efferent; SVE = special visceral efferent; GVA = general visceral afferent; SVA = special visceral afferent; SSA = special somatic afferent; GSA = general somatic afferent.

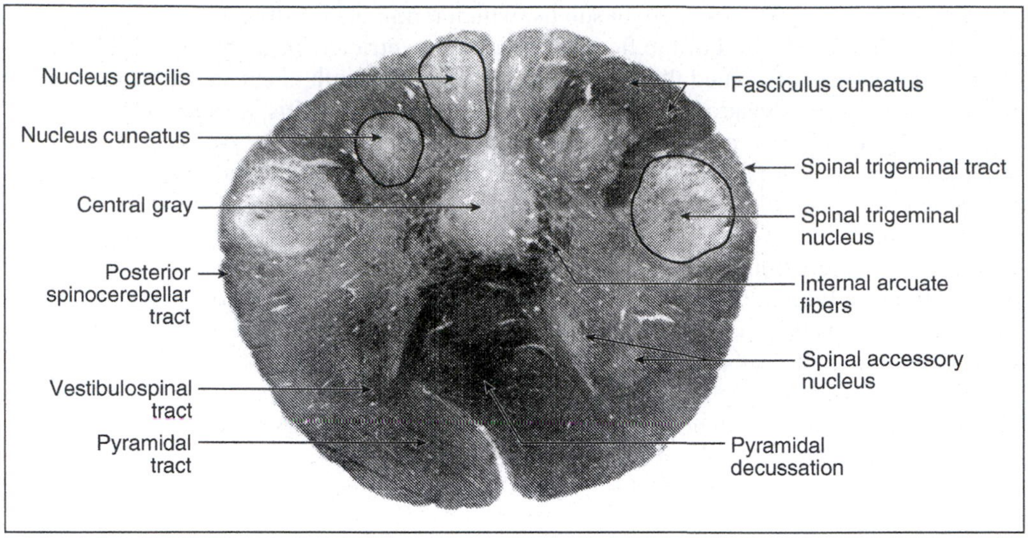

FIG. 5.8. Transverse View of the Spinomedullary Junction. This photomicrograph illustrates the pyramidal decussation and the nuclear groups in the caudal part of the medulla.

toward the lateral funiculus in the spinal cord. Nearly 90% of the fibers in the pyramidal tract cross through the decussation to provide the route by which each cerebral hemisphere controls the opposite side of the body.

Rostral to the pyramidal decussation, the pyramidal tracts proceed along the ventral surface of the medulla next to the midline. A cross section of the medulla shows each pyramidal tract lying ventral to the medial lemniscus and ventromedial to the inferior olivary nucleus (Figures 5.9 and 5.10). Because of their proximity, the pyramidal tract, medial lemniscus, and hypoglossal nerve can be damaged by a single vascular lesion (see "Inferior Alternating Hemiplegia," later in this chapter).

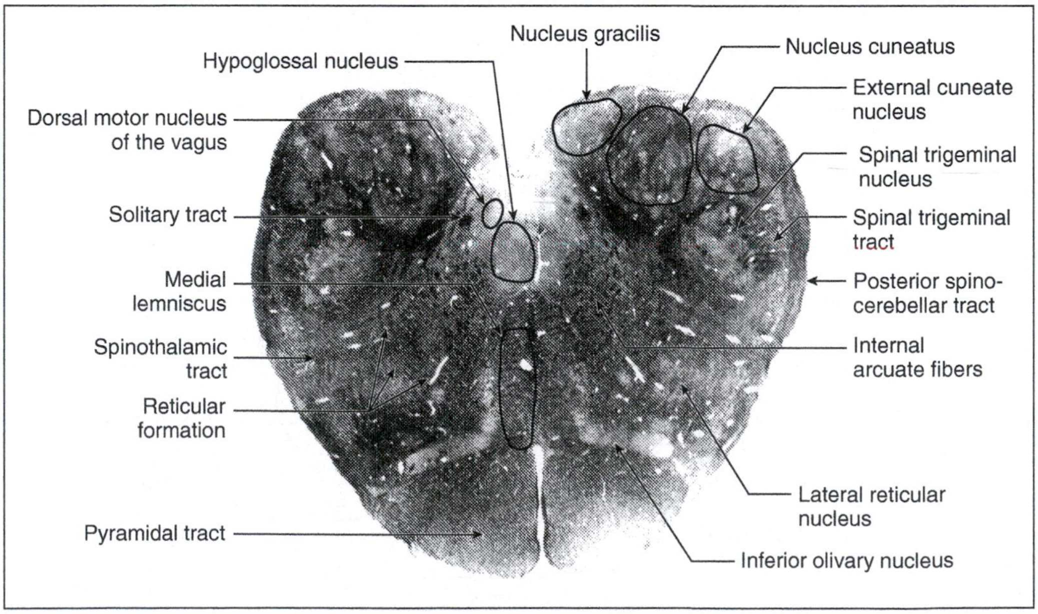

FIG. 5.9. Transverse View of the Medulla. This photomicrograph illustrates the medulla at the level of the obex and shows the position of several cranial nerve nuclei at their most caudal extent. The internal arcuate fibers and medial lemniscus are apparent in the central portion of the section.

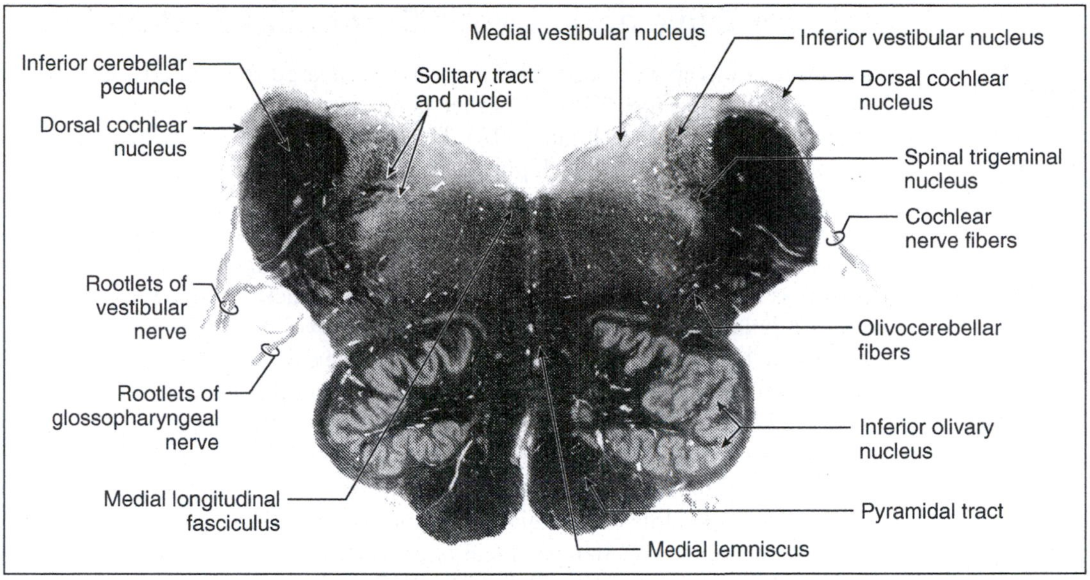

FIG. 5.10. Transverse View of the Rostral Medulla. This photomicrograph illustrates the major structures in the rostral medulla. The dorsal surface of the rostral medulla forms the floor of the fourth ventricle and contains the vestibular and cochlear nuclei. The inferior cerebellar peduncle is a collection of myelinated fibers that project into the cerebellum. The inferior olivary nucleus forms a bulge along the ventrolateral surface of the medulla.

Somatosensory Structures

The dorsal medulla contains a group of nuclei on each side of the obex that transmit somatosensory information to more rostral parts of the neuraxis. Starting at the midline, these nuclei include the nucleus gracilis, the nucleus cuneatus, the lateral (or external) cuneate nucleus, and the spinal trigeminal nucleus (Figure 5.9).

> The **nucleus gracilis** receives kinesthetic and tactile inputs from the leg.
>
> The **nucleus cuneatus** receives kinesthetic and tactile inputs from the arm.

Myelinated axons of the posterior (or dorsal) columns ascend through the caudal medulla until they terminate in either the nucleus gracilis or nucleus cuneatus. The nucleus gracilis receives inputs from primary afferent fibers that convey tactile (cutaneous sense) and kinesthetic (joint sense) information from the leg and lower trunk, whereas the nucleus cuneatus receives corresponding inputs from the arm and upper trunk. Together, these nuclei contain a somatotopic representation of the body that is maintained at higher levels of the brain by topographically organized projections. Thus, efferent axons emerge from the base of both nuclei and sweep ventromedially to form the internal arcuate fibers, which cross the midline and then ascend through the brainstem as the medial lemniscus. The decussation of the internal arcuate provides the anatomical route for transmitting somatosensory information from one side of the body to the contralateral thalamus and cerebral cortex.

The lateral (or external) cuneate nucleus, located dorsolateral to the main cuneate nucleus, receives primary afferent fibers from muscle spindles and Golgi tendon organs in the hand. The main axons from these mechanoreceptors enter the posterior columns and ascend to the lateral cuneate nucleus without synapsing in the dorsal horn of the spinal cord. Hence, the lateral cuneate nucleus is the forelimb equivalent of the dorsal nucleus of Clarke. Axonal projections from the lateral cuneate form the cuneocerebellar tract, which ascends into the cerebellum via the inferior cerebellar peduncle.

The spinal trigeminal tract contains primary afferent fibers from four cranial nerves (V, VII, IX, and X) and terminates in the spinal trigeminal nucleus. The spinal trigeminal nucleus extends into the upper cervical segments (C1-C4) of the spinal cord where it blends into the gray matter of the dorsal horn. In fact, the caudal part of the spinal trigeminal nucleus bears a striking resemblance to the substantia gelatinosa and other laminae of the dorsal horn; not surprisingly, this part of the spinal trigeminal nucleus processes pain sensations from the head.

> The **spinal trigeminal nucleus** receives pain inputs from the head.
>
> The **substantia gelatinosa** receives pain inputs from the body.

Inferior Olive and Inferior Cerebellar Peduncle

Cerebellar peduncles are massive bundles of myelinated axons that convey information to and from the cerebellum.

The inferior olivary nucleus (or inferior olive) is a large convoluted structure in the ventrolateral part of the rostral medulla that is surrounded medially and dorsally by slender accessory olivary nuclei (Figure 5.10). The inferior olive and its accessory nuclei send their axons to the cerebellum, which plays a role in many motor activities. Based on their afferent connections, however, the inferior olive and the cerebellum can be considered as sensory components in a larger network of nuclei that interact to mediate motor control. For example, the olivary nuclei receive ascending sensory inputs directly from the spinal cord as well as indirect sensory inputs from the nucleus gracilis, nucleus cuneatus, and the inferior vestibular nucleus. The inferior olive also receives descending projections from motor regions such as the red nucleus and the motor cortex. These convergent projections suggest that the inferior olive uses sensory information from the spinal cord to modify the motor commands received from higher brain levels. Most of the efferent fibers from the inferior olive cross the midline and enter the cerebellum via the inferior cerebellar peduncle. Near their termination, these olivocerebellar fibers are called climbing fibers because they literally climb the dendrites of the giant Purkinje cells in cerebellar cortex.

The **inferior cerebellar peduncle** contains four fiber groups: olivocerebellar, cuneocerebellar, posterior spinocerebellar, and vestibulocerebellar.

The inferior cerebellar peduncle is a massive fiber tract located in the dorsolateral region of the rostral medulla. Most fibers in the inferior cerebellar peduncle are olivocerebellar axons that originate from the contralateral inferior olive. The remaining fibers in the inferior cerebellar peduncle come from the posterior spinocerebellar and cuneocerebellar tracts, both of which convey information from muscle spindles and Golgi tendon organs. The inferior cerebellar peduncle is sometimes called the restiform body; fibers adjacent to the fourth ventricle that interconnect the vestibular nuclei with the cerebellum constitute the juxtarestiform body.

Cranial Nerve Nuclei of the Medulla

The medulla contains several sensory and motor cranial nerve nuclei: the hypoglossal nucleus, the supraspinal (or spinal accessory) nucleus, the dorsal motor nucleus of the vagus, the nucleus ambiguus, the nucleus of the solitary tract, and the spinal trigeminal nucleus (see Figure 5.4).

The **hypoglossal nucleus** innervates the tongue muscles.

Hypoglossal Nucleus (GSE—XII). The hypoglossal nucleus extends the entire length of the medulla and is found near the dorsal midline where it bulges into the floor of the fourth ventricle (see Figure 5.7). Axons of the large cholinergic neurons in the hypoglossal nucleus proceed ventrally between the inferior olive and pyramidal tract and emerge as a series of rootlets in the anterolateral sulcus. The hypoglossal nerves innervate the intrinsic and extrinsic muscles of the tongue to aid chewing, swallowing, and the production of speech. In addition to receiving inputs from the cerebral cortex (i.e., corticobulbar fibers), each hypoglossal nucleus receives taste inputs from the nucleus of the solitary tract and tactile inputs from the spinal trigeminal nucleus. These sensory connections help mediate reflexive movements of the tongue during the chewing and swallowing of food.

A unilateral lesion of the hypoglossal nucleus or nerve causes paralysis of the ipsilateral tongue. Consequently, patients with a hypoglossal lesion are unable to stick their tongue out straight. Instead, the tongue deviates toward the side of the lesion and, upon close inspection, the denervated side may show atrophy or fasciculations because a hypoglossal nerve lesion represents degeneration of a lower motor neuron. Hypoglossal nerve fibers are usually damaged following occlusion or hemorrhage of the tributaries arising from the anterior spinal artery.

Inferior Alternating Hemiplegia involves paralysis of the ipsilateral tongue and contralateral body.

Inferior Alternating Hemiplegia. Branches of the anterior spinal artery supply blood to the pyramidal tract, medial lemniscus, and hypoglossal nerve on one side of the medulla (Figure 5.11). Consequently, occlusion of one of these tributaries causes ipsilateral paralysis of the tongue in combination with contralateral paresis of the arm and leg. This combination of symptoms forms a distinct syndrome known as inferior alternating

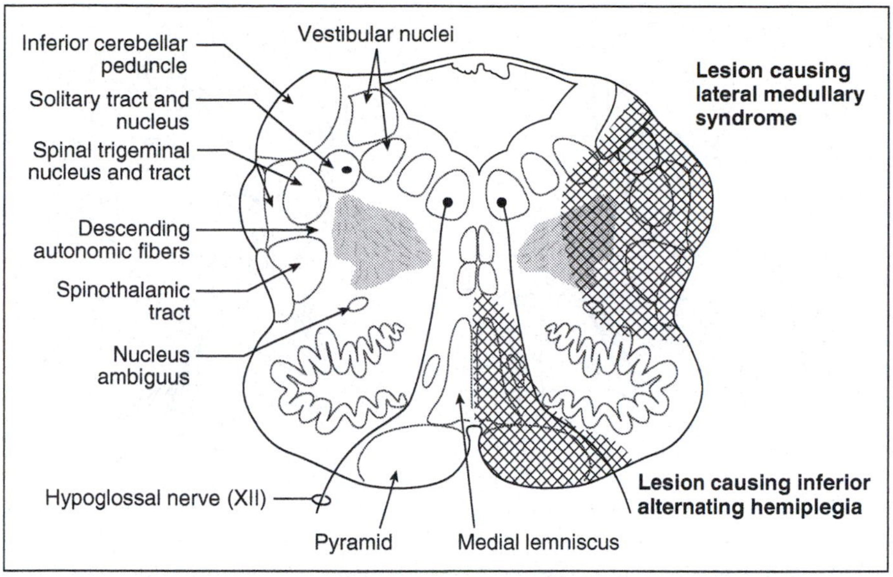

FIG. 5.11. Location of Vascular Accidents in the Medulla. This diagram indicates the structures in the medulla that can be damaged in lateral medullary syndrome or inferior alternating hemiplegia.

hemiplegia because opposite sides of the body (alternating) are paralyzed (hemiplegia) and the lesion is located at the caudal end of the brainstem (inferior). Patients with this syndrome may complain of tactile insensitivity on the contralateral body, but this symptom varies because the medial lemniscus is often spared and, even if it is damaged, other spinal pathways may compensate for the sensory loss.

Spinal Accessory Nucleus (GSE—XI). The spinal accessory (or supraspinal) nucleus is a long column of neurons that extends from the caudal medulla through the upper five or six cervical segments of the spinal cord (see Figures 5.5 and 5.8). Located near the ventral horn, the spinal accessory nucleus innervates the ipsilateral sternocleidomastoid and trapezius muscles. The sternocleidomastoid muscles are responsible for turning the head; hence, a unilateral lesion of the spinal accessory nucleus or nerve causes weakness in turning the head away from the side of the lesion. The shoulder on the lesioned side also droops noticeably because the trapezius muscle is paralyzed (Figure 5.12). These muscles are branchiomeric in origin and, for that reason, some anatomists place the spinal accessory nerve in the SVE category. Most authorities, however, think that nerve fibers exiting the spinal cord to innervate striated muscle should be classified as GSE fibers.

> The **spinal accessory nucleus** innervates the trapezius and the sternocleidomastoid muscles.

Dorsal Motor Nucleus of the Vagus (GVE—X). The dorsal motor nucleus of the vagus is a collection of small cholinergic cells that are located lateral to the hypoglossal nucleus. Efferent projections from the dorsal motor nucleus consist of preganglionic parasympathetic fibers that depart ventrolaterally and pass below the spinal trigeminal nucleus to emerge from the brainstem as part of the vagus nerve (see Figure 5.7).

The dorsal motor nucleus is the principal source of parasympathetic preganglionic fibers in the brainstem. These fibers innervate postganglionic neurons that control the glands of the pharyngeal and laryngeal mucosa as well as the smooth muscles of the thoracic and abdominal viscera. Consistent with the "rest and digest" role of the parasympathetic system, neuronal activity in the dorsal motor nucleus of the vagus slows heart rate, stimulates peristalsis and gastric acid secretion, and causes bronchial constriction. The dorsal motor nucleus of the vagus receives inputs from several brain regions that regulate autonomic functions, including the hypothalamus and reticular formation. It also receives projections from surrounding sensory nuclei, especially the caudal two-thirds of the solitary nucleus.

> The **dorsal motor nucleus of the vagus** exerts parasympathetic control of the pharyngeal and laryngeal glands, and the smooth muscles of the thoracic and abdominal viscera.

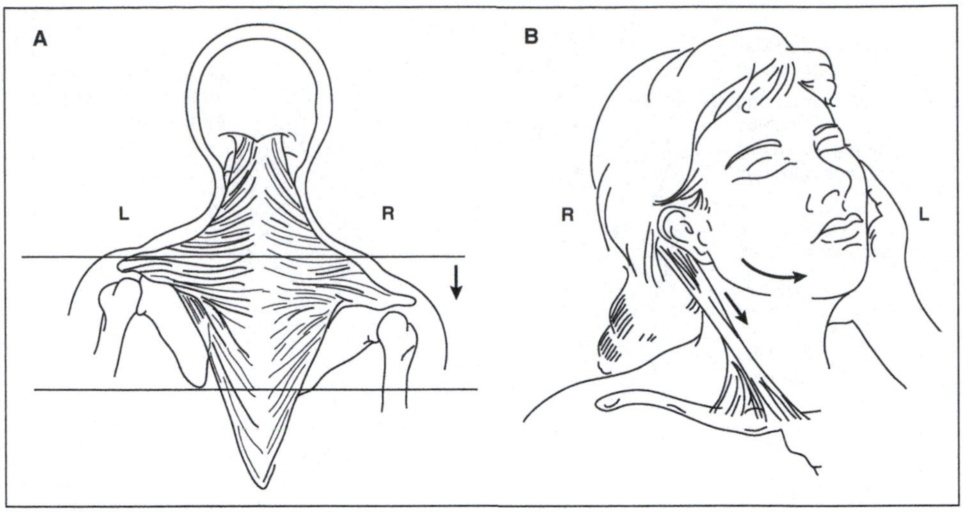

FIG. 5.12. Clinical Signs of Accessory Nerve Damage. (A) The right shoulder droops because the right spinal accessory nerve or nucleus has been damaged, and this causes paralysis of the trapezius muscle. (B) There is weakness turning the head away from the side of the lesion because the sternocleidomastoid muscles are paralyzed. (Source: Reprinted with permission from Wilson-Pauwels L, et al: *Cranial Nerves—Anatomy and Clinical Comments*. Toronto, Ontario: BC Decker, 1988:145.)

The **nucleus ambiguus** innervates the striated muscles of the pharynx and larynx

Nucleus Ambiguus (SVE—IX and X). As its name implies, the nucleus ambiguus is difficult to visualize in most histologic preparations of the brainstem. In sections stained for acetylcholinesterase, however, the nucleus ambiguus appears prominently in the lateral part of the reticular formation, halfway between the inferior olive and the spinal trigeminal nucleus. Efferent fibers from the nucleus ambiguus depart ventrolaterally and join the axons from the dorsal motor nucleus of the vagus to form cranial nerves IX and X. The nucleus ambiguus innervates the striated muscles of the pharynx and larynx, which are vital for voluntary and reflexive movements in speech, swallowing, gagging, and vomiting. Sensory inputs from the spinal trigeminal nucleus and the caudal two-thirds of the solitary nucleus are used by the nucleus ambiguus to modulate the reflexive movements of the pharynx and larynx. Voluntary movements, by comparison, are mediated by projections from the corticobulbar tract and surrounding reticular formation.

The **rostral third of the solitary nucleus** receives taste information from the oral cavity. The **caudal two-thirds of the solitary nucleus** receive cardiovascular and visceral information from the thoracic and abdominal cavities.

Nucleus of the Solitary Tract. The solitary tract is a compact bundle of SVA and GVA fibers from cranial nerves VII, IX, and X. The solitary tract, which extends the entire length of the medulla, derives its name from the fact that it is isolated from other brainstem tracts. Thus, in myelin-stained sections, the dark solitary tract is easily visualized against the pale appearance of the surrounding neurons that form the nucleus of the solitary tract (or solitary nucleus). The axons in the solitary tract terminate in different parts of the solitary nucleus according to their functional modality. The rostral third is often called the gustatory nucleus because it receives inputs from SVA fibers innervating taste buds in the tongue, whereas the caudal two-thirds of the nucleus receive inputs from GVA fibers innervating the thoracic and abdominal viscera.

Rostral Solitary Nucleus (SVA—VII, IX, and X). The gustatory part of the solitary nucleus is located in the dorsolateral part of the rostral medulla, ventral to the vestibular nuclei (see Figures 5.7 and 5.10). The gustatory nucleus receives SVA inputs from cranial nerves VII, IX, and X. The intermediate nerve, a branch of cranial nerve VII, contains SVA fibers that innervate taste buds in the rostral two-thirds of the tongue and the soft palate. The SVA fibers derived from taste buds in the caudal third of the tongue travel within cranial nerve IX. Only a few SVA fibers from cranial nerve X terminate in the gustatory nucleus, and these are derived from taste buds on the epiglottis.

The anatomic connections of the gustatory nucleus indicate the variety of functions that rely on taste information. Projections from the gustatory nucleus to surrounding motor nuclei help mediate reflexes involving the oral cavity, whereas ascending projections to the diencephalon convey the sensations of taste. Local gustatory projections to the nucleus ambiguus and the hypoglossal nucleus modulate reflexive movements of the tongue and larynx that occur during chewing, swallowing, and coughing. Eating also causes reflexive salivation, which is mediated by connections from the gustatory nucleus to the superior and inferior salivatory nuclei. Conscious appreciation of the taste of food and beverages is mediated by ascending projections from the gustatory nucleus to the ipsilateral thalamus. These second-order gustatory fibers ascend through the central tegmental tract to terminate in the parvocellular part of the ventroposteromedial nucleus (VPMpc) of the thalamus.

Caudal Solitary Nucleus (GVA—IX and X). This caudal component of the solitary nucleus extends rostrally from the level of the pyramidal decussation to the entry zone of the glossopharyngeal nerve near the obex. Afferent projections to the caudal solitary nucleus arise mainly from GVA fibers in the vagus nerve and, to a lesser extent, from GVA fibers in the glossopharyngeal nerve. These cranial nerves innervate the abdominal viscera, heart, lungs, and specialized receptors in the circulatory system. Although their innervation patterns and mechanisms of sensory transduction are poorly understood, it is generally agreed that these nerves convey pain, diffuse feelings of nausea, and related visceral sensations.

Specialized receptors sensitive to carbon dioxide, pH, and arterial blood pressure are located at critical sites in the vascular system. Baroreceptors and chemoreceptors located in the carotid sinus are innervated by the glossopharyngeal nerve, whereas those located in the aortic arch are innervated by the vagus nerve. These primary afferent fibers synapse on neurons in the caudal solitary nucleus that, in turn, project to the dorsal motor nucleus of the vagus or to thoracic and lumbar levels of the spinal cord (solitariospinal tract).

Many of the efferent connections from the caudal solitary nucleus mediate important cardiovascular reflexes and illustrate how cardiac output is closely monitored and controlled by feedback loops involving specific parasympathetic and sympathetic centers (see Chapter 13 on autonomic control). Consistent with its role in monitoring the status of the cardiovascular system, the caudal solitary nucleus projects to other brainstem regions that control ventilation. Collectively, the caudal solitary nucleus, the nucleus ambiguus, and the surrounding reticular formation comprise a medullary respiratory center that controls the breathing movements of the diaphragm and intercostal muscles by virtue of their projections to lower motor neurons in the phrenic nucleus (i.e., C3-C5) and anterior horn of the thoracic cord. This medullary region also coordinates vomiting reflexes with breathing movements to prevent aspiration of liquid or food expelled from the stomach.

> The **medullary respiratory center** is the region around the nucleus ambiguus that projects to the phrenic nucleus and other spinal regions that execute breathing.

The caudal solitary nucleus also has extensive ascending projections to the paraventricular, dorsomedial, and arcuate nuclei of the hypothalamus. These projections, along with connections to the amygdala and the pontine parabrachial nucleus, are important for integrating visceral and autonomic responses.

Lesions of the Vagus and Glossopharyngeal Nerves. Isolated lesions of the vagus or glossopharyngeal nerves are uncommon because of their close proximity. A unilateral lesion of the vagus nerve causes paralysis of the ipsilateral pharynx, larynx, and soft palate. Damage to the nucleus ambiguus results in hoarseness and dysphonia, and it impairs swallowing. Speech takes on a pronounced nasal character, and fluids enter the nasal cavity during attempted swallowing due to dysfunction of the larynx and pharynx. In these patients, the soft palate is elevated on the normal side, and the uvula deviates away from the side of the lesion. In rare instances where the vagus nerve is affected bilaterally, loss of vagal inhibition causes paralysis of the esophagus and stomach, complete loss of the carotid sinus reflex, and tachycardia. Although it is extremely rare, bilateral damage to vagal fibers

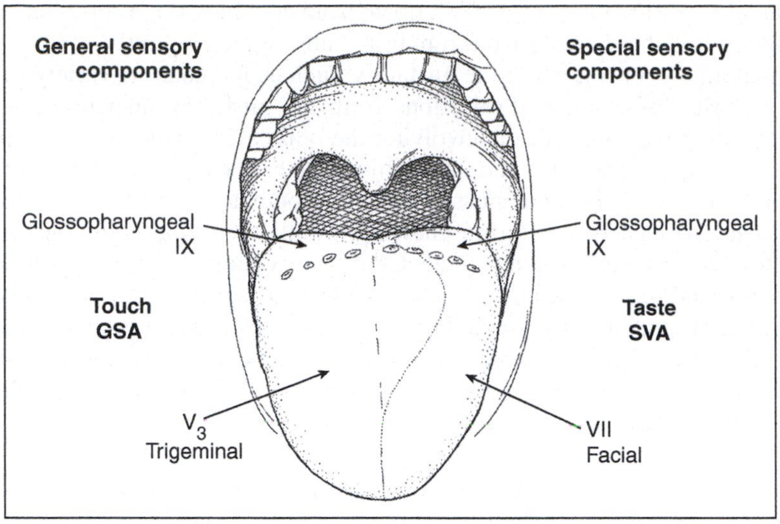

FIG. 5.13. Sensory Supply of the Tongue. The anterior third and posterior two-thirds of the tongue are innervated by different cranial nerves. (Source: Reprinted with permission from Wilson-Pauwels L, et al: *Cranial Nerves—Anatomy and Clinical Comments.* Toronto, Ontario: BC Decker, 1988:159.

Loss of the gag reflex is a clinical sign indicating a lesion of the glossopharyngeal nerve.

entering the recurrent laryngeal nerve causes complete paralysis of the pharynx and larynx. Unless a tracheotomy is performed immediately, the patient will die of asphyxiation.

Symptoms produced by isolated lesions or compression of the glossopharyngeal nerve are due mainly to loss of its sensory functions. Glossopharyngeal lesions destroy the somatosensory innervation of the posterior third of the tongue, the tonsil, the palatal arches, and the pharynx. These sensory deficits are associated with a loss of the gag reflex on the ipsilateral side. In addition, taste is also lost on the ipsilateral side of the posterior tongue, but most patients do not notice this deficit (Figure 5.13).

Trigeminal Sensory Nuclei. Somatosensory innervation of the head is mediated by primary GSA fibers of the trigeminal, facial (or intermediate), glossopharyngeal, and vagus nerves. The somatosensory components of these nerves project to three trigeminal nuclei that extend through the medulla, pons, and midbrain (see Figure 5.4). The spinal trigeminal nucleus extends from the spinal cord through the medulla and the caudal half of the pons. The main (or principal) sensory nucleus of the trigeminal nerve is a compact nucleus at the midpontine level, just caudal to the mesencephalic trigeminal nucleus, which extends into the midbrain (Figure 5.14).

The **trigeminal nuclei** contain a main sensory nucleus (cutaneous), a spinal nucleus (pain and temperature), a motor nucleus (muscles of mastication), and a mesencephalic nucleus (muscle spindles).

Most of the primary afferent fibers entering the trigeminal nuclei originate from the trigeminal nerve. The trigeminal nerve conveys tactile and nociceptive sensations from the face, the anterior two-thirds of the tongue, the cornea, the dura mater, and the mucous lining of the mouth and nose. As its name implies, the trigeminal nerve consists of three divisions: the ophthalmic, the maxillary, and the mandibular branches. After entering the pons, most first-order trigeminal fibers bifurcate and send one short collateral axon into the main sensory nucleus and a longer descending collateral axon to the spinal trigeminal nucleus. These descending collateral axons form the spinal trigeminal tract, which is located along the lateral aspect of the spinal trigeminal nucleus. The few trigeminal fibers that do not bifurcate terminate either in the main sensory nucleus or in the spinal trigeminal nucleus.

Some of the GSA fibers that enter the trigeminal nuclei originate from the facial (intermediate), glossopharyngeal, or vagus nerves. Upon entering the brain, these fibers descend through the spinal trigeminal tract and terminate in the spinal trigeminal nucleus. Some of these GSA fibers innervate the external ear and portions of the tympanic

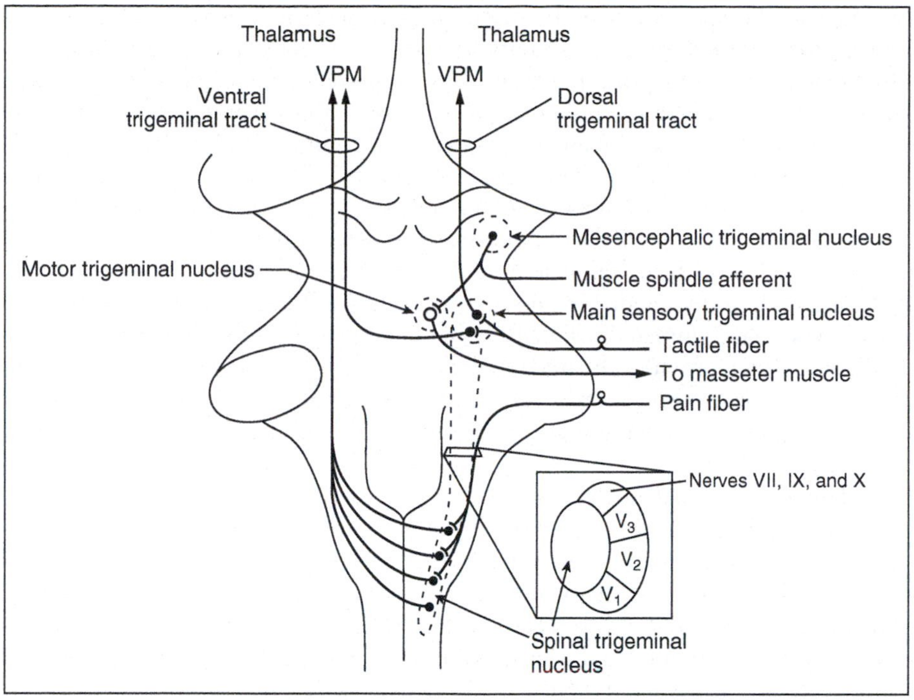

FIG. 5.14. Trigeminal Pathways. Tactile and nociceptive fibers in the trigeminal nerve project differentially to the main sensory trigeminal and spinal trigeminal nuclei, respectively. The inset indicates the somatotopic organization of the spinal trigeminal nucleus in a transverse section. VPM = ventroposteromedial nucleus of the thalamus.

membrane (VII), the posterior third of the tongue (IX), and the pharynx, larynx, and meninges of the posterior cranial fossa (X).

Spinal Trigeminal Nucleus (GSA—V, VII, IX, and X). The spinal trigeminal nucleus is the most extensive cranial nerve nucleus, largely because it receives GSA inputs from four cranial nerves (i.e., V, VII, IX, and X) that span most of the medulla and pons. The spinal trigeminal tract is somatotopically organized with the mandibular, maxillary, and ophthalmic fibers arranged in a dorsal to ventral order (Figure 5.14). As the spinal trigeminal tract descends, it becomes narrower as individual fibers depart medially to terminate in the adjacent spinal trigeminal nucleus. The spinal trigeminal tract and associated nucleus descend into upper cervical segments C2 or C3 of the spinal cord where they merge into Lissauer's tract and the underlying dorsal horn. The spinal trigeminal nucleus consists of three parts: (1) a pars caudalis that extends from the spinal cord to the level of the obex, (2) a pars interpolaris that forms the middle third of the nucleus and extends rostrally to the pontomedullary junction, and (3) a pars oralis that lies in the pons and extends to the principal (or main) sensory nucleus of the trigeminal nerve.

The transition between the spinal dorsal horn and the pars caudalis of the spinal trigeminal nucleus is imperceptible because both structures have a similar laminar organization. The most superficial layer of the pars caudalis, lamina I, receives synaptic terminals from GSA fibers containing substance P and resembles the posteromarginal layer of the spinal dorsal horn. Lamina II is immunoreactive for enkephalin and plays a role analogous to the substantia gelatinosa. Laminae III and IV contain larger neurons that form the magnocellular nucleus.

The pars caudalis of the spinal trigeminal nucleus is involved mainly in processing pain and temperature information from the head. Most of the trigeminal tract fibers projecting to the pars caudalis are small in diameter and resemble the C fibers that convey nociceptive impulses to the spinal cord. Clinical studies have shown that sectioning the

The **spinal trigeminal nucleus** contains a pars oralis (intraoral and tactile), a pars interpolaris (tactile and pain), and a pars caudalis (pain).

spinal trigeminal tract in the medulla (trigeminal tractotomy) reduces chronic pain without interfering with cutaneous sensitivity. By comparison, the pars interpolaris and pars oralis receive fewer nociceptive inputs and more large-diameter afferent fibers. In general, the neurons in the pars interpolaris process cutaneous inputs from the face, whereas neurons in the pars oralis process somatosensory inputs from the oral cavity.

Secondary trigeminal fibers depart from all levels of the spinal trigeminal nucleus and cross through the reticular formation without forming an obvious tract. After reaching the contralateral side, these secondary trigeminal fibers form the ventral trigeminothalamic tract and ascend through the brainstem in close association with the spinothalamic tract near the lateral tip of the medial lemniscus. Secondary trigeminal fibers project to several thalamic nuclei but terminate most densely in the ventroposteromedial (VPM) nucleus of the thalamus, which provides the main thalamic projection to the head and face representation of the somatosensory cortex. Hence, this subcortical pathway is critical for the perception of pain and other somatosensory stimuli involving the head, neck, face, and intraoral cavity.

The spinal trigeminal nucleus also projects to parts of the reticular formation that have multisynaptic connections with the thalamus and, thus, are analogous to the multisynaptic spinoreticulothalamic pathways. Other secondary trigeminal fibers project to motor nuclei in the brainstem to mediate a variety of cranial reflexes (Figure 5.15). Finally, some trigeminal fibers project to the cerebellum via the inferior cerebellar peduncle to convey information from the head that is analogous to the information conveyed by the spinocerebellar tracts from the rest of the body.

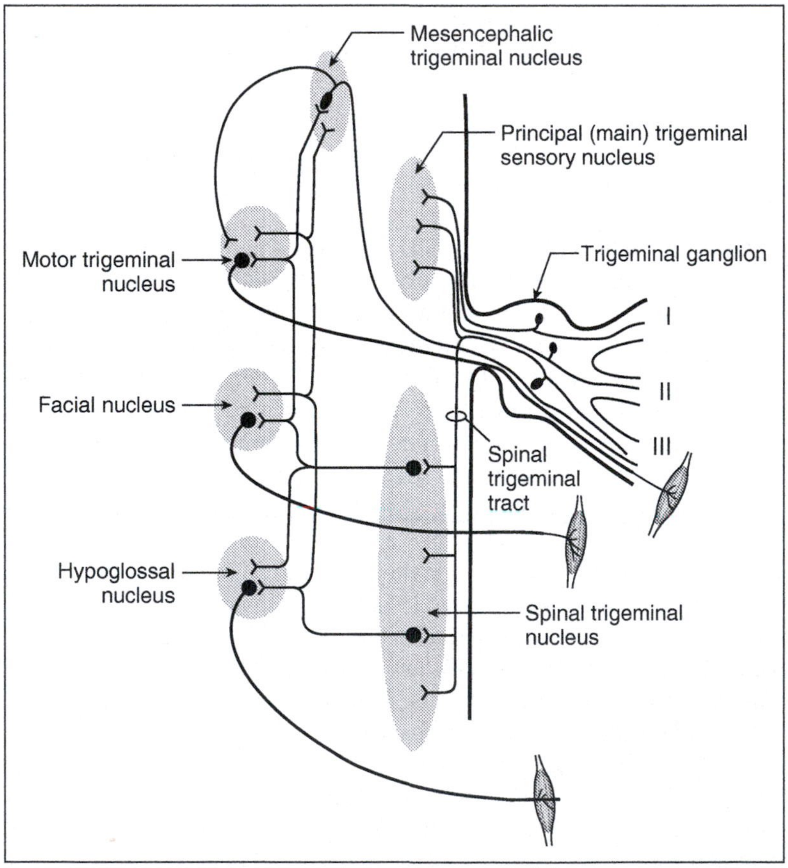

FIG. 5.15. Local Trigeminal Circuits. Synaptic connections between primary trigeminal nerve fibers, secondary trigeminal nuclei, and specific motor nuclei mediate the eye blink and other reflexes (i.e., jaw jerk and lingual).

Lateral Medullary Syndrome

The dorsolateral part of the medulla contains several somatosensory structures such as the lateral spinothalamic tract, the spinal trigeminal tract, and the spinal trigeminal nucleus. Because of the proximity of these structures, interruption of blood flow through the vertebral artery or the tributaries of the posterior inferior cerebellar artery may produce a constellation of symptoms known as the lateral medullary syndrome. This syndrome is characterized by loss of pain and temperature sensitivity on the ipsilateral face (spinal trigeminal lesion) and contralateral body (lateral spinothalamic tract lesion). Opposite sides of the head and body are affected because the spinothalamic tract is a crossed system for the body, whereas the spinal trigeminal tract and its nucleus receive inputs from the ipsilateral head. Other symptoms are usually present and may include nausea, vertigo, or dysphonia, depending on whether the damaged area includes the nucleus solitarius, the vestibular nuclei, or the nucleus ambiguus (see Figure 5.11).

Lateral medullary syndrome involves a loss of pain sensitivity on the ipsilateral face and on the contralateral body, accompanied by dysphonia, nausea, or vertigo.

PONS

Pons is a Latin word that means "bridge." This part of the brainstem is called the pons because it forms a functional bridge from the cerebral cortex to the cerebellar cortex. Thus, neurons scattered throughout the basal pons receive descending inputs from the cerebral cortex and relay this information to the cerebellum. Part of this pathway is apparent on the ventral surface of the pons where large numbers of transversely oriented fibers are seen coursing laterally and dorsally into the overlying cerebellum. These fibers originate from the pontine nuclei and cross the midline before proceeding laterally to form the middle cerebellar peduncle, which enters the cerebellum. On the lateral side of the pons, the middle cerebellar peduncle is pierced by the large trigeminal nerve.

Several cranial nerves emerge from the ventral surface of the brainstem at the pontomedullary junction (see Figure 5.5). The abducens nerve (VI) lies most medially and departs from the inferior pontine sulcus where the pyramidal tract emerges from the caudal pons. Further laterally, the facial (VII) and vestibulocochlear (VIII) nerves are attached to the brainstem at the junction of the medulla, pons, and cerebellum, which is called the cerebellopontine angle. The facial nerve consists of a large group of purely motor fibers and a smaller, more lateral group of mixed afferent and efferent fibers. This lateral group of fibers is often called the "intermediate nerve" because it lies between the eighth cranial nerve and the motor bundle of the seventh nerve. The vestibulocochlear or eighth nerve is composed of separate bundles of vestibular and cochlear SSA nerve fibers.

The fourth ventricle lies directly above the pons, its walls formed in part by the ascending fibers of the superior cerebellar peduncles. The axons in each peduncle proceed medially as they ascend the pons, and then they cross the midline after entering the midbrain. This decussation of the superior cerebellar peduncle enables each hemisphere of the cerebellar cortex to communicate with the red nucleus and the thalamus on the contralateral side.

Internal Structures of the Pons

Transverse sections through the pons indicate that this structure consists of two parts (Figures 5.16 and 5.17). The pontine tegmentum, which forms the dorsal part of the pons, represents a rostral continuation of the medullary reticular formation and contains the nuclei associated with cranial nerves V, VI, VII, and VIII, as well as a number of ascending and descending fiber tracts. The basal pons or pons proper contains a massive collection of pontine nuclei and fiber bundles that form the bulge on the ventral surface of the pons.

Pontine Nuclei and the Middle Cerebellar Peduncle

The ventral part of the pons contains numerous clusters of neurons that are interspersed among well-defined fascicles of fibers running in the transverse or longitudinal directions.

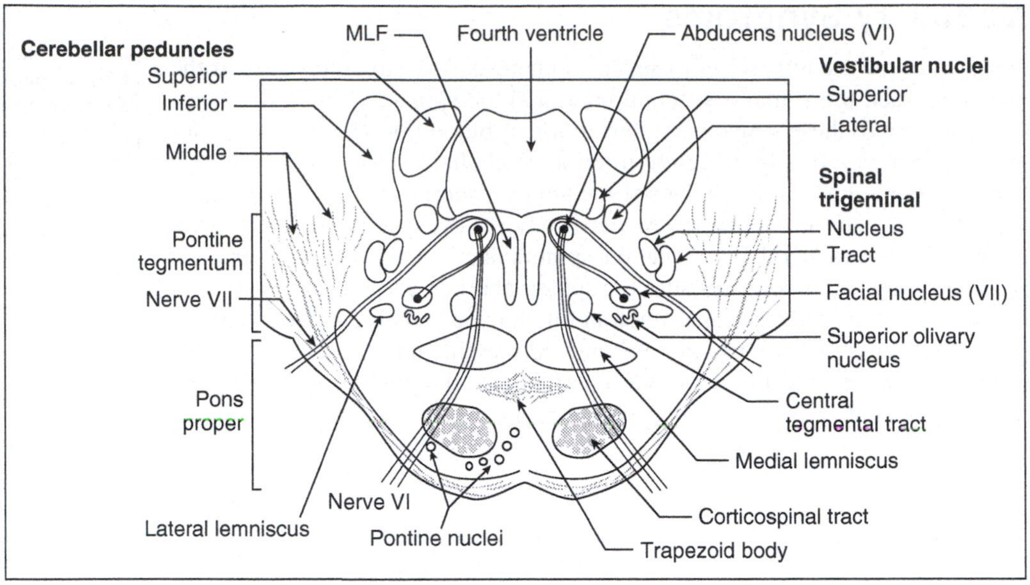

FIG. 5.16. Transverse Organization of the Pons. This drawing indicates the position of the major nuclei and fiber tracts in the pontine tegmentum and pons proper (basal pons). The cerebellum lies above the fourth ventricle and is connected to the brainstem by three fiber bundles called cerebellar peduncles. MLF = medial longitudinal fasciculus.

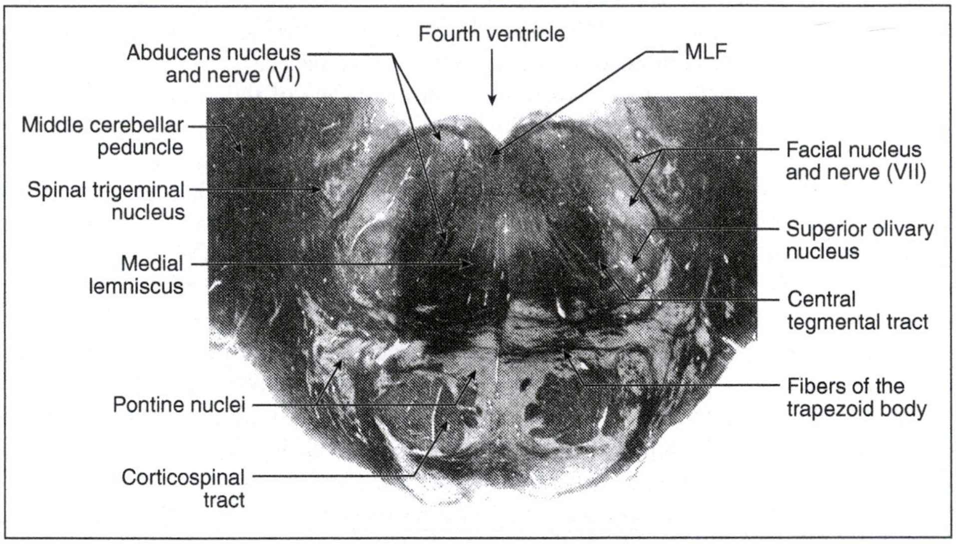

FIG. 5.17. Transverse View of the Caudal Pons. This photomicrograph illustrates the abducens and facial nuclei, as well as their cranial nerve fibers, in a section through the caudal pons. The ventral portion of the pons contains numerous pontine nuclei that surround the descending fibers of the corticospinal tract. The middle cerebellar peduncles lie laterally and have been partially cropped from view.

The **middle cerebellar peduncle** contains pontocerebellar fibers.

The longitudinal fibers are corticofugal projections that eventually terminate in the spinal cord (corticospinal), brainstem (corticobulbar), or pontine nuclei (corticopontine). Corticopontine fibers from the frontal, temporal, parietal, and occipital lobes terminate ipsilaterally on the scattered neurons comprising the pontine nuclei. The pontine nuclei give rise to pontocerebellar fibers that cross the pons in the transverse plane and project to the contralateral cerebellar cortex as the middle cerebellar peduncle. Hence, pontocerebellar fibers form the second link in the functional bridge from the cerebral cortex to the cerebellum.

Pontine Tegmentum

For many students, the medulla and pons appear to contain a bewildering array of fiber tracts and nuclei. Similar principles of organization are evident in both regions, however, and knowledge of the anatomy of the medulla provides a guide for understanding the organization of the pons.

The central part of the pontine tegmentum is dominated by the reticular formation, a region that appears to lack distinct nuclei but actually contains several nuclear clusters. In addition, the pontine tegmentum contains a large, distinctive fiber tract called the central tegmental tract (Figure 5.17). The central tegmental tract contains many functional pathways, including fibers that ascend from the reticular formation to the intralaminar nuclei of the thalamus and fibers that descend from the red nucleus to the inferior olive. Some fibers from the rostral part of the solitary nucleus also ascend through the central tegmental tract to convey taste information to the thalamus.

Central tegmental tract: rubro-olivary, reticulothalamic, and solitariothalamic fibers

The pontine tegmentum contains several motor nuclei that occupy positions similar to the motor nuclei of the medullary tegmentum. For example, the nucleus abducens is located near the dorsal midline at a site homologous to the position of the hypoglossal nuclei in the medulla. Similar to the ventral projections of the hypoglossal nuclei, axons from motor neurons in the abducens nucleus emerge from the inferior aspect of the nucleus and proceed ventrally until they exit the brainstem from the pontomedullary junction. Lateral and ventral to the abducens nucleus is the facial nucleus, which resides in approximately the same region as the nucleus ambiguus in the medulla. Facial nerve fibers are unique, however, because they emerge dorsomedially from the facial nucleus and loop around the abducens nucleus (i.e., the facial genu) before assuming a ventrolateral trajectory toward the cerebellopontine angle. More rostrally, at the midpontine level, the motor trigeminal nucleus occupies a position similar to the facial nucleus, but sends its efferent fibers laterally through the middle cerebellar peduncle.

Somatosensory Structures

In transverse sections of the medulla, the long axis of the medial lemniscus has a vertical orientation adjacent to the midline. During its ascent through the pons, however, the medial lemniscus gradually acquires a horizontal orientation at the base of the tegmentum with the arm and upper trunk representations located medially to the leg and lower trunk representations. Consistent with this topography, secondary trigeminal fibers conveying cutaneous sensations from the face and mouth cross the midline and join the medial part of the medial lemniscus. The spinothalamic tract proceeds through the ventrolateral tegmentum of the medulla and continues its ascent through the pons near the lateral tip of the medial lemniscus. The spinal trigeminal tract and nucleus occupy the dorsolateral part of the tegmentum, just medial to the middle cerebellar peduncle. More rostrally, the spinal trigeminal nucleus ends and is replaced by the main (or principal) sensory nucleus of the trigeminal nerve. The motor trigeminal nucleus is located medial to the main sensory nucleus.

Auditory and Vestibular Structures

The vestibulocochlear nerve (VIII) enters the brainstem at the pontocerebellar angle, but the vestibular and cochlear fibers separate from each other as they proceed to different central destinations. Thus, the auditory fibers terminate in the dorsal and ventral cochlear nuclei situated, respectively, near the dorsal and ventral edges of the inferior cerebellar peduncle. The vestibular nerve fibers run parallel to the auditory fibers but proceed more medially and terminate within four vestibular nuclei that reside near the lateral corner of the fourth ventricle, just medial to the inferior cerebellar peduncle and dorsal to the solitary nucleus. The medial and inferior (or spinal) vestibular nuclei are elongated structures that extend rostrocaudally through the entire medulla; the superior and lateral vestibular nuclei, by comparison, are more compact and reside just rostral to the transition between the medulla and pons.

Secondary nuclei and fiber tracts associated with the vestibulocochlear nerve are located in the pons. Immediately ventral to the base of the pontine tegmentum are the transversely oriented fibers of the trapezoid body, which contains decussating auditory fibers. Fibers of the trapezoid body terminate in a number of different nuclear targets, the most important being the superior olivary complex in the ventrolateral pontine tegmentum. Some fibers of the trapezoid body bypass the superior olive and ascend through the pons as the lateral lemniscus. Efferent fibers from the superior olive join the lateral lemniscus and ascend the brainstem until they terminate in the inferior colliculus of the dorsal midbrain.

Secondary vestibular fibers project to the cerebellum via the juxtarestiform body, a small collection of fibers that course dorsolaterally around the fourth ventricle just medial to the inferior cerebellar peduncle. Other fibers emerging from the vestibular nuclei either ascend or descend in a compact and densely myelinated tract known as the medial longitudinal fasciculus (MLF). The MLF, which is located adjacent to the midline in the dorsal tegmentum, contains some fibers that descend to the spinal cord and others that ascend to the pretectal region of the midbrain. The second-order vestibular fibers that project rostrally through the MLF terminate in motor nuclei that control the extraocular muscles; these fibers are important because they mediate vestibular-ocular reflexes.

Cranial Nerve Nuclei of the Pons

The pons and the pontomedullary junction contain several sensory and motor cranial nerve nuclei: the abducens nucleus, the facial nucleus, the vestibular nuclei, the cochlear nuclei, the trigeminal nuclei, and the salivatory nuclei. The following sections describe the central connections of these nuclei with the exception of the cochlear and vestibular nuclei, which are discussed in Chapters 8 and 9, respectively.

The **abducens nucleus** innervates the lateral rectus muscle.

Abducens Nucleus (GSE—VI). The abducens nucleus is a compact structure located adjacent to the midline below the fourth ventricle. One characteristic feature of the abducens nucleus is that it is surrounded by fibers of the facial nerve, which bulge into the fourth ventricle to form the facial colliculus.

The abducens nucleus is composed of two sets of neurons (Figure 5.18). One neuronal population is cholinergic and projects peripherally to innervate the lateral rectus muscle on the ipsilateral side. The other population consists of internuclear neurons whose axons emerge medially and cross the midline before ascending to the midbrain through the MLF. These internuclear neurons send their axons to the nucleus within the oculomotor complex that controls the medial rectus muscle. Synchronous activation of both neuronal populations in the abducens nucleus coordinates contraction of the medial and lateral recti muscles to produce smooth, conjugate horizontal movements of both eyes toward the ipsilateral side.

Horizontal eye movements are precisely controlled by neurons located in the paramedian pontine reticular formation (PPRF). The PPRF receives inputs from the frontal eye fields, a specialized motor region in frontal cortex, as well as from the superior colliculus, the vestibular nuclei, and the cerebellum. The PPRF contains different functional classes of neurons that integrate information from these regions to control the velocity and direction of conjugate eye movements. In addition to its local connections with the abducens nucleus, the PPRF sends axons through the MLF to coordinate the activities of the abducens nucleus with the trochlear and oculomotor nuclei. Similar projections from the vestibular system to the abducens, trochlear, and oculomotor nuclei coordinate eye movements that compensate for angular rotation of the head.

Lesions of the Abducens Nucleus. The clinical symptoms produced by a lesion of the abducens nucleus are different from those produced by a lesion of the abducens nerve. As indicated by Figure 5.18, such lesions affect different populations of neurons. A lesion of the abducens nucleus produces paralysis of the ipsilateral lateral rectus and paresis of the contralateral medial rectus because both populations of abducens neurons are affected. The eyes cannot be directed to the lesioned side, and the imbalance in muscle tone causes

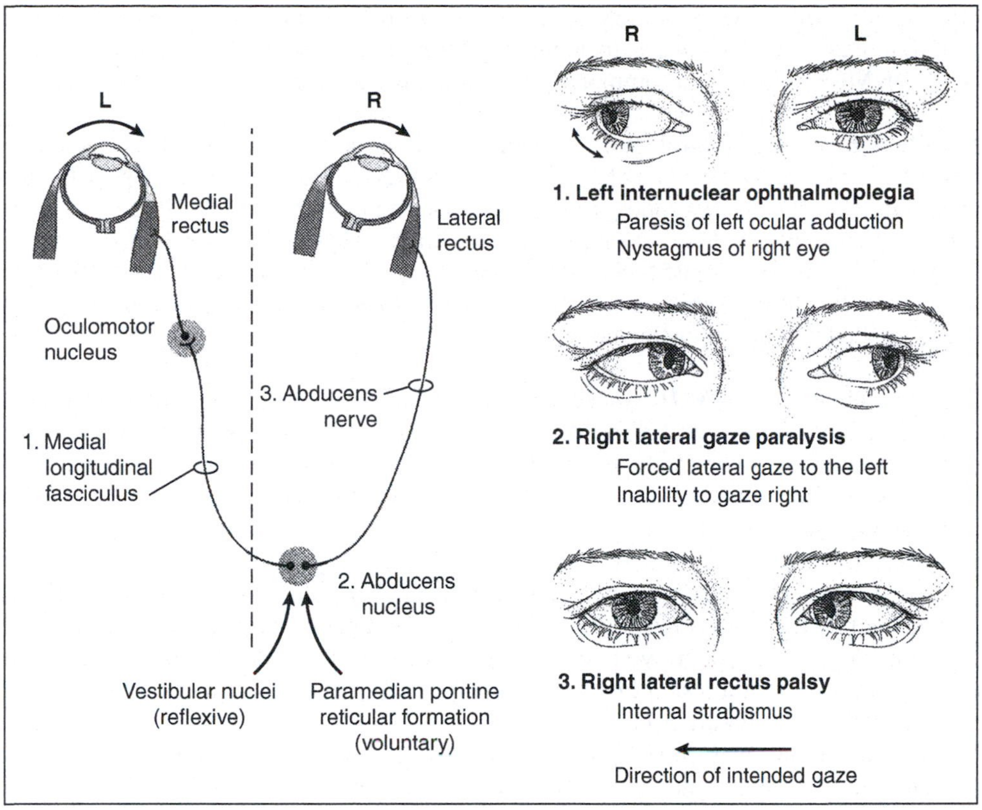

FIG. 5.18. Connections of the Abducens Nucleus. (A) The abducens nucleus contains two sets of neurons that project to the lateral rectus muscle and to the contralateral oculomotor complex. Activation of the abducens nucleus causes horizontal conjugate eye movements as indicated by the arrows. (B) Deficits in eye movements following selective damage to the numbered neural structures.

both eyes to turn toward the intact side. This set of symptoms is called lateral gaze paralysis because both eyes are turned in the same direction. The convergence response (ability to look at one's nose) remains intact, however, because the medial rectus muscle is not paralyzed and it can still respond to oculomotor commands issued by brain regions other than the abducens nucleus.

Abduction is movement toward the midline.
Adduction is movement away from the midline.

Diplopia is double vision resulting from loss of conjugate eye movements.

Lesions of the Abducens Nerve. Injury to the abducens nerve causes paralysis of the lateral rectus muscle and results in horizontal diplopia (double vision), a condition that is produced whenever both eyes are not fixated on precisely the same focal point. Following a lesion of the abducens nerve, diplopia is minimal when the patient looks straight ahead or toward the intact side but becomes maximal on attempted gaze toward the lesioned side. The affected eye is sometimes adducted because tonic activity in the intact medial rectus is unopposed, and this muscular imbalance produces an internal strabismus in which the affected eye deviates toward the midline (see Figure 5.18).

Internuclear Ophthalmoplegia. A lesion of the MLF destroys the internuclear fibers ascending from the abducens nucleus and produces a dissociation of horizontal eye movements known as internuclear ophthalmoplegia. In this event, the eye ipsilateral to the lesion fails to adduct on attempted gaze toward the contralateral side, and the abducted eye exhibits horizontal nystagmus (repetitive back-and-forth movements). The convergence response remains intact for both eyes, however, because the medial recti muscles are still innervated by neurons in the oculomotor complex, which receives some of its motor commands via input fibers that do not travel through the MLF (see Figure 5.18). Internuclear ophthalmoplegia is often seen in patients with multiple sclerosis because this viral disease destroys the myelination of many neural pathways, including the MLF. In fact, eye movement deficits associated with MLF lesions are a common sign of multiple sclerosis.

Middle alternating hemiplegia: lateral rectus palsy combined with contralateral hemiparesis

Middle Alternating Hemiplegia. The medial part of the basal pons receives oxygenated blood from the paramedian branches of the basilar artery. These tributaries supply the medial pontine nuclei, the descending root fibers of the abducens nerve, as well as fibers of the corticospinal, corticobulbar, and corticopontine tracts. Hence, a stroke of one of these tributaries on one side of the brain may damage the abducens nerve and the nearby corticospinal tract. The combination of lateral rectus palsy and contralateral hemiparesis of the body is called middle alternating hemiplegia.

The **facial nucleus** innervates the muscles of facial expression.

Facial Nucleus (SVE—VII). The facial nucleus is a large cluster of cholinergic neurons in the caudal pons at the level of the abducens nucleus. In transverse sections, the facial nucleus is located in the ventrolateral reticular formation, a position equivalent to the location of the nucleus ambiguus in the medulla. The facial nucleus is composed of several subnuclei, each of which innervates specific muscles such as the stapedius, the digastric, the platysma, the buccinator, and other muscles of facial expression. Facial motor fibers emerge from the dorsomedial aspect of the facial nucleus and loop around the abducens nucleus before coursing below the spinal trigeminal nucleus as it proceeds to the cerebellopontine angle. The proximity of the abducens nucleus to the genu of the facial nerve virtually guarantees that a lesion in the dorsal part of the pons will damage both structures simultaneously (see Figure 5.17).

The facial nucleus receives connections from the trigeminal system that enable it to mediate the clinically significant corneal reflex (see Figure 5.15). The ophthalmic division of the trigeminal nerve provides the cornea with the densest sensory innervation of any peripheral structure, making it exquisitely sensitive to specks of dust and other foreign objects. When the cornea is lightly touched, sensory impulses are transmitted along trigeminal nerve fibers to the main sensory nucleus and to the pars caudalis of the spinal trigeminal nucleus. These trigeminal nuclei project bilaterally to the facial nuclei, which control the orbicularis oculi. Hence, both eyes blink automatically in response to corneal stimulation of either eye.

The facial nucleus also receives descending projections from the motor cortex to mediate voluntary facial movements. Corticobulbar fibers originating from the motor cortex convey impulses directly to the facial nucleus. Additional projections from the motor cortex to neighboring parts of the reticular formation also convey impulses multisynaptically to the facial nucleus. In most individuals, the motor cortex sends bilateral projections to those parts of the facial nuclei that control the frontalis and other muscles in the upper face (Figure 5.19). By contrast, the parts of the facial nucleus that control the lower face receive projections only from the contralateral hemisphere. This explains why most individuals raise both eyebrows simultaneously but can exert asymmetrical control of the lower face.

Central facial palsy: an upper motor neuron lesion of the corticobulbar tract

Bell's palsy: a lower motor neuron lesion of the facial nerve

Central Facial Palsy. A small, unilateral stroke that affects corticobulbar fibers passing through the internal capsule may produce a central facial palsy. Following such an event, there is significant weakness of the lower facial muscles on the side contralateral to the lesion (Figure 5.20). Central facial palsy is often associated with hemiplegia because the damage may also affect the nearby corticospinal pathways. Lacrimation, salivation, and the corneal reflex are unaffected, however, because the lower motor neurons of the facial nerve are intact and continue to innervate the peripheral muscles and glands. Surprisingly, a patient with a central facial palsy can smile spontaneously on the weakened side because the connections that mediate facial responses to emotional stimuli are separate from the corticobulbar pathways that mediate voluntary smiling, but the exact route of this projection is not known.

Bell's Palsy. A lesion of the facial nucleus or nerve causes ipsilateral paralysis of all facial muscles (see Figure 5.20). This condition, known as Bell's palsy, is characterized

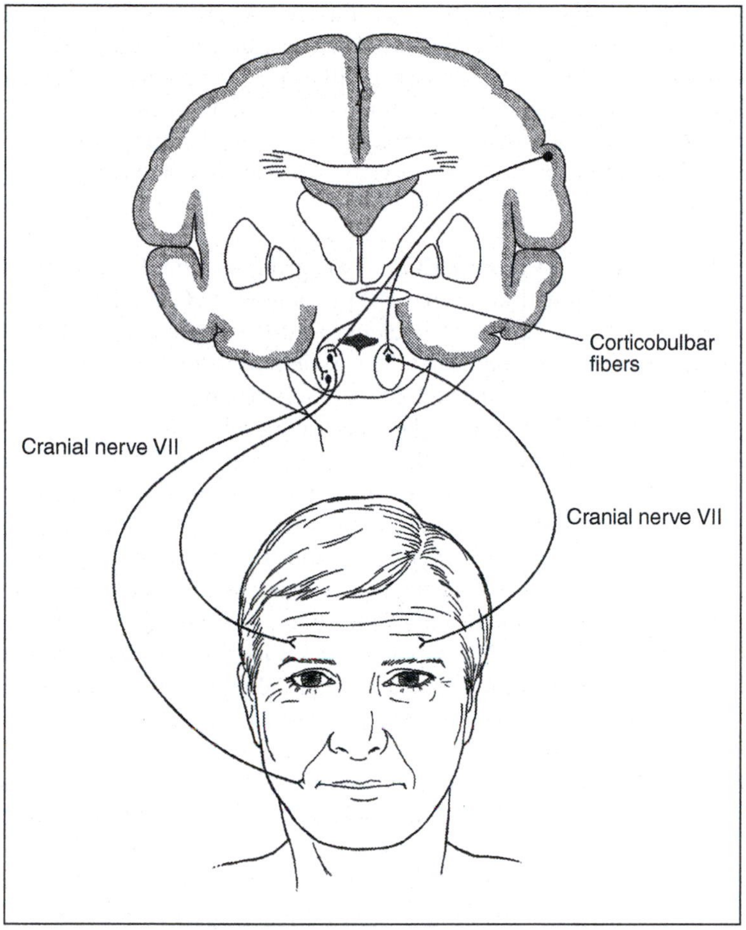

FIG. 5.19. Corticobulbar Projections to the Facial Nucleus. Each cortical hemisphere sends bilateral projections to regions of the facial nucleus controlling the upper face muscles, but only sends contralateral projections to the regions that control the lower face muscles.

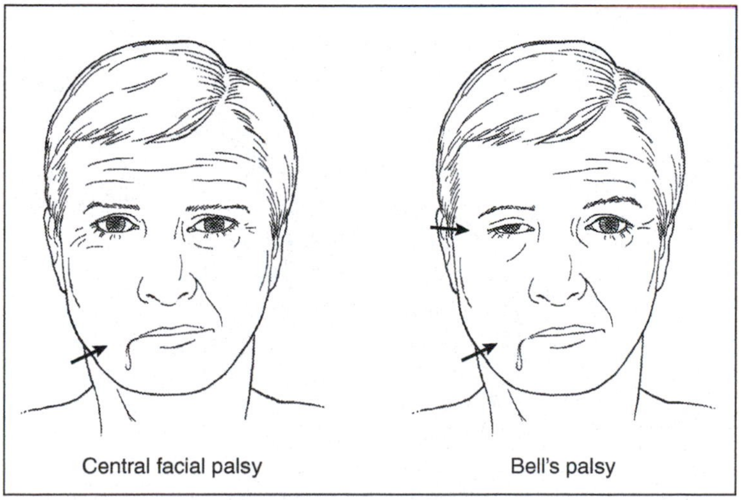

FIG. 5.20. Comparison of Central Facial Palsy and Bell's Palsy. Central facial palsy is caused by a lesion of the corticobulbar projections. Because the upper facial muscles receive bilateral innervation, only the lower facial muscles lose voluntary control. Bell's palsy affects lower motor neurons and therefore causes paralysis of both the upper and lower facial muscles.

by complete atrophy of the ipsilateral facial muscles as indicated by a flattening of the nasolabial fold, a widening of the palpebral fissure, and a droop in the corner of the mouth. Patients with Bell's palsy experience difficulty in chewing food because the buccinator muscle is paralyzed, and they are unable to close their ipsilateral eye because of denervation of the orbicularis oculi. Although facial nerve damage disables the corneal reflex, corneal sensation remains intact because afferent impulses are still conducted by the trigeminal nerve.

Salivatory Nuclei (GVE—VII and IX). Two groups of cholinergic neurons located near the pontomedullary junction give rise to preganglionic GVE fibers that control salivary secretions. The inferior salivatory nucleus is a diffuse group of neurons in the rostral medulla that lie in the lateral portion of the reticular formation. These preganglionic parasympathetic neurons project through the glossopharyngeal and lesser petrosal nerves before terminating in the otic ganglion. The postganglionic cells of the otic ganglion convey impulses to the parotid gland, which produces saliva in response to gustatory stimulation. The afferent limb of this multisynaptic reflex arc is mediated by projections from the chorda tympani nerve (leading to the intermediate nerve for taste) to the rostral solitary nucleus, which projects to both the inferior and superior salivatory nuclei.

The **inferior salivatory nucleus** controls the parotid gland. The **superior salivatory nucleus** controls the submandibular, sublingual, and lacrimal glands.

Neurons in the superior salivatory nucleus also act as relay neurons in a multisynaptic reflex arc that either releases saliva in response to tasting food or produces lacrimation in response to corneal irritation. The superior salivatory nucleus consists of a loose cluster of cholinergic, preganglionic neurons in the caudal pons. The axons of these neurons travel through the intermediate nerve and split into two groups of GVE fibers near the geniculate ganglion of the facial nerve. Some of these preganglionic fibers pass through the geniculate ganglion, enter the chorda tympani nerve, and synapse on postganglionic neurons in the submandibular ganglion, which projects to the submandibular and sublingual glands to control salivation (Figure 5.21). The remaining GVE fibers enter the greater petrosal nerve and terminate in the pterygopalatine ganglion where two groups of postganglionic neurons innervate the lacrimal gland or the mucous lining of the mouth and nose. The afferent limb of the lacrimal reflex is mediated by projections from the ophthalmic division of the trigeminal nerve to the spinal trigeminal nucleus, which projects to the superior salivatory nucleus.

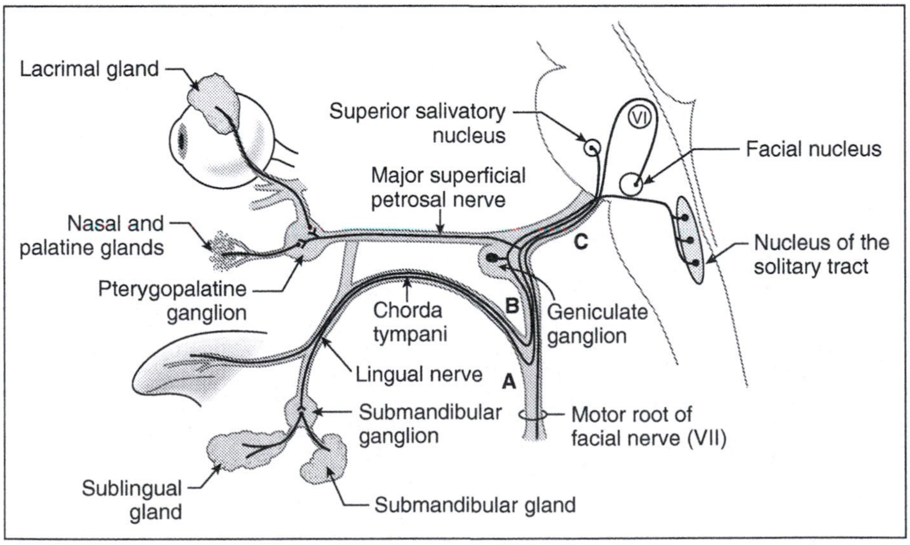

FIG. 5.21. Functional Components of the Facial Nerve. The facial nerve contains fibers connected to the facial nucleus, the nucleus of the solitary tract, and the superior salivatory nucleus. Lesions at the stylomastoid foramen (site A), distal to the geniculate ganglion (site B), or near the cerebellopontine angle (site C) produce different constellations of symptoms as described in the text.

Both the inferior and superior salivatory nuclei are controlled by descending pathways from the hypothalamus, the single most important brain region for coordinating the activities of the autonomic nervous system.

Lesions of the Facial Nerve Fibers. The superior salivatory nucleus and other brainstem nuclei contribute fibers to the facial nerve. Consequently, lesions of the facial nerve or its peripheral branches produce different constellations of symptoms that vary according to the precise location of the lesion (Figure 5.21). A lesion near the stylomastoid foramen, for example, results in Bell's palsy but no other symptoms because only the SVE fibers originating from the facial nucleus are affected. If the lesion occurs near the geniculate ganglion, however, the chorda tympani is likely to be damaged, and Bell's palsy would be accompanied by hyperacusis (paralysis of the stapedius), impaired salivation (loss of GVE fibers innervating the submandibular ganglion), and impaired taste (loss of fibers innervating the anterior two-thirds of the tongue). Finally, if a lesion occurs where the facial nerve enters the brainstem, the lacrimal reflex is lost due to interruption of GVE fibers innervating the pterygopalatine ganglion, and this disturbance accompanies all of the symptoms described above.

Main Sensory Nucleus of the Trigeminal Nerve (GSA—V). The main (or principal) sensory nucleus of the trigeminal nerve lies rostral to the spinal trigeminal nucleus and appears in transverse sections of the pons where the trigeminal nerve pierces the middle cerebellar peduncle (Figure 5.22). The main sensory nucleus receives cutaneous information from the face and, functionally, is considered the cranial equivalent to the posterior column nuclei. Large-diameter, heavily myelinated axons from all three divisions of the trigeminal ganglion enter the pons and terminate on second-order neurons of the main sensory nucleus. The somatotopic organization of the main sensory nucleus of the trigeminal nerve follows the same inverted pattern as the spinal trigeminal nucleus where the maxillary, mandibular, and ophthalmic representations are arranged in a dorsal to ventral sequence.

Secondary trigeminal projections from the main sensory nucleus ascend in two separate pathways to the thalamus (see Figure 5.14). Axons from the ventral part of the main sensory trigeminal nucleus cross the midline and join the cervical representation of the

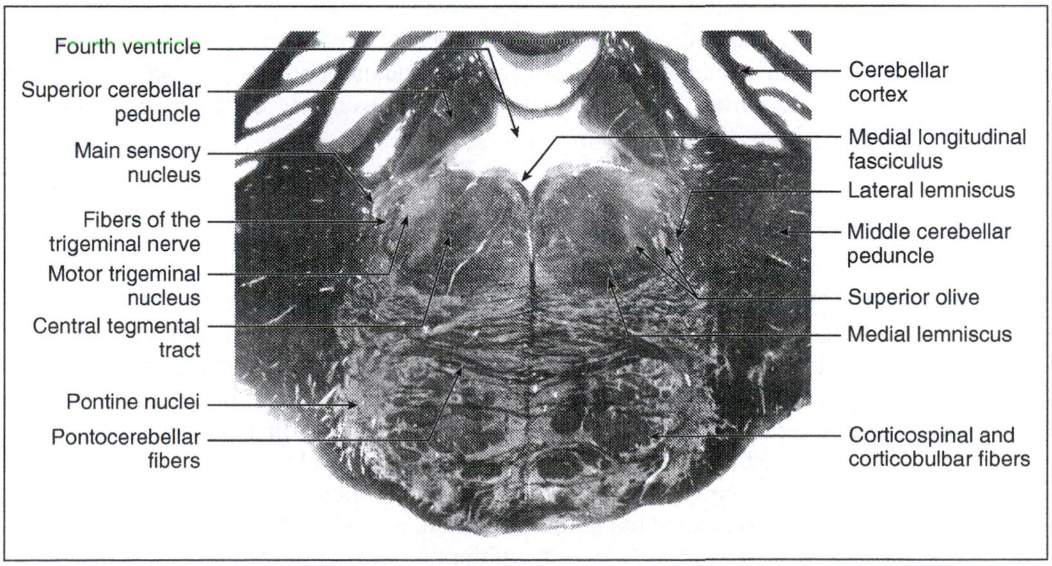

FIG. 5.22. Transverse View of the Mid Pons. This photomicrograph shows the midpontine region of the brainstem surrounded by the cerebellum dorsally and the middle cerebellar peduncles laterally. Trigeminal nerve fibers are seen in proximity to the motor trigeminal and main sensory nuclei.

medial lemniscus as it proceeds to the VPM nucleus in the thalamus. These secondary fibers represent the ventral trigeminothalamic tract, which is slightly separated from the more ventral pain-conveying fibers originating in the spinal trigeminal nucleus. The dorsal part of the main sensory trigeminal nucleus sends a small projection, the dorsal trigeminothalamic tract, to the ipsilateral VPM nucleus so that cutaneous sensations of the mouth and tongue are in register with gustatory sensations that are processed ipsilaterally in adjacent regions of the thalamus. The VPM nucleus projects to the parietal operculum where the conscious sensations of touch and pressure of the face and intraoral cavity are represented.

Tic Douloureux. Sometimes called trigeminal neuralgia, tic douloureux is characterized by repetitive, transient attacks of severe pain afflicting one or more subdivisions of the trigeminal nerve. The etiology of tic douloureux is unknown, but in susceptible individuals, it may be triggered by touching specific parts of the face or by eating. These sensitive areas are called trigger zones. In cases where the pain persists despite the use of analgesic medication, tic douloureux can be treated by cauterizing or chemically destroying the branches of the trigeminal nerve that innervate the trigger zones. Depending on the site of the surgical lesion, the patient may loose tactile sensation in the face, mouth, and cornea (along with loss of the corneal blink reflex) or may experience difficulty in chewing food if the motor component of the trigeminal nerve is affected. In some cases, a medullary tractotomy is performed to destroy the nociceptive fibers of the spinal trigeminal tract without affecting tactile sensitivity.

Motor Trigeminal Nucleus (SVE—V). The motor trigeminal nucleus is a compact group of large neurons located just medial to the main sensory trigeminal nucleus. Cholinergic fibers from the motor trigeminal nucleus emerge as a separate root that travels with the mandibular division of the trigeminal nerve to innervate the muscles of mastication (i.e., masseter, anterior digastric, mylohyoid) and the tensor tympani muscle of the middle ear. Voluntary movements of the mandible are controlled by corticobulbar fibers that project bilaterally from the motor cortex to the motor trigeminal nuclei (see Figure 5.3). Most inputs to the motor trigeminal nucleus, however, are primary afferent fibers of the trigeminal nerve or secondary fibers from the spinal trigeminal nucleus (see Figures 5.14 and 5.15). Other collateral projections from the mesencephalic trigeminal nucleus relay proprioceptive information from the masseter muscle to the motor trigeminal nucleus. This pathway enables masseter muscle spindles to activate the motor trigeminal nucleus and execute the jaw jerk reflex, a monosynaptic stretch reflex elicited by tapping the jaw. The motor trigeminal nucleus also receives auditory inputs that activate the tensor tympani muscle during loud sounds to dampen movements of the malleus and the other bony ossicles of the middle ear.

MIDBRAIN

The midbrain is the smallest subdivision of the brain. The dorsal surface of the midbrain is dominated by separate pairs of elevations that represent the superior and inferior colliculi. The superior colliculi are located more rostrally, just posterior to the pineal gland, and are near the junction between the mesencephalon and diencephalon. The inferior colliculi are located more caudally, and are just rostral to the pair of trochlear nerves (IV) that emerge from the dorsal surface of the midbrain. Collectively, the superior and inferior colliculi are called the midbrain tectum.

The ventral surface of the midbrain is characterized by a massive pair of myelinated fiber tracts, the crus cerebri, that contain descending corticospinal, corticopontine, and corticobulbar fibers. The crus cerebri represent the ventral part of the cerebral peduncles, and they surround a CSF-filled cistern called the interpeduncular fossa. The oculomotor (III) nerves emerge from the interpeduncular fossa as indicated by Figure 5.23.

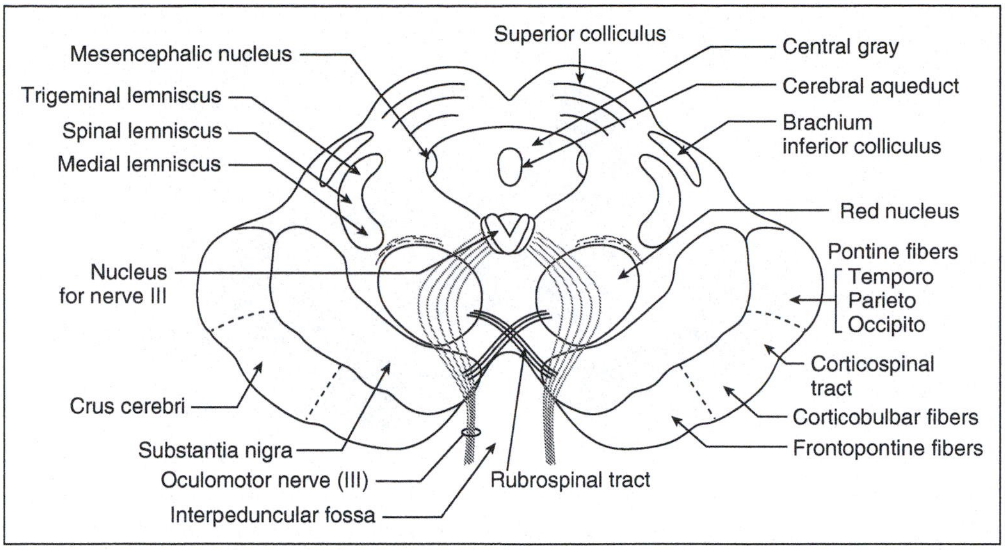

FIG. 5.23. Transverse Organization of the Midbrain. This drawing indicates the position of the major nuclei and fiber tracts in the midbrain at the level of the superior colliculus.

Internal Structures of the Midbrain

Due to its short length, transverse sections through the midbrain are capped by either the inferior or superior colliculi (Figures 5.24 and 5.25). The cerebral aqueduct perforates the midbrain below the tectum and is surrounded by a pale, homogeneous zone called the periaqueductal gray region. At the level of the inferior colliculus, the tegmentum contains fiber tracts such as the lateral and medial lemnisci, the superior cerebellar peduncles, the central tegmental tract, and the MLF. At the level of the superior colliculus, the tegmentum contains prominent nuclei, including the red nucleus, the substantia nigra, and the oculomotor nuclear complex.

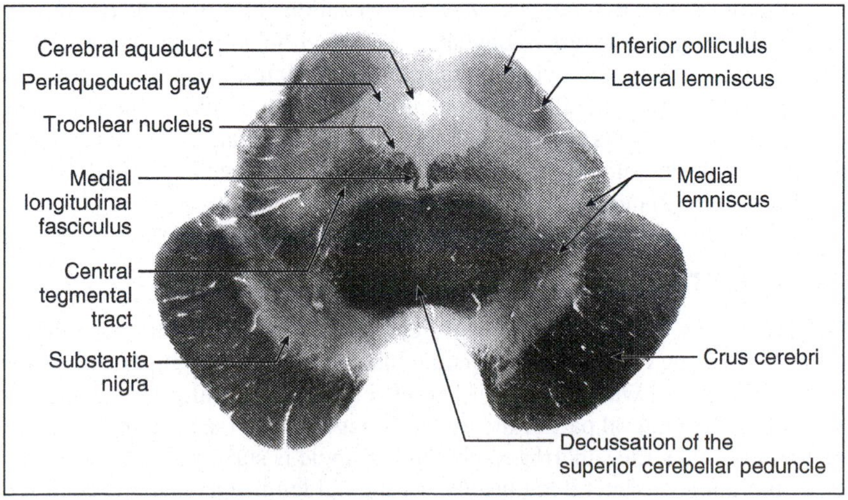

FIG. 5.24. Transverse View of the Caudal Midbrain. The caudal midbrain contains the inferior colliculus and ascending fibers of the lateral lemniscus. The decussating fibers of the superior cerebellar peduncles are prominent in the central part of the tegmentum.

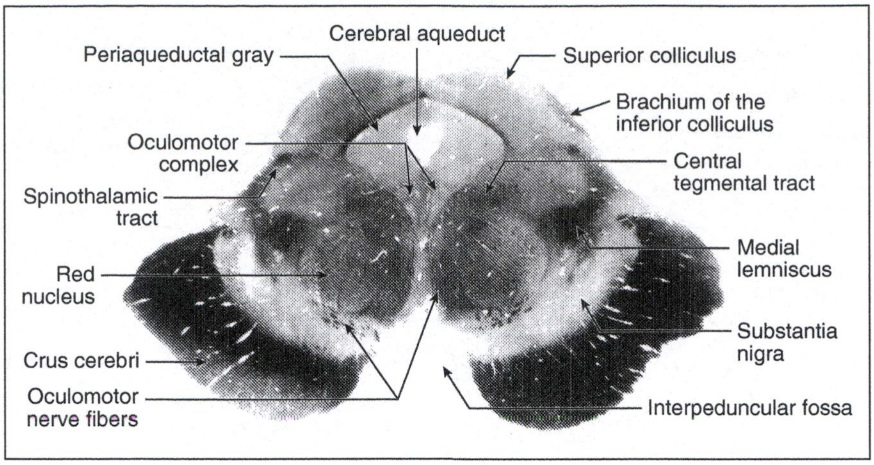

FIG. 5.25. Transverse View of the Rostral Midbrain. The rostral midbrain contains the superior colliculus, the red nucleus, the substantia nigra, and the crus cerebri. The oculomotor complex gives rise to oculomotor nerve fibers that pass through the red nucleus before entering the interpeduncular fossa.

Tectum

The midbrain tectum is sometimes called the quadrigeminal plate after its paired nuclear tenants, the inferior and superior colliculi. Located on the dorsal midbrain, the inferior colliculus receives auditory inputs from several sources in the pons including the cochlear nuclei and the superior olivary nuclei. These ascending projections form the lateral lemniscus, which originates in the caudal pons and engulfs the inferior colliculus at its rostral end (Figure 5.24). The inferior colliculus contains tonotopic representations of the cochlea and plays an important role in sound localization. The inferior colliculus sends most of its output to the medial geniculate nucleus of the thalamus, which in turn projects to the primary auditory cortex in the temporal lobe.

The superior colliculus, which lies rostral to the inferior colliculus, has a distinctive laminated structure when viewed in transverse sections (Figure 5.25). Afferent projections to the superior colliculus originate mainly in the retina (via the optic nerve and tract) and in the primary visual (striate) cortex of the occipital lobe. The upper layers of the superior colliculus detect moving targets and other salient stimuli in the peripheral part of the visual field; the deeper layers initiate and maintain tracking responses of the eyes and head. Consistent with its role in vision, the superior colliculus projects to visual nuclei in the thalamus, such as the lateral geniculate and the pulvinar, and to the prestriate visual cortex. Tracking movements of the head and eyes are mediated by efferent projections from the deeper layers of the superior colliculus to the cervical spinal cord (via the tectospinal tract) and to neurons comprising the PPRF.

Superior Cerebellar Peduncle

The **superior cerebellar peduncle,** which represents the main output pathway for the cerebellum, contains projections to the red nucleus and to the motor nuclei of the thalamus.

With few exceptions, nearly all of the efferent projections from the cerebellum ascend through the brainstem via the superior cerebellar peduncle. The superior cerebellar peduncle forms the lateral wall of the fourth ventricle in the rostral pons before continuing its ascent through the lateral part of the midbrain tegmentum (see Figures 5.22 and 5.24). In the caudal midbrain, the superior cerebellar peduncle is surrounded by other ascending fiber tracts, including the lateral lemniscus, the medial lemniscus, and the central tegmental tract. Further rostrally, at the level of the inferior colliculus, the fibers of the superior cerebellar peduncle decussate within the tegmentum and continue their ascent toward the red nucleus. Nearly a third of the crossed fibers of the superior cerebellar peduncle terminate in the red nucleus, whereas the remainder surround the red nucleus and proceed further rostrally to the ventrolateral thalamus, which projects to the motor cortex. Hence, the superior cerebellar peduncle represents the pathway by which processed information from the cerebellum reaches the red nucleus and the motor parts of the thalamus.

Periaqueductal Gray

The periaqueductal gray consists of densely packed cells surrounding the cerebral aqueduct. Although the periaqueductal gray has a uniform appearance in myelin-stained sections, it contains distinct clusters of neurons that use serotonin, enkephalin, endorphins, or other neuropeptides. Opiate receptors are densely distributed in specific parts of the periaqueductal gray, and this underscores the importance of this area in processing nociceptive information. The periaqueductal gray projects to specific parts of the reticular formation that are clinically important because they modulate nociceptive transmission in the dorsal horn of the spinal cord. Thus, many clinical studies show that electrical stimulation of the periaqueductal gray effectively ameliorates chronic pain.

Red Nucleus

The red nucleus is named after its ruddy appearance in a freshly cut brain. Located dorsal to the substantia nigra, the red nucleus is virtually encapsulated by the myelinated fibers of the superior cerebellar peduncle and the central tegmental tract. As part of the motor system, the red nucleus receives inputs from the motor cortex and sends descending projections to the ventral horn of the spinal cord via the rubrospinal tract. In addition, the red nucleus receives ascending projections from the deep cerebellar nuclei and sends descending projections to the inferior olivary nucleus via the central tegmental tract. Thus, the red nucleus is part of a larger network of feedforward and feedback pathways involved in motor control. Lesions of the red nucleus produce tremor and ataxia (lack of motor coordination) in the contralateral body, especially in the lower limbs during walking.

Substantia Nigra

The substantia nigra is located in the rostral half of the midbrain where it forms a thick nucleus along the dorsal margin of the crus cerebri. The substantia nigra is composed of two distinct layers: a ventral pars reticulata and a dorsal pars compacta. The pars reticulata contains small neurons that project to the superior colliculus and parts of the thalamus. The pars compacta is a darkly pigmented region that contains large dopaminergic neurons, which project almost exclusively to the basal ganglia, a forebrain region involved in sensorimotor integration and other aspects of motor control. The dopaminergic neurons of the substantia nigra degenerate during Parkinson's disease, a serious motor disorder characterized by rigidity, tremor at rest, and difficulty with initiating movements.

Crus Cerebri

Located on the ventral surface of the midbrain, the crus cerebri represent massive bundles of corticofugal fibers that have descended through the internal capsule and will terminate in the pons, medulla, or spinal cord. Corticospinal fibers originate mainly from the motor and parietal cortical areas and travel through the central part of the crus cerebri before collecting into the more compact pyramidal tract in the caudal pons and medulla. Corticobulbar fibers also descend through the central part of the crus cerebri, and then leave this region to terminate within specific nuclei at different levels of the brainstem. Some corticobulbar fibers innervate sensory nuclei, but most project to the motor nuclei that control the eyes, face, mouth, tongue, and larynx. The corticopontine fibers, which are located on the medial and lateral extremes of the crus cerebri, descend only as far as the pons.

Cranial Nerve Nuclei of the Midbrain

The midbrain tegmentum contains only two cranial nerve nuclei: the trochlear nucleus and the oculomotor complex. Both of these nuclei contain lower motor neurons that control the muscles associated with the eye.

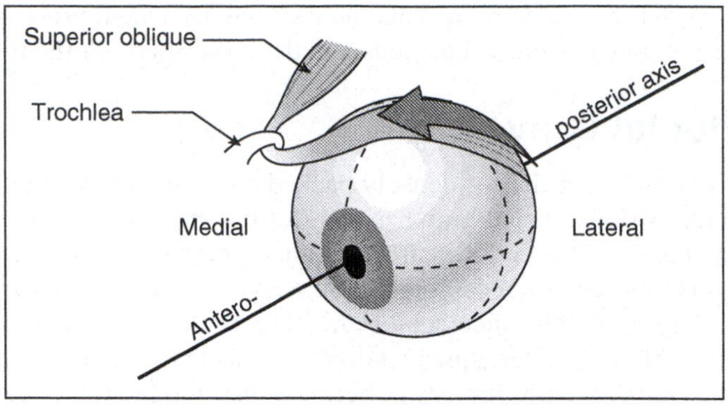

FIG. 5.26. Actions of the Superior Oblique. The superior oblique muscle passes through a bony loop, the trochlea, and attaches to the superior surface of the eyeball. Contraction of the superior oblique causes the top of the eye to rotate toward the nasal side (intortion) while simultaneously moving downward and slightly lateral. (Source: Adapted with permission from Wilson-Pauwels L, et al: *Cranial Nerves—Anatomy and Clinical Comments.* Toronto, Ontario: BC Decker, 1988:46.)

The **trochlear nucleus** innervates the superior oblique muscle.

Trochlear Nucleus (GSE—IV). The trochlear nucleus is a small oval-shaped structure that lies embedded in the MLF at the level of the inferior colliculus. Its cholinergic fibers exit the nucleus dorsally, cross the midline through the superior medullary velum, and then emerge from the dorsal surface of the midbrain immediately behind the inferior colliculus. Each trochlear nerve innervates the contralateral superior oblique muscle, which produces intortion (top of eye rotates toward the nose) and downward-lateral movements of the eyeball (Figure 5.26). To mediate voluntary contraction of the superior oblique muscle, corticobulbar fibers synapse on neurons in the adjacent reticular formation that project to the trochlear nucleus. The trochlear nucleus also receives vestibular inputs that ascend through the MLF to coordinate contractions of the superior oblique muscle with head movements.

The trochlear nerve has the longest intracranial course of all the cranial nerves and, consequently, is highly vulnerable to injury. The trochlear nerve passes around the lateral aspect of the midbrain and proceeds, with the oculomotor nerve, between the posterior cerebral and superior cerebellar arteries. Aneurysms of either of these arteries may compress or stretch the trochlear nerve. Such insults cause ocular extortion (i.e., top of the eye deviates away from midline) and impair the ability to look downward. Patients with trochlear nerve damage report difficulty in climbing down stairs, and they may compensate for ocular extortion by tilting their head toward the unaffected eye to bring the denervated eye into proper alignment (Figure 5.27).

Oculomotor Complex (GSE and GVE—III). The oculomotor complex is a collection of paired subnuclei that form a V-shaped cell column straddling the midline of the rostral midbrain. Among the subnuclei that give rise to GSE fibers, three project ipsilaterally (the dorsal, intermediate, and ventral nuclei), and one projects contralaterally (the medial nucleus). The central nucleus, which is located on the midline, innervates the levator palpebrae bilaterally, and this explains why both eyes usually blink simultaneously.

Specific subnuclei within the **oculomotor complex** innervate the medial rectus, inferior rectus, superior rectus, inferior oblique, and levator palpebra muscles.

The cholinergic GSE fibers of the oculomotor complex course ventrally through parts of the red nucleus before exiting the brain at the interpeduncular fossa. Each GSE subnucleus innervates a specific extraocular muscle (medial rectus, superior rectus, inferior rectus, inferior oblique) to produce eye movements in several directions (Figures 5.28 and 5.29). Their coordinated activities, in concert with the trochlear and abducens nuclei, enable each eye with a full range of movement.

One part of the oculomotor complex, the Edinger-Westphal nucleus, is composed of preganglionic parasympathetic neurons whose GVE fibers project to the ciliary ganglion. Postganglionic projections to the ciliary body and pupillary sphincter control the shape of

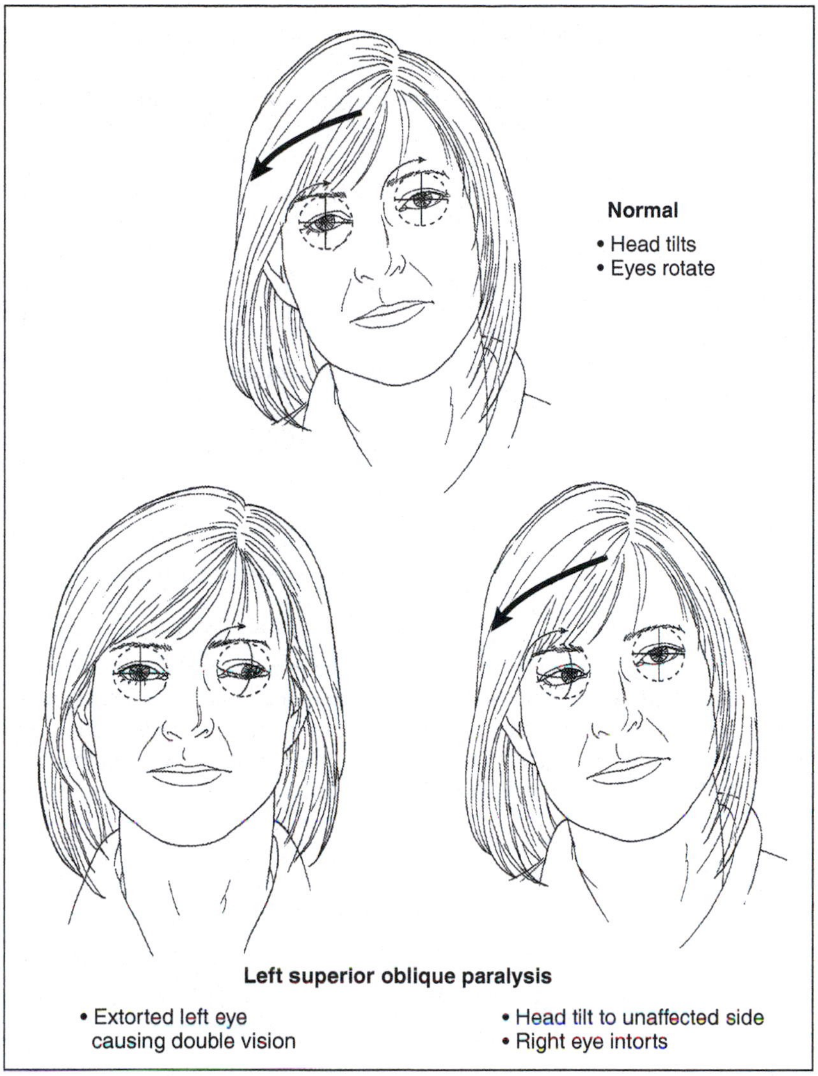

FIG. 5.27. Effects of Trochlear Nerve Damage. When the head is tilted to the side, both eyes rotate around the anteroposterior axis to maintain a vertical image on the retina. Paralysis of the superior oblique muscle causes ocular extortion, and the patient compensates by tilting the head in the opposite direction. (Source: Adapted with permission from Wilson-Pauwels L, et al: *Cranial Nerves—Anatomy and Clinical Comments*. Toronto, Ontario: BC Decker, 1988:47.)

the lens and size of the pupil, respectively. Muscle contractions in the ciliary body allow the lens to change shape so that light is refracted to a greater extent during visual fixation on nearby objects. Simultaneous contraction of the annular muscle of the pupillary sphincter causes pupillary constriction, which decreases the amount of light entering the eye. These processes occur automatically as part of the accommodation-convergence reaction when ocular fixation is shifted from distant to nearby objects. Other components of the visual system are responsible for coordinating the medial recti muscles of both eyes to produce ocular convergence.

Oculomotor Ophthalmoplegia

A complete lesion of the oculomotor nerve produces a well-defined constellation of neurologic symptoms called oculomotor ophthalmoplegia (Figure 5.30). The most obvious sign of oculomotor nerve damage is ptosis (drooping eyelid) due to paralysis of the levator palpebral muscle. A patient may attempt to compensate for ptosis by contracting the frontalis muscle to raise the eyelid. If the eyelid is gently raised during the clinical

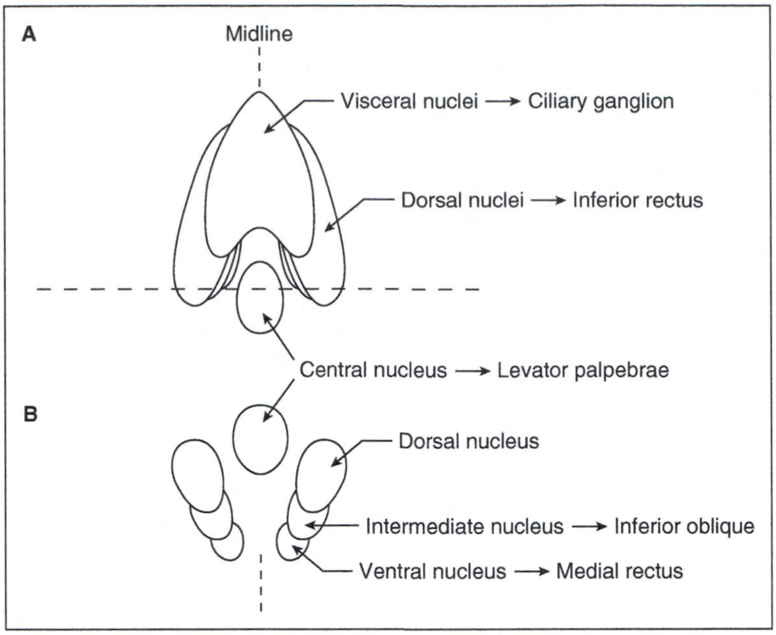

FIG. 5.28. The Oculomotor Complex. The oculomotor complex is a collection of subnuclei that innervate specific sets of extraocular muscles. (A) Horizontal view of the subnuclei within the oculomotor complex and their peripheral targets. (B) Coronal view of the oculomotor complex at the level indicated by the dashed line in panel A.

FIG. 5.29. Eye Movements Controlled by the Oculomotor Complex. This diagram shows four extraocular muscles, innervated by the oculomotor nerve, that cause the eye to adduct, gaze downward or upward, or extort. (Source: Reprinted with permission from Wilson-Pauwels L, et al: *Cranial Nerves—Anatomy and Clinical Comments*. Toronto, Ontario: BC Decker, 1988:33.)

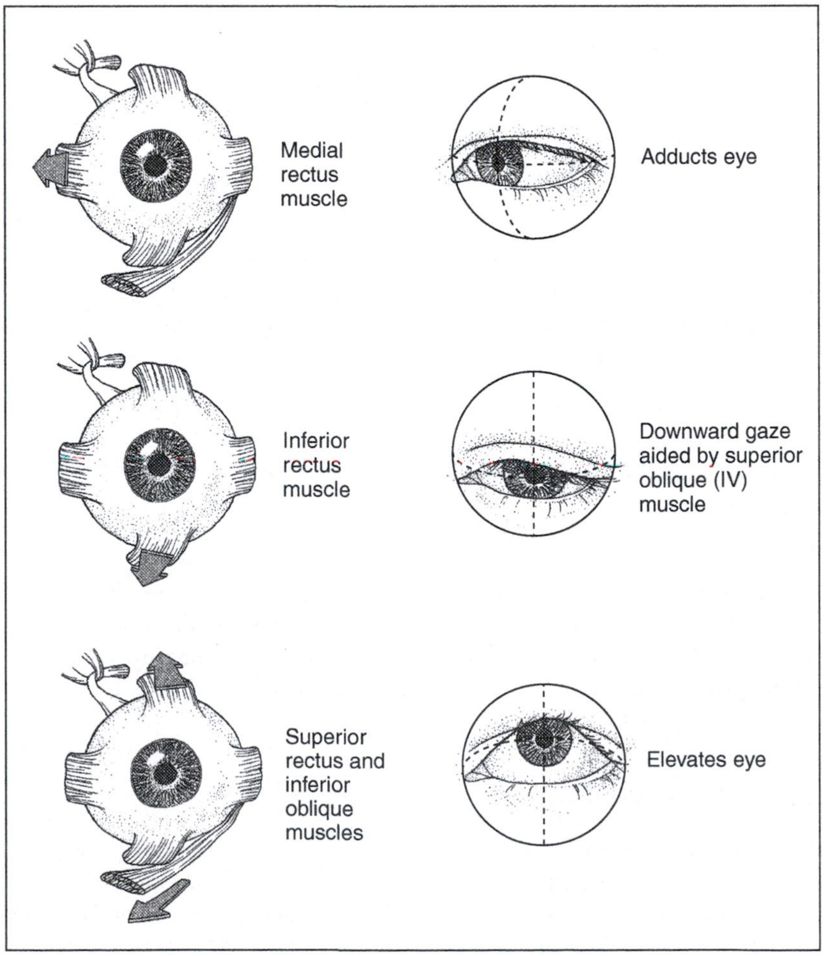

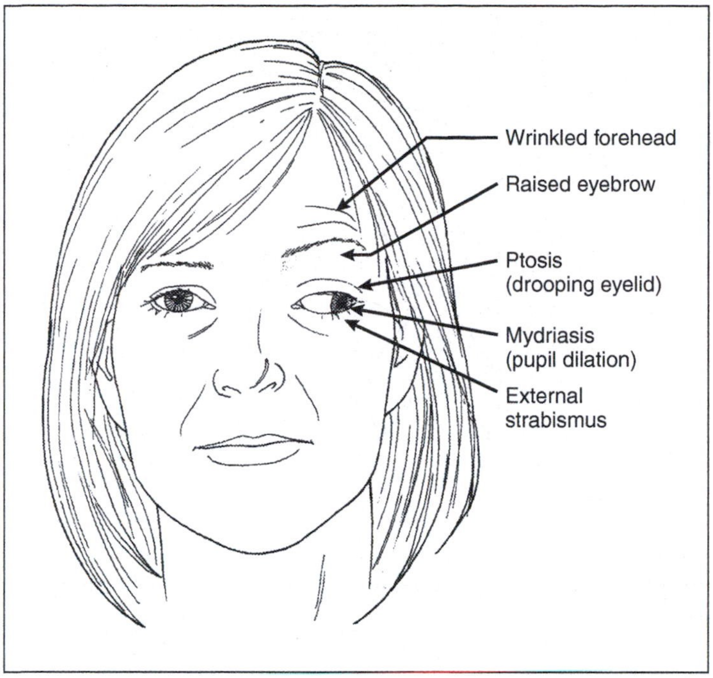

FIG. 5.30. Oculomotor Ophthalmoplegia. A lesion of the oculomotor nerve causes ptosis, mydriasis, and external strabismus. (Source: Reprinted with permission from Wilson-Pauwels L, et al: *Cranial Nerves—Anatomy and Clinical Comments*. Toronto, Ontario: BC Decker, 1988:39.)

examination, it is possible to see that the patient's eye is strongly abducted and directed downward because the tonic activities of the lateral rectus and superior oblique muscles are unopposed after the remaining extraocular muscles are paralyzed. Although external strabismus is present in oculomotor ophthalmoplegia, most patients do not experience diplopia because the drooping eyelid covers the affected eye. Finally, damage to the GVE fibers of the Edinger-Westphal nucleus causes mydriasis (pupillary dilation) due to loss of muscle tone in the pupillary sphincter and the unopposed sympathetic activation of the dilator muscles in the iris. Ocular ophthalmoplegia is often caused by compression of the oculomotor nerve produced by aneurysms of the posterior cerebral or superior cerebellar arteries.

Pupillary Light Reflex

The Edinger-Westphal nucleus and its neuronal connections are essential for constricting both pupils during increased illumination. This response, known as the pupillary light reflex, is demonstrated by flashing a light in one eye and observing the immediate constriction of the pupil in that eye (direct light reflex) and in the contralateral eye (consensual light reflex). These responses are mediated by serial connections from the retina to the midbrain and back to the eye. Although most projections from the retina terminate in the thalamus, some retinal neurons project to the pretectal olivary nucleus, which lies rostral and lateral to the superior colliculus (Figure 5.31). Reciprocal projections through the posterior commissure link the pretectal regions on each side of the midbrain. The pretectal olivary nuclei also project bilaterally to the Edinger-Westphal nuclei, which project to the ciliary ganglia. Postganglionic neurons in the ciliary ganglion innervate the pupillary sphincter, which constricts the diameter of the pupil. Hence, the pupillary light reflex is clinically significant because it provides a simple method for testing the integrity of the optic and oculomotor nerves and their central connections.

Loss of the **pupillary light reflex** indicates an insult to the optic nerve, the pretectal region, the Edinger-Westphal nucleus, or the oculomotor nerve.

A lesion of the optic nerve causes blindness in the affected eye and abolishes the direct and consensual pupillary light reflexes if light is flashed into the affected eye. If both optic nerves are intact, damage to the visceral motor fibers innervating the ciliary ganglion on one side causes an ipsilateral loss of the direct light reflex but does not interfere with the consensual reflex in the contralateral eye.

Loss of the pupillary light reflex can be produced by anything that increases intracranial pressure, including a tumor, an abscess, or an epidural hematoma caused by a blow

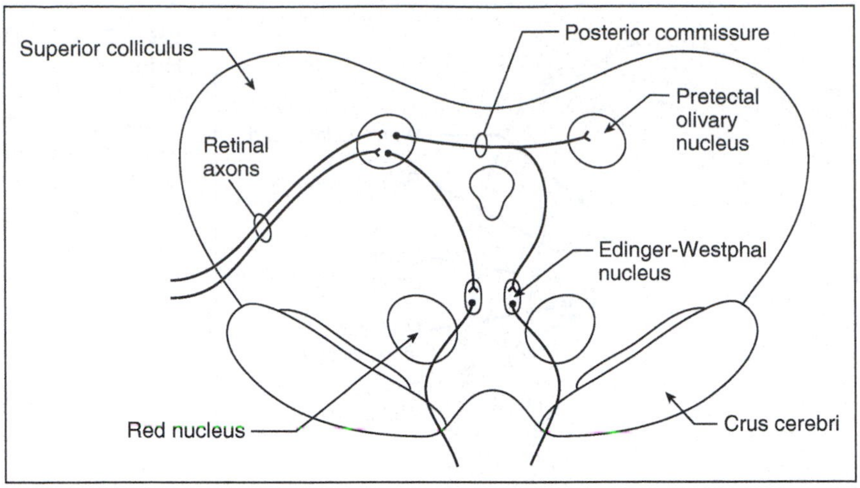

FIG. 5.31. The Pretectal Nuclei. The pretectal nuclei receive direct projections from the retina and, in turn, project bilaterally to the Edinger-Westphal nuclei, which send fibers through the oculomotor nerve to the ciliary ganglion.

to the head. When intracranial pressure increases, the uncus of the temporal lobe herniates into the tentorial notch and compresses or stretches the third cranial nerve as it travels along the medial side of the uncus and parahippocampal gyrus (Figure 5.32).

Argyll-Robertson Pupil

An Argyll-Robertson pupil is characterized by a small pupil that does not respond to light directed into the eye. Nonetheless, the pupil still exhibits an accommodation-convergence reaction (i.e., the pupil becomes smaller as the eyes converge). The intact convergence response indicates that the oculomotor nerve is intact and suggests that loss of the pupillary light reflex is caused by damage to the afferent limb of the reflex circuit, not the GVE fibers emerging from the Edinger-Westphal nucleus. Often the exact site of damage cannot be determined; in these cases the Argyll-Robertson pupil is probably caused by lesions in the pretectal region surrounding the posterior commissure.

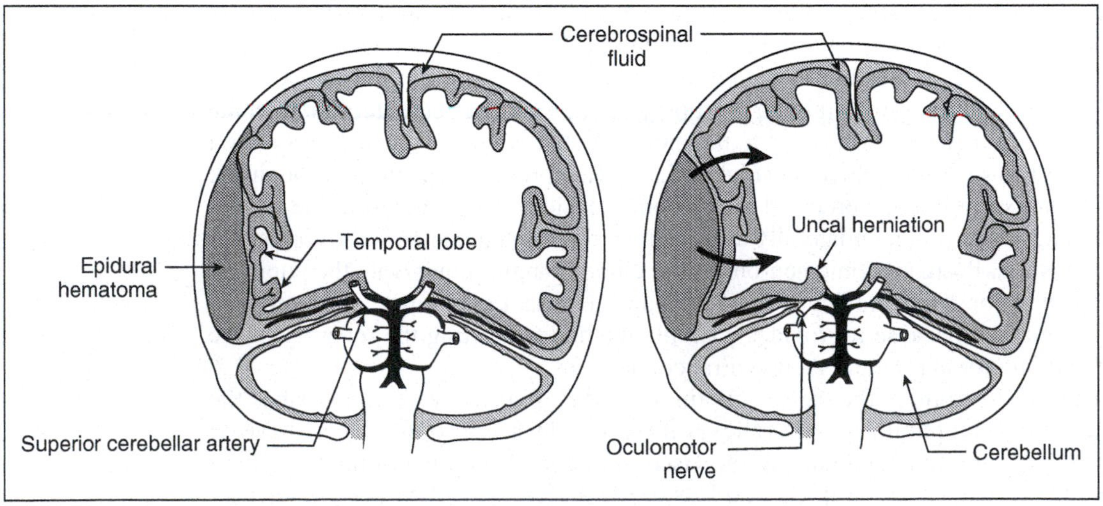

FIG. 5.32. Epidural Hematoma. (A) Trauma to the head may cause intracranial bleeding, which compresses the underlying brain. (B) Eventually, the uncus herniates through the tentorial notch and causes compression of the oculomotor nerve.

Horner's Syndrome

Horner's syndrome is characterized by miosis (small pupil), enophthalmos (sunken eye), and ptosis (a partially drooping eyelid due to loss of innervation of the superior and inferior tarsal muscles). If the lesion responsible for Horner's syndrome is preganglionic, the patient will also have anhidrosis (dryness of the skin on the ipsilateral side of the face). Lesions that cause Horner's syndrome may occur at many locations, but they always involve damage to some part of the autonomic nervous system. For example, this syndrome can be caused by lesions in the dorsolateral tegmentum that damage the autonomic fibers descending from the hypothalamus. Further caudally, damage either to the lateral horn of the cervical spinal cord or to the sympathetic preganglionic and postganglionic fibers of the superior cervical ganglion may also cause Horner's syndrome.

Horner's syndrome is caused by a loss of sympathetic innervation and results in miosis, pseudoptosis, enophthalmos, and anhidrosis.

Superior Alternating Hemiplegia

Vascular lesions involving the medial part of the cerebral peduncle may destroy the oculomotor nerve roots (lower motor neuron) as well as descending corticospinal and corticobulbar fibers (upper motor neuron). Thus, as shown in Figure 5.33, occlusion of tributaries emerging from either the posterior cerebral or superior cerebellar arteries may cause contralateral hemiparesis of the limb and facial muscles accompanied by ipsilateral oculomotor ophthalmoplegia. This set of symptoms is known as superior alternating hemiplegia because the lesion occurs in the rostral brainstem (superior) and the resulting motor deficits (including hemiplegia) affect the ipsilateral eye and the contralateral body (alternating).

Superior alternating hemiplegia is a combination of ophthalmoplegia and contralateral hemiparesis.

Benedikt's Syndrome

In Benedikt's syndrome, the lesion site involves the red nucleus and surrounding fibers of the superior cerebellar peduncle (Figure 5.33). Nearby fibers of the medial lemniscus and spinothalamic tracts are usually affected, and in some instances the lesion may damage descending fibers of the oculomotor nerve. Benedikt's syndrome is characterized by contralateral hyperkinesia, tremor, and ataxia. All of these symptoms are associated with cerebellar dysfunction caused by interruption of the ascending fibers of the superior cerebellar peduncle. Patients with this disorder may also lose cutaneous and deep sensations if the medial lemniscus is damaged or may show ophthalmoplegia if the oculomotor nerve is affected.

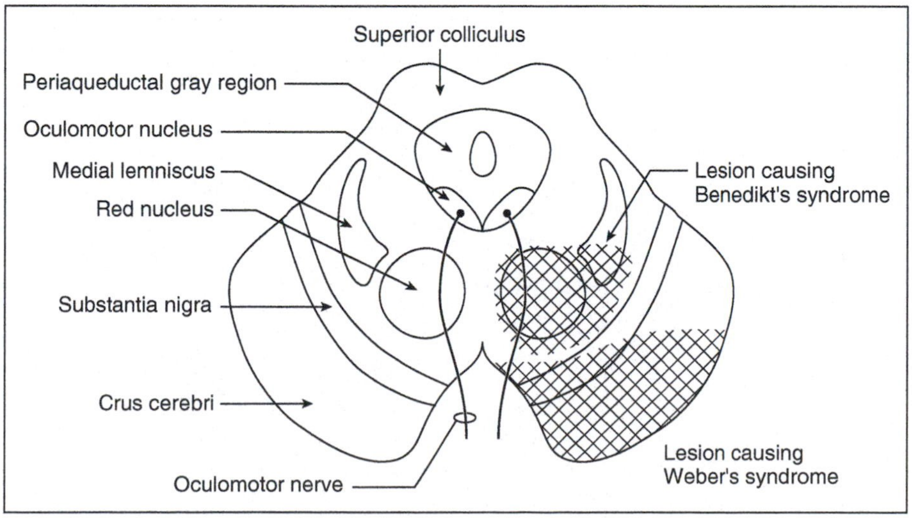

FIG. 5.33. Lesion Sites in the Midbrain. The cross-hatching indicates sites that are damaged in Benedikt's syndrome and in superior alternating hemiplegia.

RETICULAR FORMATION

The reticular formation is an extensive network of neurons in poorly differentiated nuclei that are dispersed throughout the brainstem tegmentum. Its location in the central core of the brainstem allows the reticular formation to monitor and integrate information from several brain regions involved in sensory, visceral, and limbic functions. Unlike most systems in the brainstem, however, the reticular formation is not topographically organized. Instead, it has diffuse ascending and descending projections that influence all levels of the neuraxis. Indeed, the reticular formation plays a critical role in the control of autonomic functions, the modulation of pain and muscular reflexes, and the regulation of consciousness, sleep, and behavioral arousal.

Anatomic Organization of the Reticular Formation

Initially, the term "reticular formation" was used only to indicate the diffuse network of neuronal connections that reside in the brainstem tegmentum but lie outside the well-defined cranial nerve nuclei. Although this concept remains valid to some degree, many reticular formation neurons extend beyond this classically defined region. Neurons in the reticular formation exhibit considerable diversity in their morphology, and their axons may ascend or descend long distances and send collateral projections to many parts of the neuraxis including the thalamus, cerebellum, and spinal cord. As shown by Figure 5.34, axons of some reticular formation neurons may even bifurcate into separate ascending and descending branches. Hence, it is clear that the reticular formation has an influence on widespread regions of the brain

Many neurons in the reticular formation have long dendrites that extend radially from the soma, often in a plane that is orthogonal to the longitudinal axis of the brainstem. This spatial configuration enhances the ability of these neurons to sample ascending neural inputs throughout the brainstem, and this is consistent with electrophysiologic recordings showing that neurons in the reticular formation respond to many sensory modalities.

Although the reticular formation is anatomically divided into many nuclei, conceptually it is organized into three major cell columns extending longitudinally through the brainstem and a fourth set of scattered nuclei that project to the cerebellum (Figure 5.35). The columnar organization of the reticular formation is represented by the following groups: (1) a midline group of raphe nuclei, (2) nuclei in the parasagittal medial zone, and (3) nuclei in the parasagittal lateral zone.

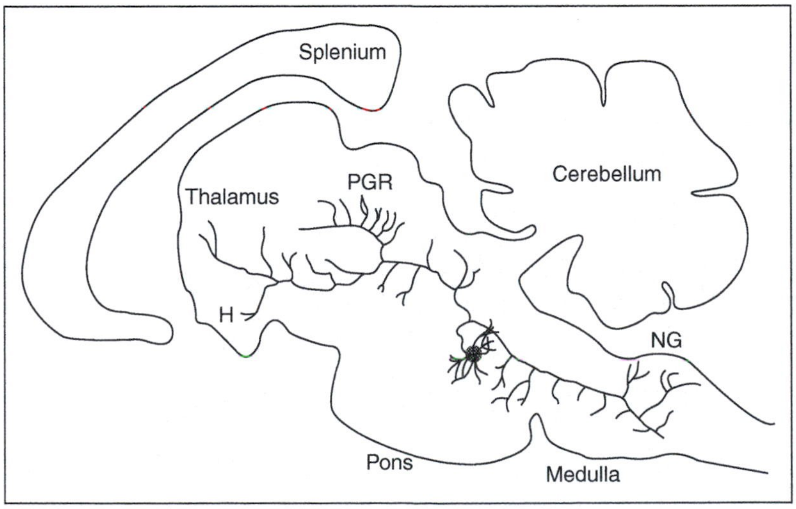

FIG. 5.34. Cellular Connections in the Reticular Formation. An example of a neuron in the reticular formation with collateral projections to the nucleus gracilis (NG), the periaqueductal gray region (PGR), the thalamus, and the hypothalamus (H).

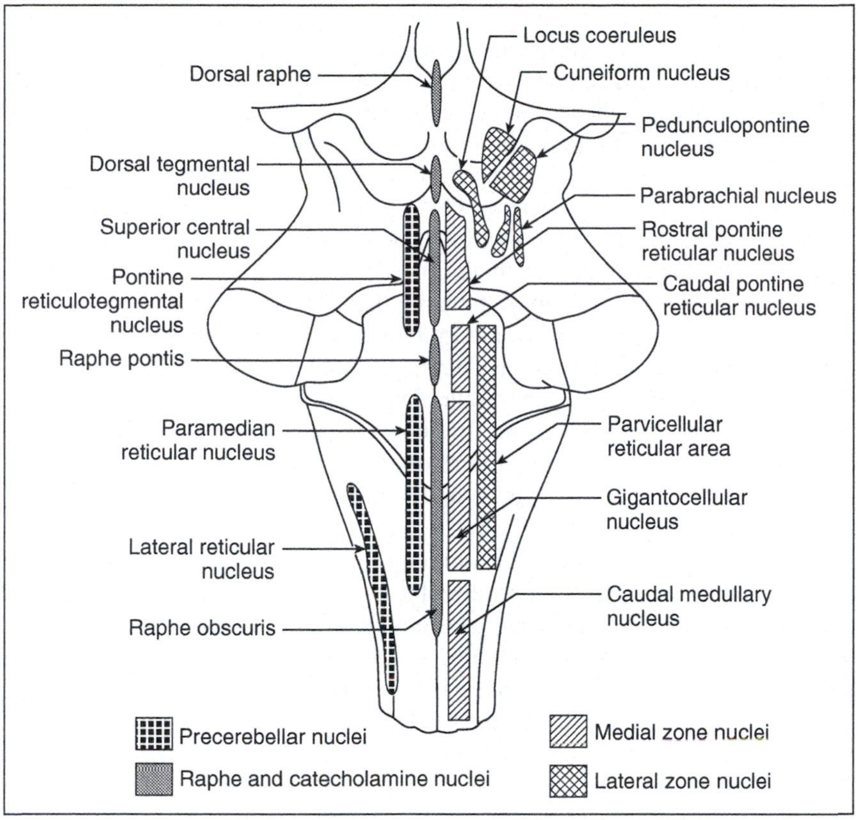

FIG. 5.35. Overview of the Reticular Formation. This diagram shows the location of the raphe nuclei, the medial nuclei, the lateral nuclei, and the precerebellar nuclei as indicated by the legend.

Raphe Nuclei. The raphe nuclei form a thin group of cells that lie in and around the midline seam of the tegmentum. Most raphe nuclei are composed of serotonergic cells, although some contain neuropeptides such as cholecystokinin. Many raphe neurons have long axons that ascend as far as the cerebral cortex or descend the length of the spinal cord. The raphe nuclei are divided into a rostral group located in the rostral pons and midbrain and a caudal group located in the caudal pons and medulla.

The raphe nuclei, which lie on the midline of the brainstem tegmentum, contain serotonergic and peptidergic neurons that project to widespread parts of the neuraxis.

The caudal raphe nuclei contain three separate neuronal populations: the raphe obscurus, the raphe pallidus, and the raphe magnus. These groups receive ascending somatosensory inputs from the spinal cord, the dorsal column nuclei, and the trigeminal nuclei, as well as descending inputs from the periaqueductal gray. Many of the ascending projections convey information related to the nociceptive qualities of a somatosensory stimulus. Complementing this role, the raphe magnus has descending projections to the spinal cord that may modulate nociceptive transmission in the dorsal horn.

The rostral raphe nuclei are composed of the raphe pontis, the superior central nucleus, the dorsal tegmental nucleus, and the dorsal nucleus of the raphe. These nuclei are involved in regulating forebrain activity, but their precise functions are not entirely understood. The raphe pontis projects to the cerebellum, whereas the other raphe nuclei project rostrally through the median forebrain bundle to the hippocampus, limbic cortex, substantia nigra, thalamus, neostriatum, and cerebral cortex. Neurons in the rostral raphe nuclei exhibit distinct discharge patterns that are highly correlated with the different stages of sleep and arousal (see Chapter 15).

Medial Reticular Zone. The medial zone is located just lateral to the raphe nuclei and includes the medial two-thirds of the reticular formation. Most of the ascending and descending projections from the reticular formation pass through the medial zone, which includes the nucleus gigantocellularis (in the medulla), the nucleus reticularis pontis (subdivided into oral and caudal parts in the pons), and the cuneiform and subcuneiform nuclei (in the midbrain). Neurons in the medial nuclei are large and have extensive dendritic and axonal arborizations, and they receive inputs mainly from the lateral reticular zone, which is activated largely by sensory modalities of a somatic or visceral origin.

The **medial reticular zone** is the effector or motor part of the reticular formation. The **lateral reticular zone** is the afferent or sensory part of the reticular formation.

Medial zone neurons have long ascending and descending axons that give off collateral projections to other parts of the reticular formation, the cranial nerve nuclei, the intralaminar nuclei of the thalamus, and the spinal cord. These connections, especially those to specific motor nuclei in the spinal cord and brainstem, suggest that the medial zone acts as the "effector" or motor part of the reticular formation.

Ascending projections from the medial zone of the reticular formation form the bulk of the ascending reticular activating system. This system ascends through the central tegmental tract and terminates in the intralaminar nuclei of the thalamus, which do not receive direct inputs from separate sensory modalities. This is consistent with the fact that the intralaminar nuclei are the only group of thalamic nuclei that have diffuse projections to all lobes of the cerebral cortex. Electrical stimulation of the intralaminar nuclei or of the reticular activating system will awaken a sleeping animal. Conversely, bilateral damage to the central tegmental tract or to the intralaminar thalamic nuclei produces an irreversible state of coma. This does not mean that consciousness resides in the reticular activating system, but that the conscious activities of the cerebral cortex depend on widespread excitatory influences from the thalamus and other subcortical regions.

There are two descending projections from the medial reticular zone that exert a powerful influence on spinal reflexes, muscle tone, and motor activity. The medullary reticulospinal tract arises from the gigantocellular reticular nucleus, descends bilaterally in the ventral part of the lateral funiculus, and terminates on interneurons in laminae VII and IX. The medullary reticulospinal system inhibits muscle tone and decreases the amplitude of myotactic reflexes. By comparison, the pontine reticulospinal system arises from the nucleus reticularis pontis, descends through the MLF in the anterior funiculus, and terminates on interneurons in laminae VII and VIII. Electrical stimulation of the pontine reticulospinal system increases the muscle tone of the antigravity muscles and facilitates spinal reflexes. Thus, the medullary and pontine reticulospinal systems have antagonistic roles that balance the inhibitory and excitatory influences on spinal circuits.

The reticulospinal tracts receive direct innervation from the cerebral cortex and may provide an alternative to the pyramidal tract for sending motor commands to spinal motor neurons. Infants born without cerebral hemispheres (anencephaly) are capable of executing simple movements such as yawning, suckling, and orienting; presumably, these actions are mediated by the reticulospinal tracts and other descending projections from the brainstem. Consistent with this view, animals whose brainstems have been transected at the midcollicular level can still display postural changes or periodic limb movements that resemble walking.

Lateral Reticular Zone. The lateral zone of the reticular formation receives sensory information used to mediate cranial nerve reflexes and basic visceral functions. This lateral zone is located in the lateral third of the tegmentum, just medial to the spinal trigeminal system (in the medulla and pons) and the superior cerebellar peduncle (in the midbrain). The lateral reticular zone includes the parvicellular nucleus (in the medulla and pons), the parabrachial nucleus (in the pons), and the pedunculopontine nucleus (in the pons). The parvicellular region is composed of small neurons that receive inputs from axonal collaterals of the ascending spinothalamic, trigeminothalamic, auditory, and vestibular pathways. The parvicellular region projects to the medial reticular zone and to the raphe nuclei, whose descending projections modulate sensory transmission and ascending projections maintain arousal. The parabrachial nuclei receive afferent projections from the caudal, visceral part of the solitary nucleus. Finally, the pedunculopontine nucleus has major projections to the substantia nigra, subthalamic nucleus, motor cortex, and raphe nuclei, all of which play an important role in motor functions.

Cerebellar Relay Nuclei

Some nuclei in the reticular formation, such as the paramedian and lateral reticular nuclei in the medulla and the reticulotegmental nucleus in the pons, project almost exclusively to the cerebellum. The lateral reticular nucleus lies dorsal to the inferior olivary nuclei and receives inputs from spinoreticular fibers, spinothalamic collaterals, and the red nucleus.

The lateral reticular nucleus projects to the cerebellum, via the inferior cerebellar peduncle, to form a part of the mossy fiber projection system. The paramedian nucleus is located near the medullary midline and receives inputs from both the cerebellum and the cerebral cortex. The reticulotegmental nucleus is located in the paramedian region of the pons (between the medial lemnisci) and receives projections from the cerebral cortex and deep cerebellar nuclei. Because these nuclei project to the cerebellum, they probably play a role in motor control, but their exact functions are unknown.

Locus Ceruleus

The group of pigmented neurons in the ventrolateral part of the periaqueductal gray that appear as a bluish spot in the freshly sectioned brain is known as the locus ceruleus (or blue spot). This nucleus contains a homogeneous group of neurons that use norepinephrine as a neurotransmitter. Neurons in the locus ceruleus innervate every level of the neuraxis from the spinal cord to the cerebral cortex. Some of the ascending axons project to a single target such as the hippocampus, but most have divergent collaterals with widely distributed terminals in the diencephalon and cerebral cortex. The diffuse noradrenergic projections from the locus ceruleus resemble the serotonergic innervation pattern of the raphe nuclei, and some evidence indicates that these neurotransmitter systems complement each other. Because its efferent projections are so widely distributed, the locus ceruleus does not relay specific information, but rather it increases the overall excitability of its postsynaptic targets in order to modulate attention and general arousal.

The **locus ceruleus** is located in the lateral part of the periaqueductal gray and uses norepinehrine to regulate arousal and attention.

RESOLUTION OF CLINICAL CASE

When conducting a neurologic examination, it is important to pay special attention to symptoms affecting opposite sides of the body because such signs are invaluable for determining the precise location of a lesion, tumor, or other event affecting the nervous system. In the clinical case presented in this chapter, decreased pain sensitivity on the right face and on the left side of the body suggest a lesion that affects both the spinothalamic tract (contralateral body) and the adjacent spinal trigeminal nucleus (ipsilateral face). Damage to the spinal trigeminal nucleus would also cause an ipsilateral loss of the corneal reflex. These symptoms are classic signs of the lateral medullary syndrome and, based on the patient's high blood pressure and other medical history, indicate that the patient has probably experienced a stroke affecting either the vertebral or posterior inferior cerebellar arteries. These arteries supply blood to many nuclei and fiber tracts in the lateral medulla, and a decrease in the blood supply to these structures can produce this constellation of symptoms. Hence, dizziness could be caused by damage to the vestibular nuclei, whereas dysphonia and a drooping soft palate would indicate that the nucleus ambiguus was affected. In addition, pseudoptosis (a partially drooping eyelid), miosis (small pupil), and anhidrosis (lack of perspiration) on one side of the face would indicate a loss of sympathetic innervation caused by the interruption of descending autonomic pathways in the lateral medulla.

REVIEW QUESTIONS

Directions: For each of the following questions, choose the **one best** answer.

1. The presence of ptosis, mydriasis, and external strabismus on one side of the face indicates a lesion of which cranial nerve?
   A. Abducens nerve
   B. Trochlear nerve
   C. Oculomotor nerve
   D. Facial nerve
   E. Optic nerve

2. Which of the following conditions is characterized by symptoms on only one side of the body?
   A. Lateral gaze paralysis
   B. Bell's palsy
   C. Superior alternating hemiplegia
   D. Inferior alternating hemiplegia
   E. Lateral medullary syndrome

3. A unilateral lesion of the medial longitudinal fasciculus (MLF) produces what?
   A. Lateral gaze paralysis
   B. Internal strabismus
   C. Impairment of convergent eye movements
   D. Dissociation of conjugate eye movements
   E. Ptosis
4. What nerve is damaged if the gag reflex is absent?
   A. Glossopharyngeal nerve
   B. Trigeminal nerve
   C. Facial nerve
   D. Spinal accessory nerve
   E. Hypoglossal nerve
5. What medullary structure remains intact following occlusion of the posterior inferior cerebellar artery?
   A. Spinothalamic tract
   B. Spinal trigeminal nucleus
   C. Hypoglossal nerve
   D. Nucleus ambiguus
   E. Nucleus solitarius
6. What function is mediated by the caudal half of the solitary nucleus?
   A. Sense of taste
   B. Saliva production
   C. Arterial baroreception
   D. Peristalsis of the esophagus
   E. Reflexive movements of the larynx during swallowing
7. The lower muscles of facial expression are paralyzed in a patient on one side. Corneal and gag reflexes are present, however, and lacrimation and salivation remain normal. What neural structure is most likely to be damaged?
   A. Facial nerve
   B. Internal capsule
   C. Hypoglossal nerve
   D. Motor trigeminal nucleus
   E. Red nucleus
8. Which pair of structures could be affected by a single focal lesion?
   A. Superior olive and inferior olive
   B. Facial nucleus and motor trigeminal nucleus
   C. Abducens nerve and spinothalamic tract
   D. Medial lemniscus and hypoglossal nerve
   E. Hypoglossal nucleus and facial nerve
9. Select the fiber system and nucleus that are associated with each other.
   A. Red nucleus—inferior cerebellar peduncle
   B. Lateral cuneate nucleus—medial lemniscus
   C. Abducens nucleus—medial longitudinal fasciculus
   D. Superior olive—spinotectal tract
   E. Inferior colliculus—central tegmental tract
10. Which pair of brainstem nuclei mediate a specific reflex?
   A. Spinal trigeminal and vestibular
   B. Abducens and facial
   C. Vestibular and salivatory
   D. Oculomotor and hypoglossal
   E. Spinal trigeminal and ambiguous

ADDITIONAL READING

Classic Literature

Carlsson A, Falck B, Hillarp NA: Cellular localization of brain monoamines, *Acta Physiol Scand* 56 (suppl 196):1–28, 1962.

Scheibel ME, Scheibel AB: On circuit patterns of the brain stem reticular core. *Ann N Y Acad Sci* 89:857–865, 1961.

Reviews and Landmark Research Papers

Baker KG, Tork I, Hornyung JP, Halasz P: The human locus coeruleus complex: an immunohistochemical and three-dimensional reconstruction study. *Exp Brain Res* 77:257–270, 1989.

Beckstead RM, Norgren R: An autoradiographic examination of the central distribution of the trigeminal, facial, glossopharyngeal and vagal nerves in the monkey. *J Comp Neurol* 184:455–472, 1979.

Brodal A: *Neurological Anatomy in Relation to Clinical Medicine*, 3rd ed. New York, NY: Oxford University Press, 1981:448–577.

Bronstein AM, Morris J, DuBoulay G, Gresty MA, Rudge P: Abnormalities of horizontal gaze. Clinical, oculographic and magnetic resonance imaging findings. I. Abducens palsy. *J Neurol Neurosurg Psychiatry* 53:194–199, 1990.

Carpenter MB, Carleton SC: Abducens internuclear neurons and their role in conjugate horizontal gaze. *J Comp Neurol* 189:191–209, 1980.

Dubner R, Bennett GJ: Spinal and trigeminal mechanisms of nociception. *Ann Rev Neurosci* 6:381–418, 1983.

Fromm GH: Trigeminal neuralgia and related disorders. *Neurol Clin* 7:305–319, 1989.

Jacobs BL, Azmitia EC: Structure and function of the brain serotonin system. *Physiol Rev* 72:165–229, 1992.

Jean A: Brain stem control of swallowing: neuronal network and cellular mechanisms. *Physiol Rev* 81:871, 2001.

Kinomura S, Larsson J, Gulyas B, Roland PE: Activation by attention of the human reticular formation and thalamic intralaminar nuclei. *Science* 271:512–515, 1996.

Mesulam M-M, Geula C, Bothwell MA, Hersh LB: Human reticular formation: cholinergic neurons of the pedunculopontine and laterodorsal tegmental nuclei and some cytochemical comparisons to forebrain cholinergic neurons. *J Comp Neurol* 281:611–633, 1989.

Moore RY, Bloom FE: Central catecholamine neuron systems: anatomy and physiology of the norepinephrine and epinephrine systems. *Ann Rev Neurosci* 2:113–168, 1979.

Morecraft RJ, Louie JL, Herrick JL, Stilwell-Morecraft KS: Cortical Innervation of the facial nucleus in the non-human primate: a new interpretation of the effects of stroke and related subtotal brain trauma on the muscles of facial expression. *Brain* 124:176–208, 2001.

Rowland LP: Treatment of Bell's palsy. *New Engl J Med* 287:1298–1299, 1972.

Savoiardo M, Bracchi M, Passerini A, Visciani A: The vascular territories in the cerebellum and brainstem: CT and MR study. *Amer J Neuroradiol* 8:199–209, 1987.

Sears ES, Franklin GM: Diseases of the cranial nerves. In *The Science and Practice of Clinical Medicine,* vol 5. New York, NY: Grune & Stratton, 1980:471–494.

Soni SR: Aneurysms of the posterior communicating artery and oculomotor paresis. *J Neurol Neurosurg Psychiatry* 37:475–484, 1974.

Steriade M, McCarley RW: *Brainstem Control of Wakefulness and Sleep*, New York, NY: Plenum Press, 1990.

Wilson-Pauwels L, Akesson EJ, Stewart PA: *Cranial Nerves: Anatomy and Clinical Comments*. Toronto, Ontario: BC Decker, 1988.

INTERNET RESOURCES

Bell's Palsy Research Foundation
http://www.bellspalsy.com/

Digital Anatomist Project
http://www9.biostr.washington.edu/da.html

Global Anatomy
Cranial Nerve Review
http://www.neuroanatomy.wisc.edu/cn/cn.htm

Neuroanatomy and Neuropathology on the Internet
A Searchable Directory for Medical Students, Residents, and Other Health Professionals
http://www.neuropat.dote.hu/

Temple University
Neuroanatomy Lab Resource Appendices
http://courses.temple.edu/neuroanatomy/lab/index.htm

Heal-National Digital Library
The Neurologic Exam
http://www.healcentral.org/services/servicesFeatures.jsp

Trigeminal Neuralgia Association
http://www.tna-support.org/

Uniformed Services University of the Health Sciences
Cranial Nerves
http://rad.usuhs.mil/cranial_nerves/

University of Florida
The Brain Stem and Cerebellum
http://medinfo.ufl.edu/year2/neuro/review/bsc.html

University of Utah
NeuroLogic Exam
http://library.med.utah.edu.neurologicexam/html/home_exam.html

Washington University
Neuroscience Tutorial
http://thalamus.wustl.edu/course/

The Whole Brain Atlas
http://www.med.harvard.edu/AANLIB/home.html

Yale University
Cranial Nerves
http://info.med.yale.edu/caim/cnerves/

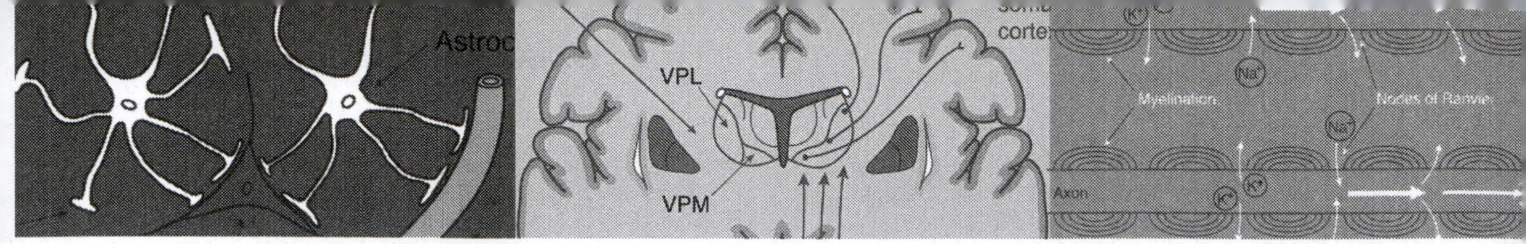

CHAPTER 6

Thalamocortical Organization

INTRODUCTION OF CLINICAL CASE

The emergency medical service was called to the home of a 79-year-old woman who had fallen and could not get up. The paramedics determined that the patient was unable to move her left arm and leg: preliminary diagnosis by the on-call physician was a stroke of the right middle cerebral artery. She was transported to the emergency department of the local hospital where a full series of computed tomography (CT) scans was conducted. Carotid and vertebral angiograms were performed the following day. During the neurologic examination she was clearheaded and cooperative. After checking the patient's vital signs, the attending physician asked her to move her left arm. Surprisingly, she protested that she had no left arm. The physician encountered the same reaction when he asked the patient to move her left leg, even though she obligingly moved her right arm and leg when asked. Testing the patient's sense of fine touch met with similar results: cooperative and accurate reports when stroking the right limbs and obstinate denial that either of her left limbs existed.

THALAMUS

The thalamus is an egg-shaped structure that forms the core of the diencephalon (Figure 6.1A–F). From its rostral border at the interventricular foramen to its caudal boundary at the posterior commissure, the thalamus makes up the wall of the third ventricle dorsal to the hypothalamic sulcus. The dorsal surface of the thalamus forms the floor of the lateral

FIG. 6.1A–E. Photomicrographs of the Human Thalamus (Weigert Stain). Figure 6.1F shows the plane of section for the slides shown in Figures 6.1A–E.

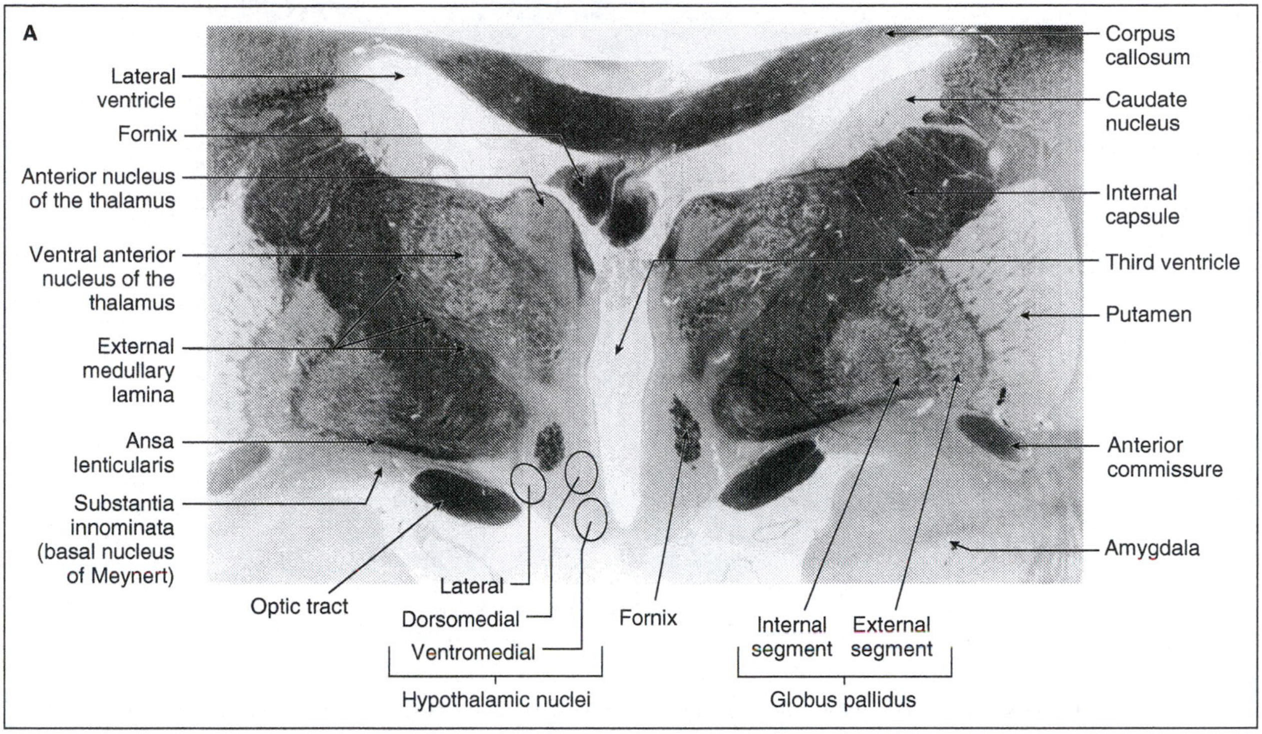

FIG. 6.1A. Coronal Section through the Rostral Thalamus at the Level of the Anterior Thalamic Nucleus.

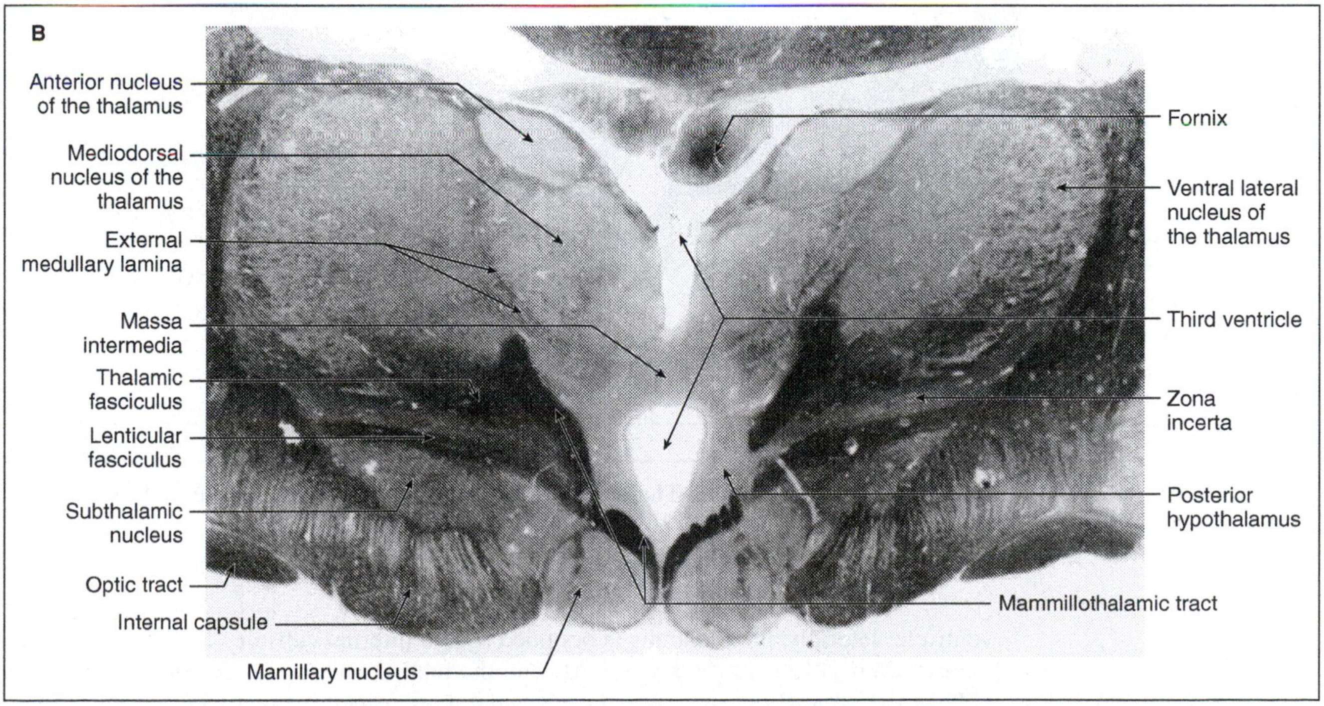

FIG. 6.1B. Coronal Section through the Thalamus at the Level of the Mediodorsal Nucleus.

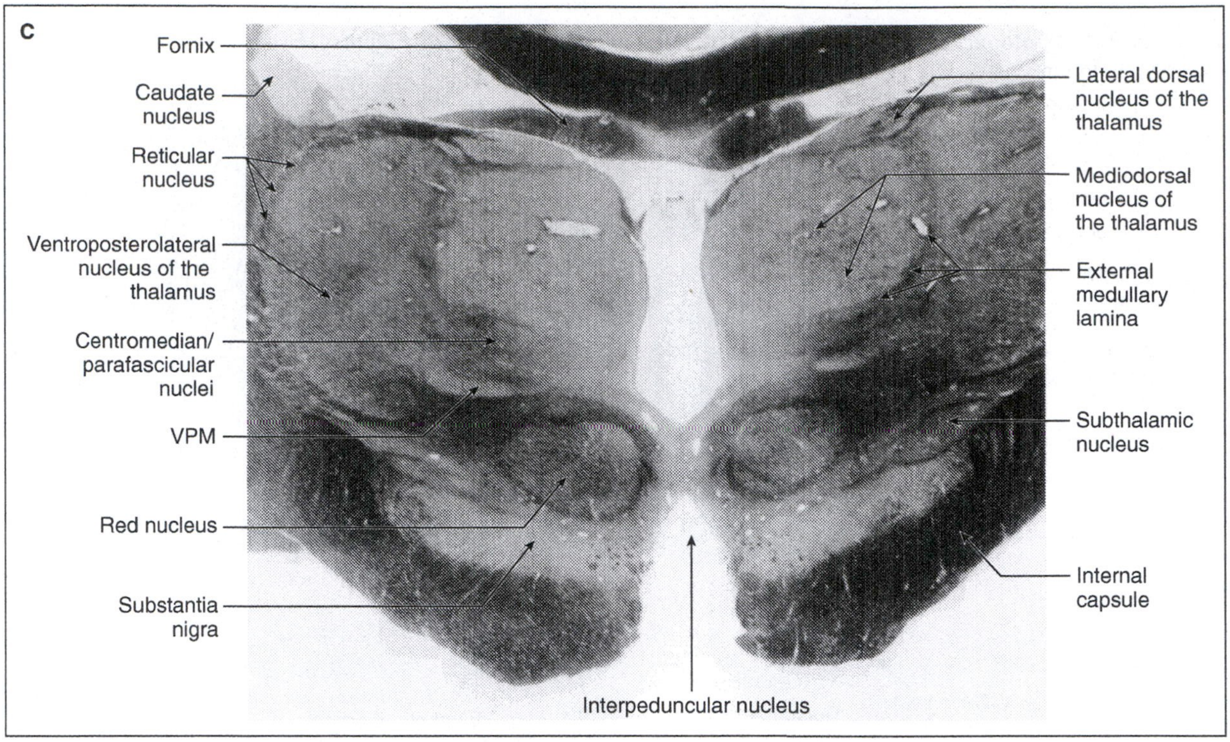

FIG. 6.1C. Coronal Section through the Thalamus near the Rostral Limit of the Ventral Posterior Nucleus. Ventroposterolateral nucleus = VPL; Ventroposteromedial nucleus = VPM.

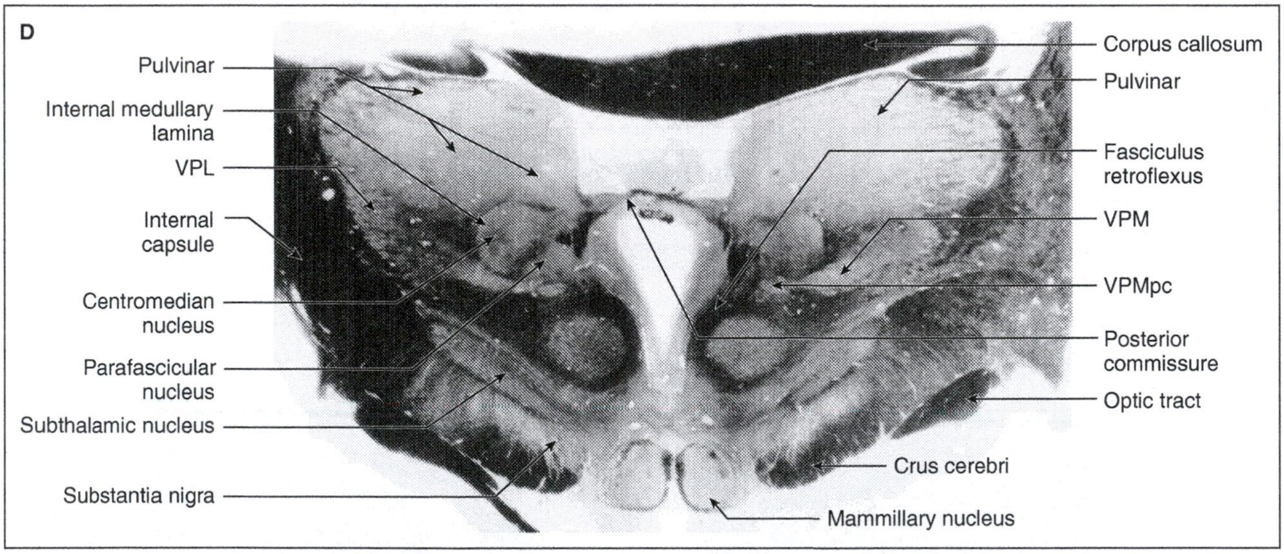

FIG. 6.1D. Near-Coronal Section through the Caudal Thalamus. VPL = ventroposterolateral nucleus; VPM = ventroposteromedial nucleus; VPMpc = parvicellular division of the VPM nucleus.

The **massa intermedia** also is called the interthalamic adhesion.

ventricle; laterally, the thalamus is bounded by the internal capsule. The caudal pole of the thalamus is formed by the pulvinar and the medial and lateral geniculate nuclei. In 80% of the population, the left and right thalami are joined by a narrow cellular bridge, the massa intermedia. There is no advantage or disadvantage conferred by having a massa intermedia.

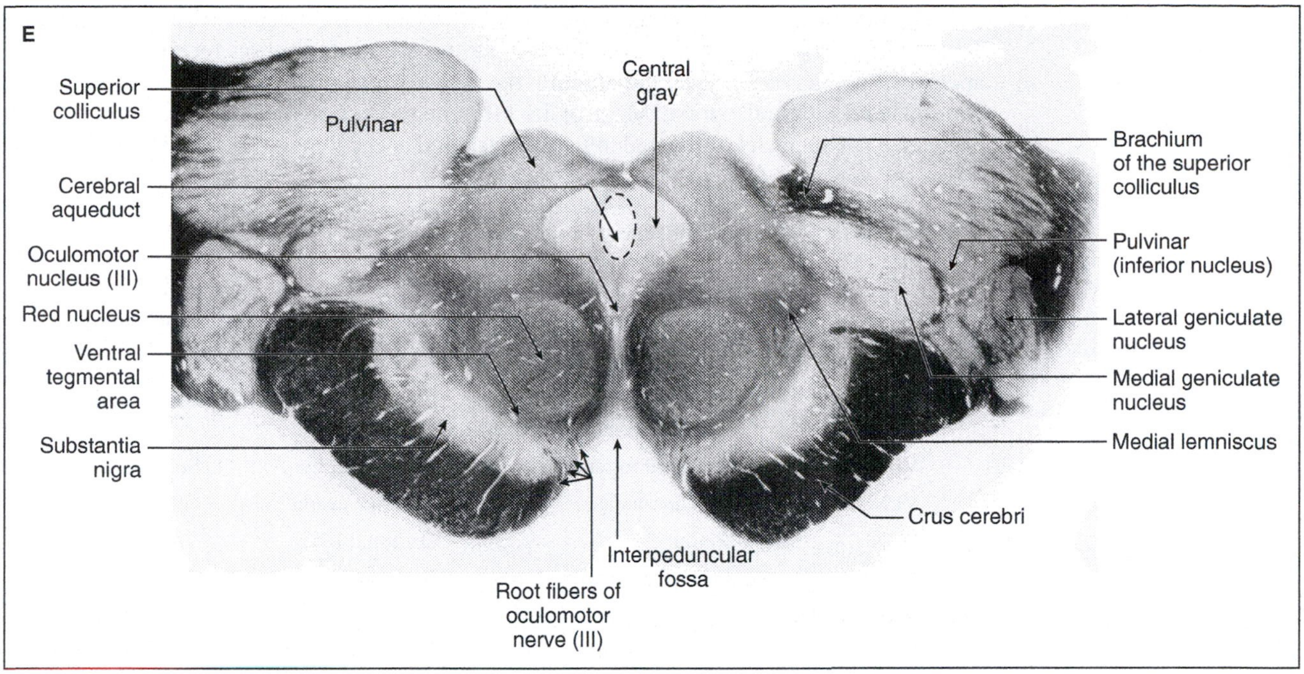

FIG. 6.1E. Near-Coronal Section through the Diencephalic-Mesencephalic Junction.

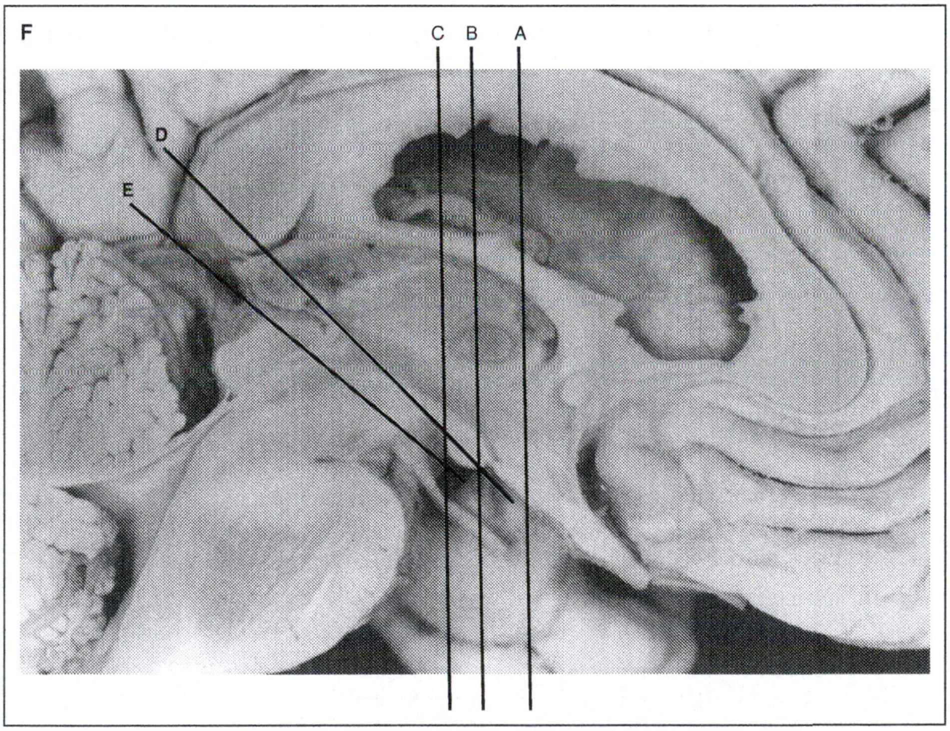

FIG. 6.1F. Midsagittal Section of the Brain Showing Planes of Section for Figures 6.1A–E.

The key landmark for understanding the organization of the thalamic nuclei is the internal medullary lamina, which divides the thalamus into anterior, medial, and lateral parts. The lateral division of the thalamus is further divided into dorsal and ventral parts. Within the caudal third of the thalamus, the internal medullary lamina splits and encapsulates several of the nonspecific nuclei, collectively known as the intralaminar nuclei (Figure 6.1D).

The **internal medullary lamina** is a key thalamic landmark.

The thalamus plays an integral role in motor, sensory, limbic, and vegetative functions. To perform these diverse functions, the thalamus uses information received from many areas of the nervous system including the spinal cord, brainstem, cerebellum, basal ganglia, and cerebral cortex. Most of its efferent projections are to the cerebral cortex (Table 6.1). The nuclei of the thalamus are classified according to their cortical projections,

TABLE 6.1 Afferent and Efferent Projections of the Major Thalamic Nuclei

Nucleus	Afferent Projections	Efferent Projections	Function
Sensory relay nuclei			
VPL	Dorsal column nuclei Spinal trigeminal nucleus	Postcentral gyrus	Somesthesis
VPM	Principal trigeminal nucleus	Postcentral gyrus	Somesthesis
VPMpc	Solitary nucleus	Anterior insula	Gustation
LGN	Retina	Occipital lobe	Vision
MGN	Inferior colliculus	Temporal lobe	Audition
Motor relay nuclei			
VA	Globus pallidus Substantia nigra	Frontal cortex Frontal eye fields	Motor planning Directed eye movements
VLo	Substantia nigra Globus pallidus	Prefrontal cortex	Motor planning
VLc	Cerebellum	Precentral gyrus	Motor accuracy
VPLo	Cerebellum	Precentral gyrus	Motor accuracy
Association nuclei			
Anterior	Mammillary nucleus	Cingulate gyrus	Memory
MD	Amygdala Parabrachial nucleus Substantia nigra Frontal cortex	Frontal cortex Frontal eye fields	Emotion/affect Olfaction Pain
LD	Hypothalamus	Cingulate gyrus	Autonomic correlates of emotion
LP	Superior colliculus	Parietal assoc. cortex	Vision
Posterior nucleus	Spinal trigeminal nucleus	Insula Cingulate gyrus Parietal and temporal association cortex	Pain
Pulvinar	Superior colliculus	Parietal, occipital, and temporal cortex	Vision
Nonspecific nuclei			
CL	Parabrachial nucleus	Cerebral cortex	Pain
CM/PF complex	Motor/premotor cortex Basal ganglia Reticular formation	Cerebral cortex Striatum	Motor integration
Midline nuclei	Reticular formation	Entire cortex	Arousal
Reticular nucleus	Cortex Thalamic relay nuclei	Thalamic relay nuclei	Selective attention EEG synchrony

Note. VPL = ventroposterolateral nucleus; VPM = ventroposteromedial nucleus; VPMpc = ventroposteromedial nucleus, parvicellular part; LGN = lateral geniculate nucleus; MGN = medial geniculate nucleus; VA = ventral anterior nucleus; VLo = ventral lateral nucleus, pars oralis; VLc = ventral lateral nucleus, pars caudalis; VPLo = ventral posterolateral nucleus, pars oralis; MD = mediodorsal nucleus; LD = lateral dorsal nucleus; LP = lateral posterior nucleus; CL = central lateral nucleus; CM/PF = centromedian/parafascicular complex; EEG = electroencephalogram.

functions, and relative location. Based on their cortical projections, the thalamus is divisible into specific sensory relay nuclei, motor relay nuclei, association nuclei, nonspecific nuclei, and intrinsic nuclei.

The specific sensory relay nuclei receive ascending projections from the somatosensory, auditory, visual, and gustatory systems and send dense projections to circumscribed areas of the cerebral cortex. By definition, the areas of the cerebral cortex that receive direct projections from the specific sensory relay nuclei are called primary sensory cortices (e.g., primary visual cortex). The motor relay nuclei receive projections from the cerebellum and basal ganglia, and like the specific sensory relay nuclei, they send axons to specific cortical areas. The thalamic association nuclei, by comparison, receive multimodal information and project to widespread association areas of the frontal and parietal lobes. By comparison, the cortical projections of the intralaminar nuclei are both diffuse and nonspecific, but they play a vital role in attention. The reticular nucleus is classified as an intrinsic nucleus because its projections remain within the thalamus.

Anterior Thalamic Nucleus

The anterior thalamic nucleus forms the anterior tubercle, which protrudes into the lateral ventricle near the interventricular foramen. Because the anterior nucleus is partially encased by the rostral part of the internal medullary lamina, it is one of the more easily recognized nuclei in the thalamus (see Figure 6.1A, B). The anterior nucleus is a key link between the limbic system and the cerebral cortex. Its largest afferent projection, the mammillothalamic tract, originates in the mammillary nucleus of the hypothalamus. Other important afferent projections from the medial temporal lobe and hippocampus arrive via the fornix. Degeneration of the anterior thalamic nucleus, often in combination with the mammillary nuclei, is the hallmark of Korsakoff's psychosis. Patients with Korsakoff's psychosis compensate for their inability to remember recent events by confabulating stories using memories from the remote past.

The **anterior tubercle** is the bulge of the anterior thalamic nuclei into the lateral ventricle.

The **anterior thalamic nuclei** form the thalamic link of the limbic system.

Medial Thalamic Nuclei

The medial thalamic nuclei include the mediodorsal (MD) nucleus and a half dozen other nuclei adjacent to the midline, some of which form the massa intermedia (see Figure 6.1B, C). The MD nucleus consists of a dorsolateral parvicellular division, a medial magnocellular division, and a thin paralaminar division pressed against the internal medullary lamina. The parvicellular division has extensive reciprocal connections with the rostral part of the frontal cortex. Patients with damage to the parvicellular MD demonstrate a flat emotional tone, transient memory loss, and anterograde amnesia (see Chapter 14). Prefrontal lobotomies, which are no longer performed, involved surgical disconnection of the MD nucleus from the frontal lobe. The magnocellular division receives afferent projections from the amygdala, the basal nucleus of Meynert, and the olfactory regions located in the temporal lobe. Olfactory information projects to the orbitofrontal cortex. By contrast, the paralaminar MD nucleus receives ascending projections from the substantia nigra and the pontine parabrachial nuclei and plays a role in eye movement and pain perception.

The **medial thalamic nuclei** project heavily to the frontal lobe.

Other nuclei in the medial thalamus represent the rostral continuation of the brainstem central gray. Like the central gray, these small and poorly differentiated regions of the medial thalamus are involved in vegetative functions. The medial thalamic nuclei receive afferent projections from numerous brainstem nuclei including the nucleus of the solitary tract, the pontine parabrachial nuclei, the periaqueductal gray, the raphe nuclei, and the locus ceruleus. The medial nuclei have weak but widespread projections to the cerebral cortex. Other projections from the medial thalamus to the amygdala and the basal ganglia link the autonomic nervous system with areas of the brain involved with emotion, memory, and movement.

Lateral Thalamic Nuclei

The lateral thalamus is divided into dorsal and ventral tiers. Whereas the dorsal tier nuclei are among the least understood nuclei in the thalamus, the ventral tier consists of specific sensory and motor nuclei whose functions are among the best understood.

The **pulvinar** is the thalamic link in the extrageniculate pathway

Dorsal Tier Nuclei. The dorsal thalamus includes, from rostral to caudal, the lateral dorsal (LD), the lateral posterior (LP), and the pulvinar nuclei (see Figure 6.1C–E). Like the anterior nucleus, the LD nucleus is encapsulated, receives projections from the mammillary nucleus, the temporal lobe, and the hippocampal formation, and projects to the cingulate gyrus. The LP nucleus, which lies posterior to the LD nucleus, is more closely aligned with its caudal neighbor, the pulvinar. The pulvinar, the largest thalamic nucleus, is located at the junction between the diencephalon and mesencephalon, dorsal to the medial and lateral geniculate nuclei. Most of the pulvinar's afferent projections originate in the superficial layers of the superior colliculus and primary occipital cortex. The pulvinar is the thalamic relay in the extrageniculate visual pathway, which projects to widespread areas of the occipital, parietal, and temporal lobes.

VA & VLo (basal ganglia); VLc & VPLo (cerebellum)

Ventral Tier Nuclei. Based on functional and connectional criteria, the ventral tier consists of three nuclei: the ventral anterior nucleus (VA), the ventral lateral nucleus (VL), and the ventral posterior nucleus (VP). The VL nucleus has oral and caudal subdivisions, VLo and VLc. The VPL nucleus consists of oral (VPLo), caudal (VPL), medial (VPM), and medial parvicellular divisions (VPMpc).

VA and VLo nuclei contribute to planning and initiation of movement.

Cortical projections from VLc and VPLo improve the accuracy of movements.

The four rostral nuclei, VA, VLo, VLc, and VPLo, contribute to motor control, but in different ways. Projections from the basal ganglia, relayed through the VA and VLo nuclei to the prefrontal and premotor cortices, participate in motor planning (Figure 6.2). Cerebellar projections to the VLc and VPLo nuclei, which project to the primary motor cortex, improve the accuracy of fine motor control. As Figure 6.2 shows, the ventral tier nuclei and the motor areas of the frontal lobe have the same rostrocaudal organization.

VPL and VPM nuclei are somatosensory relays.

VPMpc is the thalamic relay for taste.

The VPL and VPM divisions of the VP nucleus are the thalamic somatosensory relays (see Figure 6.1C, D). Somatosensory information from the body is relayed by the ventropostero*lateral* (VPL) nucleus to the medial part of primary somatosensory cortex located in the postcentral gyrus. Corresponding information from the face and oral cavity is relayed from the ventropostero*medial* (VPM) nucleus to the lateral part of the postcentral gyrus. Together, the VPL and VPM nuclei contain a topographical representation of the entire body, which can be summarized as a homunculus (Figures 6.3 and 7.10). A small, parvicellular nucleus located along the medial aspect of the VPM nucleus, VPMpc,

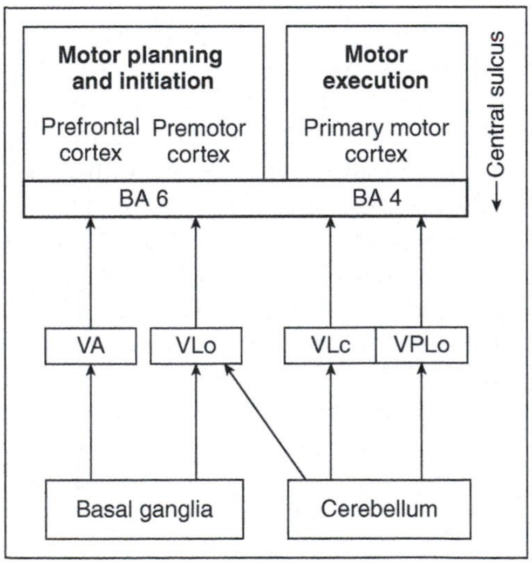

FIG. 6.2. Relationship between the Ventral Tier Thalamic Nuclei and the Frontal Cortex. The thalamic motor relay nuclei receive non-overlapping projections from the basal ganglia and the cerebellum and project to separate areas of the prefrontal and frontal cortices. Note also that these areas of the thalamus and the cerebral cortex have the same rostrocaudal sequence. BA = Brodmann area; VA = ventral anterior nucleus; VLo and VLc = ventral lateral nuclei, pars oralis and caudalis, respectively VPLo = ventroposterolateral nucleus, pars oralis.

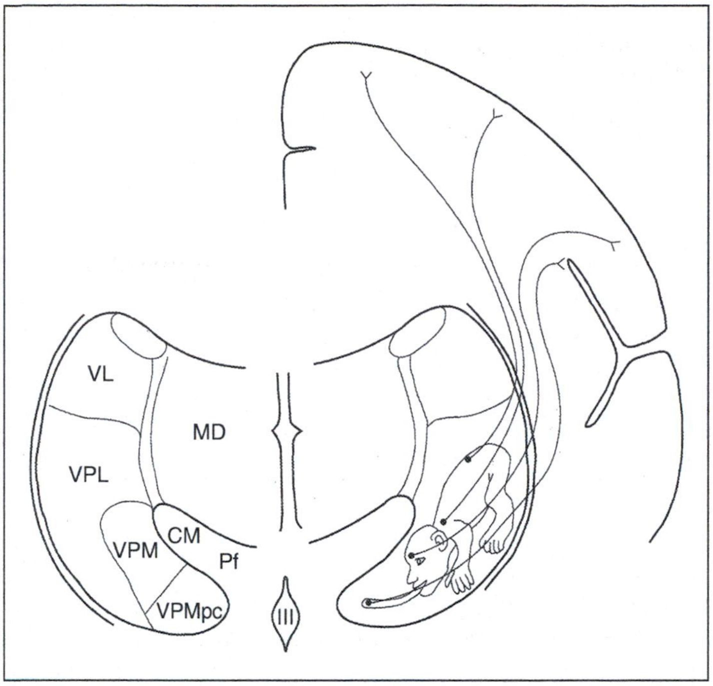

FIG. 6.3. Schematic Diagram of the Projections from the Somatosensory and Gustatory Thalamic Nuclei to the Cerebral Cortex. VLc = ventral lateral nucleus; VPL = ventroposterolateral nucleus; VPM = ventroposteromedial nucleus; VPMpc = parvicellular division of the VPM nucleus; CM = centromedian nucleus; Pf = parafascicular nucleus; MD = mediodorsal nucleus.

is the thalamic relay for gustatory information. Gustatory neurons in VPMpc project to primary taste cortex, which is located within the rostral insula.

Posterior Nucleus

The posterior thalamic nucleus is located between the VPL and the pulvinar. Although not as well understood as its neighbors, the posterior nucleus receives nociceptive input from the anterolateral system and projects to the insula, cingulate gyrus, and association cortices in the parietal and temporal lobes.

Lateral and Medial Geniculate Nuclei

LGN: vision
MGN: audition

The lateral and medial geniculate nuclei are the thalamic relays for vision and audition, respectively. The lateral geniculate nucleus (LGN) and the medial geniculate nucleus (MGN) are located side by side at the caudal pole of the thalamus, ventral to the pulvinar (see Figure 6.1E). In transverse sections, the LGN is horseshoe-shaped and consists of six layers. The LGN projects to the primary visual cortex located along the banks of the calcarine sulcus. The lamination of the MGN, though present, is not readily apparent because the interlaminar bands are unmyelinated. Ascending projections to the MGN originate in the inferior colliculus; efferent projections of the MGN form the auditory radiations, which terminate in primary auditory cortex.

Intralaminar Nuclei

In the caudal third of the thalamus, the internal medullary lamina splits and forms an oval pocket that encapsulates several nuclei, which are appropriately called the intralaminar nuclei (see Figure 6.1D). The largest of the intralaminar nuclei are the centromedian (CM) and the parafascicular (Pf) nuclei. The CM nucleus receives projections from the primary motor cortex, the basal ganglia, and the brainstem reticular formation. The afferent projections of the Pf originate in the premotor cortex. Both nuclei have light, widespread projections to the cerebral cortex as well as dense projections to restricted areas of the basal ganglia (CM → putamen; Pf → caudate nucleus). These projections, along with

FIG. 6.4. **Afferent and Efferent Projections of the Reticular Nucleus.** The reticular nucleus receives excitatory projections from the cerebral cortex and the thalamus. Inhibitory projections from the reticular nucleus to the thalamus contribute to selective attention and electrical synchrony of the cerebral cortex.

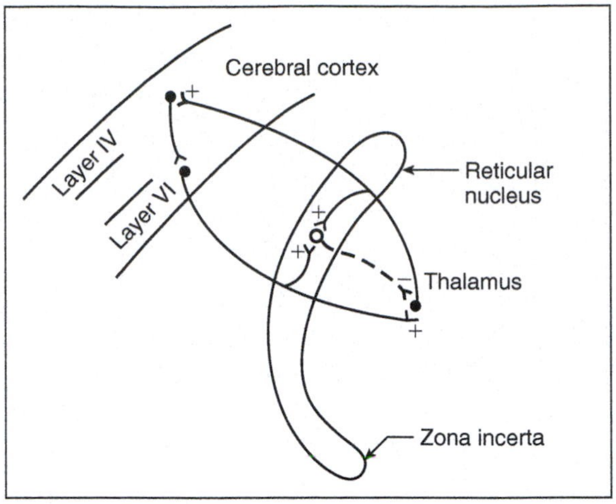

others to the subthalamic nucleus, the substantia nigra, and the globus pallidus, suggest that the CM and Pf nuclei integrate cortical and subcortical aspects of movement.

The central lateral (CL) nucleus is one of the small intralaminar nuclei located further rostrally. The CL nucleus is a sliver-shaped cluster of cells in the seam between MD and VPL. Input to CL originates in the spinothalamic tract, the deep cerebellar nuclei, and the pontine parabrachial nucleus. Its projections to the cerebral cortex and the striatum suggest that CL plays a role in state-dependent arousal of the cerebral cortex and perception of pain.

Reticular Nucleus

GABAergic neurons in the **reticular nucleus,** which has no cortical projections, provide recurrent inhibition of the thalamic relay nuclei.

The reticular nucleus is a thin shell of GABAergic neurons sandwiched between the external medullary lamina and the internal capsule that plays a key role in selective attention (see Figure 6.1C, D). From its position near the lateral and rostral edges of the thalamus, the reticular nucleus modulates the two-way neural traffic between the thalamic relay nuclei and the cerebral cortex. The reticular nucleus receives excitatory projections from the thalamus and the cerebral cortex but sends inhibitory projections only to the thalamus (Figure 6.4). These recurrent inhibitory projections sharpen sensory transmission by facilitating thalamocortical signals related to the task at hand and suppressing others. This neural circuit enables us to attend to a single modality (e.g., vision; reading a book) while ignoring other sensory modalities (e.g., audition; music, extraneous noises). The ebb and flow of the excitatory and inhibitory loops between the thalamic relay nuclei and the reticular nucleus contribute to the synchronized and desynchronized patterns of cortical electroencephalogram (EEG) activity that signal periods of sleep and increased attentiveness, respectively.

INTERNAL CAPSULE

The **genu of the internal capsule** joins the anterior and posterior limbs.

The internal capsule consists of reciprocal connections between the thalamus and cortex as well as projections from the cerebral cortex to the brainstem and spinal cord. In horizontal sections, the internal capsule resembles a boomerang with its two long anterior and posterior limbs joined at the genu near the interventricular foramen (Figure 6.5). The genu contains descending corticonuclear fibers that terminate in the facial and oral motor nuclei of the brainstem. The anterior limb of the internal capsule, located between the lentiform nucleus (globus pallidus and putamen; see Figure 6.5) and the head of the caudate nucleus, consists of thalamic projections to the frontal cortex and descending frontopontine fibers. Axons interconnecting the motor and somatosensory areas of the thalamus and cortex form the superior thalamic radiations, which travel within the posterior limb of the internal capsule. The posterior limb of the internal capsule forms a thick barrier between the lentiform nucleus and the thalamus. Corticospinal projections

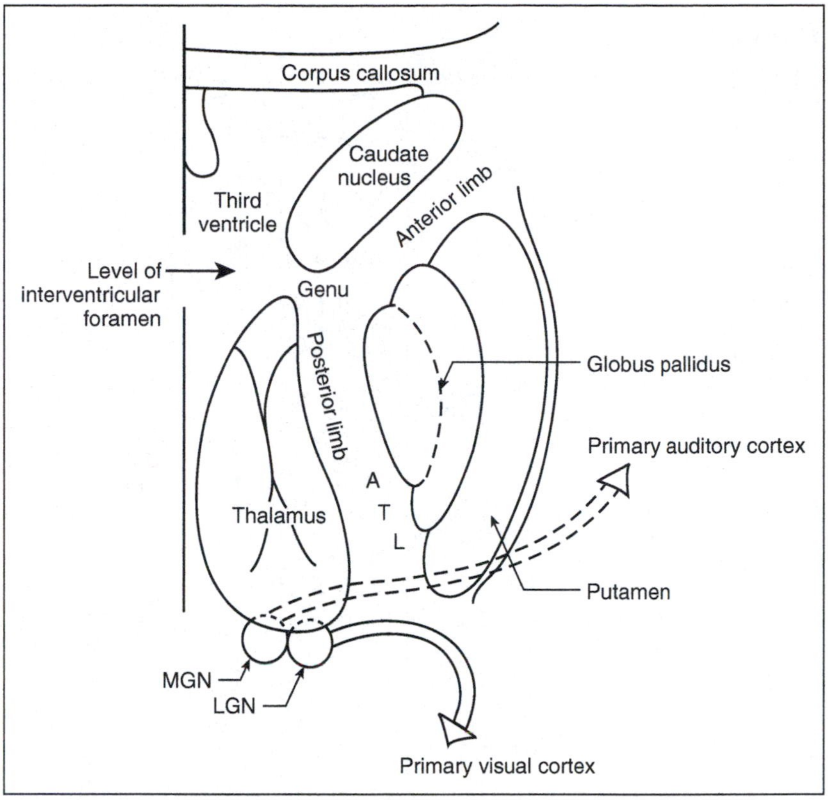

FIG. 6.5. Diagram of the Internal Capsule (Horizontal Plane). A = arms; T = trunk; L = legs; LGN = lateral geniculate nucleus; MGN = medial geniculate nucleus.

to the motor neurons that control the arms, trunk, and legs are arranged in a rough rostrocaudal sequence near the caudal end of the posterior limb. The relative proximity of the corticospinal axons to the ascending somatosensory, optic, and auditory projections makes this area of the brain unique—and damage to this region particularly devastating. Patients with damage in the vicinity of the caudal internal capsule may experience contralateral analgesia and paresis, as well as visual and auditory deficits.

CEREBRAL CORTEX

The cerebral cortex is the laminated shell of neurons, axons, dendrites, and glia that forms the surface of the telencephalon. As the crowning achievement of the central nervous system (CNS), the cerebral cortex is the structure that distinguishes humans from each other and from other animals. In its role as the organ of thought, large parts of the cerebral cortex are dedicated to personality, strategic planning, sensory perception, volitional movement, and language.

Cortical Anatomy

Two classes of cortex are found in the telencephalon: allocortex and neocortex. Allocortex, a primitive, three-layered cortex, is found in the hippocampal formation (archicortex) and the olfactory cortex (paleocortex). Neocortex, which contains six layers, is found throughout the rest of the telencephalon.

> Neocortex: 6 layers
> Allocortex: 3 layers

Cell Types. Pyramidal and granule (stellate) cells are the most common neurons in the cerebral cortex. Pyramidal cells, named for their pyramid-shaped soma (10-70 μm in diameter),

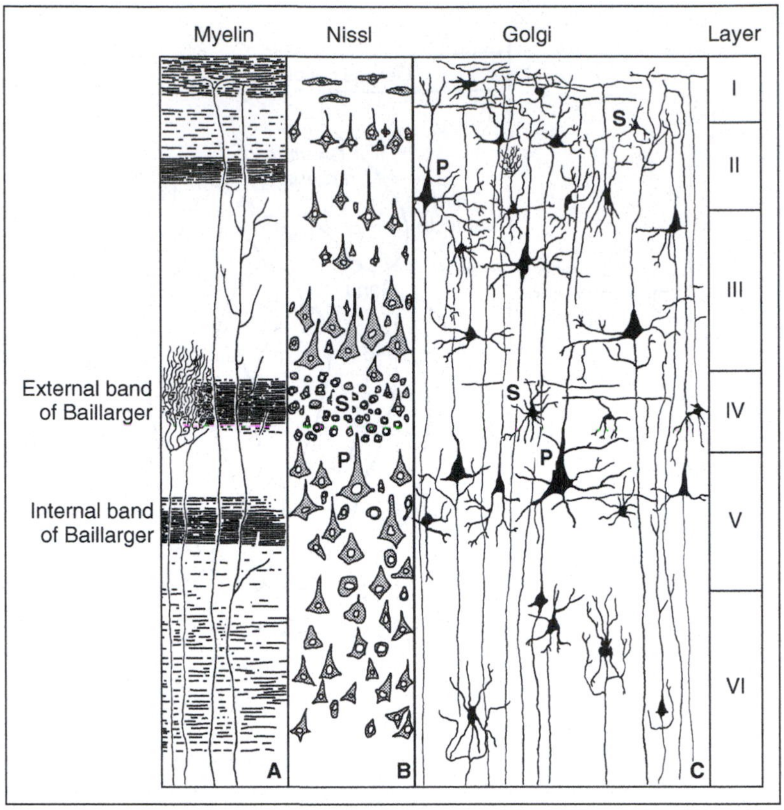

FIG. 6.6. Cross Section of the Cerebral Cortex. (A) A myelin stain shows the horizontally and vertically oriented fibers that connect different parts of the cerebral cortex. The internal and external layers of Baillarger are the largest bands of horizontal fibers in the cerebral cortex. (B) A cresyl violet stain binds to the endoplasmic reticulum of the cell bodies. (C) By permeating the entire neuron, Golgi stains highlight cell bodies, axons, and dendrites. P = pyramidal neuron; S = stellate neuron. (Reprinted with permission. Ranson SW and Clark, SL. *The Anatomy of the Nervous System*. Philadelphia, PA: W. B. Saunders, 1966:437.)

have a prominent apical dendrite, short basal dendrites, and a lone basal axon (Figure 6.6). Unlike other neurons, a pyramidal cell has a consistent orientation in which its apical dendrite extends to the superficial cortical layers and its shorter basal dendrites ramify within the deeper cortical layers. The lone basal axon usually projects to remote cortical and subcortical targets, but it often has collateral branches that innervate local neurons. Granule cells, by comparison, have much smaller, star-shaped somas (5-15 μm in diameter) and shorter processes that rarely project beyond the cortical mantle. Spiny granule cells are excitatory, and nonspiny granule cells are inhibitory; both have short axonal and dendritic processes that form local cortical circuits.

Pyramidal cells are the efferent neurons of the cerebral cortex.

Laminar Organization. The cerebral cortex varies in thickness from 2 mm across the crowns of the gyri to 4 mm in the depths of the sulci. Differences in cell type, cell size, and cell-packing density give the cerebral cortex its laminated appearance.

The six layers of neocortex are numbered consecutively from the pial surface (see Figure 6.6):

- Layer I, the molecular layer, is composed of horizontally oriented axons and the terminal arborizations of apical dendrites of cortical neurons located in the deeper cortical layers.
- Layer II, the external granular layer, consists primarily of small, closely packed granule cells. These neurons have short dendritic and axonal processes that form an integral part of the local cortical circuits.
- Layer III, the external pyramidal layer, is a relatively thick layer dominated by small and medium-size pyramidal cells. Many local intracortical projections originate from layer III, whereas the longer subcortical projections derive from the larger pyramidal neurons located in layer V.
- Layer IV, the internal granular layer, consists of densely packed spiny and aspiny granule cells that receive ascending thalamocortical projections. Layer IV also contains a dense plexus of horizontal axons, the external band of Baillarger. Neurons in layer IV

project to both infragranular (V) and supragranular (II and III) layers, but primarily the latter. The internal granular layer is thick in the primary sensory cortices and virtually nonexistent in primary motor cortex.

- Layer V, the internal pyramidal layer, is the primary output layer of the cerebral cortex. Layer V is composed of medium and large pyramidal neurons and contains a prominent swath of horizontally oriented axon collaterals called the internal band of Baillarger. The internal pyramidal layer is thicker in primary motor cortex than in other parts of the cerebral cortex.
- Layer VI, the multiform layer, contains an assortment of cell types including pyramidal, granule, and spindle-shaped fusiform cells. Pyramidal cells in layer VI project to the thalamus.

Six layers of neocortex:
I. Molecular layer
II. External granular layer
III. External pyramidal layer
IV. Internal granular layer
V. Internal pyramidal layer
VI. Multiform layer

Columnar Organization. Abundant research has shown that cortical neurons in the sensory cortices are arranged into vertical columns. The first electrophysiological description of cortical columns was made by Mountcastle, who reported that single neurons in the postcentral gyrus that respond to tactile stimulation of one body area (e.g., thumb) typically form a column of cells oriented perpendicularly to the pial surface. Electrode penetrations parallel to the pial surface, on the other hand, encounter neurons whose receptive fields gradually shift across the periphery. Subsequent research by Hubel and Wiesel in the visual system and Abeles and Goldstein in the auditory system confirmed the generality of this concept. Columns in the primary visual cortex contain neurons that respond to the same part of the visual field and have similar response properties (e.g., eye dominance or orientation). Cortical columns have not been identified in the gustatory or olfactory system, but neither sensory system has been studied thoroughly enough to rule out their existence. In the senses known to have columns, the cerebral cortex contains a coherent, but usually distorted, map of the peripheral receptor sheet (i.e., the skin, the retina, or the inner ear).

The **receptive field** of a neuron is the circumscribed part of the receptive sheet where stimulation activates the cell.

Conceptually, a cortical column represents a processing module interposed between specific sets of input and output connections. The complexity of an individual column is astounding because multiple inputs may be integrated and multiple outputs generated. Inputs for a single column may arrive from the thalamus, various brainstem areas (e.g., the raphe nuclei), or other cortical areas. The outputs from an individual cortical column terminate in a variety of subcortical regions, neighboring areas of the cerebral cortex, or corresponding regions of the opposite hemisphere. Even though most of what we know about the circuitry of cortical columns has been learned in the sensory cortices, columns are presumed to be the fundamental processing unit for the entire neocortex.

The **cortical column** is the functional unit of the sensory cortex.

Regional Differences. Even though there is general agreement that the cerebral cortex consists of six layers, regional variations in the laminar pattern are common and represent the basis for subdividing the cerebral cortex into separate areas. The cytoarchitectonic map of the cerebral cortex proposed by Brodmann in 1909 remains the most widely used partition of the cerebral cortex (Figure 6.7). Brodmann assumed that regional variation in cortical lamination reflects functional heterogeneity. Among the 47 distinct Brodmann areas, slightly more than a dozen are used routinely to designate brain areas with well-known functions (Table 6.2).

Brodmann areas: function follows form

Some Brodmann areas are synonymous with a specific function.

Neurotransmitters. Cortical neurons contain an assortment of inhibitory and excitatory neurotransmitters. The inhibitory neurotransmitter γ-aminobutyric acid (GABA) is found in nonspiny granule cells, which are the most common inhibitory neurons in the cerebral cortex. The two most common excitatory neurotransmitters in the cerebral cortex, glutamate and aspartate, are found in the synaptic terminals of pyramidal and spiny granule neurons. Pyramidal neurons are the cells of origin for the long intracortical and subcortical (e.g., corticostriate, corticopontine, corticospinal) projections. Glutamate and aspartate also are found within the axon terminals of thalamocortical neurons.

Glutamate and **aspartate** are the two most common neurotransmitters in the cerebral cortex

Other neurotransmitters in the cerebral cortex arise from neurons located in remote locations such as the raphe nuclei (serotonin), the locus ceruleus (norepinephrine), the basal nucleus of Meynert (acetylcholine), and the mesolimbic system (dopamine). These

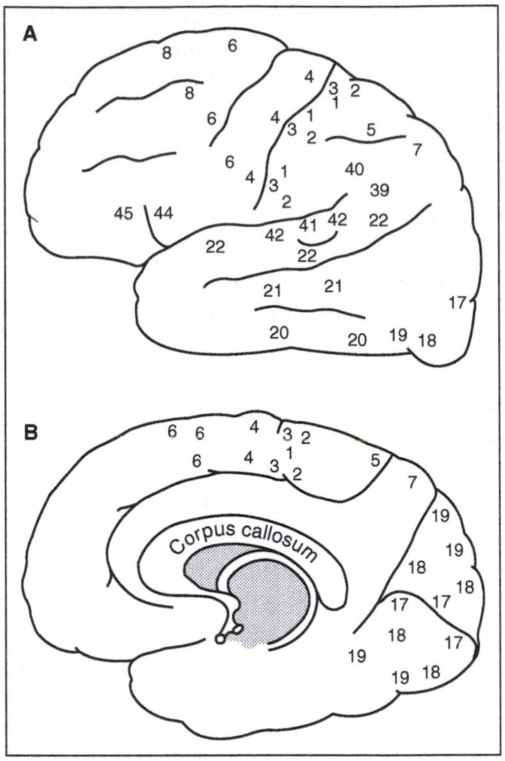

FIG. 6.7. Brodmann Areas. Major cytoarchitectural divisions of the lateral (A) and medial (B) surfaces of the cerebral cortex based on the divisions of Brodmann (1909).

neurotransmitters modulate the actions of other neurotransmitters in the cerebral cortex. Serotonergic projections from the raphe nuclei terminate primarily in cortical layers III and IV, which are the layers that receive thalamic input. For this reason, serotonin is believed to act as a sentinel that sharpens sensory processing by the cerebral cortex. Serotonin also has been implicated in sleep and pain perception. The noradrenergic projections from the locus ceruleus also may play a role in the sleep-wake cycle, but because many of these terminals are located in the deeper layers of the cerebral cortex, they may modulate cortical output as well. Widespread regions of the cerebral cortex receive cholinergic projections from the basal nucleus of Meynert, a group of medium and large neurons located ventral to the anterior commissure. Because the basal nucleus of Meynert degenerates in patients with Alzheimer's disease, it is possible that acetylcholine plays an important role in cortically mediated processes such as learning and memory. Dopaminergic projections to the cerebral cortex from the ventral tegmental area are important for normal cognitive function. Because excessive levels of dopamine may be partly responsible for affective disorders such as schizophrenia, the most effective antipsychotic drugs are dopamine antagonists.

TABLE 6.2 Selected Brodmann Areas of the Cerebral Cortex

Brodmann Area	Location	Function
17	Banks of the calcarine sulcus	Primary visual cortex
18, 19	Medial aspect of occipital lobe	Secondary visual cortex
5, 7	Posterior parietal cortex	Sensory association cortex
3, 1, 2	Postcentral gyrus	Primary somatosensory cortex
4	Precentral gyrus	Primary motor cortex
6	Superior and middle frontal gyri	Premotor cortex
44, 45	Inferior frontal gyri	Language
41, 42	Superior temporal gyrus	Auditory cortex

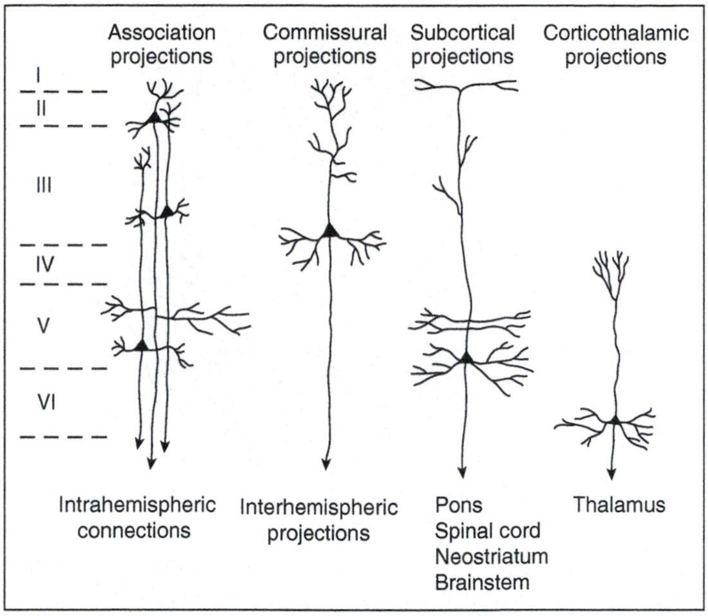

FIG. 6.8 Laminar Origins of Corticofugal Projections.

Cortical neurons also contain a variety of neuroactive peptides, including cholecystokinin, vasoactive intestinal polypeptide, neuropeptide Y, somatostatin, substance P, and corticotropin-releasing factor. These peptides, like many of the neurotransmitters just described, modulate the activity of other neurotransmitters in the cerebral cortex.

Cortical Projections. Axons emanating from the cerebral cortex are classified as association fibers, commissural fibers, or projection fibers (Figure 6.8).

Association pathways are *intra*hemispheric.

Association Fibers. Association fibers provide intrahemispheric connections and, depending on their length, are classified as either short or long. Short association fibers are U-shaped because they connect adjacent gyri (Figure 6.9). Long association fibers connect different lobes within the same hemisphere. Five of the more notable long association pathways are

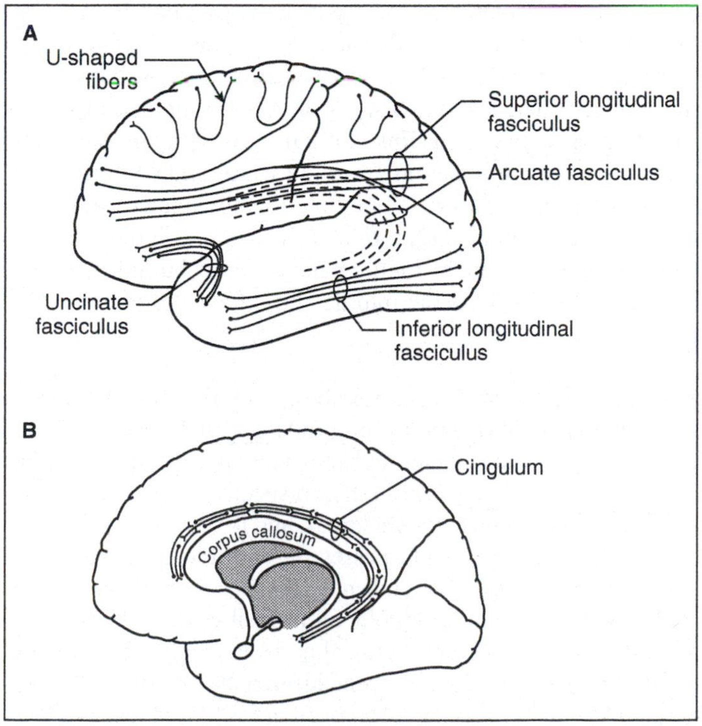

FIG. 6.9. Intracortical Pathways. (A) Phantom of the cerebral cortex showing the superior and inferior longitudinal fasciculi, the arcuate fasciculus, and the U-shaped fibers of the intracortical pathways. Note that the fibers of the arcuate fasciculus are intermixed with the axons of the superior longitudinal fasciculus. (B) Phantom showing the location of the cingulum relative to the corpus callosum.

FIG. 6.10. Anterior and Posterior Forceps of the Corpus Callosum.

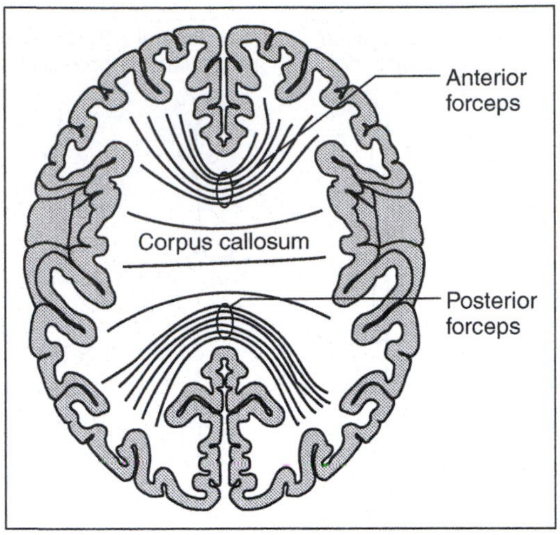

the uncinate fasciculus, the arcuate fasciculus, the superior and inferior longitudinal fasciculi, and the cingulum. The uncinate fasciculus is a curved pathway that connects the inferior and middle temporal gyri with the orbital gyri of the frontal lobe. The arcuate fasciculus conveys information from the superior temporal gyrus to the middle and inferior frontal gyri. Whereas the uncinate fasciculus carves out a relatively direct pathway between the insula and the temporal lobe, the arcuate fasciculus takes a longer, sweeping trajectory around the insula. Fibers of the arcuate fasciculus intermingle with those of the superior longitudinal fasciculus, which courses between the occipital and frontal lobes. The inferior longitudinal fasciculus interconnects the occipital, parietal, and temporal lobes. The cingulum, which is buried within the cingulate gyrus, is a large, bidirectional pathway between the frontal and parietal lobes and the parahippocampal gyrus and adjacent temporal lobe.

Commissural pathways are *inter*hemispheric.

The **corpus callosum** consists of the rostrum, genu, body, and splenium.

Commissural Fibers. Commissural pathways connect the two hemispheres and probably enable them to share information and function as a unit. The corpus callosum, the largest and most important commissural pathway, forms the floor of the longitudinal fissure and the roof of the lateral ventricles (Figure 6.10; see also Figures 6.9, 3.6, 3.8). The corpus callosum consists of four parts, the rostrum, genu, body, and splenium. Because the corpus callosum does not extend to the rostral or caudal pole of the brain, fibers originating in these areas of cortex form arcs called the anterior and posterior forceps that cross in the rostrum and splenium, respectively. There are two types of commissural connections: homotypic and heterotypic. Homotypic connections link cortical areas with predominantly midline representations, such as the somatosensation from the trunk and central vision. Heterotypic connections link anatomically different but functionally related areas. For example, reading requires the cooperation and coordination of the right occipital lobe with the language areas of the left hemisphere. A much smaller band of fibers buried within the telencephalon, the anterior commissure, connects the middle and inferior temporal gyri of the left and right hemispheres.

Cortical projection pathways target subcortical and spinal neurons.

Projection Fibers. Projection fibers exit the cerebral cortex and descend to subcortical structures, including the thalamus, the basal ganglia, the brainstem, and the spinal cord. As cortical projection fibers descend through the corona radiata and the internal capsule, individual corticostriate and corticothalamic axons terminate within their respective target nuclei (Figure 6.11). The entire cerebral cortex is connected to the thalamus, and in some cases, to multiple nuclei of the thalamus. After the internal capsule passes through the diencephalon, it assumes a new name, the crus cerebri (see Figure 5.24) and enters the mesencephalon. Cortical projection fibers terminate in the superior and inferior colliculi as well as the pontine nuclei (corticopontine fibers) and all of the sensory and motor cranial nerve nuclei (corticobulbar or corticonuclear fibers) in the brainstem. After this long descent through the brainstem, the only fibers left in this once majestic pathway are those of the corticospinal tract (see Figure 4.28).

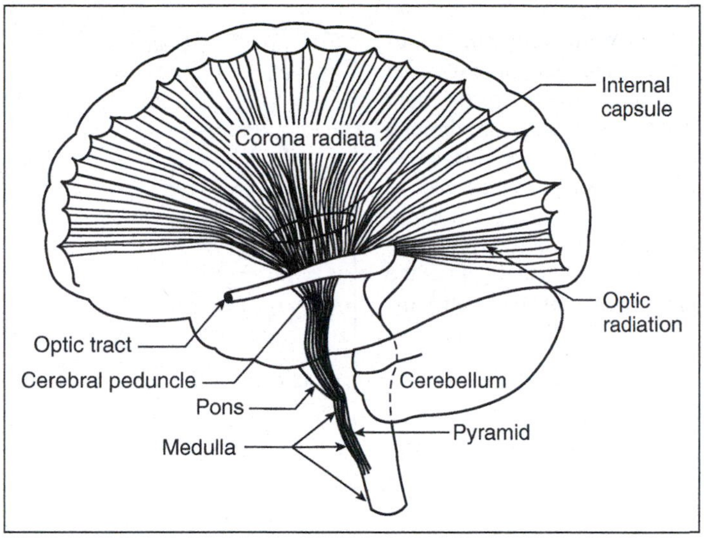

FIG. 6.11. Corticofugal Pathways. Dissection of the telencephalon reveals the fibers of the corona radiata. As the fibers of the internal capsule exit the telencephalon, they form the crus cerebri, pass through the mesencephalon, and then become the pyramidal tracts on the ventral surface of the medulla.

Functional Specialization and Bilateral Symmetry

The concept of functional specialization within the cerebral cortex dates to antiquity, but it lacked empirical support until 1861 when Paul Broca linked damage to a small region of the frontal cortex with a profound language deficit. The concept of functional specialization was bolstered by the discovery of specific sensory and motor areas related to the contralateral side of the body. Even though functional specialization is the rule rather than the exception in the cerebral cortex—and in the entire brain for that matter—it would be a mistake to view the central nervous system as a patchwork of compartments exclusively dedicated to a specific motor skill, sensory attribute, or personality trait.

Broca's discovery that language functions were located in the left hemisphere of his right-handed patient suggested that the two cerebral hemispheres are not functionally equivalent despite their apparent anatomic similarity. Although the hemispheric asymmetry of language is striking, for most other skills the differences between the two hemispheres are subtle and not fully appreciated despite decades of study.

The discovery of functional asymmetries between the two hemispheres led to the concept of a dominant and a nondominant hemisphere. Handedness is used to identify the dominant hemisphere, but the implications of this designation extend to language, perception, and emotion. Despite its widespread use, the notion of a dominant hemisphere is antiquated, inadequate, and often inaccurate. The concept of hemispheric dominance arose when neuroscientists lacked the sophistication to identify the subtle but important functions of the so-called nondominant hemisphere. More importantly, the locus of language is highly correlated with handedness only in right-handed individuals. As more is learned about the functions of the so-called nondominant hemisphere, this nomenclature may disappear along with the obvious implication that the functions of the nondominant hemisphere are less important than those controlled by the other side.

Broca's rule states that language is located in the left hemisphere of right-handed individuals.

We speak with the left hemisphere.

Split-Brain. The lateralization of hemispheric functions has been revealed by studies of patients with traumatic brain injury, surgeries on epileptic patients, and studies using noninvasive brain-imaging techniques. All three have provided valuable insight, but the most definitive data are those obtained from epileptic patients whose interhemispheric connections

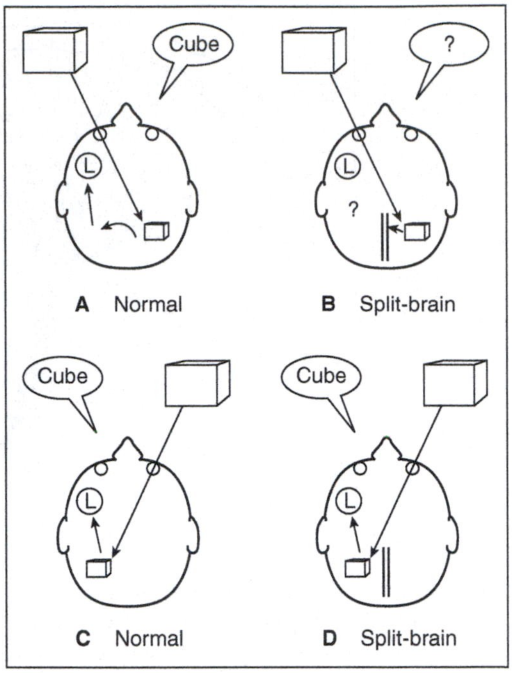

FIG. 6.12. Hemispheric Transfer of Information Following Commissurotomy. (A) The visual image of a cube projected onto the left visual field of the left eye crosses and is processed by visual cortex in the right hemisphere. After the information is returned to the left hemisphere through the corpus callosum, the patient is able to report verbally that the image was a cube. (B) Following a commissurotomy, visual information that ascends to the right hemisphere is unable to reach the language areas in the left hemisphere, so the patient is unable to describe the stimulus verbally. (C and D) When the visual image of a cube is projected onto the right visual field of the right eye, both the normal and commissurized patient are able to identify the stimulus verbally.

Commissurotomies prevent interhemispheric transfer of seizures—and information.

have been severed. Surgical disconnection of the cerebral hemispheres, called a commissurotomy, is the procedure of last resort for epileptic patients whose seizures resist pharmacologic control. A commissurotomy involves sectioning the corpus callosum and the anterior commissure; the optic chiasm, the hippocampal commissure, and the posterior commissure are not cut. Although a commissurotomy prevents seizures from spreading from one hemisphere to the other, it also prevents the two hemispheres from sharing information. In a commissurized patient, sensory information that reaches one hemisphere is unable to cross to the opposite side. Thus, somatosensory, visual, and perhaps even gustatory and olfactory information presented to one side of the body, retina, and so on are able to reach only one cerebral hemisphere; the opposite hemisphere would not be privy to this information.

Roger Sperry, whose pioneering work on commissurized patients earned him the Nobel Prize, has given us tremendous insight into how different skills are lateralized within the brain. In a typical experiment, a visual image is projected onto half of a patient's visual field. In Figure 6.12A, the image was projected onto the left visual field of a normal, right-handed subject. This image is transmitted to the visual areas in the opposite (right) hemisphere; note that the language areas are located in the left hemisphere. (To fully understand Figure 6.12, it may be necessary to consult Chapter 11, which describes visual fields and the partial decussation that occurs in the optic chiasm.) The normal subject in Figure 6.12A is able to report that a cube was presented because the information was transmitted through the corpus callosum to the language areas in the left hemisphere. Following section of the corpus callosum, however, the image of the cube reaches the right hemisphere, but not the left (Figure 6.12B). This patient with the "uninformed" left hemisphere is unable to identify the object verbally. If the same image were presented to the right visual field of the right eye, the commissurotomy would be irrelevant because this information projects directly to the left hemisphere (Figures 6.12C, D).

Handedness is not a perfect predictor of the cortical locus of language, even for right-handed patients.

Hemispheric Dominance. Studies on commissurized patients have shown that the most profound interhemispheric differences are in the association areas rather than in the primary sensory or motor areas of the cerebral cortex. In addition, the degree to which skills are lateralized to one hemisphere is related to handedness. Most skills in right-handed individuals are strongly, but not completely, lateralized; in left-handed and ambidextrous individuals, however, there is better balance between the two hemispheres. For this reason, accurate generalizations about hemispheric specialization can be made only for right-handed individuals (approximately 88% of the population).

As a rule, the left hemisphere in right-handed individuals is specialized for the comprehension and production of language, symbolic representation, and analysis of temporal order and duration. Thus, the left hemisphere is better-suited for sequential analysis of discrete items or events that have temporal continuity. For example, words retain their individuality, even when embedded in a sentence; for this reason the left hemisphere plays a key role in semantic memory. Bilateral motor planning and control is also under the jurisdiction of the left hemisphere. The right hemisphere, by comparison, is more holistic and thus better suited for perception of space, synthesis of sensory information into a unified form (e.g., music, form, color, faces), and perception and expression of emotion. Perception of faces, attending to our bilateral personal and extrapersonal spaces, and episodic memory are also performed by the right hemisphere. The motor aspects of language (i.e., speech, writing) are strongly lateralized to the left hemisphere, whereas its emotive components are located primarily in the corresponding area of the right hemisphere. Cerebral dominance is determined by genetic and environmental (i.e., in utero) factors.

Left hemisphere: sequential analysis of discrete items

Right hemisphere: holistic analysis

In right-handed individuals, there is a strong but not perfect relationship between handedness and language. Language processing occurs in the left hemisphere of 98% of right-handed persons; the percentage of left-handed or ambidextrous persons with language areas in the left hemisphere is in dispute. Recent studies claim the percentage is above 90%; older reports put the figure as low as 50%. Because handedness is not a perfect indicator for language lateralization, the location of the speech areas must be determined with certainty prior to neurosurgical procedures involving the temporal lobe or inferior frontal cortex. The accepted method for locating the dominant hemisphere for language is the Wada test in which a quick-acting barbiturate (e.g., amobarbital) is injected into one of the carotid arteries. As the injection is made, the patient raises both arms and begins counting. When the injection is made in the artery ipsilateral to the language area, counting is interrupted; an injection in the carotid artery on the opposite side has no effect on the verbal task. If the drug has affected only one hemisphere, only the arm contralateral to the injected artery falls.

The **Wada test** is used to determine the hemispheric locus of language.

Language. Communication in the animal kingdom is common, but humans are the only species that communicates with language. Other animals such as insects (e.g., bees, termites), fish, cetaceans, birds, and nonhuman primates (monkeys, apes) communicate with chemical (pheromones), visual (display), and auditory (barks, chirps, calls) signals that lack the complexity of human language. Language is creative, virtually unlimited in its range, and independent of the mode of production and comprehension; communication by other animals, besides being limited in scope, is stereotypic in form.

Without a satisfactory animal model, research on the central organization of language has relied on patients who have suffered some type of neurologic accident. Such studies have shown that language is controlled by subcortical (e.g., thalamus, basal ganglia) and cortical structures. Patients with damage to the thalamus and basal ganglia are often mute, but the precise roles these structures play in language are not known. At the cortical level, language consists of sensory, cognitive, and motor components distributed across the temporal, parietal, and frontal lobes. Focal cortical lesions in these regions produce specific deficits in the production and comprehension of language.

Aphasias and the Cortical Organization of Language. In 1861, Paul Broca described a right-handed patient with a circumscribed lesion in the left inferior frontal gyrus who had difficulty speaking, but was able to comprehend spoken and written language. Despite the proximity of the lesion to the primary motor cortex, this patient had full control of his oral musculature. The damaged area within the inferior frontal gyrus, now known as Broca's area, contains motor templates that control the facial and respiratory components of speech.

Broca's area, located on the inferior frontal gyrus of most right-handed individuals, contains the motor templates for speech.

In 1874, Carl Wernicke reported that damage to the temporal lobe interferes with language comprehension, but not the ability to speak. Wernicke's observation effectively separated language into motor and cognitive components. The language comprehension

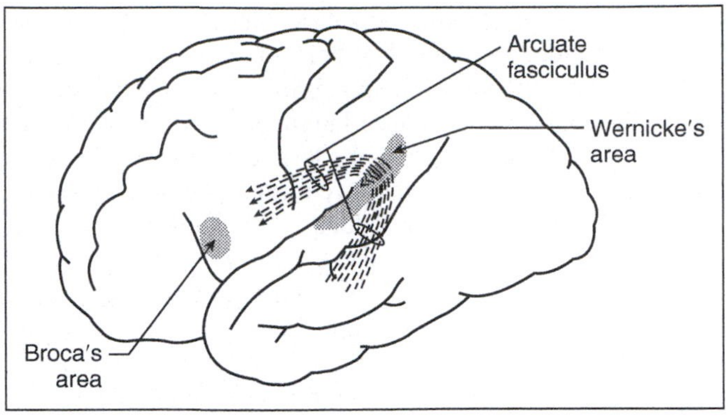

FIG. 6.13. Arcuate Fasciculus. The arcuate fasciculus, which courses around the perimeter of the insula and joins the superior longitudinal fasciculus, connects the language areas in the parietal (Wernicke's area) and frontal (Broca's area) lobes.

Wernicke's area interprets what we hear and selects the words we speak.

area, now known as Wernicke's area, includes the posterior aspect of the temporal lobe and part of the inferior parietal lobule (Figure 6.13). Projections from the visual, auditory, and somatosensory cortices to Wernicke's area enable written, spoken, and tactile (i.e., Braille) signals to be interpreted for linguistic content. Wernicke's area also interprets symbols that have linguistic meaning. For example, the symbols "B-U-G" should conjure up images of insects and perhaps memories of past encounters with insects. Other areas of the brain that associate insects with descriptive (brown, crawly), emotional (disgusting), and cognitive (infectious) labels create a detailed and personalized mental image. By comparison, a series of arbitrary symbols (e.g., ♋•♎♐♑) that have no linguistic meaning do not generate mental images or stir memories or emotions. Following damage to Wernicke's area, words and sounds that should have meaning lie stranded within sensory cortex along with other meaningless sensations.

Broca's aphasia is a nonfluent aphasia.

The language deficits associated with damage to Broca's area and Wernicke's area are strikingly different. Broca's aphasia is characterized by slow, labored, and poorly articulated speech. Sentences are telegraphic—that is, they include nouns and attributes of objects but usually omit small words such as "is" and "if." Patients with Broca's aphasia also have difficulty writing. Because their speech is labored and technically poor, Broca's aphasia is referred to as a nonfluent aphasia.

Wernicke's aphasia is a fluent aphasia.

In Wernicke's aphasia, speech is effortless with well-preserved rhythm and melody. Speech may be a little more rapid than normal and have normal grammatical structure, but comprehension is poor and accompanied by severe reading and writing disabilities. Patients who have trouble finding the right word may compensate by making up words (neologisms), substituting one word for another (paraphasia), or creating a meaningless word salad (jargon aphasia). Patients with Wernicke's aphasia are noteworthy for their fluent speech, but lack of comprehension.

Damage to the arcuate fasciculus, the pathway that connects Wernicke's area with Broca's area, causes a conduction aphasia. Patients with conduction aphasias are fluent and have good comprehension because Broca's area and Wernicke's area are intact, but disconnected. Naming is severely impaired, and there is some word substitution; writing, spelling, and reading aloud are severely impaired.

Wernicke's description of language as a serial process is both simplistic and incomplete, but nevertheless remains credible because it accounts for many of the language and speech disorders observed in the clinic.

Cortical asymmetry is the norm for language areas, not the exception.

Central Correlates of Language. Broca's lasting contribution to the study of language was the link he forged between left hemispheric control of language and right-handedness. Lateralization of language has several neuroanatomic correlates, but the most pronounced is the size of the planum temporale (PT). The PT is a wedge-shaped area at the caudal end of the superior temporal gyrus that includes part of Wernicke's area (see Figures 6.13 and 6.14). The PT is larger on the left side in 89% of the population and, on average, is 40% larger than the right side; in extreme cases, the left PT may be 10 times larger. Enlargement of the PT in the left hemisphere is accompanied by lengthening of the

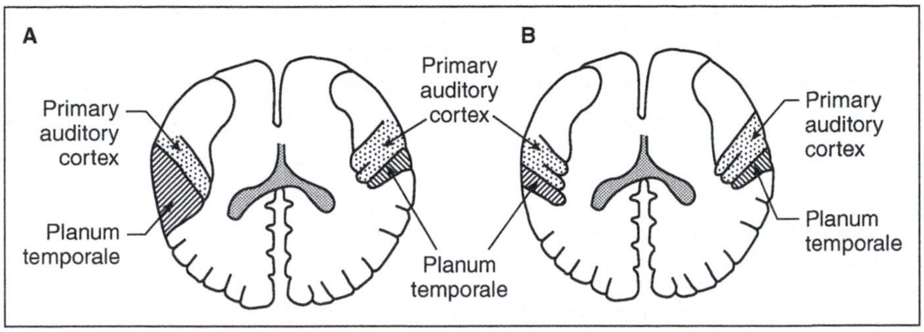

FIG. 6.14. Superior Surface of the Temporal Lobe Exposed by Dissection. The PT (planum temporale) is located posterior to the primary auditory cortex. (A) In the normal brain, the left PT is significantly larger than the right PT. (B) In dyslexic patients, the PTs of the left and right hemispheres are nearly equal in size.

Sylvian fissure. The larger size of the left PT is accompanied by a higher concentration of choline acetyltransferase, which suggests a high level of neural activity. Broca's area and the angular gyrus (Brodmann area 39) are also larger on the left side.

Dyslexia. The hallmarks of developmental dyslexia are an inability to read proficiently and an impaired directional sense. Developmental dyslexia is a diagnosis of exclusion, which means that a reading disorder is attributed to dyslexia after all other neurologic, motivational, and sociologic causes have been ruled out. The incidence of developmental dyslexia is about 3%. Postmortem examination of the brains of dyslexic individuals has shown both gross and microscopic abnormalities within the PT and auditory cortex on the left side. At the gross level, the left and right PTs are symmetrical in size, unlike normal brains in which the left PT is noticeably larger. The PT of dyslexic patients also may show micropolygyria and thinning of the parietal corpus callosum, which connects the left and right PTs. At the microscopic level, the planum temporale and inferior frontal gyrus (Broca's area) have dysplasic (abnormal) lamination and ectopic (misplaced) cell groups.

> **Dyslexia** is characterized by left-right confusion and a failure to read with normal proficiency.

> **Micropolygyria** are numerous pathologically small gyri that lack normal lamination.

Albert Galaburda of Harvard has suggested that dyslexia, left-handedness, cortical symmetry, and certain immune disorders are caused by in utero mutagenesis induced by endogenous testosterone. Although the evidence for this view is circumstantial, it is appealing because it explains the high correlation of these phenomena, which are more prevalent in males. According to Galaburda, testosterone prevents the left hemisphere from reaching its normal, exaggerated size by delaying its maturation. This delay would make the left hemisphere vulnerable to in utero mutagenic agents capable of causing the gross and microscopic anomalies found in the left hemisphere of dyslexia patients.

> **Dyslexia** is associated with left-handedness, diabetes, rheumatoid arthritis, and ulcerative colitis.

Plasticity of Language. Recovery of language function following a middle cerebral artery stroke or resection of a tumor varies tremendously between individuals. Because language in most right-handed individuals is strongly lateralized, a stroke in the dominant hemisphere is likely to produce a severe and persistent language deficit. The degree of language recovery depends on the locus and size of the injury as well as the age of the patient. Although the prospects for recovery are best with children and decrease with age, some improvement is possible in all patients.

A bilateral representation for language may predispose otherwise healthy people to dyslexia, but it also may provide a neural substrate for recovery of language function following damage to the dominant hemisphere. Normally, language functions resident in the nondominant hemisphere are suppressed by the dominant side. Damage to the dominant hemisphere, however, releases the normally silent hemisphere, which enables it to "speak" for the first time. This interpretation is consistent with the observation that dyslexic and non-right-handed stroke patients, whose language skills are often represented

> **Left-handed and dyslexic individuals** have better recovery of language function than right-handed, nondyslexic individuals.

bilaterally, show better language recovery than right-handed patients following damage to the left hemisphere. Because the tendency for language to be located bilaterally extends to right-handed individuals who either are dyslexic or have relatives who are non-right-handed or dyslexic, these patients also have a better prognosis for recovery than strong right-handed persons.

Association Cortex

A person with an **agnosia** would not be able to identify a comb by sight or touch.

A person with an **apraxia** would not know how to use a comb.

The primary sensory and motor areas constitute about 25% of the cerebral cortex; the remainder is classified as association cortex. Even though the functions of the association cortices have been more difficult to decipher than the primary motor and sensory areas, some general statements can be made. First, cortical association areas process the output of the primary areas. Second, neurons in cortical association areas respond to more complex stimuli than the sensory and motor cortices. Last, damage to association cortex produces more complex deficits than seen in patients with lesions in primary sensory or motor areas. For example, damage to association cortex may not interfere with sensory processing per se, but rather with the ability to use that information in a meaningful way. These deficits, which take many forms, are classified as agnosias and apraxias. An *agnosia* is an inability to recognize or attach meaning to an object despite the patient having normal intellect, memory, and sensory abilities. An *apraxia* is an inability to engage in purposeful movement that cannot be attributed to motor paralysis or sensory loss, per se (Table 6.3).

The **posterior parietal lobe** constructs our immediate extrapersonal space.

Parietal Lobe. The parietal lobe can be divided on functional grounds into anterior and posterior parts. Primary somatosensory cortex (Brodmann areas 3, 1, and 2) is located in the anterior parietal lobe, adjacent to the postcentral gyrus. The association areas are located in the inferior and superior parietal lobules of the posterior parietal lobe. The inferior parietal lobule, which consists of the supramarginal (Brodmann area 40) and angular (Brodmann area 39) gyri, forms part of Wernicke's area, whose role in language comprehension was discussed in the previous section. Brodmann areas 5 and 7 constitute the superior parietal lobule. The inferior and superior parietal lobules are ideally situated to assemble sensory information from the adjacent parietal, temporal, and occipital lobes into a complex multimodal map of our immediate extrapersonal space. Patients with parietal lobe damage are often unable to construct an accurate map of their extrapersonal space and, consequently, get lost in familiar surroundings (topographagnosia). They also have trouble moving and interacting within their extrapersonal space because this spatial map is the foundation for planning and coordinating movements.

TABLE 6.3 Parietal Cortex Deficits

Disorder	Greek or Latin Derivation	Deficit
Abulia	No will or drive	General slowing of the intellect
Acalculia	No calculations	Simple arithmetic calculations
Agnosia	Lack of knowledge	Object recognition
Agraphia	No writing	Writing letters or words
Akinetopsia	No knowledge of movement	Seeing moving objects
Alexia	No reading	Reading
Anosognosia	No knowledge of disease	Denial of disease
Apraxia	Lack of action	Familiar, purposeful movements
Asomatognosia	No knowledge about the body	Sensory and motor neglect
Prosopagnosia	No knowledge of faces	Facial recognition
Simultanagnosia	No knowledge of items occurring together	Perception of multiple items
Topographagnosia	No knowledge of place	Navigation in familiar areas

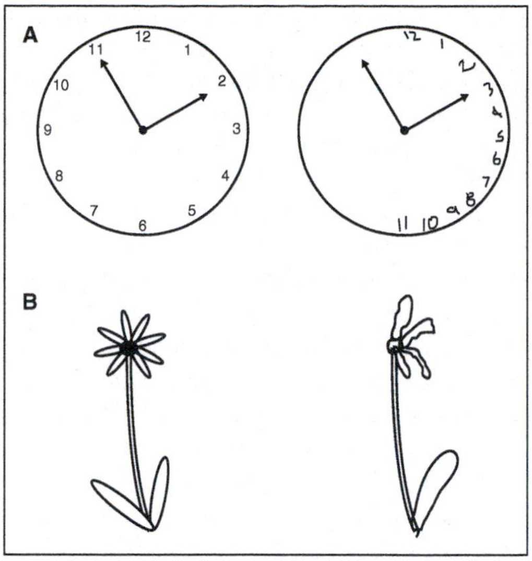

FIG. 6.15. Drawings of a Clock Face and Flower by a Patient with Sensory Neglect. The model appears on the left and the patient's copy on the right. Note that the patient has squeezed all twelve numbers of the clock face onto the right side. Similarly, the patient's drawing of the flower has petals only on the right side.

Neurophysiologic experiments in monkeys and clinical observations in human patients have provided a two-tiered understanding of the function of the parietal association cortex. Single neurons in the superior parietal lobule respond when a monkey reaches for or grasps an object or visually tracks a moving object. Passive manipulation of the hand or arm activates neurons in the primary somatosensory cortex, but not in the superior parietal cortex. Thus, the superior parietal lobule responds to behaviorally relevant stimuli that are actively engaged within the immediate extrapersonal space. Data from human patients suggest that the posterior parietal cortex links perception of the extrapersonal space with motor execution. Patients with damage to the posterior parietal cortex on the nondominant side not only fail to engage the local environment, but also ignore it. Patients with sensory neglect ignore objects that enter the contralateral space and, in extreme cases, will deny ownership of their contralateral limbs (asomatognosia). Because hemineglect usually occurs following damage to the right (i.e., nondominant) hemisphere, it is believed that the right parietal lobe attends to the environment on both the left and right sides, and the left hemisphere attends only to the contralateral side. Not surprisingly, these patients have trouble dressing themselves (dressing apraxia) and copying pictures (constructional apraxia). Their portrayals of other inanimate objects are similarly affected (Figure 6.15). Some patients with apraxias are able to identify an object (e.g., a comb or spoon), but are unable to use the object properly.

Gerstmann's syndrome, characterized by damage to the angular gyrus in the dominant hemisphere, is marked by left-right confusion and an inability to perform simple arithmetic calculations (acalculia), write down thoughts (agraphia), and name fingers (finger agnosia).

Gerstmann's syndrome is caused by damage to the angular gyrus.

Damage further posteriorly at the parieto-occipital border produces Balint's syndrome, which affects visual perception and visually guided movements. Patients with Balint's syndrome struggle to attend to more than one object at a time (simultanagnosia), which affects their ability to interpret a complex scene or perceive the relationship between multiple items in their field of view. These patients are also unable to use visual guidance to grasp an object. Although patients with Balint's syndrome retain their ability to make spontaneous or reflexive eye movements, they lack the ability to gaze at a target on command. Some patients have trouble breaking fixation from a target that remains within view. Balint's syndrome is rare because it is typically found in patients with bilateral damage, but it is important as a pedagogical tool because it illustrates how the parietal lobe enables us to engage our immediate extrapersonal space.

Temporal Lobe. The temporal lobe contains primary auditory cortex, higher-order auditory and visual cortices, important language areas (PT and part of Wernicke's area), and primitive cortical areas that work in conjunction with the hippocampal formation in memory acquisition.

The higher-order visual association cortex of the temporal lobe represents a rostral extension of the visual areas in the occipital lobe. Analysis of visual images, which began in the retina, is completed in the visual association areas of the temporal and parietal lobes. Both laboratory and clinical data demonstrate that sophisticated visual analysis takes place in the temporal lobe. For example, neurons in the inferior temporal lobe of the monkey respond when the subject is shown a picture of a face. These "face-neurons" are less responsive to other visual stimuli whose shape or luminance only vaguely resembles the effective face stimulus. Similarly, the effectiveness of a stimulus is reduced if the facial features are inverted, obscured, or scrambled. The faces that prove to be most effective stimuli are "generic faces"; that is, they have all of the features of a face but do not depict specific or familiar people. If neurons in the temporal lobe play a role in facial recognition, one might predict that temporal lobe damage in humans would interfere with the ability to recognize faces. This disorder, known as prosopagnosia, is a form of object agnosia caused by damage to Brodmann areas 20 and 21, which are located on the inferior temporal and the occipitotemporal gyri. Although prosopagnosia is usually caused by a lesion in the right temporal lobe, it may accompany unilateral damage of the left hemisphere. Patients with prosopagnosia are unable to recognize their own friends and family; in extreme cases, they may not recognize themselves. In other forms of object agnosia, patients struggle to identify members of other classes, such as houses, cars, or boats. Some patients with object agnosias can compensate for their specific deficit if cues from other sensory modalities are available. A patient unable to recognize the face of a friend, for example, may be able to identify that person by voice, clothes, or gait.

Prosopagnosia is an inability to recognize faces.

The medial inferior aspect of the temporal lobe, which includes the parahippocampal gyrus, is a staging area for sensory information bound for the underlying hippocampal formation. Damage to the parahippocampal gyrus impairs acquisition of new memories but leaves retrieval of existing memories relatively unimpaired.

Frontal Lobe. Unlike the parietal, temporal, and occipital cortices, the functions of the frontal lobe are difficult to summarize with one or two descriptive labels. The functional complexity of the frontal lobe derives, in part, from its elaborate set of reciprocal connections with the rest of the brain. In general, the frontal lobe is intimately involved with higher-order thought processes, personality, reward, and planning and execution of behavior. The frontal lobe, more than any other area of the brain, is what makes us human.

On functional grounds, the frontal lobe consists of motor and association areas located caudally in Brodmann areas 4, 6, and 8. These motor areas are critically important for initiation and execution of skilled movements. The association areas, by comparison, contribute to distinctly human activities such as planning, memory, problem-solving ability, and proper social conduct. Although research on nonhuman primates has provided some insight into the function of the prefrontal cortex, the most revealing data have come from clinical cases involving traumatic injury, disease, and neurosurgical intervention.

The association areas of the frontal lobe, known as prefrontal cortex, consist of ventromedial, dorsomedial, and dorsolateral parts.

Damage to the **ventromedial part of the frontal lobe** causes changes in mood and affect.

The ventromedial area encompasses all of the orbital cortex and the ventral part of the medial surface of the frontal lobe. Damage to the ventromedial area produces profound changes in mood and affect that may be accompanied by impulsive and improper behavior. The first major insight into the function of the prefrontal area was provided by the case of Phineas T. Gage, a railroad worker whose unfortunate accident in 1848 has earned him a permanent position in the annals of neurology. Mr. Gage was a railroad foreman entrusted with setting the dynamite charges used to blast the right-of-way through the stony Vermont countryside. Setting the charge involved pouring gunpowder into a predrilled hole, covering it with sand, and compressing it with the flat end of a tamping iron. One day as Mr. Gage bent over a blasting hole and tamped the powder into place, the charge ignited prematurely, propelling the tamping iron out of the hole. The tamping rod pierced Mr. Gage's face just below the cheek bone, drove through his left eye orbit and cranial vault before finally exiting the top of his skull (Figure 6.16). Mr. Gage survived this accident, but his personality was permanently altered. Prior to the accident Mr. Gage was serious, intelligent, conscientious, and polite; afterwards, he was impatient, childish, crude, and irresponsible.

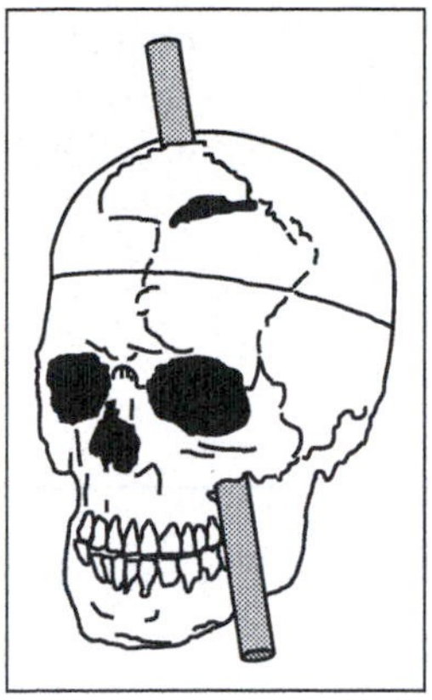

FIG. 6.16. Drawing of Phineas Gage's Skull with the Tamping Iron Shown as It Passed through His Skull. The most severe damage was sustained by the left frontal lobe and the orbital gyri. Because Mr. Gage's language functions remained unimpaired, it would appear that Broca's area was not seriously damaged.

Although Mr. Gage is an extreme example, his post-traumatic loss of socially appropriate behavior is the hallmark of damage to the frontal lobe. Other clinical cases have confirmed that damage to the frontal lobe causes flattened affect as well as a loss of social inhibition, initiative, and empathy. Many patients with frontal lobe damage are unable to plan a course of action, despite having normal intellect, memory, and sensory-motor function. Frontal lobe damage neutralizes pain; that is, patients report that they can feel pain, but they are relieved of the suffering. This constellation of symptoms is now referred to as frontal lobe syndrome.

These clinical data, together with several lesion experiments in nonhuman primates, prompted Egas Moniz to suggest that frontal lobotomies could be used to treat psychiatric disorders (e.g., depression, anxiety) and intractable pain in human patients. The first frontal lobotomies were performed in the 1940s. A less radical surgery, the prefrontal leucotomy, was introduced in an effort to minimize the undesirable side effects of the frontal lobotomy. The prefrontal leucotomy preserved the frontal lobe but severed the fibers connecting it with the thalamus. Both surgeries achieved the desired effects but left the patients withdrawn and without sufficient initiative and drive to lead independent and productive lives. The use of lobotomies and leucotomies waned in the late 1950s when newly discovered tranquilizers proved to be safer, more effective, and more acceptable treatments for psychiatric disorders.

The dorsomedial prefrontal area is an important site for personal characteristics such as introversion and extroversion. Our ability to comprehend the emotional tone of others and generate appropriate emotions of our own reside in the dorsomedial region. Patients with damage to this area may lack the proper level of arousal and alertness to initiate or maintain behavior (akinesia), a condition referred to as abulia. Not surprisingly, mutism often accompanies abulia. A patient with abulia may answer the telephone but be unable to continue the conversation. These patients are also unable to adapt their behavior to changing task conditions. This phenomenon, called perseveration, has been studied extensively in monkeys with focal lesions in the superior medial prefrontal cortex. These monkeys are taught a task, lesioned, and then retested with the same task. Their performance on the task is not affected by the lesion, but if the task is changed so that the monkeys must adopt a new strategy, they perseverate with the old, now maladaptive strategy. Hence, damage to the dorsolateral prefrontal cortex impairs the ability to develop new strategies, but beyond that, little else is known with certainty.

RESOLUTION OF CLINICAL CASE

The initial diagnosis of a stroke involving the right middle cerebral artery was correct, but even though the patient was unable to move, she was not paralyzed. This patient exhibited the classic symptoms of asomatognosia, or sensory neglect. Patients with asomatognosia do not move their limbs on one side of the body, because they do not recognize that the limbs belong to them. Similarly, they do not report somatosensory stimulation applied to that side of their body. In this case the patient suffered a stroke of the right middle cerebral artery, which supplies the posterior parietal cortex. Sensory neglect of the left side of the body ensued.

REVIEW QUESTIONS

Directions: For each question, choose the **one** best answer.

1. Which symptom is characteristic of patients with damage in Wernicke's area?
   A. Nonfluent aphasia
   B. An inability to hum a melody
   C. Fluent aphasia
   D. Language comprehension, but an inability to speak smoothly
   E. Labored, telegraphic speech

2. A neurosurgeon is considering surgical intervention on a 31-year-old right-handed male epileptic patient. Which of the following results from the Wada test would indicate that language in this patient is *not* located in the hemisphere that controls his preferred hand?
   A. The patient is unable to speak following injection of the right carotid artery.
   B. The patient is unable to speak following injection of the left carotid artery.
   C. Injection of the left carotid artery produces paralysis of the right arm.
   D. Injection of the left carotid artery produces paralysis of the left arm.
   E. The patient is unable to sing following injection of the right carotid artery.

3. Which symptom is characteristic of patients with damage to the prefrontal cortex?
   A. Flattened affect
   B. An inability to recognize faces of familiar people
   C. Nonfluent aphasia
   D. Neglect of objects in their immediate extrapersonal space
   E. The ability to recognize, but not use, an object (e.g., a nail file)

4. What is the most useful structure for understanding the anatomical organization of the thalamus?
   A. Pulvinar
   B. Reticular nucleus
   C. Ventroposteromedial nucleus (VPM)
   D. Internal medullary lamina
   E. Anterior thalamic nucleus

5. Which of the following pathways connects corresponding areas of the left and right hemispheres?
   A. Superior longitudinal fasciculus
   B. Uncinate fasciculus
   C. Internal capsule
   D. Anterior commissure
   E. Cingulum

6. Which of the following disorders is characterized by an inability to recognize faces?
   A. Gerstmann's syndrome
   B. Broca's aphasia
   C. Prosopagnosia
   D. Asomatognosia
   E. Balint's syndrome

7. The arcuate fasciculus and the uncinate fasciculus are similar in which of the following respects?
   A. Damage to either pathway will produce a conduction aphasia.
   B. Both funnel information to the hippocampus.
   C. Both connect parts of the temporal lobe with the frontal lobe.
   D. Both are important commissural pathways.
   E. The importance of both pathways has diminished over the course of phylogenetic development.

8. Your chances of recovering language function following a stroke are best if which of the following is true?
   A. You are right-handed
   B. You are right-handed and dyslexic
   C. You are ambidextrous
   D. You have a severe stutter
   E. You are left-handed

9. Which of the following thalamic nuclei receives a projection from the mammillary nucleus?
   A. Anterior nucleus
   B. Posterior nucleus
   C. VPL
   D. Pulvinar
   E. Reticular nucleus

10. A single lesion produces contralateral paresis and anesthesia, hearing loss, and visual impairment. Where is the damage?
    A. Frontal lobe
    B. Genu of the internal capsule
    C. Posterior internal capsule
    D. Intralaminar nuclei
    E. Temporal lobe

ADDITIONAL READING

Classic Literature

Brodmann K: *Vergleichende Lokalisation lehre der Grosshirnrinde in ihren Prinzipien dargestellt auf Grund des Zellenbaunes*. Leipzig, Germany: J. A. Barth, 1909:324.

Geschwind N: Disconnection syndromes in animals and man II. *Brain* 88:585–644, 1965.

——: The organization of language and the brain. *Science* 170:940–944, 1970.

Harlowe JM: Passage of an iron bar through the head. *Boston Med Surg J* 39:389–393, 1848.

Sperry R: Consciousness, personal identity and the divided brain. *Neuropsychologia* 22:661–673, 1984.

Sperry RW: Cerebral organization and behavior. *Science* 133:1749–1757, 1961.

Reviews and Landmark Research Articles

Abeles M, Goldstein MH, Jr: Functional architecture in cat primary auditory cortex: columnar organization and organization according to depth. *J Neurophysiol* 33:172–187, 1970.

Annett M: Laterality and types of dyslexia. *Neurosci Biobehav* Rev 20:631–636, 1996.

Damasio H: The return of Phineas Gage: clues about the brain from the skull of a famous patient. *Science* 264:1102–1105, 1994.

Driver J, Mattingley JB: Parietal neglect and visual awareness. *Nat Neurosci* 1:17–22, 1998.

Galaburda AM, Sherman GF, Rosen GD, Aboitiz F, Geschwind N: Developmental dyslexia: four consecutive patients with cortical anomalies. *Ann Neurol* 18:222–233, 1985.

Gazzaniga MS: Cerebral specialization and interhemispheric communication: does the corpus callosum enable the human condition? *Brain* 123:1293–1326, 2000.

Hubel DH, Wiesel TN: Receptive fields, binocular interaction, and functional architecture in the cat's visual cortex. *J Physiol* 160:106–154, 1962.

Mountcastle VB: Modality and topographic properties of single neurons of cat's somatic sensory cortex. *J Neurophysiol* 20:408–434, 1957.

Pedersen PM, Jorgensen HS, Nakayama H, Raaschou HO, Olsen TS: Hemineglect in acute stroke—incidence and prognostic implications: the Copenhagen Stroke Study. *Am J Phys Med Rehabil* 76:122–127, 1997.

Pinault D: The thalamic reticular nucleus: structure, function and concept. *Brain Res Rev* 46:1–31, 2004.

Stuss DT, Knight RT: *Principles of Frontal Lobe Function*. Oxford, UK: Oxford University Press, 2002.

Tonnessen FE: Testosterone and dyslexia. *Pediatr Rehabil* 1:51–57, 1997.

INTERNET RESOURCES

American Speech-Language-Hearing Association Aphasia
http://www.asha.org/public/speech/disorders/Aphasia.htm

Comparative Mammalian Brain Collections
Human Brain Sections
http://www.brainmuseum.org/Specimens/primates/human/index.html

California State University-Chico
Neuropathologies of Language and Cognition
Unit 7. Specific Syndromes: The Nonfluent Aphasias
http://www.csuchico.edu/~pmccaffrey//syllabi/SPPA336/336unit7.html

National Aphasia Association
http://www.aphasia.org/

National Institute on Deafness and Other Communication Disorders
Aphasia
http://www.nidcd.nih.gov/health/voice/aphasia.htm

National Institute of Neurological Disorders and Stroke
Gerstmann's Syndrome
http://www.ninds.nih.gov/disorders/gerstmanns/gerstmanns.htm
Prosopagnosia
http://www.ninds.nih.gov/disorders/prosopagnosia/Prosopagnosia.htm

Prosopagnosia Research Centers at Harvard University and University College London
http://www.faceblind.org/index.html

University of Colorado-Boulder
Hemispatial Neglect Syndrome
http://www.members.aol.com/_ht_a/mazdakh/index.html

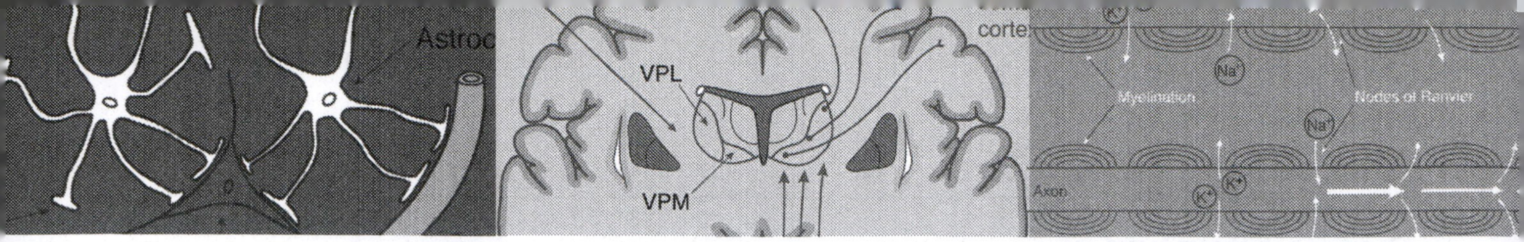

CHAPTER 7

Somesthesis

INTRODUCTION OF CLINICAL CASE

A 45-year-old woman with severe face pain was examined at the pain clinic because she was suffering from recurrent episodes of intense, stabbing pain in the center of her left cheek. These attacks occurred three or four times a day, each episode lasted at least 10 minutes, and the pain had a sharp, searing quality that was accompanied by involuntary twitching movements in the maxilla. The attacks had a sudden onset and were often triggered by eating or by touching the center of her cheek. Consequently, to prevent triggering these attacks, the woman minimized facial movements by not smiling and by skipping meals to avoid chewing movements. In fact, after losing 25 lbs in the last 6 months, her weight was in the bottom quartile for someone of her age and height. Despite this significant loss of weight, the woman was generally healthy, and a dental exam indicated that her teeth and gums were free of disease.

INTRODUCTION TO THE SOMATOSENSORY SYSTEM

The somatosensory system detects stimuli that directly contact the body. In addition to mediating the sensations of touch and temperature that are produced by innocuous stimuli, it mediates the sensations of pain that are produced by injury or disease. The somatosensory system also monitors skeletal movements and mediates the kinesthetic sensations that signal limb position.

To perform these tasks, the somatosensory system has thousands of peripheral nerve fibers (i.e., general somatic afferent fibers) that innervate the skin, muscles, and joints to convey tactile, kinesthetic, and nociceptive information to the central nervous system (CNS). Somatosensory nerve fibers also innervate the meninges, the surfaces of the nasal and oral cavities, and many organs in the thoracic and abdominal cavities. These afferent nerve fibers project to specific nuclei in the spinal cord or brainstem that project to the forebrain.

The dorsal column-medial lemniscal system conveys tactile and kinesthetic information and is segregated from the anterolateral system, which is primarily responsible for conveying pain and temperature information. These two systems were briefly described in Chapters 4 and 5, and this chapter completes the discussion of these systems and their relationship to cutaneous sensation and pain. Although the peripheral receptors, nerves, and central pathways that convey information from the muscles and tendons to the cerebellum are considered part of the somatosensory system, they do not mediate conscious sensations and are not discussed here.

SKIN FUNCTIONS

The skin, or integument, is a major organ of the body and performs many vital functions. In a typical adult, the skin has an area ranging from 1.5 to 2.5 m^2 and a thickness that varies from 1.5 to 4.0 mm, thus forming approximately 8% of total body mass. In addition to its sensory function, it provides a formidable barrier against microbes and protects the organism from a variety of mechanical, chemical, thermal, and photic stimuli. Although the skin prevents dehydration, it may excrete or absorb limited amounts of fluid. Furthermore, because the skin is highly vascularized, changes in its blood flow are an important mechanism for regulating body heat. Many aspects of health and aging are reflected in skin appearance, which may indicate certain pathologic conditions such as jaundice, shingles, or chicken pox.

The skin contains a high density of free nerve endings and specialized cutaneous receptors that supply the CNS with a rich source of sensory information. Tactile information is essential for making skilled hand movements and for discriminating the size, shape, and texture of objects. The sense of touch provides an avenue for social communication and is critical for establishing intimacy and engaging in sexual behavior. Furthermore, the skin is a versatile sensory organ that may substitute for loss of other sensory modalitites; blind or deaf individuals learn to rely on the somatosensory system to acquire information that would otherwise be unavailable to them.

Some of the afferent fibers that innervate the skin, muscles, or joints are responsible for detecting intense mechanical, thermal, or chemical stimuli that are potentially damaging. These nociceptive fibers usually mediate pain sensations that are well localized and have specific sensory qualities. Other nociceptive fibers innervate the visceral organs and give rise to the noxious sensations associated with myocardial infarction, appendicitis, gastric reflux, or other visceral events.

INNERVATION OF THE SKIN

The skin is formed by two tightly opposed layers of tissue: epidermis and dermis. The epidermis is located superficially and is composed of stratified epithelial cells. Directly below the epidermis is the dermis, which is composed of moderately dense connective tissue. Most peripheral fibers innervating the skin terminate in the dermis or in the lower part of the epidermis (Figure 7.1).

When discussing the neural innervation of the skin, it is useful to distinguish between glabrous skin and hairy skin. Glabrous skin is devoid of hairs and covers the surface of the palms, the soles of the feet, and the flexor surfaces of the digits and toes; the remainder of the body is covered by hairy skin. Glabrous skin has a series of small papillary ridges or grooves, which provide friction for manipulating objects or for gaining traction during

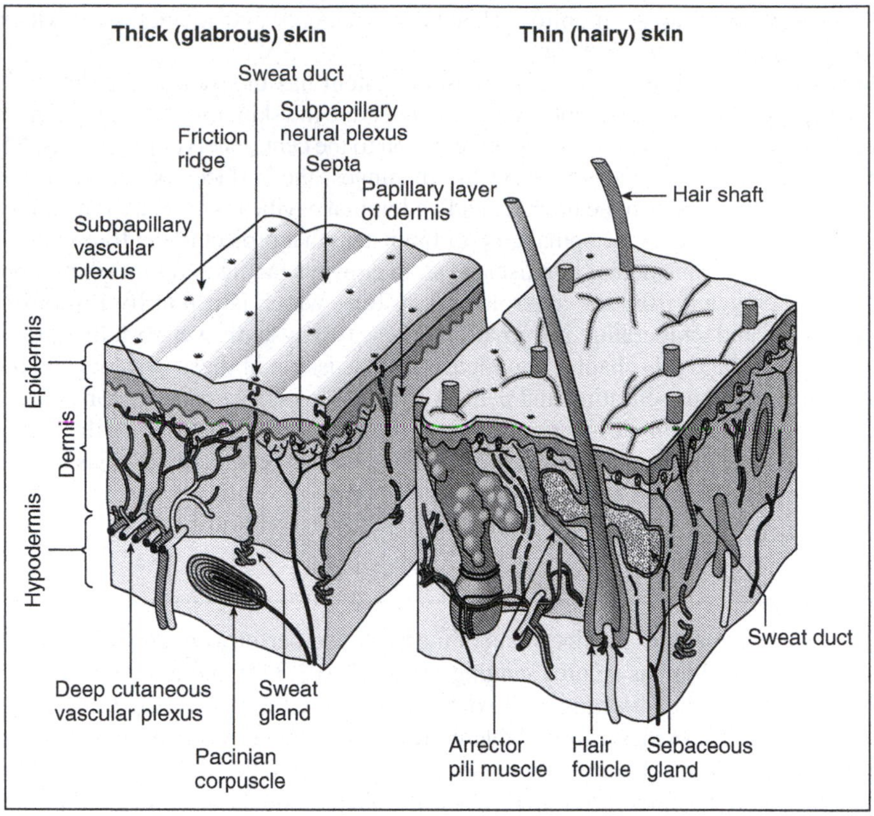

FIG. 7.1. Structure of the Skin. Diagram showing the organization of glabrous and hairy skin. The innervation of the glabrous skin is shown in more detail in Figure 7.3.

locomotion. Glabrous skin is much thicker than hairy skin and has a greater density of sweat glands to help cool the skin. Although sensory endings in both the glabrous and hairy skin are extremely sensitive to cutaneous stimulation, only the glabrous skin on the hand is used for fine tactile discrimination.

Rapidly adapting fibers respond to vibration.

Slowly adapting fibers respond to constant indentation.

Afferent fibers in the skin are categorized according to the physical stimulus that optimally activates their receptive endings. Thus, somatosensory nerve fibers are classified as mechanoreceptive, thermoreceptive, or nociceptive, but the usefulness of this classification is limited because many fibers respond to more than one sensory modality.

Sensory fibers in the skin are also defined by their rate of adaptation during a constant stimulus (Figure 7.2). Fibers that respond continuously to steady indentation are called

FIG. 7.2. Sensory Adaptation. Peripheral mechanoreceptors and their nerve fibers show different rates of adaptation to maintained indentation of the skin. Rapidly adapting mechanoreceptors adapt quickly to changes in skin position; slowly adapting mechanoreceptors continue to respond during the plateau portion of the skin indentation.

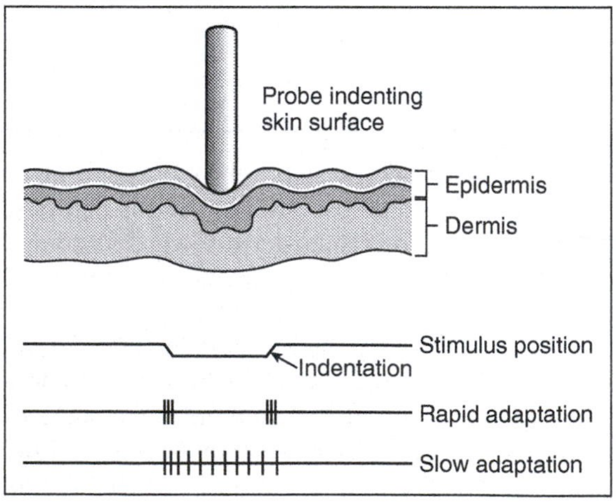

slowly adapting fibers. Rapidly adapting fibers, by comparison, respond to changes in stimulus position or during the onset and offset of a stimulus. Rapidly adapting fibers respond best to vibrations or to the phasic components of a stimulus, whereas slowly adapting fibers respond to steady pressure.

Somatosensory fibers are also identified by the morphology of their terminal endings. Most mechanoreceptive fibers have either an encapsulated ending or terminals that are juxtaposed against other cellular specializations. By comparison, most nociceptive and thermoreceptive fibers are called free nerve endings because they do not have encapsulated terminals.

Tactile Mechanoreceptors

Four classes of cutaneous mechanoreceptors have been identified in human skin: Merkel corpuscles, Meissner corpuscles, Pacinian corpuscles, and hair receptors (Figure 7.3). These mechanoreceptors differ according to their location, morphology, and response to mechanical stimulation. Another class, known as Ruffini endings, has been proposed on the basis of physiology studies of the human hand, but encapsulated receptors that correspond to the Ruffini endings seen in animal tissue have not been seen in human skin.

For most cutaneous mechanoreceptors, stimulation of the skin deforms or stretches the receptor membrane and causes a change in its ionic permeability. The flow of positive ions into the receptor produces a depolarizing potential that spreads passively along the nerve ending until it reaches a trigger site and evokes an action potential. The process of converting external mechanical energy into a series of neural impulses is known as sensory transduction. Different types of mechanoreceptors vary in their ability to transduce specific types of mechanical energy because of structural differences in their encapsulated endings. Despite these differences, all cutaneous mechanoreceptors are innervated by large-diameter A-β fibers, which conduct impulses rapidly to the CNS.

Sensory transduction is the process of converting physical energy into neural impulses.

Merkel Corpuscles. Merkel corpuscles are located in the epidermis immediately under the papillary ridges of the glabrous skin. A Merkel corpuscle is innervated by a single myelinated nerve fiber that branches into several collateral endings, each of which forms a

Merkel corpuscles: slowly adapting, small receptive fields

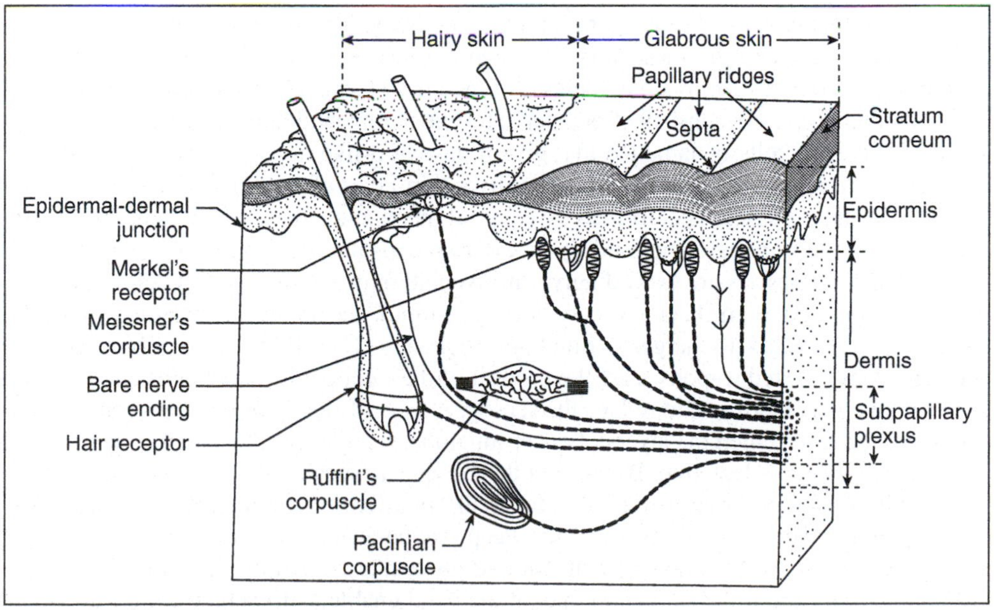

FIG. 7.3. Innervation of the Glabrous Skin. The glabrous skin is innervated by a plexus of nerve fibers that terminate in a variety of cutaneous mechanoreceptors, including Meissner corpuscles, Pacinian corpuscles, and Merkel corpuscles.

very small disk-shaped terminal or Merkel disk that is closely apposed to the basal membrane of an overlying Merkel cell (see Figure 7.3). Thus, a cluster of 5 to 10 Merkel cells are innervated by a single myelinated nerve fiber that branches into a corresponding number of disk-like endings. Merkel cells lie in the basal epidermis and have spike-shaped processes that protrude into the surrounding epithelium. Large dense-core vesicles (80-120 μm) in the Merkel cells contain neuropeptides that may modulate the activity of the nerve ending.

Merkel corpuscles comprise at least one-fourth of the mechanoreceptors of the hand and are densest in the fingertips, lips, and external genitalia. The high density of Merkel corpuscles in these regions is closely related to their tactile sensitivity. Consistent with their close proximity to the papillary ridges in the glabrous skin, the receptive fields of fibers innervating Merkel corpuscles are small, perhaps 2-4 mm in diameter. Merkel corpuscles exhibit slowly adapting responses to punctuate indentations of the skin and mediate sensations of light pressure required to code local form, edges, texture, and other surface features of objects manipulated by the hand.

Meissner corpuscles: rapidly adapting (10-50 Hz), small receptive fields

Meissner Corpuscles. Meissner corpuscles are large receptors (30 μm by 80 μm) that occupy the grooves between the dermal papillae of the glabrous skin (Figure 7.3). They have a cylindrical shape with their long axis oriented perpendicular to the surface of the skin. The corpuscle is comprised of an outer capsule surrounding a central core of arborized nerve fibers. The outer capsule is formed by a layer of connective tissue that is continuous with the perineurium of the afferent nerve fibers. Usually two or three myelinated nerve fibers invade the interior of the capsule to form a coiled bundle of processes among a dense collection of flattened cells known as lemmocytes.

The dense layers of connective tissue and lemmocytes surrounding the nerve terminals endow Meissner corpuscles with specific filtering properties. Meissner corpuscles are rapidly adapting mechanoreceptors, which discharge best during vibratory stimulation in the range of 10-50 hertz (Hz). Like Merkel corpuscles, Meissner corpuscles have small receptive fields because they are located close to the surface of the epidermis. Approximately 40% of the mechanoreceptors in the hand are Meissner corpuscles and, consistent with their sensitivity to low-frequency vibrations, they detect stimulus movement across the skin and are important for controlling hand force when grasping an object.

Pacinian corpuscles: rapidly adapting (100-300 Hz), large receptive fields

Pacinian Corpuscles. Pacinian corpuscles are located in the subcutaneous tissue directly underneath the dermis and in deeper regions of the body, including the interosseous membranes, the joints, and the mesentery. Pacinian corpuscles are oval or spherical in shape and may extend up to 2 mm along the axis of the nerve terminal. The encapsulated ending of a Pacinian corpuscle consists of one nerve terminal surrounded by a concentric arrangement of flattened cells or lamellae that give it an onion-like appearance (see Figure 7.3). The lamellae are separated from each other by a thin layer of fluid that flows between the lamellae as the corpuscle is deformed by external mechanical forces. The lamellae and the afferent nerve terminal are enclosed by an external capsule of elastic fibrous tissue.

Pacinian corpuscles are exceedingly sensitive and may respond to skin deformations of a few microns. As such, Pacinian corpuscles are rapidly adapting mechanoreceptors that transmit phase-locked discharges during high-frequency (100-300 Hz) skin vibrations (Figure 7.4). Phase-locked responses are the product of the multiple layers of cells and fluid that surround the nerve terminal to reduce the sensory effects of steady pressure and slow indentations of the skin. When the layers of encapsulation are removed, the naked nerve fiber exhibits a slow rate of adaptation. Because of their exquisite sensitivity and their deep location in the skin, Pacinian corpuscles respond to small vibrations transmitted through the subcutaneous tissue. Their sensitivity and their deep, subcutaneous location endow them with large receptive fields that often span an entire digit or a large part of the palm (Figure 7.5). Pacinian corpuscles in the skin and joints of the hand enable us to perceive high-frequency vibrations that are transmitted through probes or objects that are gripped by the hand.

Hair Receptors. Several hair types have been classified according to the thickness, length, and structure of the hair follicle. Most hairs are innervated by free nerve endings that enter

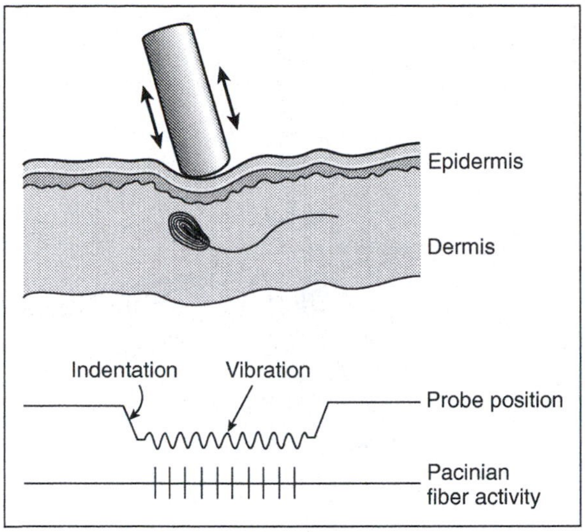

FIG. 7.4. Phase-Locked Responses of Pacinian Corpuscles. Rapid vibrations of the skin (i.e., 100-300 Hz) cause Pacinian receptors to discharge in the same part of the vibratory phase during successive stimulus cycles.

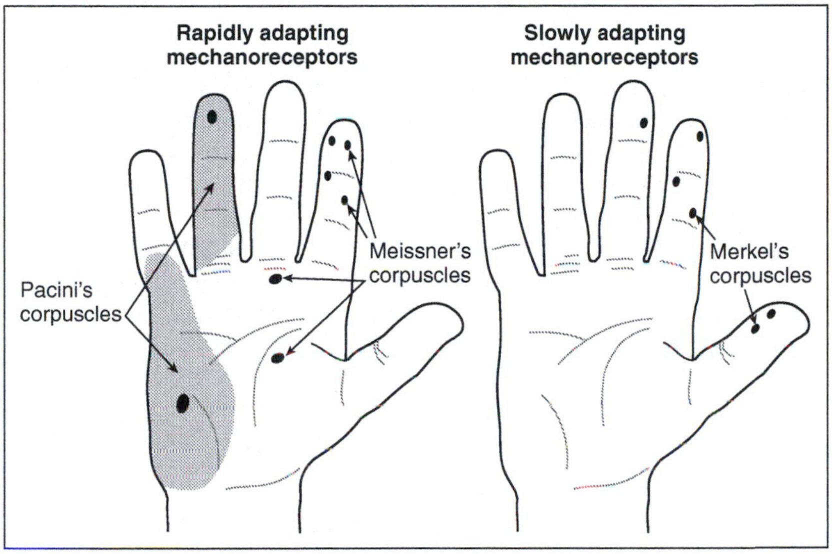

FIG. 7.5. Cutaneous Receptive Fields. Comparison of receptive fields for different classes of rapidly and slowly adapting mechanoreceptors. Meissner and Merkel corpuscles, which are located superficially, have small receptive fields. Pacinian corpuscles, which are in the subdermal layers, have highly sensitive receptive fields (small dots) that are surrounded by larger regions of reduced sensitivity (shading).

the hair follicle and encircle the hair at its base, at an intermediate level, or superficially just below the epidermis (Figure 7.6). Some of the afferent fibers form palisade endings that run along the length of the follicle. In addition, nerves that innervate Merkel corpuscles may send collaterals around the neck of the hair follicle, just below the epidermis.

Depending on the type of hair that is innervated and the morphology of its afferent ending, hair fibers may exhibit rapidly adapting or slowly adapting responses. Most afferent hair fibers respond to lever-like movements of the hair. Although some animals possess whiskers or vibrissal hairs that are actively moved during exploration, human skin hairs act passively to detect the part of the body that has been touched.

Kinesthetic and Nociceptive Endings

Some receptors in the somatosensory system are specialized to detect stimuli affecting the muscles, joints, or other deep tissues of the body. Most of these receptors are responsible for the perception of kinesthesia or pain.

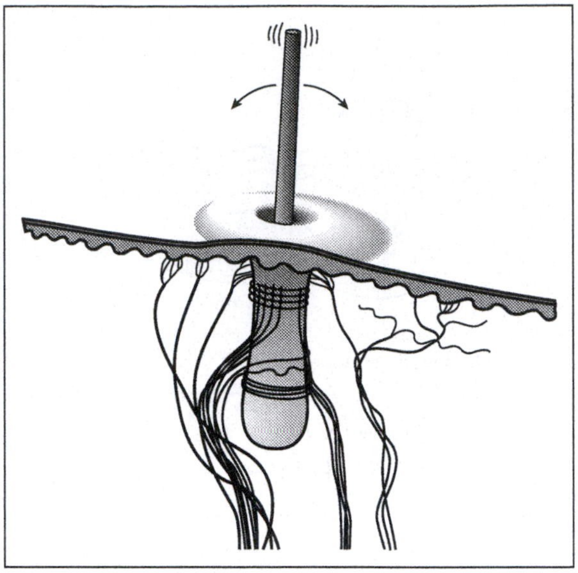

FIG. 7.6. Innervation of a Hair Follicle. Free nerve endings encircling the follicle are activated by lever-like movements of the hair.

Slowly adapting joint receptors signal limb position.

Rapidly adapting joint receptors signal limb movement.

Joint Receptors. Several types of joint receptors have been identified in various parts of the joint capsule. Most joint receptors are encapsulated endings that resemble Pacinian corpuscles or Golgi tendon organs, and these are innervated by myelinated nerve fibers (Figure 7.7). These encapsulated joint receptors are distributed throughout the fibrous joint capsule and in the intrinsic and extrinsic ligaments.

Encapsulated joint endings are basically tension receptors that respond to stretching of the tissues in the joint. Some of these receptors are slowly adapting, and their rate of activity indicates the angle of the joint. Other joint receptors are rapidly adapting and encode the speed or acceleration of joint movement. Collectively, joint receptors help individuals

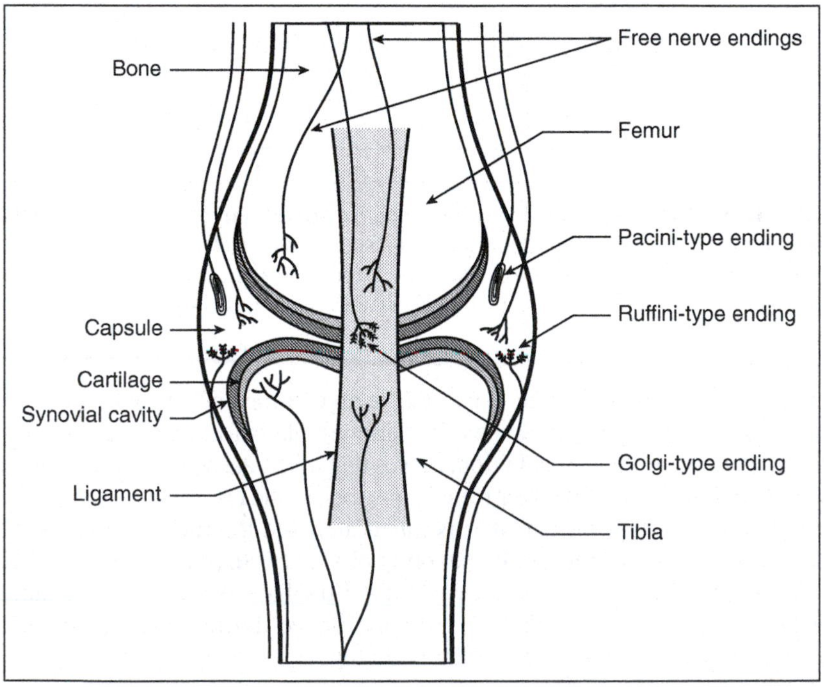

FIG. 7.7. Joint Receptors. Schematic diagram of a joint and its sensory innervation. Joint capsules are innervated by free nerve endings and by encapsulated nerve terminals that resemble Pacinian corpuscles. Ligaments are innervated by free nerve endings and by encapsulated nerve terminals that resemble Golgi tendon organs.

recognize the position of their limbs at rest and during movement. This proprioceptive function is augmented by cutaneous and muscle afferent fibers that innervate the regions surrounding the joints; this explains why patients maintain kinesthetic sense even after total joint replacement.

In addition to encapsulated joint receptors, the joints are also innervated by the free nerve endings of unmyelinated fibers (see below). In the joints, free nerve endings usually terminate as an arborized plexus within the joint capsule, the subsynovial capsule, the ligaments, or the fat pads associated with the joint. These endings mediate the sensations of joint pain produced by trauma or arthritis.

Free Nerve Endings. Nerve terminals in the skin and subcutaneous tissues that lack encapsulated endings are called free nerve endings. In the skin, these highly branched endings terminate in the layers below the epidermal-dermal junction (see Figure 7.3). Free nerve endings also innervate ligaments, tendons, blood vessels, the meninges, the periosteum, the cornea, the respiratory tracts, and the capsules enclosing organs in the thoracic and abdominal cavities. Finally, free nerve endings innervate the joint tissues and all types of muscles (i.e., striated and smooth), including the myocardium.

Regardless of the tissue that is innervated, most free nerve endings convey impulses related to the perception of pain or temperature. The small-diameter axons of free nerve endings conduct impulses more slowly than the fibers that terminate in encapsulated mechanoreceptors. Some free nerve endings are classified as thermoreceptors because they convey innocuous sensations of warmth or cold. Other free nerve endings have high thresholds and respond only to noxious mechanical stimulation or to extreme temperatures. These nociceptive fibers are subdivided further depending on whether they respond best to tissue damage, extreme temperatures, or chemical stimulation. Even though nociceptive fibers have free nerve terminals, different fibers convey different sensations depending on the types of ion channels located in their terminal membranes.

Tactile Discrimination

The surface of the body is not uniformly sensitive to tactile stimulation, and this property is easily demonstrated in a two-point discrimination test. In this task, a pair of calipers is used to stimulate two points on the skin simultaneously, and subjects are asked to report whether they detect one or two stimuli. The distance between the two points is varied from one trial to the next until the minimum distance required to distinguish the pair of stimuli has been determined. In normal individuals, the skin of the digits, palm, or face can resolve two stimuli that are separated by a few millimeters (Figure 7.8). By comparison, separate sites on the leg or trunk cannot be distinguished unless they are separated by several centimeters.

Tactile sensitivity increases with the density of nerve fibers that innervate a given area of skin.

The threshold for two-point discrimination varies with the density of afferent fibers that supply a given skin region. For example, a large number of dorsal root fibers innervate the fingertip, but each nerve fiber supplies only a few papillary ridges. By comparison, a region of the same size on the trunk is innervated by a small number of dorsal root fibers so that each fiber supplies a large area that overlaps with the receptive fields of adjacent fibers. For example, when the fingertip is indented by two pins separated by 5 mm, two different sets of peripheral fibers are activated to produce the perception of two points on the skin. When the skin on the trunk is indented by the same pins, however, each pin activates the same set of peripheral fibers, and this creates the sensory impression of a single point.

The ability to recognize different textures depends on several factors besides the high density of nerve endings in the digits. To discriminate silk from velvet, for example, rubbing each fabric with the fingertips produces a unique pattern of activity in the peripheral fibers. Thus, actively touching and rubbing the fabric activates several populations of different mechanoreceptors (i.e., Meissner, Pacinian, Merkel) to produce a continuous flow of neural impulses in the peripheral fibers. This activity ascends the neuraxis and produces a complex spatiotemporal pattern of activity within multiple cortical areas. Although the mechanism of texture discrimination is not completely understood, the

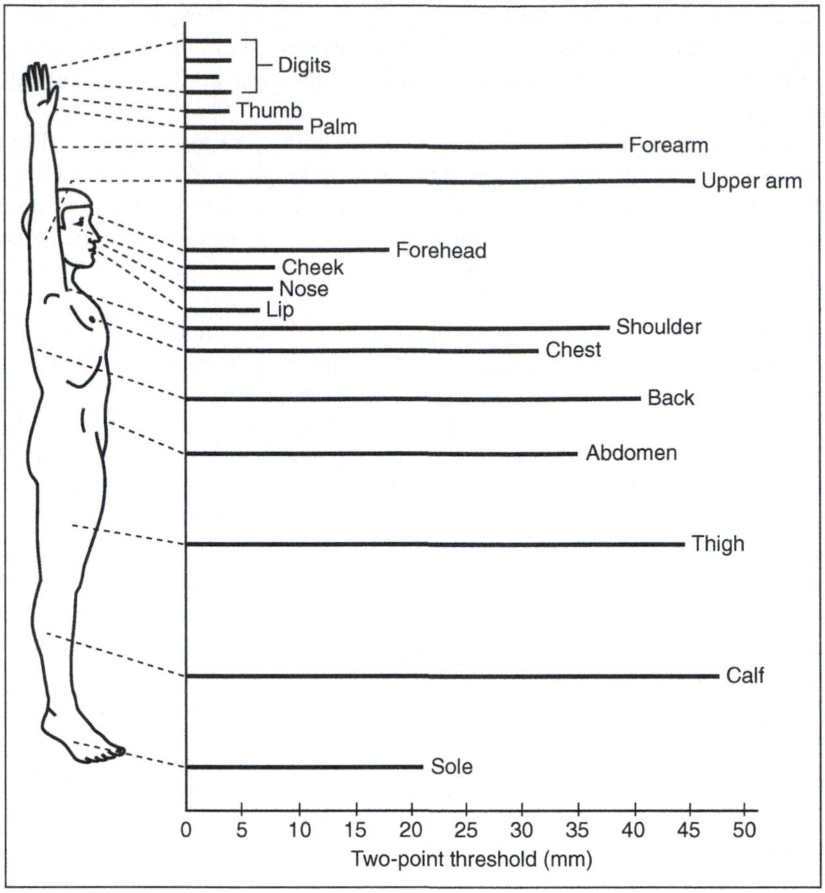

FIG. 7.8. Distribution of Tactile Sensitivity. Different parts of the body vary in their sensitivity, as measured by the two-point discrimination test.

sensations of smoothness and other distinct textural qualities are mediated by unique patterns of cortical activity that are evoked by each texture.

Dorsal Column-Medial Lemniscal and Trigeminothalamic Systems

The spinal nerves and their ascending axons in the dorsal columns of the spinal cord convey cutaneous and kinesthetic information from all parts of the body to the nucleus gracilis and nucleus cuneatus (Figure 7.9). Axons from these dorsal column nuclei cross the midline and ascend through the medial lemniscus before terminating in the ventroposterolateral (VPL) nucleus of the thalamus. Axonal projections from the VPL nucleus proceed through a massive bundle of myelinated fibers, the internal capsule, before terminating in the postcentral gyrus of the cerebral cortex.

Cutaneous information from the face and mouth is conveyed by the ophthalmic, maxillary, and mandibular divisions of the trigeminal nerve to the principal (or chief) sensory nucleus and to the rostral part of the spinal trigeminal nucleus. The efferent projections of these trigeminal nuclei cross the midline and ascend the brainstem as the ventral trigeminothalamic tract. This tract is associated with the medial part of the medial lemniscus before it terminates in the ventroposteromedial (VPM) nucleus of the thalamus. Like the VPL nucleus, the VPM nucleus projects to the postcentral gyrus of the cerebral cortex via the internal capsule.

The dorsal column-medial lemniscal system and the trigeminothalamic pathways transmit cutaneous information from the periphery to the cerebral cortex by a series of

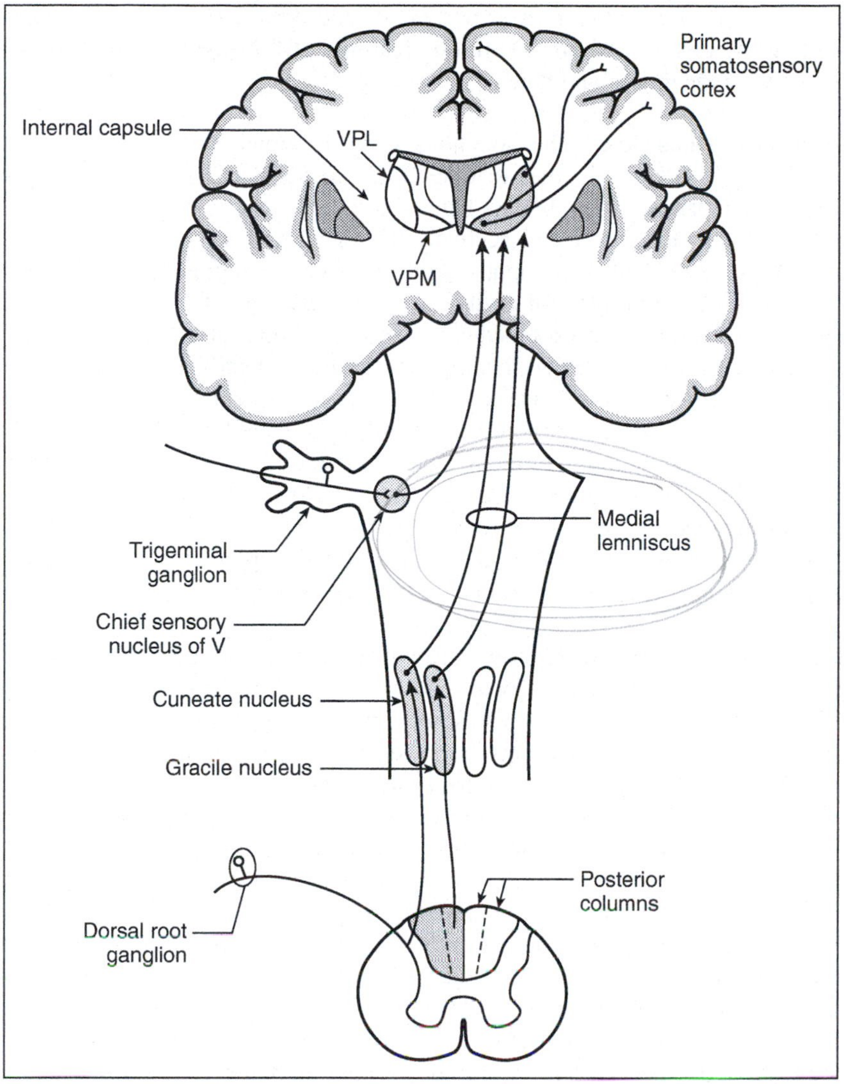

FIG. 7.9. Cutaneous Pathways. Summary of the pathways that convey cutaneous sensation to the thalamus and cerebral cortex. The trigeminothalamic system and the dorsal column-medial lemniscal system conduct cutaneous information from the face and body, respectively. VPL = ventroposterolateral nucleus; VPM = ventroposteromedial nucleus.

three neurons and their intervening synapses. Because these pathways consist of large-diameter fibers that are heavily myelinated, cutaneous information is transmitted rapidly to the cerebral cortex where conscious perception of touch takes place.

Topographical Organization. Each neuron in the somatosensory system responds to external stimulation within a discrete peripheral region known as the receptive field. The dorsal column nuclei and the trigeminal nuclei are topographically organized so that adjacent neurons have neighboring receptive fields on the body. This somatotopic organization is preserved at subsequent levels of the somatosensory system by a precise point-to-point set of projections to the thalamus and cortex. Collectively, the topographic organization of neurons in each region forms a complete representation, or neural map, of the head and body. Somatotopic maps are not isomorphic representations of the body; they contain prominent distortions that reflect the differential distribution of peripheral receptors throughout the body. For example, the thalamic and cortical representations of the mouth and hand occupy a disproportionately large part of the neural map because these body regions are more densely innervated than other body parts. The large amount of cortex devoted to representing these body parts endows them with exquisite sensitivity for assessing the texture and other stimulus features of food or other objects that come into contact with the mouth and hand.

Cutaneous mechanoreceptors project to the central core of VPM and VPL.

Joint and **muscle receptors** project to the surrounding shell.

Somatosensory Thalamus. The somatosensory thalamus is subdivided into medial (VPM) and lateral (VPL) nuclei that, together, form the ventrobasal complex. This region is somatotopically organized such that the leg and arm representations occupy the lateral and medial parts of the VPL nucleus, respectively. The head representation occupies the entire VPM nucleus such that cutaneous inputs from the face are represented laterally, whereas those from the tongue and intraoral cavity are located medially. Gustatory sensations from the tongue are processed in the most medial part of the ventrobasal complex (see Chapter 10).

Different parts of the ventrobasal complex respond to specific submodalities. Neurons in the central part of the ventrobasal complex respond to gentle, cutaneous stimulation. This central cutaneous representation is surrounded by a shell of neurons that respond to joint movement or manipulation of the muscles and other deep tissues. The segregation of cutaneous and proprioceptive submodalities indicates that information from the Merkel, Meissner, and Pacinian receptors is transmitted predominately to the central part of the ventrobasal complex, whereas information from muscle spindles, Golgi tendon organs, and encapsulated joint receptors terminate in the outer shell.

Cutaneous mechanoreceptors project to Brodmann areas 3b and 1.

Joint and **muscle receptors** project to areas 2 and 3a, respectively.

Primary Somatosensory (SI) Cortex. Relay neurons in the ventrobasal thalamus send topographically organized projections to the SI cortex, which is located in the postcentral gyrus. The SI cortex contains a complete somatotopic map of the body such that the medial part of the postcentral gyrus represents the lower limb and lower trunk, the middle third of the gyrus represents the upper trunk and arm, and the lateral third of the gyrus represents the face and head. Intraoral structures are represented near the parietal operculum (Figure 7.10).

The SI cortex is subdivided into four cytoarchitectonic regions known as Brodmann areas 3a, 3b, 1, and 2. Each area contains a complete neural map of the body, which is based on differential projections from the core and shell regions of the ventrobasal thalamus (Figure 7.11). Some projections from the shell region convey proprioceptive information from the muscles to area 3a; other neurons in this region convey kinesthetic information from the joints to area 2. Neurons in the core region convey cutaneous information to areas 3b and 1. Consistent with these projection patterns, cortical lesions restricted to areas 3b and 1 impair texture discrimination, whereas lesions of area 2 impair the ability to discriminate the size or shape of hand-held objects.

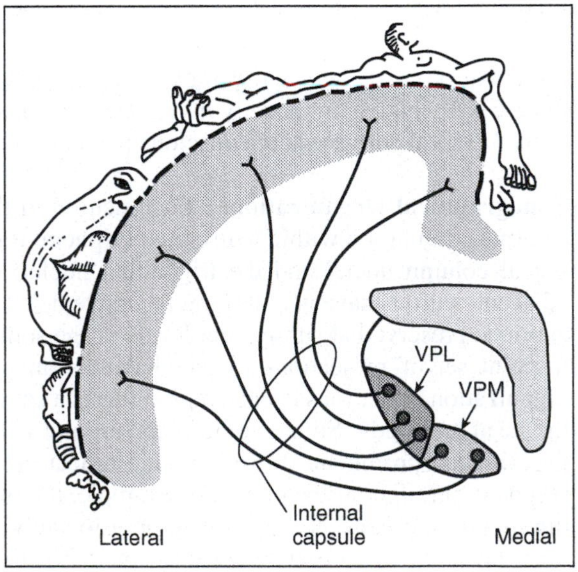

FIG. 7.10. Map of Primary Somatosensory (SI) Cortex. The somatotopic organization of the SI cortex is determined by the pattern of projections from the ventroposteromedial (VPM) and ventroposterolateral (VPL) nuclei of the thalamus.

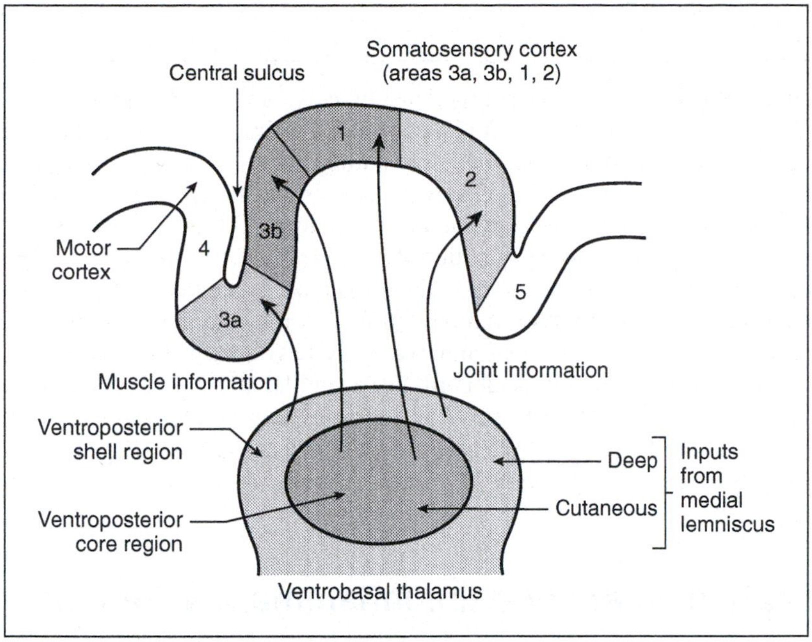

FIG. 7.11. Central Projections of Deep and Cutaneous Submodalities. Cutaneous information is transmitted from a core region in the VPL nucleus to Brodmann areas 3b and 1 in the primary somatosensory cortex. Information from deep tissues (i.e., muscles and joints) is transmitted from the shell region of the VPL nucleus to areas 3a and 2.

Secondary Somatosensory (SII) Cortex. The SII cortex is located in the upper bank of the Sylvian or lateral sulcus. Substantial evidence indicates that somatosensory information is processed in the SI cortex before it is transmitted to the SII cortex. Although a few neurons in the ventral part of the ventrobasal complex project directly to the SII cortex, the majority of somatosensory projections from the thalamus terminate in the SI cortex. Hence, most somatosensory information that is processed by SII cortex originates from SI cortex, not the thalamus. Consistent with this anatomical pattern, selective lesions of the SI cortex cause SII neurons to become unresponsive to tactile stimulation; similar lesions of the SII cortex, however, have little effect on SI responsiveness. These findings indicate a hierarchical organization in which somatosensory information is processed sequentially by the ventrobasal thalamus, SI cortex, and then SII cortex.

Several facts indicate that SII cortex is involved in higher-order processing of somatosensory information. For example, SII neurons have much larger receptive fields than SI neurons that represent similar parts of the body. Furthermore, SII neurons are more responsive to peripheral stimulation if attention is directed to the part of the body that is stimulated. Neurons in the SII cortex project to the insula, which, in turn, projects to limbic structures such as the amygdala and hippocampus. This serial pathway enables SII cortex to form tactile memories, perhaps for recognizing textures and other features of hand-held objects.

Somatosensory Connections to the Motor Cortex. The posterior part of the SI cortex (Brodmann areas 1 and 2) projects to the motor and premotor cortex, which consist of Brodmann areas 4 and 6, respectively. The motor cortices send feedback connections to somatosensory cortical areas 1, 2, and 3a. These corticocortical projections interconnect topographically matched regions in the somatosensory and motor cortical areas. Thus, the digit representations in sensory and motor areas are reciprocally connected. These cortical interconnections allow tactile information to modulate efferent signals from the motor cortex, a role that is consistent with the use of somatosensory information for guiding hand movements during object manipulation.

NEURAL BASIS OF PAIN

The treatment of pain is an important aspect of clinical practice that requires an understanding of the pain pathways and their neural mechanisms. Pain sensations indicate that peripheral nerve fibers have been activated by tissue damage or by irritating stimuli that produce inflammation. In many cases, the cause of pain is easily identified. Pain caused by toothache, earache, sore throat, or skin trauma, for example, is well localized. In other cases, however, the intensity and sensory qualities of pain vary widely and depend on several factors. Pain originating from the musculoskeletal system has a dull, aching character that is poorly localized. Visceral pain is even more diffuse and may radiate away from the affected organ because the visceral organs are innervated by few afferent fibers that are dispersed across multiple segments of the spinal cord. For example, afferent fibers that innervate the heart send divergent projections to cervical, thoracic, and lumbar segments of the spinal cord. Although visceral pain may reflect irritation or disease at a specific site, the pain may extend across a broad part of the body. Determining the locus and cause of visceral pain may require several diagnostic tests.

Nociceptive Fibers and the Inflammatory Response

C fibers convey slow pain with a burning or throbbing quality.

A-δ fibers convey fast pain with a sharp and stabbing quality.

Pain is considered a sensory modality in the somatosensory system because specific classes of nociceptive fibers convey noxious sensations. Peripheral nociceptive fibers are classified into two groups on the basis of axon diameter and conduction velocity. The thinly myelinated A-δ fibers have conduction velocities of 10–40 meters per second (m/s) that convey immediate sensations of intense, sharp pain. Another class of nociceptive fibers, the C fibers, conduct impulses at a much slower velocity (1-2 m/s) and convey sensations that are often characterized by a dull, throbbing, or burning quality. The pain sensations mediated by C fibers are called "slow pain" because they occur after a noticeable time delay. It should be noted, however, that not all C fibers transmit pain information. In fact, a subset of C fibers have been identified that respond exclusively to innocuous stimulation, but their behavioral functions have not been determined.

Tissue damage causes a cascade of local chemical changes that sensitize nociceptors to subsequent stimulation (Figure 7.12). Following skin injury, for example, many substances are released from the skin tissue including bradykinin, serotonin, prostaglandins, and protons (H^+). These chemicals excite the free nerve endings of nociceptive fibers and cause them to transmit action potentials both to the spinal cord and to local collaterals. The latter route represents an axon reflex that releases substance P and calcitonin gene-related peptide (CGRP), which cause nearby mast cells to release histamine. Local diffusion of histamine causes further activation of the nociceptive fibers, and this leads to additional release of substance P and CGRP; hence, the axon reflex is a positive feedback loop that sensitizes the skin to subsequent stimulation. Substance P also causes local capillaries to dilate, and the resultant increase in blood flow leads to edema, which causes further release of bradykinin and other chemicals.

Allodynia is increased sensitivity to stimuli that normally are innocuous. **Hyperalgesia** is increased sensitivity to stimuli that cause moderate pain.

In addition to activating nociceptive nerve fibers, these inflammatory responses lower the threshold of the nerve endings to subsequent stimulation. Consequently, stimuli that are normally innocuous become painful (allodynia) and more intense stimuli become extremely noxious (hyperalgesia). Although these local responses increase the intensity of the perceived pain, they are essential for the healing process because they facilitate recovery by encouraging the patient to protect the injured area from additional trauma.

Anti-inflammatory Medications

Several pharmacological treatments are effective in treating the acute pain that is produced by inflammation. The most commonly used agents are nonsteroidal anti-flammatory drugs (NSAIDs) such as aspirin, ibuprofen, and naproxen. These drugs act by blocking the enzyme, cyclooxygenase, which synthesizes prostaglandins. Prostaglandins promote the inflammatory

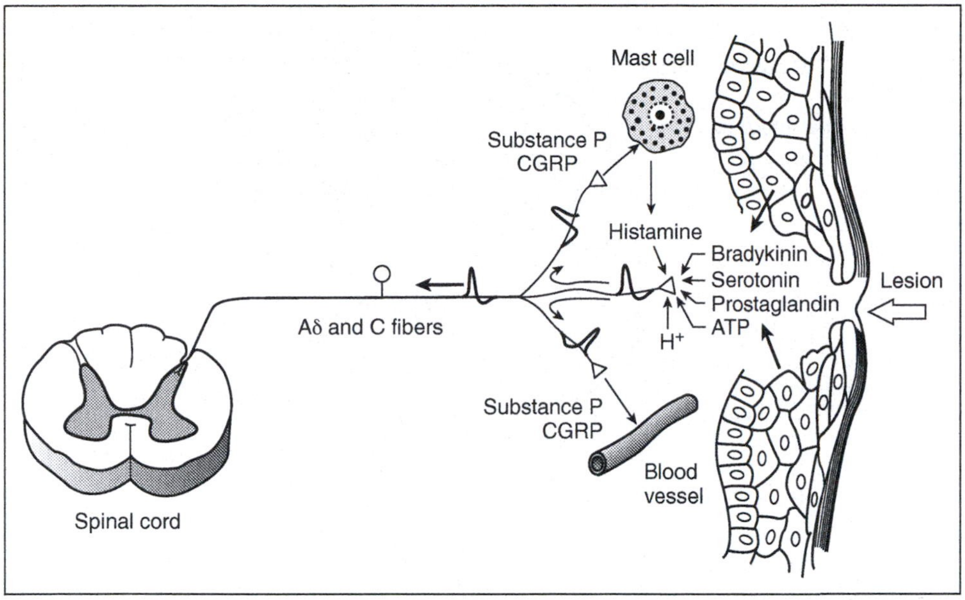

FIG. 7.12. Axon Reflex and Peripheral Sensitization. Tissue damage causes surrounding skin cells to release chemicals that excite the nociceptive fibers and cause them to release substance P and other neuropeptides in an axon reflex. Substance P triggers histamine release from mast cells and promotes vasodilation, effects that cause additional release of bradykinin and prostaglandins. This mechanism of peripheral inflammation increases the sensitivity of nociceptive fibers to subsequent stimulation (allodynia and hyperalgesia).

response (see above) but are also needed to protect the stomach lining and to form platelets for clotting the blood. Hence, by lowering the prostaglandin concentration at the site of an injury, the inflammatory response is weakened and the nociceptive fibers do not become sensitized.

Some NSAIDs, known as Cox-2 inhibitors (e.g., Celebrex), are more selective than aspirin in blocking the form of cyclooxygenase that promotes inflammation (Cox-2) but do not affect the form of the enzyme that protects the stomach lining. Consequently, Cox-2 inhibitors are much more potent in blocking the inflammatory response without producing side effects such as stomach ulcers. However, because these drugs have cardiovascular effects that increase the risk of stroke and heart attack, many Cox-2 inhibitors are no longer prescribed.

Inflammatory responses are also treated by compounds that have another pharmacologic basis for desensitizing peripheral nociceptive fibers. Capsaicin, for example, is used increasingly as an analgesic and anti-inflammatory agent to relieve the pain produced by arthritis and neuralgia. Originally isolated as the active ingredient responsible for the pungent taste of hot peppers, research has shown that capsaicin opens vanilloid (VR-1) channels that permit the entry of Na^+ and Ca^{2+} into the endings of the nociceptive fibers. If initially administered in high concentrations, capsaicin produces a burning pain. With repeated application of low doses, however, capsaicin desensitizes nociceptive endings and reduces the concentration of substance P and other neuromodulators that mediate the inflammatory response.

Anterolateral and Trigeminothalamic Systems

As discussed in Chapters 4 and 5, the central pathways for pain and temperature information are segregated from those that conduct cutaneous information. Most nociceptive information coming from the body is conducted through the spinal cord and brainstem by the anterolateral system. Unlike the dorsal column-medial lemniscal system, the anterolateral system has several groups of fibers (i.e., spinothalamic, spinohypothalamic, spinoreticular, spinomesencephalic, and spinotectal) that terminate in different regions of the brainstem and diencephalon (Figure 7.13).

The **anterolateral system** consists of spinothalamic, spinoreticular, spinomesencephalic, and spinotectal fibers.

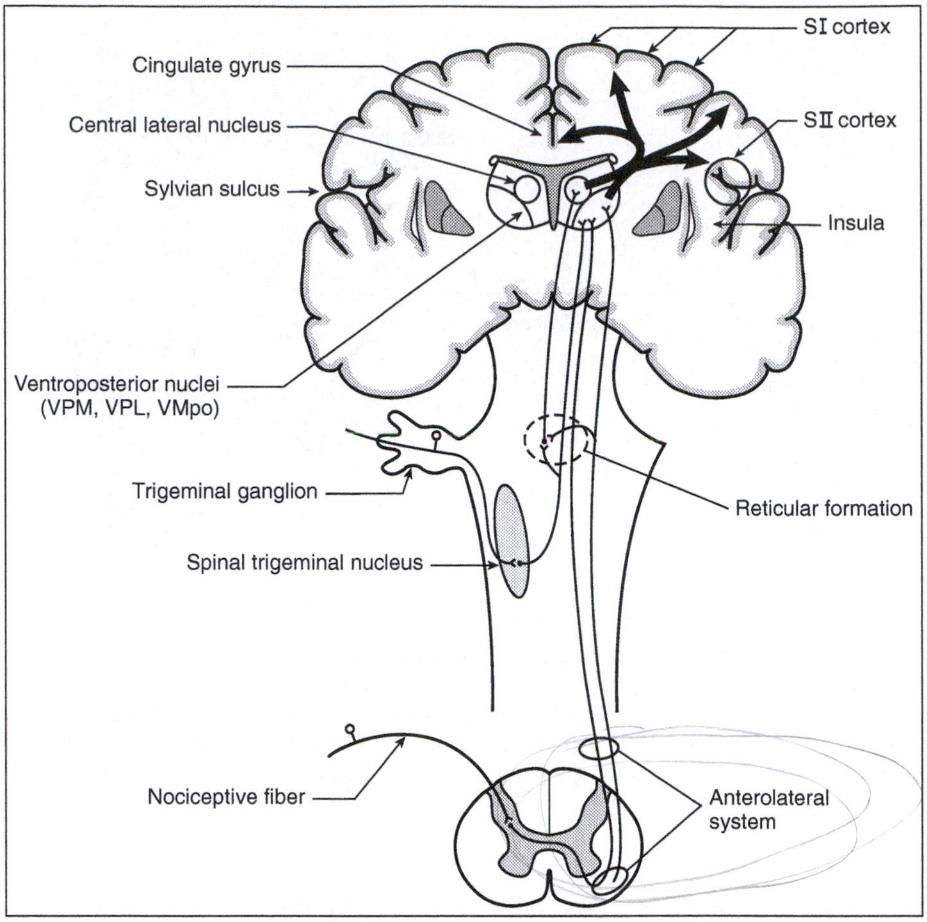

FIG. 7.13. Ascending Pain Pathways. Summary of the pathways that convey pain and temperature information to the brainstem, thalamus, and cerebral cortex. The fibers of the anterolateral system terminate in the ventrobasal complex and the posterior part of the ventral medial nucleus (VMpo). Other fibers terminate in the reticular formation that, in turn, sends ascending projections to the central lateral nucleus. Pain-sensitive regions in the thalamus project to a variety of cortical regions, including the anterior cingulate gyrus, the insula, and the primary (SI) and secondary (SII) somatosensory cortices.

Nociceptive and thermoreceptive nerve fibers from the body enter the spinal cord through the dorsal roots and terminate on neurons in the dorsal horn. Glutamate is the major neurotransmitter that is released by these primary afferent fibers onto the second-order neurons in the dorsal horn. The anterolateral system originates mainly from projection neurons in laminae I, IV, V, and, to a lesser extent, laminae VI and VII. Neurons in these laminae send axons across the midline via the white commissure and then ascend the spinal cord through the ventrolateral part of the lateral funiculus. As the anterolateral system ascends through the lateral part of the brainstem, many fibers peel away from the main tract and terminate in the reticular formation, the periaqueductal gray (PAG), or the superior colliculus. Most of the remaining fibers in the anterolateral system eventually terminate in the VPL nucleus of the thalamus. This latter group of fibers, known as the lateral spinothalamic tract, conveys thermal and nociceptive information from both A-δ and C fibers. The thalamus, especially the intralaminar nuclei, also receives polysynaptic projections from the reticular formation, and these projections convey nociceptive information received from ascending spinal fibers in the anterolateral system. Although the exact function of the reticulothalamic pathway is not known with certainty, many investigators believe these projections play a role in general arousal and in the affective components of pain.

The trigeminothalamic system transmits nociceptive information from one side of the brainstem to the contralateral thalamus. Nociceptive information from the face and head enter the brainstem primarily through the trigeminal nerve. A few fibers of cranial nerves VII, IX, and X also innervate the ear, tongue, throat, and meninges. All of these primary afferent fibers descend through the spinal trigeminal tract and synapse on neurons at different levels in the spinal trigeminal nucleus of the medulla. Second-order neurons in the spinal trigeminal nucleus send axons across the midline and then ascend to the VPM nucleus of the thalamus via the trigeminothalamic tract (or trigeminal lemniscus).

Referred pain is visceral pain with a cutaneous component.

Referred Pain Sensations

Pain sensations arising from the viscera are not only difficult to localize, but may have cutaneous qualities that originate from sites other than the affected organ. This type of pain sensation, known as "referred" pain, occurs because the projection neurons of the anterolateral system, which are located in the dorsal horn of the spinal cord, receive convergent inputs from nociceptive fibers in superficial tissues (e.g., skin) and visceral organs (e.g., heart, stomach; Figure 7.14). In this situation, the brain is confused about the source of the pain because the projection neurons are normally activated by stimulating the skin.

In making a clinical diagnosis, it is helpful to know that visceral pain arising from a specific organ produces a well-defined pattern of referred sensations. For example, insufficient blood flow to the myocardium produces angina, a form of referred pain characterized by the sensation of extreme pressure on the upper chest that is often accompanied by pain radiating into the arms, shoulders, neck and, in some cases, the jaw and teeth. Referred pain is also produced by nociceptive fibers innervating the gallbladder (pain in the upper abdomen and, less often, the scapula), the kidney (pain in the lower abdominal wall), the appendix (pain in the anterior abdominal wall around the umbilicus), or the prostate gland (pain in the abdominal wall, lower back, or upper legs).

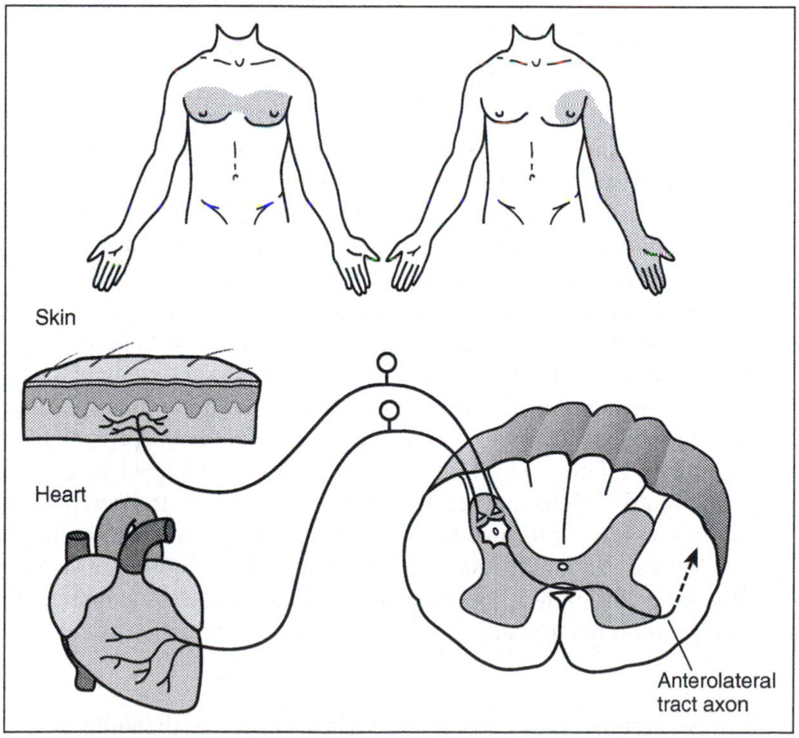

FIG. 7.14. Referred Pain Sensations. The projection neurons of the anterolateral system receive convergent inputs from two sets of nociceptive fibers: those that innervate the visceral organs and those that innervate the skin. Hence, activation of the projection neurons by myocardial infarction may evoke the perception of cutaneous sensations.

Forebrain Structures Involved in Pain

Many parts of the thalamus and cerebral cortex receive ascending nociceptive projections from the anterolateral system and reticular formation. The exact mechanisms by which pain is processed in the forebrain are not understood, but they appear to involve a complex network of thalamic and cortical regions that control the autonomic and affective responses to pain.

In general, the term "nociception" denotes the detection and transmission of information related to tissue injury. Therefore, nociception is mediated by peripheral nerves, spinal pathways, and the brainstem pathways that transmit nociceptive information to the thalamus and cortex. The perception of pain, including its locus, intensity, and other qualities (e.g., burning or cramping) is mediated by the forebrain regions that receive nociceptive inputs. Moreover, pain has an emotional impact or affective component that depends both on its context and the cultural experiences of the individual. Undoubtedly, the affective component of pain is strongly influenced by limbic regions in the forebrain.

Thalamic Representation of Pain

The **ventrobasal complex** is involved in discriminative aspects of pain.
The **central lateral nucleus** is involved in affective components of pain.

The ascending fibers of the lateral spinothalamic tract terminate in several thalamic nuclei, and this finding has generated controversy about the role of the thalamus in the perception of pain. Projections from the dorsal horn of the spinal cord and the spinal trigeminal nucleus have dense terminations in the ventrobasal complex (VPM and VPL). Some neurons in this part of the thalamus, especially those located most caudally in the ventrobasal complex, may respond exclusively to nociceptive stimulation. Most of the neurons, however, are activated by cutaneous and noxious stimulation, and their discharge rate is related to the intensity of the stimulation. This response pattern resembles the wide dynamic responses in the dorsal horn of the spinal cord (see Figure 4.10), which underscores the view that cutaneous and noxious information are both conveyed by the anterolateral system. These results also suggest that the rate of neuronal activity in VPM and VPL encodes the intensity of pain. The ability to localize pain to specific body parts, however, is probably mediated by the precise spatial organization in the VPM and VPL nuclei and their topographically arranged connections with the cortex. Thus, the ventrobasal complex has a well-defined topographic organization that encodes the location of noxious stimulation.

Spinothalamic fibers also terminate in thalamic regions that lack topographic organization. Ascending spinothalamic projections from the deep layers of the dorsal horn terminate in the intralaminar complex of the thalamus, especially in the central lateral nucleus. A second, indirect pathway supplements this direct route to the intralaminar complex. Thus, nociceptive neurons in the reticular formation send polysynaptic projections to the intralaminar nuclei. These pathways, however, do not mediate the discriminative aspects of pain perception that are represented by stimulus quality, intensity, and location. Neurons in the intralaminar complex have enormous receptive fields that make them unsuitable for localizing pain. Because the intralaminar nuclei receive convergent inputs from many brain regions and send diffuse projections to the cerebral cortex, it is more likely that nociceptive information received from the reticulothalamic pathways is used to regulate cortical excitability and behavioral arousal. Therefore, instead of conveying the discriminative sensations of nociceptive stimulation, the intralaminar nuclei probably modulate the emotional aspects of suffering and other affective components of pain perception.

Central pain is caused by lesions that produce abnormal neural activity in the nociceptive pathways of the CNS.

Thalamic Pain Syndrome. Lesions in the ventral posterior thalamus may produce a form of central pain that is associated with abnormal and unpleasant somatic sensations. The thalamic pain syndrome is characterized initially by analgesia that, after several weeks or months, is replaced by paresthetic sensations such as burning, prickling, or lacerating pain. Thalamic pain and other central pain syndromes are also associated with allodynia (i.e., pain evoked by stimulation that is normally considered innocuous).

Although the exact mechanism of central pain is unknown, the sequence of analgesia followed by paresthesia suggests that a lesion-induced loss of neurons is followed by sprouting of inappropriate neuronal connections that increase the activity of the remaining nociceptive neurons. Central pain is not alleviated by morphine or other opioids because the syndrome is produced by lesions in brain regions that lack a high concentration of opioid receptors. Pharmacologic agents that suppress overall neuronal activity (e.g., antiepileptic drugs) are the most successful agents for treating central pain.

Cortical Representation of Pain

The importance of the cerebral cortex in pain perception was disputed for many years because most physiologic studies found few nociceptive neurons in the SI or SII cortex. In addition, electrical stimulation of the SI cortex rarely caused human patients to perceive pain, and removal of the SI cortex did not prevent the perception of pain. By comparison, many neurons in the ventral posterior thalamus respond to intense thermal or noxious stimulation. Moreover, electrical stimulation of the thalamus produces pain responses in humans and animals. Hence, for many years, the available evidence prompted the view that pain perception was mediated by processes in the thalamus.

Noninvasive imaging studies, however, indicate substantial increases in blood flow to specific cortical areas during intense thermal or noxious stimulation. The largest increases in cortical blood flow are observed in the insula and in the anterior part of the cingulate gyrus. These results are consistent with anatomical studies showing that the ventrobasal and intralaminar regions of the thalamus project to the anterior cingulate gyrus, whereas SI and SII project to the insula and may supplement the direct thalamic projections to insular cortex (see Figure 7.13). The insula and anterior cingulate gyrus are part of the limbic system, and activation of these regions by noxious stimuli may contribute to the affective components of pain. The anterior cingulate cortex is a vital component in the neural system that directs attention to sensory stimuli, and this cortical region may perform a similar function in response to pain.

The somatosensory cortex is activated by noxious stimulation, but to a lesser degree than the insula or the anterior cingulate cortex. The SI and SII cortices receive direct and indirect projections from the thalamic ventrobasal complex that enable the discriminative aspects of pain perception. Indeed, removal of SI or SII cortex impairs the ability to localize painful stimulation but does not completely prevent the perception of pain because other cortical areas (i.e., insula, anterior cingulate gyrus) receive substantial inputs from the ventroposterior thalamus.

Phantom Limb Pain. Following removal of an arm or leg, many patients report sensations from the missing limb. The most vivid sensations arising from the missing or phantom limb usually involve the distal structures (e.g., hand and foot) that received the highest density of innervation (Figure 7.15). For some patients, the phantom limb seems normal in size, whereas other patients perceive the distal hand or foot extending directly from the proximal stump. Phantom sensations, though commonly associated with limbs, may arise following denervation of any part of the body. For example, some women report phantom breasts after mastectomy, and paralyzed individuals may perceive phantom sensations from body parts located below the level of the transected spinal cord. Phantom sensations can also be induced by local anesthesia; patients undergoing arm surgery frequently report false impressions about the position of their limb during anesthetic block of the brachial plexus. Phantom sensations can be relatively benign, or they can be characterized by serious debilitating pain. Nearly 70% of all limb amputees experience burning or cramping pain. Phantom limb pain is not managed with narcotics, however, because the aberrant activity occurs in somatosensory cortex, which contains few opioid receptors.

Phantom pain originates from distorted and unregulated patterns of neuronal activity in the somatosensory cortex and related brain regions. When somatosensory cortex is deprived of sensory inputs because the limb is missing, the cortical map becomes reorganized so that the deprived region responds to body parts that are represented in surrounding

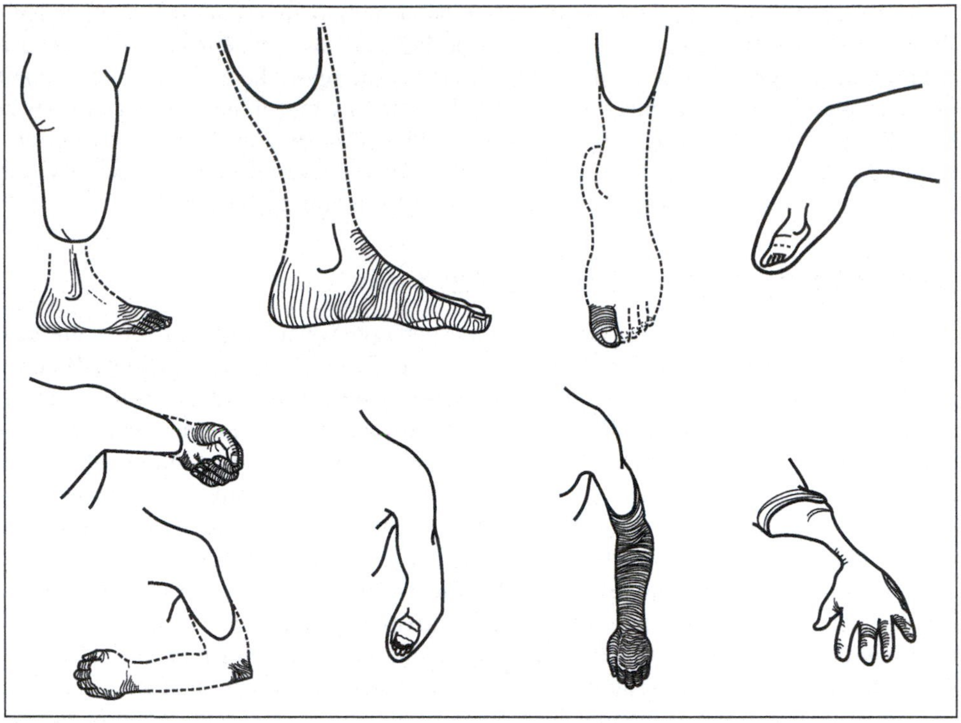

FIG. 7.15. Phantom Sensations. Illustration of phantom limb sensations following amputation of the arm or leg. Dashed lines indicate the outlines of the missing part of the limb; shading indicates the perceived location of the phantom sensations.

cortical regions. This occurs, in part, because the cortical sites that represent the intact body parts have some connections with the sites that had represented the missing limb, and an increase in the synaptic strength of these connections permit new somatotopic responses to arise in the deprived region. The spatiotemporal patterns of activity in the deprived cortical region are abnormal, however, and may resemble patterns associated with burning pain. Similarly, cramping pain may arise because the somatosensory cortex sends the motor cortex a signal to move the phantom limb. In the absence of a true limb, the message to move the limb may become progressively stronger until the cramping sensation intensifies and becomes painful.

Phantom limb sensations and pain can be managed to some degree by fitting the patient with a prosthetic limb. In time, patients acquire the feeling that the prosthetic limb is real or "fleshed out" because the mechanoreceptors in the stump retain their sensibility and are activated whenever the prosthetic limb is moved or perturbed. Moreover, correspondence between these tactile inputs and the visual image of the prosthesis helps to reestablish some of the normal thalamocortical and corticocortical inputs to the deprived cortical region.

Phantom sensations can be managed by prosthetic devices or mirror therapy.

Phantom limb pain is also relieved by using behavioral techniques that exploit the projections of commissural and long association fibers to the somatosensory cortex and surrounding cortex in the parietal-occipital-temporal junction. In this therapy, which was developed by Ramachandran in the 1990s, amputees insert their intact limb into an enclosure with a mirror and visualize the mirror image that corresponds to the missing limb (Figure 7.16). While doing this, they imagine that "both arms" occupy symmetrical positions and that they are making identical finger movements in "both hands." Hence, they can see and feel the finger movements of the intact hand in synchrony with the finger movements of the mirror image that represents the missing hand. Because they can see symmetrical finger movements while imagining the movement of both hands, inputs from the visual cortex converge with commissural inputs from the intact hand representation to reestablish normal activity in the deprived somatosensory cortex.

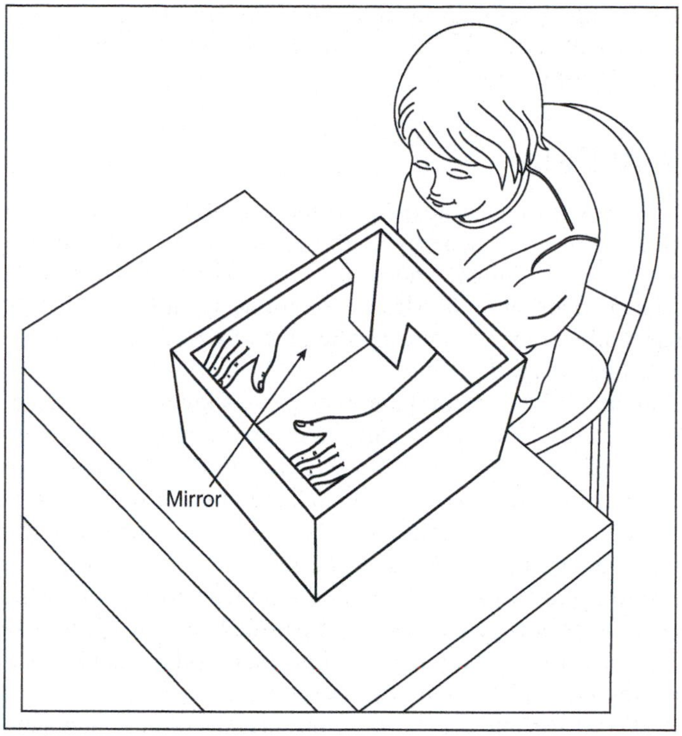

FIG. 7.16. Mirror Therapy. Patients with phantom limb pain can relieve the painful cramping sensations if they imagine that they are making symmetrical finger movements in the intact and phantom hands while they visualize the mirror image of the intact hand.

Migraine Headache. Severe recurring headache pain that is preceded by light sensitivity or visual hallucinations denotes the classic feature of a migraine headache. Visual sensations are common before the onset of a migraine headache, and they usually expand from one part of the visual field to another as the dysfunctional zone moves across the visual cortex. The visual symptoms, which are described as flashing or shimmering lights, may occur without headache pain on occasion. Consistent with these findings, migraine headache is correlated with a decrease in vascular perfusion of the occipital lobe, but this is probably secondary to changes in neuronal activity.

The majority of patients with migraine headaches also suffer from cutaneous allodynia. Thus, lightly touching the face or brushing the hair can be extremely painful during a migraine attack. Somatosensory involvement suggests that the trigeminal nerve fibers and the neurons in the trigeminal nucleus become hypersensitive during the course of a migraine headache. According to this view, a migraine headache is due to inflammation of the dura, and the trigeminal pain represents secondary activation of the nociceptive nerve fibers that innervate the dura and nearby blood vessels. The caudal part of the spinal trigeminal nucleus receives convergent inputs from fibers that innervate the skin as well as those that innervate the meninges covering the brain. Hence, the cutaneous component of migraine pain may represent a form of referred pain.

The exact cause of migraine headache is unknown, but several findings suggest that serotonergic projections from the brainstem play a critical role. Migraine headache is usually alleviated by sleep, and sleeping is correlated with a reduction in the activity of serotonergic neurons in the dorsal raphe nuclei (see Chapter 15). Consistent with these findings, electrical stimulation of the dorsal raphe nuclei can produce migraine-like headaches. Ascending projections from the dorsal raphe nuclei terminate in the lateral geniculate nucleus, in the superior colliculus, in the visual cortex, and on cerebral arteries. Hence, raphe projections to any of these sites could trigger the visual and circulatory symptoms associated with migraine headaches.

Although narcotics can relieve chronic headaches, they are employed only as a last resort. Consistent with a serotonergic mechanism, migraine headaches are treated by drugs (e.g., sumatriptan or ergotamine) that act selectively at certain types of serotonergic receptors to inhibit the firing of dorsal raphe neurons. To be effective, however, these drugs must be administered at the onset of the abnormal sensory sensations, especially before the pain becomes excruciating. After cutaneous allodynia is present, the trigeminal nerve and its central nuclei have already become sensitized and are less responsive to drugs that modulate serotonergic transmission.

Central Modulation of Pain

The perception of pain often depends on the context of events surrounding the injury as well as the cultural and social experiences of the individual. Perhaps the most striking example of this is illustrated by soldiers in combat, who ignore their wounds and deny having pain until they are out of danger. During such extreme situations, the ability to inhibit pain is highly adaptive because it allows an individual to attend to other stimuli and make appropriate behavioral responses for survival.

Endorphin means endogenous morphine.

The influence of social and cultural factors on pain perception suggests that higher-order regions in the CNS must interact with descending nociceptive-modulatory pathways to reduce the perception of pain during intense, stressful conditions. The existence of such neural systems was long suspected because morphine and opium exert powerful analgesic effects that are mediated by specific receptors in the brain. Consistent with this view, the discovery of opioid receptors in the 1970s suggested that some endogenous opioid-like compound must be released from specific neural pathways to regulate pain. This hypothesis was eventually supported by studies that identified several opioid-like compounds that were highly concentrated in brainstem regions that modulated pain perception. For example, enkephalins, endorphins, and other neuropeptides are concentrated in the periaqueductal gray (PAG) of the midbrain, which produces profound analgesia when it is electrically stimulated by implanted electrodes. Further experiments have shown that PAG stimulation inhibits neurons in the spinal dorsal horn, even though very few neurons in the PAG project directly to the dorsal horn.

Descending Modulatory Systems. As illustrated in Figure 7.17, the cerebral cortex, hypothalamus, amygdala, and PAG control the activity of specific regions in the medulla that project to the spinal cord. These descending projections from the medulla can either suppress or facilitate nociceptive transmission in the dorsal horn, and most of these projections originate from the rostral ventromedial medulla (RVM). Those that suppress nociceptive transmission ("off" cells) descend through the dorsolateral funiculus of the spinal cord and terminate in Rexed laminae II and III of the dorsal horn where they activate the inhibitory interneurons in the substantia gelatinosa. Projections from the RVM that facilitate nociceptive transmission ("on" cells) descend in more anterior parts of the lateral funiculus and terminate in the dorsal horn. Although the precise circuit mechanisms are unknown, the net effect of activating the "on" cells is to increase the activity of the dorsal horn neurons that give rise to the anterolateral system.

In order to develop drugs that activate the descending modulatory systems, substantial effort has focused on identifying the neurotransmitters used by the RVM projections. Although serotonin and noradrenalin have been identified in some of the fibers in this projection pathway, growing evidence indicates that the serotonergic projections are less effective than the noradrenergic projections in modulating nociceptive transmission. Other neurotransmitters, such as acetylcholine and GABA, are also present in the descending projections from the RVM and are likely to modulate nociceptive transmission in the dorsal horn.

Neurons in the RVM are regulated by descending projections from the PAG of the midbrain. The PAG contains a variety of neurotransmitters, including serotonin, glutamate, and all three classes of opioid neuropeptides (i.e., enkephalins, endorphins, and dynorphins) and their receptors. Descending projections from the PAG can activate the "off" cells in the RVM, and electrical stimulation of the PAG or RVM regions produce similar analgesic effects. Only a small fraction of neurons in the PAG project directly to the spinal trigeminal nucleus or the spinal dorsal horn; these projections use substance P and cholecystokinin to activate interneurons in lamina II of those neural processing centers.

Several studies indicate that direct electrical stimulation of the descending modulatory systems produces analgesia in both humans and animals. Currently, the use of

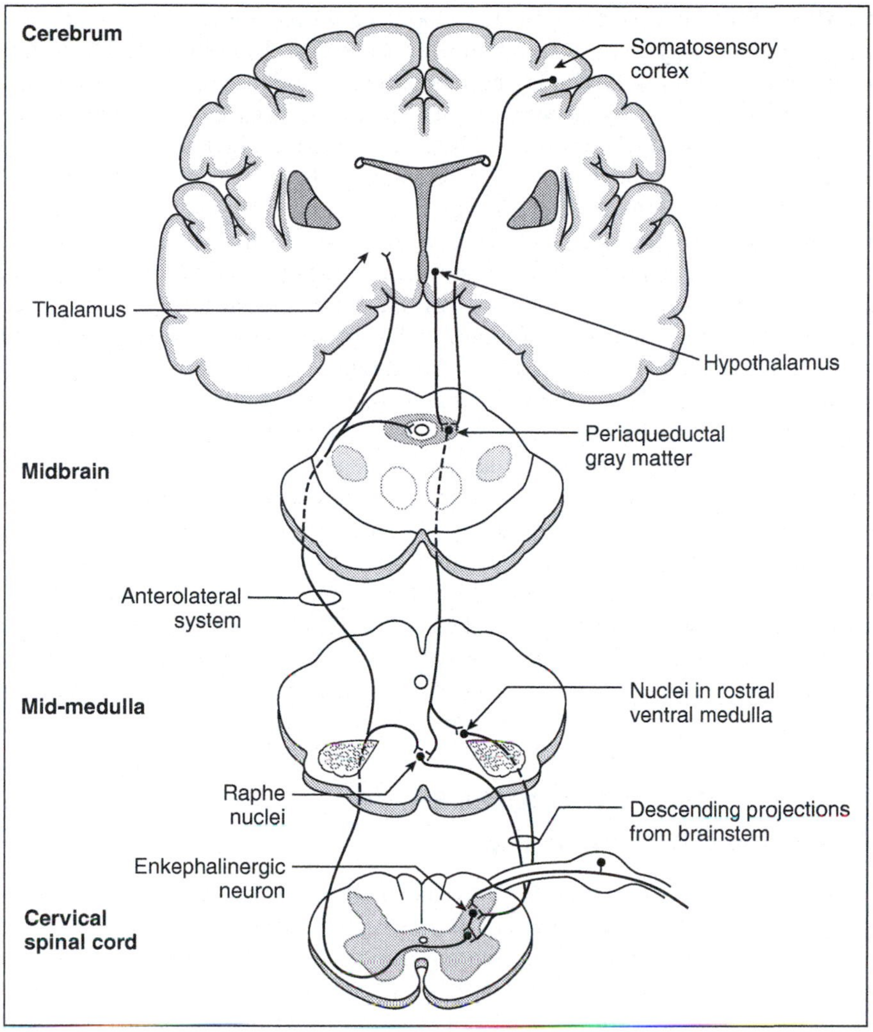

FIG. 7.17. Pain Modulating Pathways. The periaqueductal gray (PAG) receives ascending inputs from the anterolateral system and descending inputs from the hypothalamus, amygdala, and cerebral cortex. In response to these inputs, descending projections from the PAG activate neurons in the rostral ventromedial medulla (RVM) and surrounding regions, which then activate inhibitory interneurons in the spinal trigeminal nucleus of the brainstem and in the dorsal horn of the spinal cord.

electrical brain stimulation to treat chronic pain remains investigational in the United States and has not been approved by the Food and Drug Administration for pain control. Nonetheless, clinical tests on patients indicate that many have obtained relief from chronic pain by electrical brain stimulation of the PAG and related brain regions. After the electrodes are chronically implanted, the patient determines when brief pulses of electrical current are sent through the electrodes to produce brief periods of analgesia.

In the absence of direct electrical stimulation, the descending modulatory systems can be engaged by neural mechanisms. For example, some fibers in the ascending anterolateral system terminate in the ventrolateral medulla and PAG region, and these connections provide a route by which ascending pain impulses can activate these modulatory systems. In addition, enkephalinergic projections from the hypothalamus to the PAG provide a route by which autonomic arousal may suppress pain during emergency conditions. Furthermore, the prefrontal and somatosensory cortices also project to the PAG region, and these pathways provide another route by which pain perception can be influenced by environmental context, social experience, personality, or other psychological factors.

Neural Basis for the Placebo Effect. One reliable technique for activating the descending modulatory systems is to administer a placebo. Based on the Latin word that means "I am pleasing," a placebo is pharmacologically inert, but in the appropriate context it may produce measurable physiological responses that have beneficial effects. A placebo is most effective when it is administered to a patient in a context in which multiple cues simulate the administration of an actual drug. In the treatment of pain, for example, hypodermic injections of inert substances by medical personnel who inform the patient that they are receiving a painkiller can reduce the incidence and intensity of many types of postoperative pain. Moreover, controlled studies have shown that the placebo effect is prevented by naloxone or other drugs that block opioid receptors. For these reasons, clinical testing of a new drug requires that its therapeutic outcome be compared against the effects of a placebo in a double-blind randomized study.

Placebo, from Latin, means "I am pleasing."

The placebo effect is a psychobiological response to a specific psychosocial context and may involve different neural mechanisms, including both opioid and non-opioid pathways. Studies that used noninvasive imaging to examine the neural systems activated by a placebo have shown that both opioid drugs and a "painkilling" placebo activate the same brain regions, especially the rostral part of the anterior cingulate cortex (rACC), the orbital frontal cortex (OFC), and the anterior insula. In these studies, activation of these forebrain regions was highly correlated with activity in the lower pons and medulla. Given that the rACC and OFC project to the PAG and RVM, the mere expectation and anticipation of analgesia is sufficient to produce detectable activation of the descending pain-modulating systems. In other circumstances, placebo administration has been used to activate the immune system, the dopamine pathways, and other neural systems.

Use of Tricyclic Antidepressants to Alleviate Chronic Pain

Both clinical and basic research studies have shown that tricyclic antidepressants are reliable and effective for treating many forms of chronic pain. Tricyclic antidepressants are commonly used to alleviate the burning or searing pain produced by nerve injury or the neuropathic pain associated with diabetes or post-herpetic neuralgia (e.g., shingles). These drugs treat depression by blocking the reuptake of serotonin and norepinephrine, but the mechanisms by which they alleviate pain have not been established. If the serotonergic and noradrenergic projections to the spinal cord inhibit nociceptive transmission, blocking the presynaptic reuptake of these neurotransmitters in the dorsal horn should produce analgesic effects. Unfortunately, antidepressants such as fluoxetine (Prozac) that act exclusively by blocking serotonin reuptake have no therapeutic value in treating chronic pain and have prompted skepticism about the role of serotonin in modulating nociceptive transmission.

The tricyclic antidepressants that are most effective for managing pain (e.g., amitriptyline, imiprimane, desipramine) are efficacious at doses much lower than those needed to treat depression. Recent data suggest that tricyclic antidepressants may reduce pain by blocking certain types of sodium channels that become chronically open during neuropathic pain. Regardless of the precise mechanism, tricycle antidepressants must be taken for several weeks before they reduce pain. This suggests that a time-dependent metabolic process, such as synaptic plasticity, is responsible for the analgesic effects produced by antidepressants.

RESOLUTION OF CLINICAL CASE

This case illustrates trigeminal neuralgia, a pain disorder that affects one or more branches of the trigeminal nerve. Also known as tic douloureux, this disorder is characterized by recurring paroxysms of sharp, penetrating pain in the lips, cheek, or other parts of the face. The pain typically affects one side of the face, usually within the territory of the maxillary division of the trigeminal nerve. Involuntary facial movements or ipsilateral lacrimation often accompanies the pain. Attacks vary in frequency, and the episodic or periodic nature of these attacks distinguishes them from the steady throbbing pain that accompanies tooth disease or sinus infection. The painful attacks produced by trigeminal neuralgia can be provoked by touching trigger zones on the face or by facial movements (e.g., smiling, chewing, brushing teeth). For this reason, patients suffering from trigeminal neuralgia often skip meals to avoid triggering an attack and may become undernourished.

Trigeminal neuralgia is attributed to excessive neuronal activity in the spinal trigeminal nucleus, but the cause of this remains unknown. Trigeminal neuralgia may occur secondary to brainstem lesions produced by multiple sclerosis, yet it is unusual to detect noticeable damage in the trigeminal nerve or in the trigeminothalamic pathways. Finally, many have argued that trigeminal neuralgia is the result of anomalous blood vessels compressing the fifth cranial nerve.

Trigeminal neuralgia is usually treated with anticonvulsant agents, such as carbamazepine, phenytoin, or baclofen. These drugs are not analgesics and thus are ineffective in treating most types of pain. If these pharmacologic interventions fail to produce relief, surgery is often employed to decompress the trigeminal nerve by separating it from surrounding blood vessels. Alternatively, the nociceptive fibers can be destroyed by radiofrequency stimulation that affects the small-diameter pain fibers while sparing the less vulnerable large-diameter fibers.

REVIEW QUESTIONS

Directions: For each of the following questions, choose the **one best** answer.

1. Vibratory sensations are mediated by which mechanoreceptors?
A. Pacinian corpuscles
B. Hair receptors
C. Merkel corpuscles
D. Encapsulated joint receptors
E. Muscle spindles

2. What pain is best treated with opiate narcotics?
A. Phantom limb pain
B. Trigeminal neuralgia
C. Childbirth pain
D. Central (thalamic) pain
E. Migraine headache

3. Which brain region is most responsive to light touch?
A. Anterior cingulate gyrus
B. Periaqueductal gray (PAG) region
C. Substantia gelatinosa
D. Secondary somatosensory (SII) cortex
E. Nucleus raphe magnus

4. What neural tract conveys cutaneous information to the ventroposteromedial (VPM) nucleus?
A. Spinal trigeminal tract
B. Trigeminothalamic tract
C. Medial lemniscus
D. Central tegmental tract
E. Lateral spinothalamic tract

5. Which of the following fibers are found in the posterior columns?
A. Spinocerebellar fibers
B. Axonal projections from the nucleus proprius
C. A-δ fibers from nociceptors
D. C fibers from the leg
E. Spinothalamic fibers

6. Two-point discrimination is impaired by lesions of what neural structure?
A. Spinothalamic tract
B. Periaqueductal gray
C. Spinocerebellar tracts
D. Cuneocerebellar tract
E. Posterior columns

7. Which brain region might be a suitable target for implanting stimulating electrodes to alleviate chronic pain?
A. Primary somatosensory cortex
B. Ventral anterior nucleus of the thalamus
C. Intralaminar nuclei of the thalamus
D. Periaqueductal gray region
E. Parabrachial nucleus

8. What type of pain is mediated by the convergence of different sets of afferent fibers?
A. Referred pain
B. Phantom limb pain
C. Chronic pain
D. Paresthetic sensations
E. Headache

9. What neural pathway is necessary to recognize letters traced on the arm?
A. Lateral spinothalamic tract
B. Spinoreticular tract
C. Posterior spinocerebellar tract
D. Cuneocerebellar tract
E. Fasciculus cuneatus

ADDITIONAL READING

Classic Literature

Beecher HR: Pain in men wounded in battle. *Ann Surg* 123:96, 1946.

Melzack R, Wall PD: Pain mechanisms: a new theory. *Science* 150:971–979, 1965.

Reviews and Landmark Research Articles

Akil H, Mayer DJ, Liebeskind JC: Antagonism of stimulation-produced analgesia by naloxone, a narcotic antagonist. *Science* 191:961–962, 1976.

Bagheri SC, Farhidvash F, Perciaccante VJ: Diagnosis and treatment of patients with trigeminal neuralgia. *J Am Dent Assoc* 135:1713–1717, 2004.

Basbaum AI, Fields HL: The origin of descending pathways in the dorsolateral funiculus of the spinal cord of the cat and rat: further studies on the anatomy of pain modulation. *J Comp Neurol* 187:513–531, 1979.

——: Endogenous pain control systems: brainstem spinal pathways and endorphin circuitry. *Ann Rev Neurosci* 7:309–338, 1984.

Bittar RG, Kar-Purkayastha I, Owen L, Bear RE, Green A, Wang S, Aziz TZ: Deep brain stimulation for pain relief: a meta-analysis. *J Clin Neurosci* 12:515–519, 2005.

Burstein R, Collins B, Jakubowski M: Defeating migraine pain with triptans: a race against the development of cutaneous allodynia. *Ann Neurol* 55:19–26, 2004.

Cannon JT, Liebeskind JC: Analgesic effects of electrical brain stimulation and stress. Brain stem mechanisms. *Pain Headache* 9:283–294, 1987.

Colloca L, Benedetti F: Placebos and painkillers: is mind as real as matter? *Nat Rev Neurosci* 6:545–552, 2005.

Craig AD, Bushnell MC, Zhang ET, Blomqvist A: A thalamic nucleus specific for pain and temperature sensation. *Nature* 372:770–772, 1994.

Darian-Smith I: The sense of touch: performance and peripheral neural processes. In: Brookhart JM, Mountcastle VB, eds. *Handbook of Physiology: The Nervous System.* vol III. Bethesda, MD: American Physiological Society, 1984:739–788.

Fields HL: Pain modulation: expectation, opioid analgesia and virtual pain. *Prog Brain Res* 122:245– 253, 2000.

Gebhart GF: Descending modulation of pain. *Neurosci Biobehav Rev* 27:729–737, 2004.

Hughes J, Smith TW, Kosterlitz HW, Fothergill LA, Morgan BA, Morris HR: Identification of two related pentapeptides from the brain with potent opiate agonist activity. *Nature* 258:577–580, 1975.

Johnson KO: The roles and functions of cutaneous mechanoreceptors. *Curr Opin Neurobiol* 11:455–461, 2001.

Jones EG: Cortical and subcortical contributions to activity-dependent plasticity in primate somatosensory cortex. *Annu Rev Neurosci* 23:1–37, 2000.

Kosterlitz HW, Hughes J: Opiate receptors and endogenous opioid peptides in tolerance and dependence. *Adv Exp Med Biol* 85B:141–154, 1977.

Kuhar MJ, Pert CB, Snyder SH: Regional distribution of opiate receptor binding in monkey and human brain. *Nature* 245:447, 1973.

Mayer DJ, Wolfe TL, Akil H, Carder Liebeskind JC: Analgesia from electrical stimulation in the brainstem of the rat. *Science* 174:1351–1354, 1971.

Millan MJ: Descending control of pain. *Prog Neurobiol* 66:355–474, 2002.

Munger BL, Ide C: The structure and function of cutaneous sensory receptors. *Arch Histol Cytol* 51:1–34, 1988.

Petrovic P, Kalso E, Petersson KM, Ingvar M: Placebo and opioid analgesia—imaging a shared neuronal network. *Science* 295:1737–1740, 2002.

Pons TP, Garraghty PE, Friedman DP, Mishkin M: Physiological evidence for serial processing in the somatosensory cortex. *Science* 237: 417–420, 1987.

Ramachandran VS, Hirstein W: The perception of phantom limbs. The D. O. Hebb lecture. *Brain* 121:1603–1630, 1998.

Ramachandran VS, Rogers-Ramachandran D: Synaesthesia in phantom limbs induced with mirrors. *Proc Biol Sci* 263:377–836, 1996.

Sindrup SH, Jensen TS: Efficacy of pharmacological treatments of neuropathic pain: an update and effect related to mechanism of drug action. *Pain* 83:389–400, 1999.

Talbot JD, Marrett S, Evans AC, Meyer E, Bushnell MC, Duncan GH: Multiple representations of pain in human cerebral cortex. *Science* 251:1355–1358, 1991.

Wall PD, Melzack R: *Textbook of Pain.* New York, NY: Churchill Livingstone, 1989.

Willis WD, Haber LH, Martin RF: Inhibition of spinothalamic tract cells and interneurons by brain stem stimulation in the monkey. *J Neurophysiol* 40:968, 1977.

Willis WD, Zhang X, Honda CN, Giesler CJ: A critical review of the role of the proposed VMpo nucleus in pain. *J Pain* 3:79–94, 2002

INTERNET RESOURCES

American Chronic Pain Association
http://www.theacpa.org/

American Pain Foundation
http://www.painfoundation.org/

American Pain Society
    http://www.ampainsoc.org/

Arthritis Foundation
    http://www.arthritis.org/

ArthritisInsight.com
    http://www.arthritisinsight.com/

Bandolier "Evidence-based thinking about neuropathic pain and antidepressants"
    http://www.jr2.ox.ac.uk/bandolier/band65/b65-2.html

International Association for the Study of Pain
    http://www.iasp-pain.org/

National Headache Foundation
    Educational Resources
    http://www.headaches.org/consumer/educationindex.html

National Institute of Arthritis and Musculoskeletal and Skin Diseases
    http://www.niams.nih.gov/

National Institute of Neurological Disorders and Stroke
    Chronic Pain
    http://www.ninds.nih.gov/disorders/chronic_pain/chronic_pain.htm

National Institute of Neurological Disorders and Stroke
    Trigeminal Neuralgia
    http://www.ninds.nih.gov/disorders/trigeminal_neuralgia/trigeminal_neuralgia.htm

Trigeminal Neuralgia Association
    http://www.tna-support.org/

Womenshealth.gov
    Migraine Headaches
    http://www.4woman.gov/faq/migraine.htm

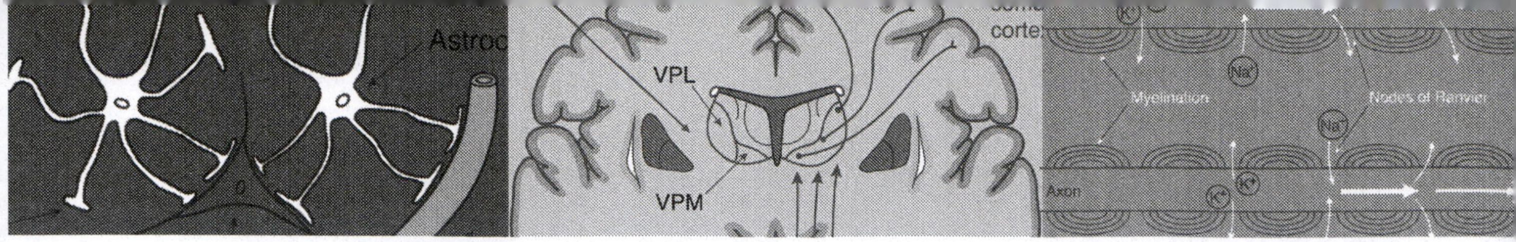

CHAPTER 8

Auditory System

INTRODUCTION OF CLINICAL CASE

A 50-year-old man stayed home from work for several days with flu-like symptoms: vertigo, headache, nausea, and vomiting. There was little improvement in his condition during this time, so after he began showing signs of an unsteady gait, his wife scheduled an appointment with his primary care physician. The patient was still unsteady when he arrived in the doctor's office. When his history was taken, he admitted having more headaches than usual over the last 6 months. Examination of the patient revealed nystagmus to the right side and mild weakness of the left facial muscles, accompanied by mild facial analgesia. His corneal reflex was diminished only on the left side, and there was mild papilledema bilaterally. The patient disputed his wife's claim that his hearing had deteriorated over the last few years, but he admitted having trouble understanding voices over the telephone. A taste test revealed that saline perception was weaker on the left side of the anterior tongue.

OVERVIEW

Hearing is important because speech is the most common medium for language and communication. Severe hearing deficits isolate patients socially and have a tremendous impact on their quality of life. Identification of a hearing loss is a sign of a disease and not a diagnosis; the key to diagnosis is having a solid understanding of the physics of sound as well as the anatomy and physiology of the auditory system. After the correct diagnosis has been made and the proper treatment initiated, most types of hearing loss can be improved, and in some cases normal function can be restored.

12% of the population will experience hearing loss during their lifetime.

PHYSICAL PROPERTIES OF SOUND

Sounds are evoked by oscillations or vibrations of a medium, such as air, water, or bone. For pure tones, the oscillations are both periodic and sinusoidal, but most sounds, including speech, involve complex, aperiodic fluctuations in pressure that the auditory system decomposes into simple sine waves (Figures 8.1 and 8.2). Because the increases (compression) and decreases (rarefaction) in pressure constitute vibrations, the adequate stimulus for audition is mechanical energy, which explains why a vibrating tuning fork placed on the base of the mastoid process of the temporal bone can be heard. The perceived pitch of a sound is related to the number or frequency of pressure oscillations each second, expressed in Hertz (Hz).

The range of human hearing is usually cited as 20-20,000 Hz, but this is true only for children. It is normal for the upper frequency limit to recede with age, typically at the rate of 300 Hz per year, beginning at age 20. Loudness, the perceptual correlate of sound intensity, is measured as the peak-to-trough difference in sound pressure level. Loudness is expressed on a logarithmic scale devised by Alexander Graham Bell, appropriately named the decibel (dB) scale.

The dynamic range for hearing spans almost 12 logarithmic units, or 120 dB, from a lower limit close to the physical background of thermal energy (Brownian movement) up to the point of pain where physical injury may occur. Despite this tremendous operating range, human subjects can distinguish between two sounds that differ by as little as 0.5 dB. Figure 8.3 illustrates the decibel rating of some familiar sounds. As Figure 8.4 shows, threshold sensitivity varies significantly across the audio spectrum and is lowest from 2000-4000 Hz. Most conversational speech is based on frequencies from 250 to 4000 Hz, the range within which our sensitivity is good.

Presbycusis: the progressive loss of high-frequency sound with age

Frequency: measured in Hz and perceived as pitch

Sound intensity: measured in dB and perceived as loudness

Every 20-dB increase in loudness reflects a 10X increase in physical energy.

Peak sensitivity: 2000-4000 Hz

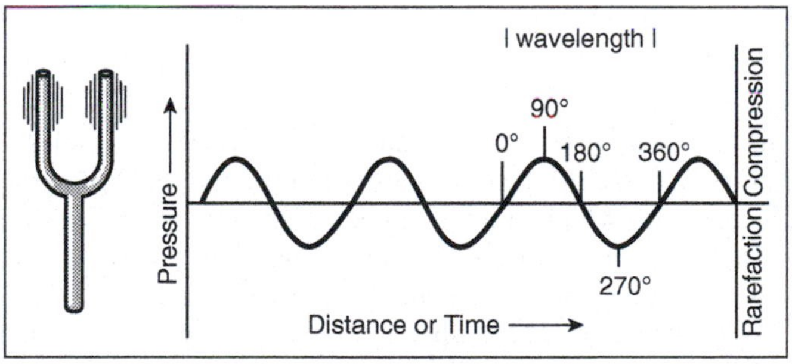

FIG. 8.1. Compression and Rarefaction of Air Molecules Associated with a Pure Tone. Vibrations from a tuning fork are transmitted through the media (e.g., air, water, bone) as a series of oscillatory molecular compressions and rarefactions. The frequency of these oscillations determines the perceived pitch of the tone; the magnitude of the pressure wave is correlated with loudness. Loudness is independent of pitch.

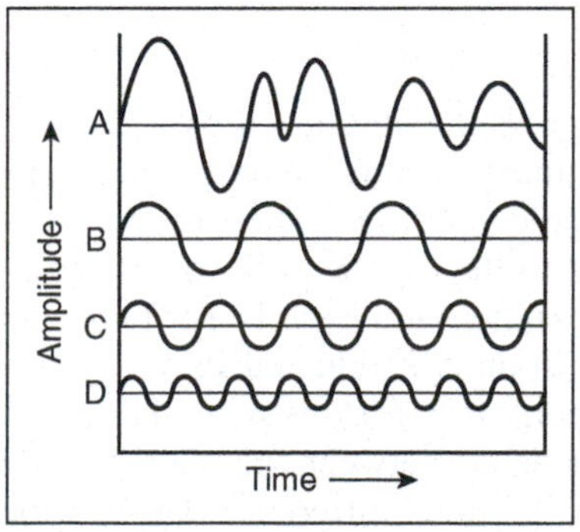

FIG. 8.2. Relationship between Complex Sounds and Pure Tones. Most natural sounds, including speech, consist of complex pressure waves (trace A) rather than periodic, sinusoidal oscillations. However, complex waves can be decomposed into a series of sine waves that vary in amplitude, frequency, and phase through a process that is not well understood but is reminiscent of Fourier analysis (traces B, C, and D).

FIG. 8.3. Decibel Ratings of Familiar Sounds.

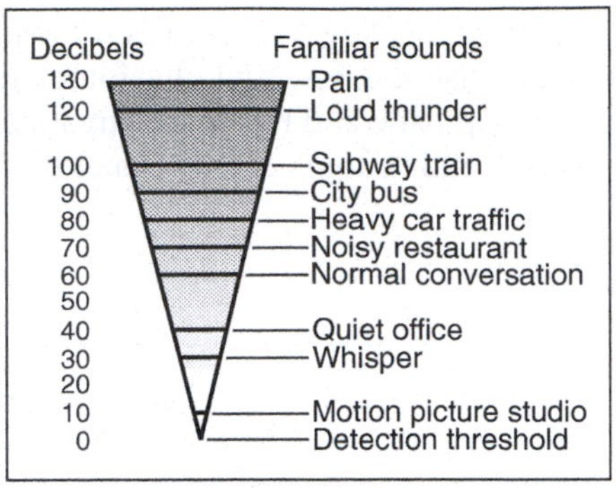

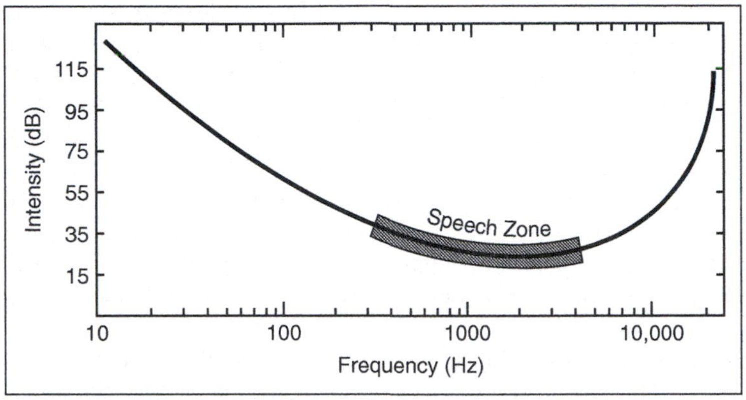

FIG. 8.4. Human Detection Thresholds. Monaural detection thresholds expressed as a function of frequency.

PERIPHERAL AUDITORY APPARATUS

The peripheral auditory apparatus has three parts: the outer ear, the middle ear, and the inner ear.

Outer Ear

The outer ear consists of the auricle (pinna) and the external auditory meatus, which together gather vibrations in the air (i.e., acoustic stimuli) and funnel them to the tympanic membrane (Figure 8.5). The efficacy with which animals gather sounds varies depending on the size of their ears and on whether they can orient their ears toward the sound source. Although the pinna acts as a passive receptacle for sound in humans, it makes other important contributions to hearing. The complex shape of the pinna favors midrange frequencies that dominate normal vocalization. In addition, the pinna helps differentiate sounds originating from behind from those arising directly in front of us.

Middle Ear

Hammer→ anvil → stirrup

The middle ear: impedance matching

Vibrations of the tympanic membrane are transmitted across the middle ear by a chain of three ossicles or bones. The first bone, the malleus (hammer), is attached to the inner surface of the eardrum (Figure 8.6). Movement of the malleus is transmitted to the incus (anvil) and then to the stapes (stirrup), which is attached to the oval window of the fluid-filled inner ear. Transmission of the acoustic signal across the middle ear is a critical step in sound transduction because normally 99.9% of the sounds conducted in air are reflected at the transition to a fluid medium. Partial compensation for this potential loss is achieved by the ossicular chain, which matches the impedance between the outer ear and the inner ear. The basis for the impedance match is the 22:1 areal difference between the

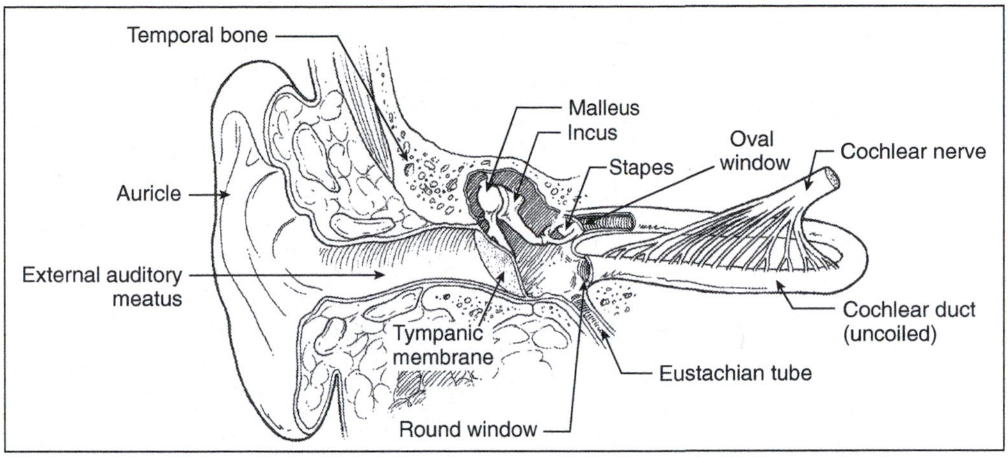

FIG. 8.5. The Peripheral Auditory Apparatus. The parts of the outer, middle, and inner ear are shown. The cochlea is "unfolded" to illustrate the continuity of the scala vestibuli and the scala tympani between the oval and round windows.

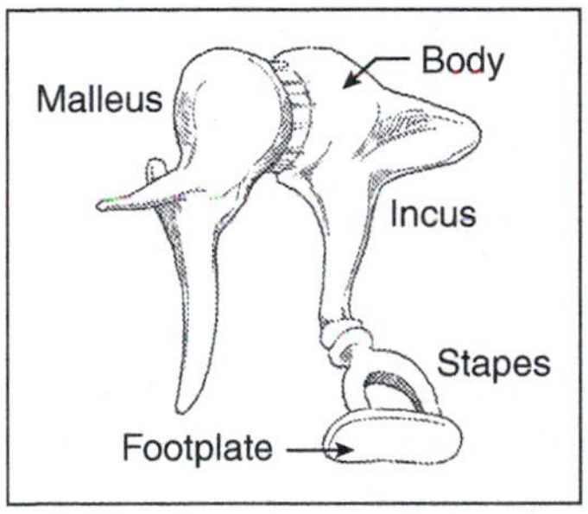

FIG. 8.6. The Ossicles of the Middle Ear. The three ossicles of the middle ear are the malleus, incus, and stapes. The tympanic membrane (not shown) would be located to the left of the malleus.

tympanic membrane and the oval window, which enables the ossicles to act like an "energy funnel." A smaller contribution to impedance matching is the lever action created by movement of the ossicles.

Patients with otosclerotic restriction of stapedic motion experience a clinically significant 20-30 dB loss of sensitivity. In addition to the muffled sound transmission though the middle ear, these patients continue to hear sounds conducted to the inner ear through the bones of the skull.

Eustachian tube: equalizes pressure between the middle ear and the outside world

The middle ear is filled with air, which makes the tympanic membrane susceptible to pressure differentials between the middle ear and the environment. For example, the passenger compartment of commercial airliners flying at an altitude of 35,000 ft is pressurized to an altitude of 8000 ft. At this altitude, the pressure in the middle ear is greater than the cabin pressure, so the eardrum is pushed outward. Mild deformation of the tympanic membrane impedes its motion, which muffles sounds. Extreme pressure differentials are painful and may burst the eardrum. Equalizing the pressure across the tympanic membrane ("popping" your ears) restores normal hearing and alleviates the pain. Pressure differentials across the eardrum are normally dissipated through the Eustachian tube, which connects the middle ear with the nasopharynx. The Eustachian tube is usually closed but opens during swallowing. Scuba divers experience more extreme pressure differentials because they are immersed in water, which is much heavier than air. The ability to equalize the ears is an absolute prerequisite for diving. Failure to equalize the pressure across the tympanic membrane during descent will burst the eardrum and allow cold water to enter the middle ear. The cold water will create strong convection currents in the semicircular canals and trigger reflexive postural gyrations that could put the diver at further risk (see COWS in Chapter 9).

Two muscles within the middle ear, the tensor tympani and stapedius, protect the delicate structures of the inner ear from excessively loud sounds. The tensor tympani

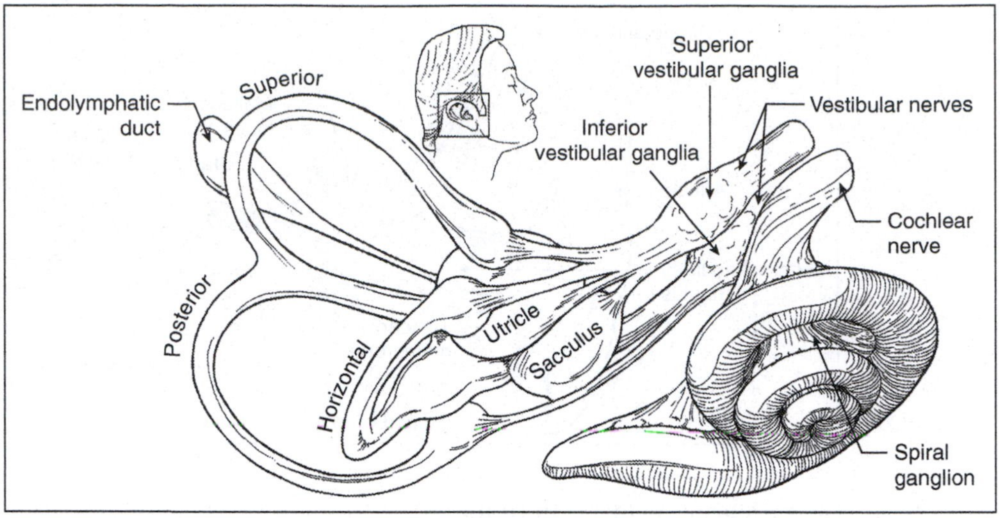

FIG. 8.7. Auditory and Vestibular Components of the Inner Ear. The cochlea, the vestibule (saccule and utricle), and the three semicircular canals are shown in this figure. The bones of the middle ear (not shown) would be located to the left of the cochlea. The inset illustrates the in situ location and orientation of the inner ear.

Tensor tympani = trigeminal (TT = T)
Stapedius = facial

muscle, which is innervated by neurons in the trigeminal motor nucleus, limits the excursions of the tympanic membrane. The stapedius muscle is innervated by the facial motor nucleus and restricts movement of the stapes. One of the presenting symptoms of damage to the facial nerve is hyperacusis, the perception that normal sounds are too loud. Like the pupillary reflex, contractions of the tensor tympani and the stapedius muscles are consensual. The response latency for the stapedius and tensor tympani muscles is about 10 ms, making these protective reflexes more effective for sustained, rather than for brief, percussive sounds. Both of these muscles also play a role in the suppression of auditory transmission during self-vocalization.

Inner Ear

The inner ear consists of membranous sacs and ducts encased in bony chambers and canals within the petrous portion of the temporal bone. Based upon anatomic and functional considerations, the inner ear is divisible into two parts: the cochlea and the vestibular apparatus. The cochlea is concerned with hearing, and the vestibular apparatus detects changes in balance and movement (Figure 8.7).

Cochlea. The cochlea is a fluid-filled tube coiled two and a half times around itself to resemble a snail shell (see Figure 8.7). The vestibular (Reissner's) and basilar membranes partition the cochlea into three chambers (Figure 8.8). The scala (*pl.* scalae) vestibuli and scala tympani flank the middle chamber, the scala media (cochlear duct), which contains the specialized epithelium of the organ of Corti, where sound transduction takes place. The scalae vestibuli and tympani are filled with a cerebrospinal-like fluid called perilymph and are continuous with one another at the helicotrema, a small opening located at the apex of the cochlear coil. The scala media is filled with endolymph, a clear fluid with a high potassium (K^+) concentration that is secreted by the stria vascularis, a layer of vascular tissue located on the outer wall of the cochlea duct. Endolymph perfuses the scala media as well as the semicircular canals and otolith organs of the inner ear.

Cochlea, from Latin, means snail.

The piston-like action of the footplate of the stapes against the oval window creates a pressure wave in the perilymph of the scala vestibuli that travels through the helicotrema and into the scala tympani. Compliance of the round window at the basal end of the scala tympani enables the pressure wave to be transmitted through the cochlea rather than

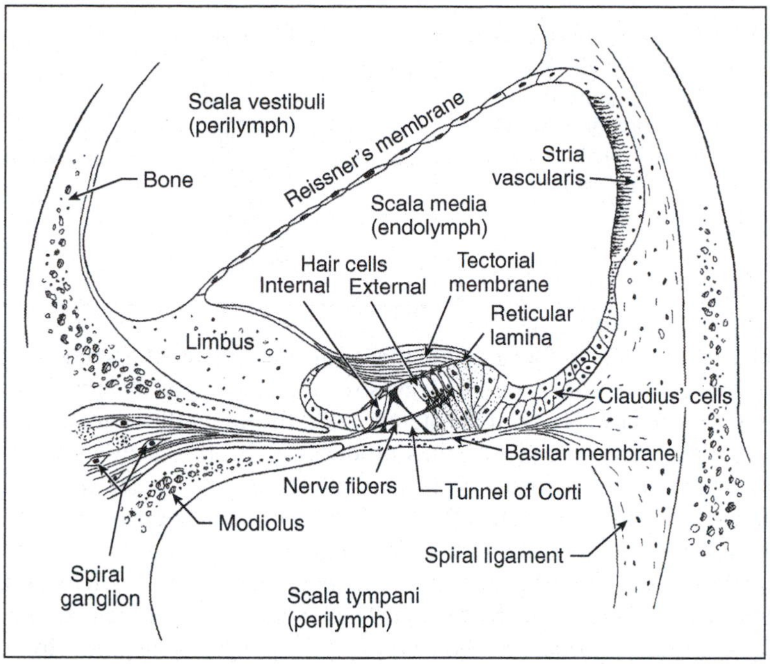

FIG. 8.8. Cross Section of the Cochlea. The three main chambers of the cochlea—the scala vestibuli, the scala tympani, and the scala media—are seen when the cochlea is viewed in cross section. Sound transduction takes place at the hair cells of the organ of Corti, which is located along the basilar membrane.

reflected at the oval window by the incompressible perilymph. As these pressure waves distort the vestibular and basilar membranes, movement is transmitted, in turn, to the endolymph of the scala media, the organ of Corti, and the tectorial membrane suspended above the organ of Corti from its point of attachment at the limbus.

Scala vestibuli
Scala media
Scala tympani

Organ of Corti. The basilar membrane suspended between the modiolus and the spiral ligament is the platform for the organ of Corti, which consists of the inner and outer hair cells and their adjacent support cells (see Figure 8.8). Sound transducton takes place at the organ of Corti. The inner hair cells form a single row on the basilar membrane adjacent to the modiolus, and the outer hair cells form three rows on the opposite side of the tunnel of Corti. All four rows run the entire length of the cochlea. The stereocilia of the outer hair cells are arranged in a chevron pattern (Figure 8.9). Both inner and outer hair cells have an apical tuft of 30-200 stereocilia of graded height emerging from a tough

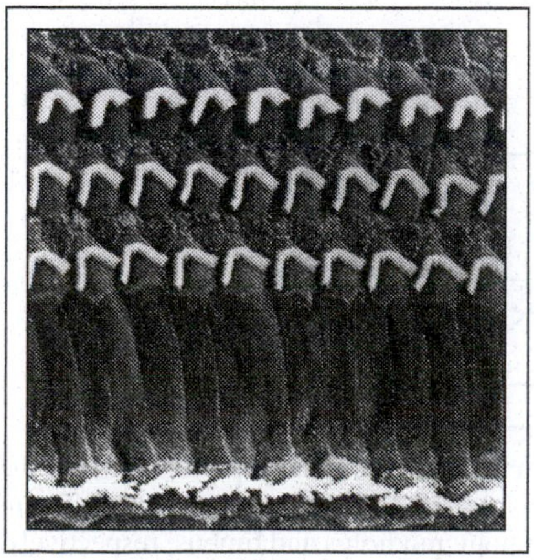

FIG. 8.9. Scanning Electron Micrograph of the Organ of Corti. The organ of Corti contains a single row of inner hair cells and three rows of outer hair cells. In this photomicrograph, the hair cells are viewed from above. The tectorial membrane has been removed. (Reprinted with permission from Lewis ER, et al: *The Vertebrate Inner Ear*. Boca Raton, FL: CRC Press, 1985:21.)

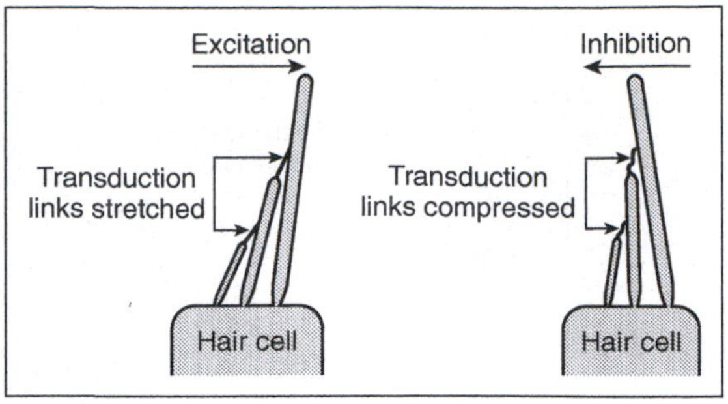

FIG. 8.10. Ciliary Cross-Links. The cross-links between adjacent stereocilia may provide the trigger mechanism for the electrochemical events associated with sound transduction. This diagram illustrates how movement of the hair cell stereocilia in one direction stretches the cross-links secured to adjacent stereocilia, which enables its K^+ channels to open. Movement of the stereocilia in the opposite direction relaxes the cross-links and closes the ion channels.

Auditory hair cells transduce sound.

Shearing forces amplify the mechanical stresses that bend stereocilia.

cuticular plate (Figure 8.10). Because the tips of the inner hair cell stereocilia contact the overlying tectorial membrane, pressure waves within the cochlea that displace the basilar and tectorial membranes also bend the stereocilia. Movement of the tectorial and basilar membranes on their different pivot points produces a shearing action on the stereocilia that amplifies the receptor potential of the hair cells (Figure 8.11; see also Figure 8.9).

The stereocilia of the outer hair cells, unlike those of the inner hair cells, are embedded within the overlying tectorial membrane. In addition, the outer hair cells contain actin-myosin complexes that enable the cells to increase or decrease their length by as much as 5% during mechanical and electrical stimulation. The kinetic ability of the outer hair cells and their attachment to the tectorial membrane may serve two functions. First, by securing the basilar membrane to the tectorial membrane, the outer hair cells may limit the shearing force produced by sounds loud enough to damage the inner hair cells. Second, the kinetic action of the outer hair cells may enable the tectorial membrane to resonate with the auditory stimulus and reinforce the oscillations of the basilar membrane. These functions would not only justify the large number of outer hair cells and their highly convergent synaptic arrangement (see below), but they would also explain why these cells act in unison.

Sound Transduction. Basilar and tectorial membrane displacement bends the hair cells of the organ of Corti at their attachment to the cuticular plate. The stereocilia move as a unit because their tips are linked to their taller neighbors (see Figure 8.10). Bending a stereocilium in one direction stretches its cross-links to the adjacent stereocilia and opens a protein channel that allows endolymphatic K^+ to flow down its concentration gradient and depolarize the cell. Activation of an inward calcium (Ca^{2+}) current and an outward K^+ current releases neurotransmitter from the base of the hair cell. Bending the

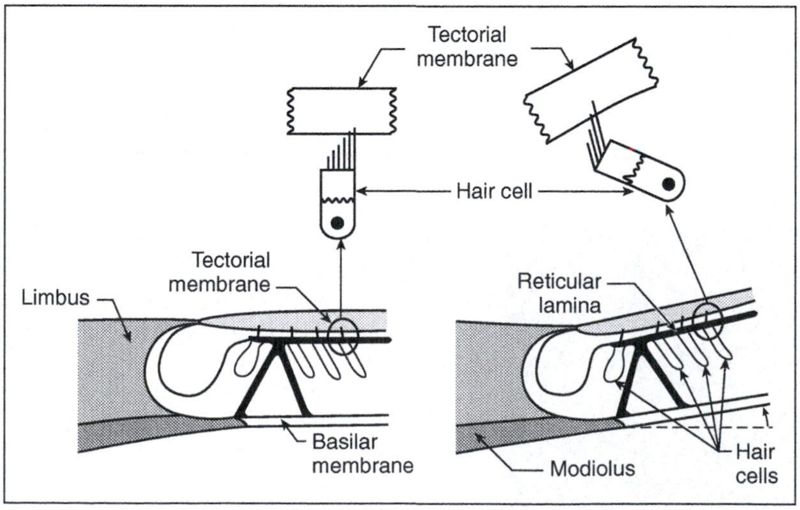

FIG. 8.11. Shearing Force within the Organ of Corti. Diagrammatic representation of the shearing force applied to the tips of the hair cell cilia. The shearing force is caused by the different pivotal points of the basilar and tectorial membranes on the bony modiolus and limbus, respectively.

stereocilia in the opposite direction releases the tension on the cross-links and closes the K^+ channels. Oscillations in K^+ and Ca^{2+} fluxes produce an electrochemical resonance in the stereocilia that follows the mechanical action of the basilar membrane and produces sharper tuning of the auditory signal.

Bass is not at the base; it is at the apex.

Coding of Pitch. Despite active discussion and debate for over a century, there is no consensus regarding the mechanisms responsible for pitch perception. Presently, there is partial support for both place and frequency theories of pitch perception. Place theories maintain that perception of pitch varies according to the locus of excitation along the basilar membrane. The earliest place theory dates to the mid-19th century when Helmholtz suggested that the fibers of the basilar membrane resonate like a harp. According to Helmholtz's resonance theory, high and low tones differentially stimulate the base and apex of the basilar membrane, respectively (Figure 8.12). Experiments conducted decades later by von Bekesy demonstrated that the resonance theory was untenable because the fibers of the basilar membrane are cross-linked to one another and lack sufficient tension to resonate as suggested by Helmholtz. In addition, auditory stimuli distort large portions of the basilar membrane, not focal areas as required by the resonance theory. Although the mechanical properties postulated by Helmholtz were wrong, the general concept of the place theory was correct and today forms the basis for the tonotopic organization that begins in the cochlea and is observed at every level of the auditory system, including the cerebral cortex.

Sound-induced vibrations of the basilar membrane are the basis for frequency transduction.

Von Bekesy also demonstrated that an auditory tone produces one region of maximal displacement as it travels from the base to the apex of the basilar membrane. The locus of maximal displacement is determined by the mechanical characteristics of the basilar membrane, the fluid dynamics of the cochlea, and the frequency of the auditory stimulus. Basilar membrane displacement is largest near the base of the cochlea for high-pitched tones; low tones preferentially displace the apex of the basilar membrane

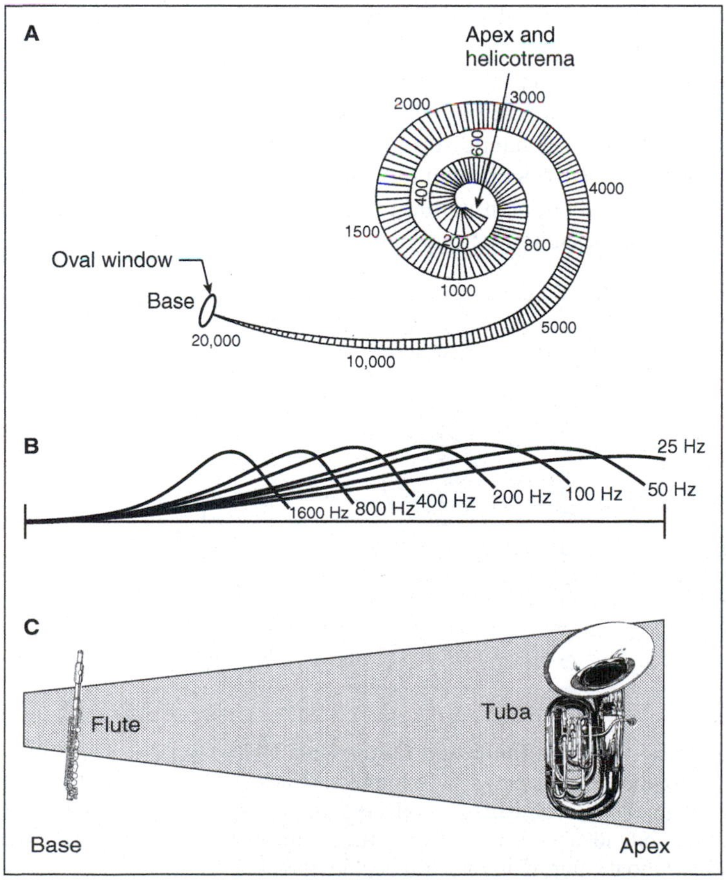

FIG. 8.12. Tonotopic Organization of the Cochlea. (A) Transduction of high frequencies takes place near the oval window; cells that respond to low frequencies are located near the helicotrema at the apex of the cochlea. (B) Vibrations conducted from the oval window to the cochlea produce traveling waves that move from the base to the apex. Maximal displacement of the basilar membrane occurs within a restricted region that varies as a function of auditory frequency. (C) High tones produce maximal displacement near the oval window, where the basilar membrane is relatively narrow. Maximal displacement of the basilar membrane takes place near the apex during stimulation with low tones. Note that as the width of the basilar membrane progressively increases from the base to the apex, the thickness and tension of the basilar membrane decreases.

(see Figure 8.12). The crest of the traveling wave, however, is too broad to allow fine discrimination of pitch, especially at low frequencies. Von Bekesy suggested that the locus of peak displacement is sharpened by lateral inhibition. More recently, it has been suggested that rhythmic changes in the length of the outer hair cells amplifies receptor potentials that originate in the area of peak displacement.

In the late 19th century, Rutherford proposed the telephone theory of pitch perception. This frequency theory, as originally conceived, postulated that the basilar membrane vibrates as a whole, with each vibration triggering one action potential. As the field of neurophysiology matured, it became apparent that neurons are unable to fire at frequencies above 800-1000 Hz. The frequency theory fell into disfavor, but it received a partial reprieve when Wever suggested that auditory neurons might keep pace with auditory frequencies above 1000 Hz by responding to every 2nd, 3rd, or *n*th beat of the basilar membrane. The demonstration that some axons of the cochlear nerve fire in synchrony with basilar membrane movement has provided support for Wever's "volley theory," at least for tones up to 5000 Hz. At present, it is believed that the frequency and place theories combine to span the entire auditory spectrum. According to this duplex theory, low tones (i.e., <5000 Hz) are encoded by the frequency of action potentials and high tones (i.e., >5000 Hz) are encoded by the location of the active hair cells.

Cochlear Nerve (VIII)

All axons in VIII terminate in the cochlear nuclei.

Both inner and outer hair cells synapse on the distal dendrites of the first-order neurons of cranial nerve VIII, but differences in their innervation patterns suggest that they have different roles in sound transduction. Approximately 20,000 outer hair cells converge onto 3000 cochlear nerve fibers. Convergence increases the certainty of synaptic transmission at the expense of locus specificity along the basilar membrane. For this reason, it is unlikely that the output of the outer hair cells is used by the central nervous system (CNS) for frequency discrimination. By comparison, roughly 3000 inner hair cells synapse onto 20,000 cochlear nerve fibers (Figure 8.13). This divergent pattern ensures that the location and output of individual inner hair cells is accurately reported to the CNS where frequency discrimination takes place.

The cell bodies of the auditory branch of the vestibulocochlear nerve (VIII) are located within the spiral ganglion of the inner ear (see Figures 8.7 and 8.8). The distal processes of these bipolar neurons synapse on the basolateral surfaces of the inner and outer hair cells, and the central processes course to the CNS through the internal auditory meatus. Fibers of VIII enter the brainstem at the cerebellopontine angle, immediately lateral, dorsal, and caudal to the root of the vestibular branch of cranial nerve VIII (see Figure 5.10).

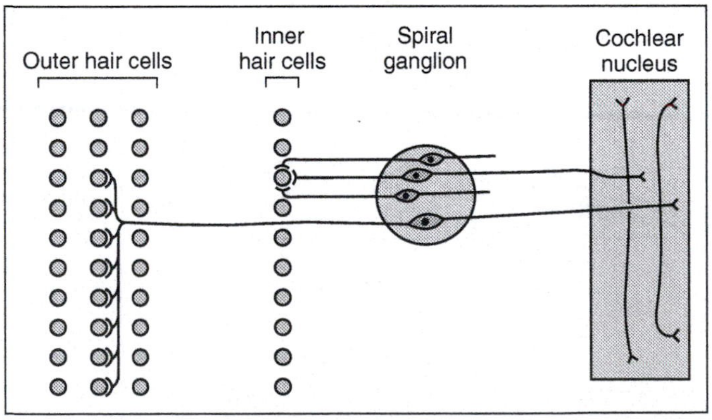

FIG. 8.13. Innervation Patterns of the Inner and Outer Hair Cells. The divergent innervation of the inner hair cells provides redundancy, which improves transmission fidelity. The central projections of the outer hair cells, by comparison, converge onto single spiral ganglion cells, which causes the identity of the individual cells to be lost. Afferent information arising from both inner and outer hair cells projects to the dorsal and ventral cochlear nuclei.

CENTRAL ANATOMY

Cochlear Nuclei

The cochlear nerve fibers bifurcate after entering the brain and terminate in the dorsal and ventral cochlear nuclei (see Figure 5.10). The dorsal and ventral cochlear nuclei are located on the surface of the pontomedullary brainstem, along the lateral aspect of the inferior cerebellar peduncle. Primary auditory fibers terminate in the cochlear nuclei in an orderly fashion that preserves the tonotopic organization of the organ of Corti. Neurons in the lateral half of the cochlear nuclei respond to low frequencies; high frequencies are represented medially.

Second-order fibers from the cochlear nuclei ascend bilaterally, but the contralateral pathway predominates. The efferent projections of the dorsal cochlear nuclei form three pathways: the dorsal, intermediate, and ventral acoustic striae (Figure 8.14). The most important of these is the ventral acoustic stria, which originates in the ventral cochlear nucleus. As the ventral and intermediate acoustic striae cross the pontine tegmentum within the trapezoid body, some fibers terminate bilaterally within the superior olivary nuclei, the nuclei of the

Tonotopic map of the cochlear nuclei:
- Low Lateral (LL)
- High Medial

Tonotopic is to hearing as **somatotopic** is to touch.

The **ventral acoustic stria** is the main efferent pathway from the cochlear nuclei.

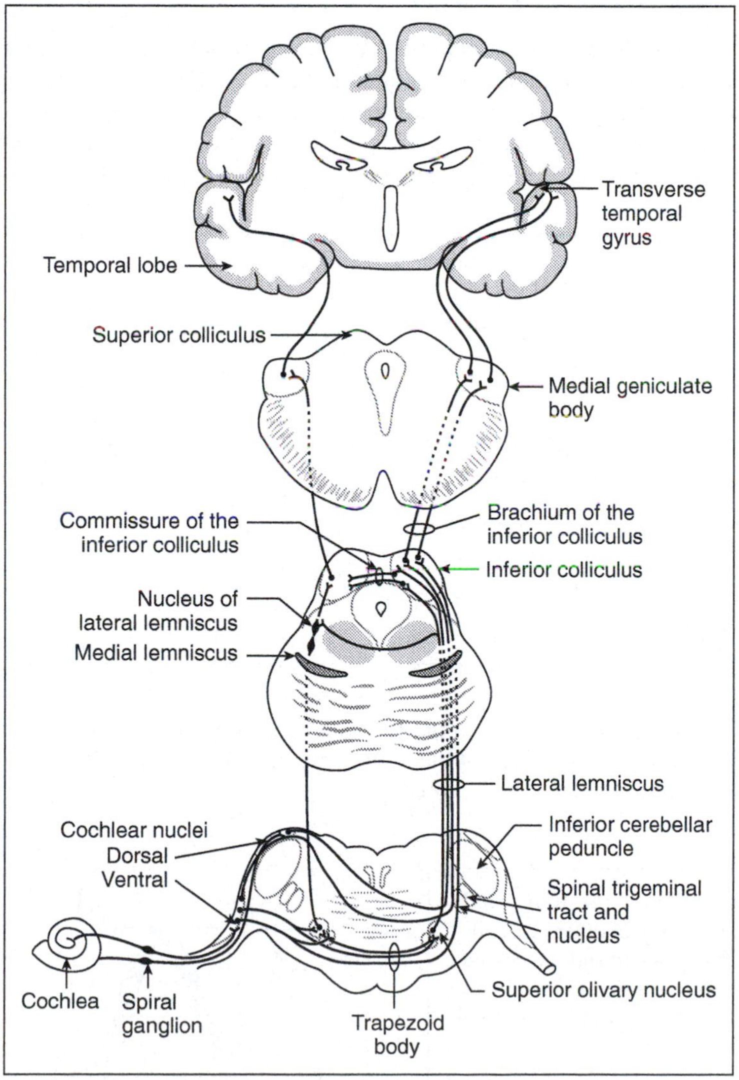

FIG. 8.14. Diagram of the Auditory System. The auditory pathway is illustrated in these selected sections through the medulla, pons, midbrain, and forebrain. Note that auditory information ascends bilaterally, with contralateral dominance.

trapezoid body, and the adjacent reticular formation (see Figures 5.16, 5.17, and 5.22). The remaining fibers of the ventral acoustic stria and the efferent projections of the superior olive form the contralateral lateral lemniscus and ascend to the inferior colliculus.

Most auditory information ascends **contralaterally.**

The dorsal acoustic stria originates in the dorsal cochlear nucleus, crosses the pontine tegmentum, and like the other two auditory pathways, joins the lateral lemniscus and terminates in the inferior colliculus. The dorsal stria does not project to the superior olivary complex and its associated nuclei, however.

Superior Olivary Nuclei

Sound localization is based on interaural differences in loudness, phase angle, and time of arrival.

The superior olivary complex consists of two small nuclear groups and a halo of periolivary neurons (see Figures 5.17 and 5.22). Located in the ventral tegmentum near the descending root fibers of the abducens nerve, the superior olive receives binaural input from the ventral cochlear nuclei. Interaural differences in sound intensity, arrival time, and phase angle enable the olivary nuclei to determine if a sound originated from the left or right side. Projections from the superior olive join the lateral lemniscus and ascend bilaterally.

Efferent Control of Auditory Input

Cholinergic neurons located in the superior olivary complex protect the cochlear hair cells from loud sounds and tune them for maximal sensitivity (Figure 8.15). Protection is afforded by olivocochlear fibers that terminate on the basal surfaces of the outer hair cells, which are believed to limit the excursions of the tectorial membrane caused by loud sounds (Figure 8.16). These projections also may optimize sound transduction by synchronizing

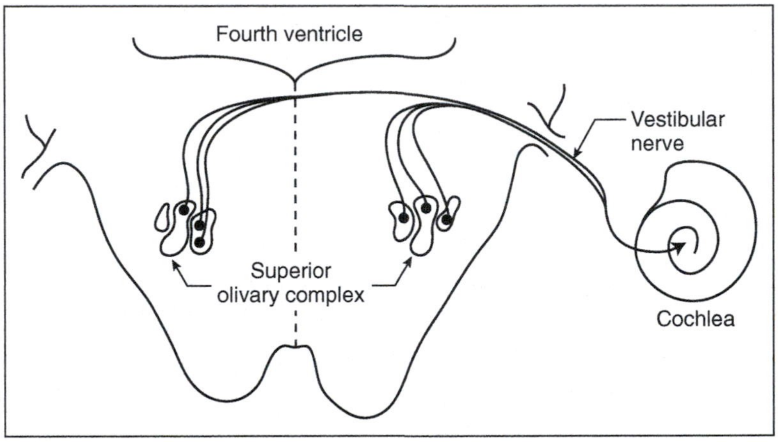

FIG. 8.15. Efferent Projections to the Cochlea. The cells of origin for the efferent projections to the inner and outer hair cells of the cochlea are located in the periolivary nuclei. Efferent modulation of hearing is reflexive and consensual.

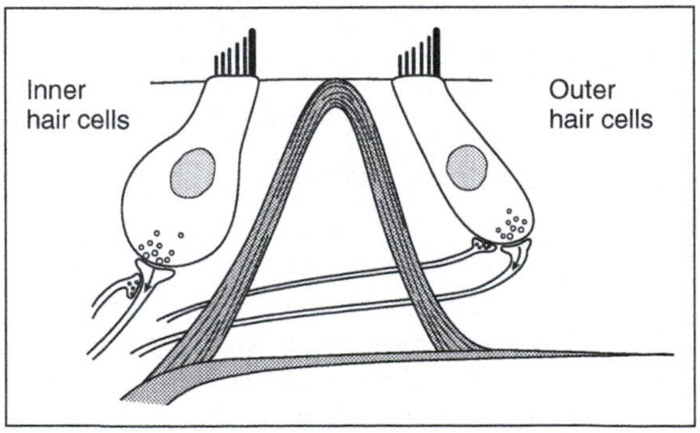

FIG. 8.16. Afferent and Efferent Innervation of the Inner and Outer Hairs. Axosomatic synapses located at the base of outer hair cells enables periolivary neurons to sharpen sound transduction and protect the inner hair cells from acoustic trauma. Afferent information from the inner hair cells may be modulated by efferent axodendritic synapses located near the distal end of the cochlear nerve fibers.

TABLE 8.1 Neural Components of the Lateral Lemniscus

Lateral Lemniscus Contains	Origin of Neurons
Second-order neurons	Ventral cochlear nucleus (contralateral)
Third-order neurons	Ventral cochlear nucleus (ipsilateral and contralateral)
	Dorsal cochlear nucleus (contralateral)
Fourth-order neurons	Superior olivary nuclei (ipsilateral)
Fifth-order neurons	Nuclei of the lateral lemniscus

the movements of the basilar and tectorial membranes. Additional protection is provided by cholinergic neurons of the superior olive that project to the facial motor nucleus (not shown), which executes the stapedial reflex during sustained loud sounds.

Lateral Lemniscus

The lateral lemniscus contains ascending auditory axons that originate in the cochlear nucleus and the superior olivary nuclei bilaterally. The presence of second-, third-, fourth, and fifth-order fibers in the lateral lemniscus illustrates the complexity of the ascending auditory pathway (Table 8.1). From its origin lateral to the superior olivary nucleus, the lateral lemniscus ascends through the pons in close proximity to the anterolateral system. In the midbrain the lateral lemniscus resembles a flattened ribbon along the lateral edge of the superior cerebellar peduncle. Some collateral fibers depart the lateral lemniscus and terminate in the nuclei of the lateral lemniscus; the remaining fibers assume a goblet-like appearance that embraces the base of the inferior colliculus as its axons terminate within its central nucleus (Figure 8.17).

The **lateral lemniscus** contains second-, third-, fourth-, and fifth-order neurons.

Inferior and Superior Colliculi

The inferior and superior colliculi receive projections from auditory relays of the lower brainstem, but each processes this information for a different end. The inferior colliculus serves as the primary mesencephalic relay for pitch and loudness information bound for the forebrain (see Figure 5.24). The superior colliculus consists of a superficial visual region and a multimodal core; only the latter participates in auditory functions. The inferior and superior colliculi warrant separate discussion.

The inferior colliculus is divided into three parts based upon cytologic, connectional, and functional criteria: the central nucleus, the external nucleus, and the pericentral

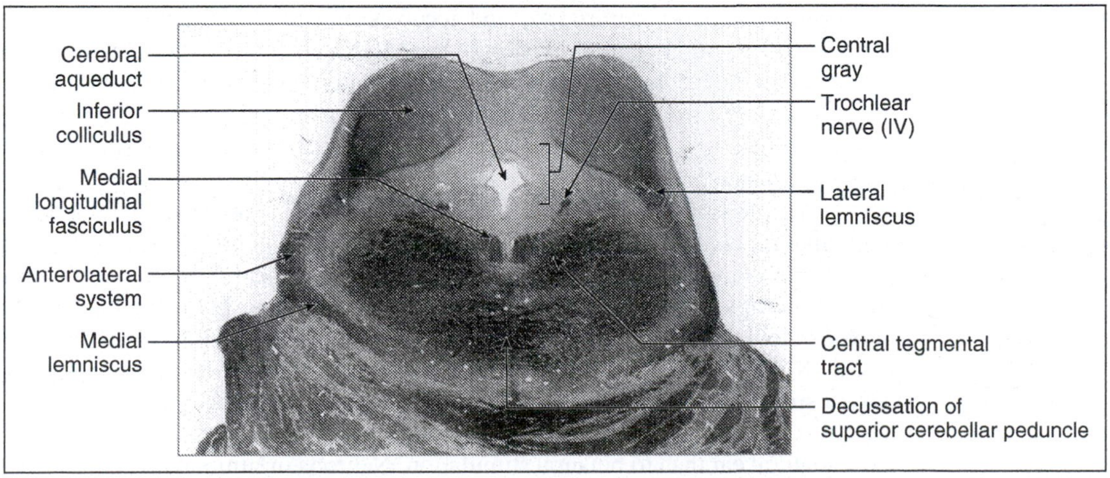

FIG. 8.17. The Caudal Mesencephalon. The lateral lemniscus, which resembles a narrow ribbon during its ascent through the pons, becomes wider as it approaches the inferior colliculus. (Weigert stain)

Music and speech are relayed through the central nucleus (core) of the inferior colliculus.

Belt area: acousticomotor reflexes

nucleus. The central nucleus, located in the core region of the inferior colliculus, receives direct, tonotopically organized projections from the cochlear nuclei and the superior olivary complex. Neurons responsive to high frequencies are located more superficially than neurons that respond to low frequencies.

The external and pericentral nuclei that form the belt region of the inferior colliculus receive projections from the central nucleus, the cochlear nuclei, and the primary and secondary auditory cortices, as well as input from nonauditory sources such as the dorsal column nuclei and the parietal cortex. This pattern of afferent projections and the fact that weak electrical stimulation produces orientation of the head, eyes, and pinna to the contralateral side suggest that the belt areas of the inferior colliculus mediate acousticomotor reflexes.

The deep layers of the superior colliculus receive afferent projections from the belt areas of the inferior colliculus as well as from parts of the periolivary nuclei, the auditory cortex, the posterior column nuclei, and the frontal eye fields. Auditory, visual, and somatosensory information that reaches the deep layers of the superior colliculus contributes to reflexive postural adjustments of the head and neck by the tectospinal tract.

Medial Geniculate Nucleus

Music and speech are relayed through the ventral (core) MGN.

The inferior colliculus and the MGN have core and belt regions.

Axons originating from the inferior colliculus form the brachium of the inferior colliculus, a robust tract perched on the outside of the midbrain that terminates in the medial geniculate nucleus (MGN) of the thalamus (see Figures 5.24, 5.25, and 6.1E). The MGN is located in the caudal diencephalon ventral to the pulvinar and medial to the lateral geniculate nucleus. The MGN consists of ventral, dorsal, and medial subdivisions. The ventral division is the largest part and the core projection area for fibers ascending from the central nucleus of the inferior colliculus. Like the central nucleus of the inferior colliculus, the ventral MGN contains a precise tonotopic organization, with high and low frequencies arranged mediolaterally. The ventral MGN projects to the primary auditory cortex where auditory discrimination takes place.

The dorsal and medial divisions of the MGN are belt areas that receive projections from the belt nuclei of the inferior colliculus. Auditory information ascending through the belt areas may direct attention to auditory cues in the environment or link auditory cues with objects detected by the visual or somatosensory systems.

Auditory Cortex

Auditory cortex: the transverse gyri of Heschl

Auditory cortex is located along the transverse gyri of Heschl and the adjacent dorsomedial and dorsolateral aspects of the superior temporal gyrus (see Figures 3.7 and 6.14). Like the midbrain and thalamic auditory relays, the auditory cortex is organized into core and belt regions. The core region, located in Brodmann area 41 (see Figure 6.7), represents the primary auditory cortex (AI) and receives ascending projections from the thalamic auditory core within ventral division of the MGN. The higher-order auditory cortex (AII) is located in the belt region (Brodmann area 42) along the lateral border of AI and receives most of its input from the dorsal and medial subnuclei of the MGN. Both sets of thalamocortical projections exit the MGN laterally and pass through the sublenticular part of the internal capsule on their way to the temporal lobe.

Suppression column: contralateral > binaural

Summation column: binaural > monaural

Neurophysiologic experiments conducted mostly in cats have identified isofrequency and binaural columns within AI. Isofrequency columns contain neurons that respond best to a narrow range of frequencies. The orderly arrangement of isofrequency columns creates a tonotopic organization that is similar across primates. In the marmoset, a New World monkey, low frequencies are represented further rostrally in AI than high frequencies (Figure 8.18). Although human data are limited, positron emission tomography studies indicate a similar organization. Binaural columns are classified as suppression or summation columns. Neurons in suppression columns respond better to monaural stimulation of the contralateral ear than to binaural stimulation. Neurons in summation columns respond better to binaural stimulation than to monaural stimulation of either ear. Alternating bands of suppression and summation columns are superimposed upon the isofrequency columns of AI. Because neurons in AI receive binaural input, unilateral cortical damage does not produce deafness in either ear.

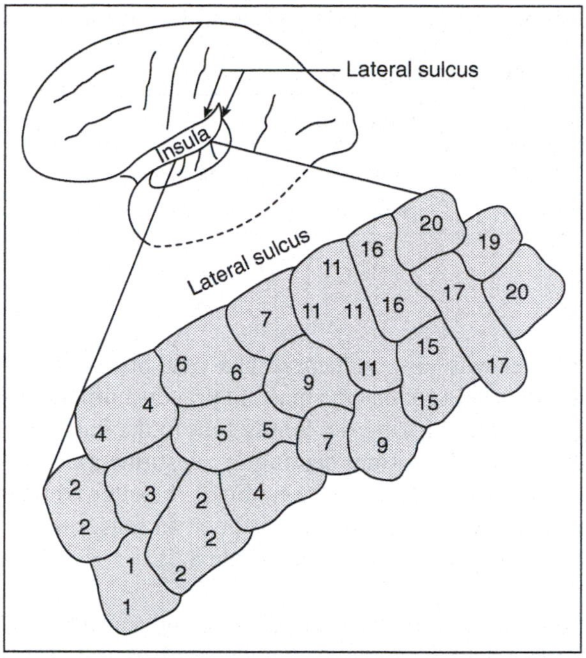

FIG. 8.18. Tonotopic Organization of Primary Auditory Cortex. In the top panel, the AI has been exposed by opening the lateral sulcus. Electrophysiologic recordings in the monkey reveal columnar and tonotopic organizations in AI. The cellular columns are oriented perpendicularly to the cortical surface. Each area outlined in the lower panel represents a column; the number indicates the preferred frequency (in kHz) of the auditory neurons located in that column. Low frequencies are located within the rostral part of AI.

The belt region of the left hemisphere includes the planum temporale, which forms part of Wernicke's area, whose role in language was discussed in Chapter 6. Patients with damage in Wernicke's area have fluent speech but struggle to comprehend spoken or written words.

CLINICAL ASPECTS

Auditory deficits are either conductive or sensorineural.

Approximately 12% of the population has some form of hearing disorder. Although the incidence of auditory problems increases with age and are common in the elderly, even children and infants can be affected. Hearing disorders vary from mild to profound, often involve only part of the audible spectrum, and may be accompanied by an unpleasant ringing in the ears called tinnitus (Table 8.2). Auditory deficits are caused by congenital and environmental (e.g., noise) factors as well as trauma, disease, and aging (presbycusis). Despite the wide range of symptoms and causative factors, hearing loss falls into two general categories: conductive or sensorineural. Conductive hearing loss is caused by obstructions (e.g., ear wax), infections (e.g., otitis media with effusion), or damage within the middle ear that prevents airborne vibrations from reaching the inner ear. Sensorineural hearing loss reflects damage to the cochlea, the VIIIth cranial nerve, or the brain.

Diagnostic Tests

The distinction between conduction and sensorineural deafness is determined in the clinic with two simple air and bone conduction tests. As a general rule, auditory threshold deficits greater than 40 dB are usually of sensorineural origin.

TABLE 8.2 Categories of Hearing Loss

	Magnitude of Hearing Loss (dB)
Normal	0–20
Mild	20–40
Moderate	40–60
Severe	60–80
Profound	>80

TABLE 8.3 Differential Diagnosis of Sensorineural and Conductive Hearing Loss

	Type of Hearing Loss	
Test	**Sensorineural**	**Conductive**
Rinne	Air conduction > bone conduction	Bone conduction > air conduction
Weber	Sound is heard in the normal ear.	Sound is heard in the affected ear.

Rinne's test: on the mastoid process

Rinne's Test. Normal patients hear better with air conduction than with bone conduction. In Rinne's test, a vibrating tuning fork is held against the mastoid process until the patient signals that the sound is no longer audible. Moving the tuning fork to the outside of the pinna reinstates the sound in individuals with normal hearing or sensorineural deafness. Patients with conduction deafness, however, can hear the tuning fork better while it is applied to the mastoid process because middle ear conduction is poor. In sensorineural hearing loss, air conduction and bone conduction are both weak (Table 8.3).

Weber's test: on the forehead

Weber's Test. Weber's test is used to distinguish between conduction and sensorineural deafness in patients with unilateral deafness. Patients with conduction deafness report that the sound evoked by a vibrating tuning fork held against the forehead is louder in the affected ear; in patients with sensorineural deafness, the sound lateralizes to the normal ear.

Auditory Evoked Potential Testing. Patients with sensorineural hearing loss may require extensive audiometric and electrophysiologic testing, and in some cases MRI scans, to determine the locus of the problem. In many patients the integrity of the auditory pathway can be evaluated with surface electrodes that measure the electrical potentials evoked by a brief, acoustic stimulus (Figure 8.19). Using this technique, individual potentials are recorded from each level of the auditory brainstem. Changes in the latency and amplitude of brainstem auditory evoked potentials (BAEP) provide diagnostic information about acoustic neuromas, multiple sclerosis, the progression of postsurgical edema, and even the probability of recovery from coma. The anatomical precision of BAEP testing is high in the auditory nerve and the lower brainstem, but it gradually decreases further rostrally because the second-order to fifth-order auditory neurons overlap within the lateral lemniscus (see Table 8.1).

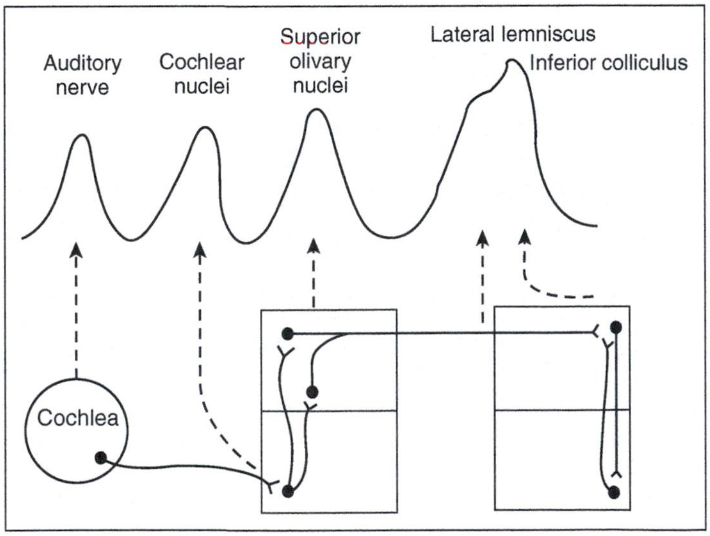

FIG. 8.19. Auditory Evoked Potentials. Diagram showing auditory evoked potentials from the auditory nerve, the cochlear nuclei, the superior olivary nuclei, the lateral lemniscus, and the inferior colliculus.

Conductive Hearing Loss

Conductive hearing loss is caused by mechanical interference of sound transmission through the outer and middle ear. Otitis media, when accompanied by effusion, is accompanied by pressure changes within the middle ear that impair hearing by impeding movement of the tympanic membrane. Chronic cases of otitis media in children should be treated aggressively to ensure that normal speech and language development continues during this critical period.

Conductive hearing loss: within the outer and middle ear

Perforated Tympanic Membrane. Most perforations of the eardrum are caused by middle ear infections (otitis media), but injuries due to local trauma (e.g., aggressive cleaning of the ear canal with a cotton-tipped applicator), an open-handed slap to the ear, or barotrauma during scuba diving are not uncommon. Mild hearing loss is common until the tympanic perforation heals.

Otosclerosis. Otosclerosis is a degenerative disease of unknown origin that attacks the bones of the middle ear of young adults. As the mineralized bones soften, the effectiveness of the ossicular chain gradually decreases and hearing deteriorates. Mineral deposits at the footplate of the stapes ultimately freezes ossicular motion. The treatment of choice is a stapedectomy, in which all or part of the stapes is replaced with a metallic prosthesis. Stapedectomy restores normal hearing in most patients.

Sensorineural Hearing Loss

Sensorineural hearing loss is caused by damage to the cochlear hair cells, the cochlear nerve, or the brain. Four common causes of sensorineural hearing loss are ototoxicity, trauma caused by prolonged exposure to loud sounds, Meniere's disease, and acoustic neuroma.

Sensorineural hearing loss: between the oval window and cortex

Ototoxicity. Transient and permanent episodes of tinnitus, vertigo, and deafness can be caused by aminoglycoside antibiotics (e.g., streptomycin, gentamycin), antineoplastic agents (e.g., cisplatin), various heavy metals, and overdoses of quinine or aspirin, which damage the hair cells of the inner ear.

Hair Cell Trauma. Excessively loud sounds bend and break stereocilia and ultimately destroy hair cells within the organ of Corti. Excessive auditory stimulation within a narrow frequency range damages the region along the basilar membrane where transduction of those frequencies takes place. Hair cell regeneration has been reported in birds, but not in humans.

Meniere's Disease. Meniere's disease is a disorder of the inner ear characterized by episodic, unpredictable attacks of vertigo, tinnitus, and permanent hearing loss. Hearing loss begins unilaterally, but after a few years becomes bilateral. The symptoms of Meniere's disease are caused by distortion of the membranous labyrinth by endolymphatic hydrops, an excessive accumulation of endolymph. Hydrops is caused by impaired resorption rather than overproduction of endolymph. Spontaneous remission of Meniere's disease is common and is probably caused by fistulization between the endolymphatic and perilymphatic compartments, which permits excess endolymph to drain. When severe symptoms persist, the excess endolymph can be drained with a surgically installed shunt. The etiology of Meniere's disease is unknown.

Meniere's disease: endolymphatic hydrops

Meniere s disease is caused by inadequate resorption of endolymph.

Acoustic Neuroma. Hearing loss is a common symptom associated with acoustic neuromas that engulf cranial nerve VIII within the cerebellopontine angle. Although the phrase "acoustic neuroma" is used almost universally, it a misnomer for two reasons: First, the tumors originate on the vestibular branch of cranial nerve VIII, not the acoustic branch. Second, these slow-growing, benign tumors are actually schwannomas, or tumors originating on the myelin-producing Schwann cells. Because these tumors may become very large

Acoustic neuromas are actually schwannomas.

before they are diagnosed, hearing loss is often accompanied by vertigo, ataxia, and loss of taste as the tumor compresses the vestibular branch of VIII, the inferior cerebellar peduncle, and the facial nerve (VII). Surgical removal is the treatment of choice. Early treatment is essential because large tumors are likely to cause irreversible hearing loss.

Correction of Hearing Loss

Many forms of conductive and sensorineural hearing loss can be improved and in some cases returned to normal.

Hearing Aids. Hearing aids benefit patients with conductive hearing loss and some types of sensorineural deficits by amplifying the sounds that reach the outer ear. In patients with conductive hearing loss, amplification compensates for poor sound conduction through the outer and middle ear. Amplification may also compensate for the partial loss of hair cells in the cochlea or impaired neural conduction in the CNS auditory pathways.

Cochlear Implants. Partial restoration of hearing is possible for patients with severe loss caused by damage within the middle or inner ear. Cochlear implants use a microphone to gather airborne vibrations, a microprocessor to convert them into electrical pulses, and a series of microscopic wires that stimulate the auditory nerve with those pulses. Even though cochlear implants do not restore normal hearing, they help patients engage their auditory world and may be a useful supplement to lip reading.

RESOLUTION OF CLINICAL CASE

The patient has an acoustic neuroma. Acoustic neuromas are slow-growing tumors that begin on the vestibular division of cranial nerve VIII at the cerebellopontine angle, infiltrate the internal auditory meatus, and gradually envelop the auditory and vestibular divisions of VIII and the facial nerve (VII). In extreme cases, acoustic neuromas may involve the trigeminal nerve (V). Because small tumors are typically asymptomatic, large tumors that displace the pons and cerebellum are common. This patient's headaches were caused by increased intracranial pressure, as indicated by papilledema in both eyes. He also had a progressive hearing loss but failed to recognize (or admit) the deficit. Some patients do recognize, however, that they hear conversations better over the telephone if they hold the receiver to one ear rather than the other. It is not uncommon for patients with acoustic neuromas to seek medical treatment initially for symptoms other than hearing loss. The patient's vertigo and ataxia were caused by entrapment of the vestibular division of VIII and physical displacement of the inferior cerebellar peduncle and the cerebellum. Focal testing revealed a taste deficit on the front of the tongue, which is innervated by the chorda tympani nerve, a branch of VII. Because taste is subserved by three different cranial nerves, few patients recognize that they have a gustatory deficit. Entrapment of the facial nerve produced a diminished corneal reflex and weak facial musculature on the left side. Spread of the tumor rostrally affected the root of the trigeminal nerve, causing facial anesthesia on the ipsilateral side.

REVIEW QUESTIONS

Directions: For each question, choose the **one** best answer.

1. Which auditory region receives monaural input?
- **A.** Ventral cochlear nucleus
- **B.** Inferior colliculus
- **C.** Superior olivary nucleus
- **D.** Medial geniculate nucleus
- **E.** Auditory cortex

2. What causes hyperacusis?
- **A.** Paralysis of the tensor tympani muscle
- **B.** Faulty modulation of the inner and outer hair cells by the olivocochlear tract
- **C.** Obstruction of the Eustachian tube
- **D.** Damage to the facial nerve
- **E.** Fusion of the ossicles

3. What is the relationship between the tonotopic organization within the CNS and the peripheral auditory apparatus?
   A. The tonotopic organization within the CNS reflects the orderly arrangement of the acoustic spectrum along the basilar membrane.
   B. The tuning properties of the ossicles define the tonotopic organization of the CNS.
   C. The tonotopic organization of the CNS is responsible for peak hearing sensitivity falling in the 2000-4000 Hz range.
   D. The relative insensitivity of the cochlea to high and low frequencies shapes the tonotopic organization of the CNS.
   E. The tonotopic organization of the CNS is the basis for sound localization.

4. Which symptom is observed in patients with an acoustic neuroma?
   A. Paresis of the contralateral leg
   B. Weakness on the ipsilateral face
   C. Paresis of the contralateral arm
   D. Loss of sensation from the contralateral face
   E. Loss of the gag reflex

5. Which of the following auditory relays is the first to receive binaural input?
   A. Ventral cochlear nucleus
   B. Inferior colliculus
   C. Superior olivary nucleus
   D. Medial geniculate nucleus
   E. Dorsal cochlear nucleus

6. What membrane contacts the distal tips of the inner hair cell stereocilia?
   A. Basilar membrane
   B. Reissner's membrane
   C. Endolymph
   D. Cupula
   E. Tectorial membrane

7. Damage to which structure causes unilateral deafness?
   A. Trapezoid body
   B. Primary auditory cortex
   C. Lateral lemniscus
   D. Cochlear nucleus
   E. Inferior colliculus

8. Which of the following would cause conductive hearing loss?
   A. Rupture of the round window
   B. Treatment with streptomycin
   C. Prolonged exposure to loud noise
   D. Acoustic neuroma
   E. Otosclerosis

9. A patient undergoing Rinne's test reports that the sound of the tuning fork disappears when it is removed from his mastoid process. What does the patient have?
   A. Damage to the cochlear hair cells
   B. Normal hearing
   C. An acoustic neuroma
   D. Conductive hearing loss
   E. Sensorineural hearing loss

ADDITIONAL READING

Classic Literature

Abeles, M, Goldstein MH: Responses of single neurons in the primary auditory cortex of the cat to tones and to tone pairs. *Brain Res* 42:337–352, 1972.

Hudspeth AJ: How the ear's works work. *Nature* 341:397–404, 1989.

Jeffries LA: A place theory of sound localization. *J Comp Physiol Psych* 41:35–39, 1948.

von Bekesy G: *Experiments in Hearing*. New York, NY: McGraw-Hill, 1960.

Reviews and Landmark Research Articles

Bilecen D, Scheffler K, Schmid N, Tschopp K, Seelig J: Tonotopic organization of the human auditory cortex as detected by BOLD-fMRI. *Hear Res* 126:19–27, 1998.

Clark GM: The multiple-channel cochlear implant: the interface between sound and the central nervous system for hearing, speech, and language in deaf people—a personal perspective. *Phil Trans R Soc B* 361:791–810, 2006.

Furness DN, Hackney CM: Cross-links between stereocilia in the guinea pig cochlea. *Hear Res* 18:177–188, 1985.

Jia S, He DZ: Motility-associated hair bundle motion in mammalian outer hair cells. *Nat Neurosci* 8:1028–1034, 2005.

Kaas JH, Hakett TA: Subdivisions of auditory cortex and processing streams in primates. *Proc Nat Acad Sci, U S A* 97:11793–11799, 2000.

Kinney SE, Sandridge SA, Newman CW: Long-term effects of Meniere's disease on hearing and quality of life. *Am J Otol* 18:67–73, 1997.

Knudsen EI, Konishi M: A neural map of auditory space in the owl. *Science* 200:795–797, 1978.

LeMasuirer M, Gillespie PG: Hair-cell mechanotransduction and cochlear amplification. *Neuron* 48:403–415, 2005.

Monsell EM, Teixido MT, Wilson MD, Hughes GB: Nonhereditary hearing loss. In: Hughes GB, Pensak ML, Jung KI,

Yanagisawa E, eds. *Clinical Otology.* New York, NY: Thieme, 1997:289–312.
Pickles JO: *An Introduction to the Physiology of Hearing.* 2nd ed. New York, NY: Academic Press, 1988:163–204.
Ricci AJ, Crawford AC, Fettiplace R: Mechanisms of active hair bundle motion in auditory hair cells. *J Neurosci* 22:44–52, 2002.
Schonwisner M, von Cramon DV, Rubsamen R: Is it tonotopy after all? *Neuroimage* 17:1144–1161, 2002.
Shepherd GM: *Neurobiology.* 2nd ed. New York, NY: Oxford University Press, 1988:304–325.
Webster DB: An overview of mammalian auditory pathways with an emphasis on humans. In: Webster DB, Popper AN, Fay RR, eds. *The Mammalian Auditory Pathway: Neuroanatomy.* New York, NY: Springer-Verlag, 1992:1–22.
Winer JA: The functional architecture of the medial geniculate body and the primary auditory cortex. In: Webster DB, Popper AN, Fay RR, eds. *The Mammalian Auditory Pathway: Neuroanatomy.* New York, NY: Springer-Verlag, 1992:222–409.

INTERNET RESOURCES

American Hearing Research Foundation
Barotrauma
http://www.american-hearing.org/disease/barotrauma.html
Cornell University, Weill Medical College
Stapedotomy
http://www.nycornell.org/ent/otosclerosis.html
Healthtouch Online
Otosclerosis
http://www.healthtouch.com/bin/Econtent_HT/hdShowLfts.asp?lftname=HHIRR007& cid=HTHLTH
National Institute on Deafness and Other Communication Disorders
Otosclerosis
http://www.nidcd.nih.gov/health/hearing/otosclerosis.asp
National Institutes of Health (MedlinePlus)
http://www.nlm.nih.gov/medlineplus/ency/article/000778.htm
University of British Columbia (David R. Stapells)
Auditory Evoked Potentials
http://www.audiospeech.ubc.ca/haplab/aep.htm
University of Buffalo
http://serous.med.buffalo.edu/hearing/index.html
University of California at San Diego, Department of Surgery
Acoustic Neuroma (Vestibular Schwannoma)
http://health.ucsd.edu/specialties/Surgery/otolaryngology/Ear/acoustic.htm
Meniere's Disease
http://health.ucsd.edu/specialties/Surgery/neuro/cnd/meniere.htm
Otosclerosis
http://health.ucsd.edu/specialties/Surgery/otolaryngology/Ear/otosclerosis.htm
University of Regensburg
Audiology and Hearing Disability
http://www.uni-regensburg.de/Fakultaeten/Medizin/HNO/audiowww.htm
University of Virginia Health System
Acoustic Neuroma
http://www.healthsystem.virginia.edu/uvahealth/adult_ent/acoustic.cfm
The Washington University School of Medicine
Auditory and Vestibular Pathways
http://thalamus.wustl.edu/course/audvest.html
Inner Ear Anatomy
http://oto.wustl.edu/cochlea/intro1.htm

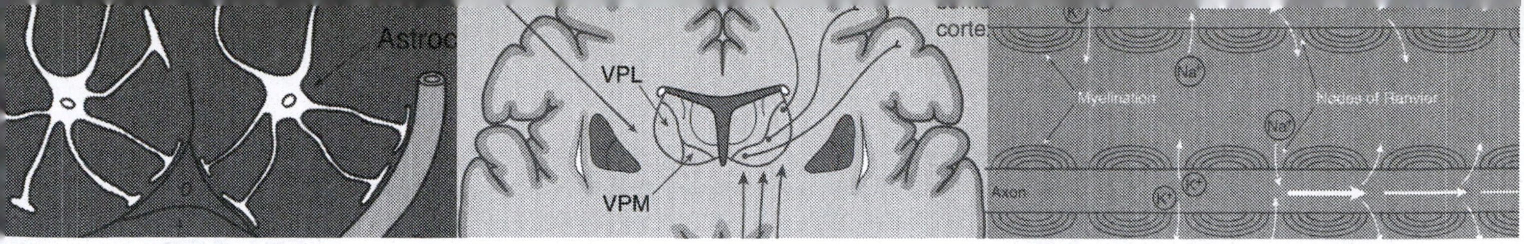

CHAPTER 9

Vestibular System

INTRODUCTION OF CLINICAL CASE

A 68-year-old woman scheduled an appointment with her primary care physician after experiencing brief but recurrent episodes of vertigo. Most of these attacks were triggered by rolling over in bed, bending down, or getting up quickly. Several episodes that began when she rolled over in bed ended abruptly when she rolled back to the first side. None of the attacks lasted longer than 1 minute. Physical examination showed an otherwise healthy woman whose physical and mental condition was appropriate for her age. Visual examination of the auditory meatus and the tympanic membrane was unremarkable; hearing appeared normal. During the examination, the physician was able to trigger a vertigo attack by having the patient sit on the examination table, turn her head to the right side, and quickly lie down on her left side. Confident of his diagnosis, the physician suggested that the patient perform a series of head and neck exercises each day and predicted that these attacks would stop within a few weeks.

OVERVIEW

Unlike small movements of the hands and fingers, larger movements that involve the arms, legs, or torso often change the body's center of balance and force a repositioning of the head. Reflexive, compensatory musculoskeletal adjustments initiated by the vestibular apparatus prevent a loss of balance following a change in the center of gravity. The

FIG. 9.1. Vestibular Apparatus in Perspective. The diameter of the membranous labyrinths and cochlea is less than the diameter of a penny.

vestibular system also stabilizes images on the retina by coordinating head and eye movements. In the absence of movement, the vestibular system contributes to muscle tone and maintenance of posture. Normally, the actions of the vestibular system do not enter the conscious sphere; following injury, however, symptoms may emerge that are obvious and disabling, at least in the short term. The importance of the vestibular apparatus should not be gauged by its small size (Figure 9.1).

PERIPHERAL ORGANIZATION

The auditory and vestibular parts of the inner ear are interconnected by the ductus reuniens.

The vestibular apparatus consists of a series of fluid-filled membranous cavities suspended within the bony labyrinths of the petrous portion of the temporal bone. Although continuous with and in many ways similar to the auditory apparatus of the inner ear, the vestibular apparatus is anatomically and functionally independent.

The vestibular apparatus consists of two parts, the otolith organs and the semicircular canals (Figure 9.2). Receptors located within the otolith organs respond to linear acceleration in the vertical and horizontal planes and tilting of the head (i.e., gravity). Receptors in the semicircular canals, by comparison, respond to angular acceleration (i.e., turning of the head). The otolith organs and the semicircular canals, like the cochlea, are bathed in endolymph and have sheets of specialized hair cells that respond to mechanical stimulation. Unlike the auditory system, the adequate stimulus for vestibular transduction is the inertial flow of endolymph caused by head movement.

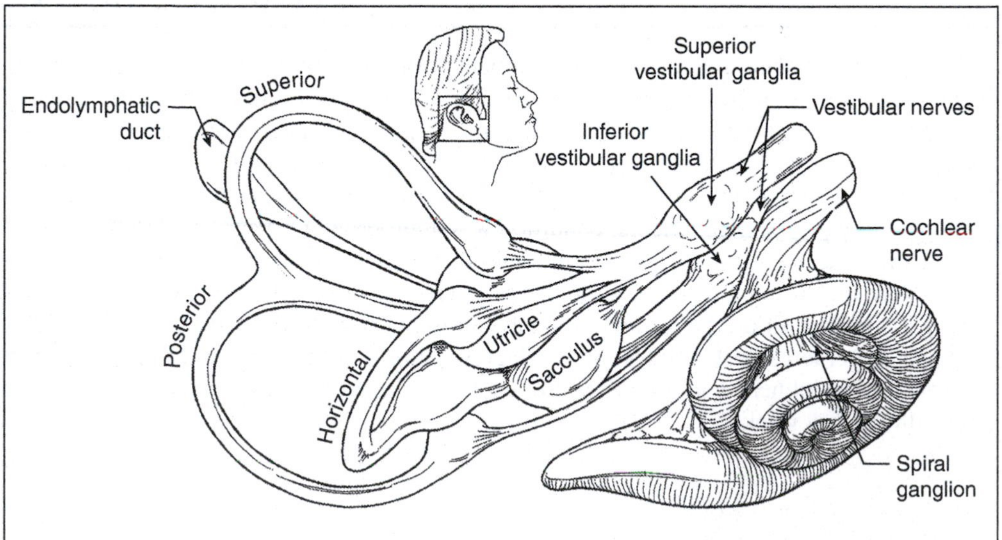

FIG. 9.2. Auditory and Vestibular Components of the Inner Ear. The orthogonal arrangement of the superior, posterior, and lateral semicircular canals ensures that angular acceleration in the x-axis, y-axis, and z-axis will be detected. Note that all three semicircular canals attach to the vestibule and that the posterior and superior canals have a common section.

Otolith Organs

The utricle and the saccule are located within the vestibule, the large chamber that separates the semicircular canals from the cochlea. With the head tilted down at approximately a 30° angle, the utricle is oriented horizontally and ideally positioned to respond to head tilt and movement along the horizontal plane. In that position, the vertical orientation of the saccule on the medial wall of the vestibule responds to dorsoventral excursions (Figure 9.3). Although movement at an oblique angle provides suboptimal stimulation of both otolith organs, it is their combined activation that signals movement at intermediate angles. The utricle and the saccule each have a 1-mm^2 patch of sensory neuroepithelium called the macula where sensory transduction takes place. The maculae contain hair cells, similar in some respects to those of the auditory system. Vestibular hair cells have a tuft of 40-110 apical stereocilia arranged like a pipe organ placed against a single kinocilium (Figure 9.4). The arrangement of stereocilia along one side of the kinocilium gives each hair cell an asymmetrical appearance and the ability to respond differentially to movements in various directions. Hair cell sensitivity is amplified because the tips of the stereocilia are embedded in an overlying otolithic membrane. The otolithic membrane is covered with a gelatinous matrix containing dense crystals of calcium

The orderly arrangement of the hair cells to the curved striola ensures that the otolith organs can work in all planes.

Otoconia, from Latin, means "ear stones."

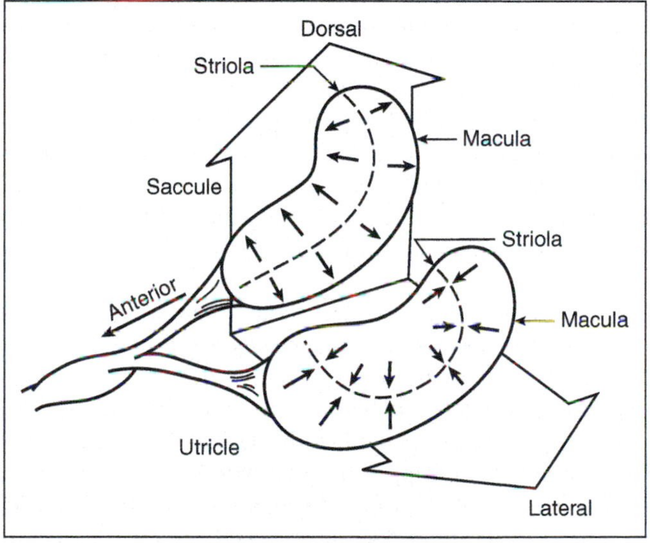

FIG. 9.3. Orientation of the Otolith Organs. The saccule and utricle are oriented perpendicularly to one another in the vestibule of the inner ear. The utricle, which is located on the floor of the vestibule, responds to head tilt or linear acceleration in the horizontal plane. The saccule, which forms part of the medial wall, responds to motion in the dorsoventral plane.

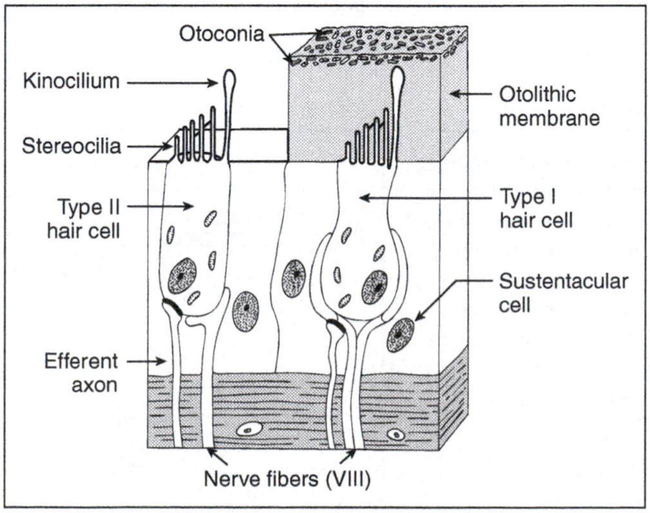

FIG. 9.4. Vestibular Receptor Cells. Vestibular hair cells are classified as either Type I or Type II cells. Type I cells (right) are goblet-shaped and have large chalice-type synapses with the primary afferent neurons. Efferent modulation of afferent activity is suggested by the presence of axodendritic synapses at the distal end of the afferent process. Type II cells (left) are columnar and have multiple small synapses at the base of the cell. Efferent projections to Type II cells terminate on the basal surface. Responses of Type I hair cells are phasic, whereas those of Type II cells are tonic. The hair cells of the otolith organs are covered by a gelatinous substance called the otolithic membrane. Calcium carbonate crystals that stud the surface of the otolithic membrane make the entire structure top-heavy, unstable, and thus more responsive to small changes in either tilt or linear acceleration.

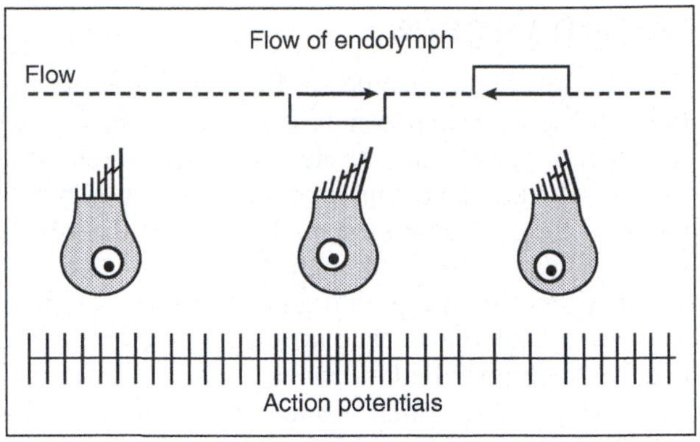

FIG. 9.5. Functional Polarity of the Vestibular Hair Cells. The high spontaneous rate of the vestibular receptor cells enables them to either increase or decrease their activity during movement. Bending of the stereocilia toward the kinocilium depolarizes the receptor cell and increases the firing rate of first-order vestibular fibers. The firing rate of primary vestibular fibers decreases when endolymph flows away from the kinocilium.

carbonate called otoconia or otoliths. These crystals make the otolithic membrane top-heavy, which provides additional leverage on the underlying stereocilia during head movement.

Bending the stereocilia toward the kinocilium results in depolarization. Bending the stereocilia away from the kinocilium results in hyperpolarization.

Transduction. The adequate stimulus for transduction is deflection or bending of the stereocilia. Bending of the stereocilia toward the kinocilium depolarizes the cell, whereas deflection away from the kinocilium causes hyperpolarization (Figure 9.5). Thus, movement of the stereocilia signals both direction and intensity of movement. As in the auditory system, fine links between the taller stereocilia and their shorter neighbors trigger ion flow that generates the hair cell receptor potentials. Movement of the stereocilia toward the kinocilium increases the influx of potassium ions (K^+). The increase in K^+ current depolarizes the hair cell, which creates a secondary influx of calcium ions (Ca^{2+}) and neurotransmitter release from the base of the cell (Figure 9.6). Movement of the stereocilia away from the kinocilium hyperpolarizes the cell by reducing the influx of K^+. The high spontaneous firing rate of the vestibular receptor cells enables them to increase or decrease their activity accordingly.

The stereocilia of vestibular hair cells, like their auditory counterparts, are damaged by systemic administration of aminoglycosides such as streptomycin and gentamicin. Aminoglycoside ototoxicity is best avoided by using short-term, low-dose treatment regimens. The early signs and symptoms of ototoxicity such as nausea, vomiting, dysequilibrium, vertigo, and a positive Romberg sign (see Chapter 12) indicate that hair cell damage has begun. When treatment is discontinued promptly, the symptoms usually resolve. Permanent impairment indicates that irreversible hair cell degeneration has taken place. Because the central vestibular components are moderately plastic, some degree of compensation may take place over the next 2 years, but over the long term, patients with permanent damage rely on visual and proprioceptive feedback for visual tracking and balance.

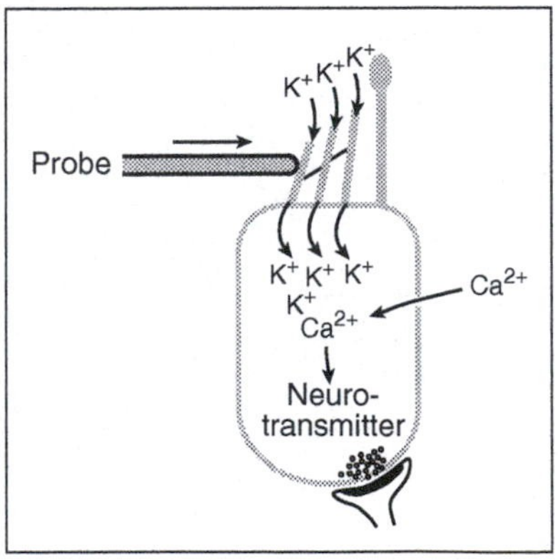

FIG. 9.6. Transduction of Vestibular Movement. Transduction begins when the stereocilia bend and distort the apical surface of the hair cell. When the stereocilia bend toward the kinocilium, the potassium (K^+) channels open, and K^+ flows down its concentration gradient and into the cell. Depolarization of the hair cell triggers an influx of calcium ions (Ca^{2+}), which releases the cell's neurotransmitter. Repolarization begins as the intracellular concentration of Ca^{2+}increases, causing K^+ to exit through the base of the cell.

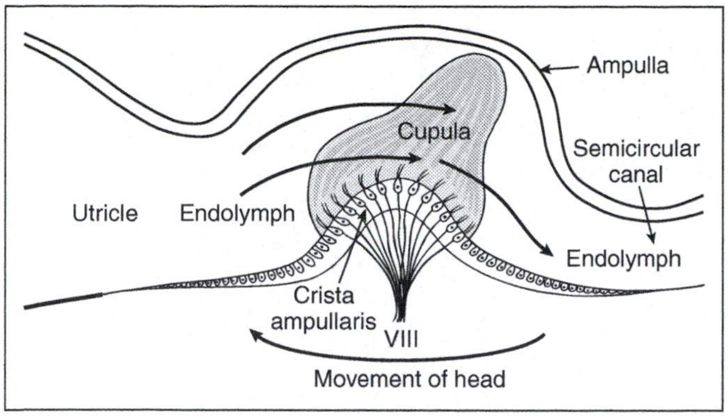

FIG. 9.7. Flow of Endolymph through the Ampulla. The cupula, by almost completely blocking the lumen of the ampulla, bends as endolymph flows past it.

Role of Hair Cell Polarity in Response Specificity. The hair cells of the utricle straddle a curved, shallow depression called the striola, which runs through the center of the macula (see Figure 9.3). Because each hair cell is arranged with its kinocilium oriented toward the curved striola, the macula is able to detect linear acceleration or head tilt in any direction in the horizontal plane. In the saccule, the hair cells are oriented away from the curved striola, ensuring that all movements in the vertical plane will be perceived.

Roll is rotation around the *x*-axis (e.g., log rolling). **Pitch** is rotation around the *y*-axis (e.g., leaning forward). **Yaw** is rotation around the *z*-axis (e.g., scanning the horizon).

Semicircular Canals

There are three semicircular canals oriented perpendicularly to one another so that head rotation in the *x*-axis, *y*-axis, or *z*-axis causes inertial flow of the endolymph through at least one canal (see Figure 9.2). One end of each canal contains an enlarged region, the ampulla, where the flow of endolymph provides the mechanical stimulus for sensory transduction (Figure 9.7). The floor of the ampulla contains a ridge of specialized hair cells, the crista ampullaris, which is capped by a towering mass of gelatin, the cupula. Endolymph flowing through the ampulla pushes the cupula, whose lever action bends the underlying stereocilia of the hair cells. The hair cells of the crista ampullaris have the same structure as those of the otolith organs and are arranged in a polarized fashion with respect to the utricle. All hair cells in the horizontal canal are polarized toward the utricle; those in the anterior and posterior canals are polarized away from the utricle. The polarity of the hair cells in the ampulla enables the semicircular canals to accurately report the direction of angular rotation to the brain.

Turn left, depolarize left; turn right, depolarize right.

In the horizontal canal, all hair cells are oriented toward the utricle. In the anterior and posterior canals, the hair cells are oriented away from the utricle.

CENTRAL ORGANIZATION

Projections of the Vestibular Apparatus

The hair cells of the crista ampullaris and the maculae are innervated by the vestibular branch of cranial nerve VIII. The cell bodies of these first-order neurons form the vestibular or Scarpa's ganglion, which is located in the internal auditory meatus. The central processes of these cells enter the brainstem at the cerebellopontine angle immediately caudal to the auditory fibers (see Figure 5.10). Vestibular fibers, after coursing dorsomedially between the inferior cerebellar peduncle and the spinal trigeminal tract, bifurcate into ascending and descending branches and terminate in the vestibular nuclei.

Four vestibular nuclei are clustered along the floor of the fourth ventricle (Figure 9.8; see also Figure 5.10). The lateral vestibular nucleus is a spherical nucleus located in the lateral tegmentum at the pontomedullary junction. The lateral vestibular nucleus consists of a ventral part that receives projections from the utricle and semicircular canals and a dorsal part whose afferent projections originate in the spinal cord and cerebellum (Figure 9.9). At its caudal end near the entry level of the vestibular nerve, the lateral vestibular nucleus abuts the rostral pole of the inferior vestibular nucleus, which descends almost as far as the

The lateral vestibular nucleus (Deiters' nucleus) is located at the point of entry for the vestibular branch of VIII.

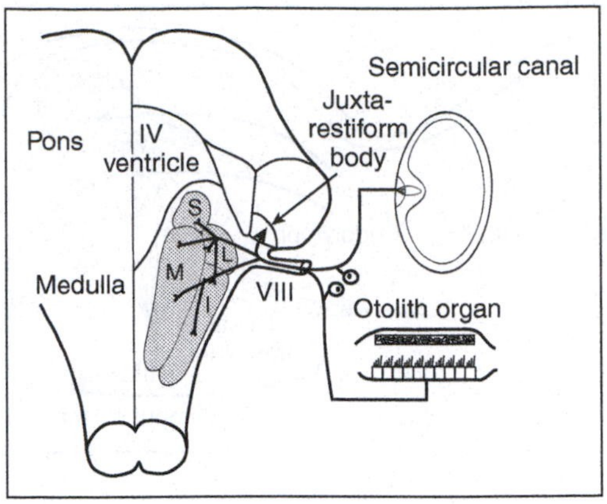

FIG. 9.8. Vestibular Nuclei. Four vestibular nuclei line the floor of the fourth ventricle. In this diagram, the fibers of the vestibulocochlear nerve enter the brainstem at the cerebellopontine angle, traverse the lateral vestibular nucleus, and distribute to all four vestibular nuclei. S = superior vestibular nucleus; M = medial vestibular nucleus; L = lateral vestibular nucleus; I = inferior (spinal or descending) vestibular nucleus.

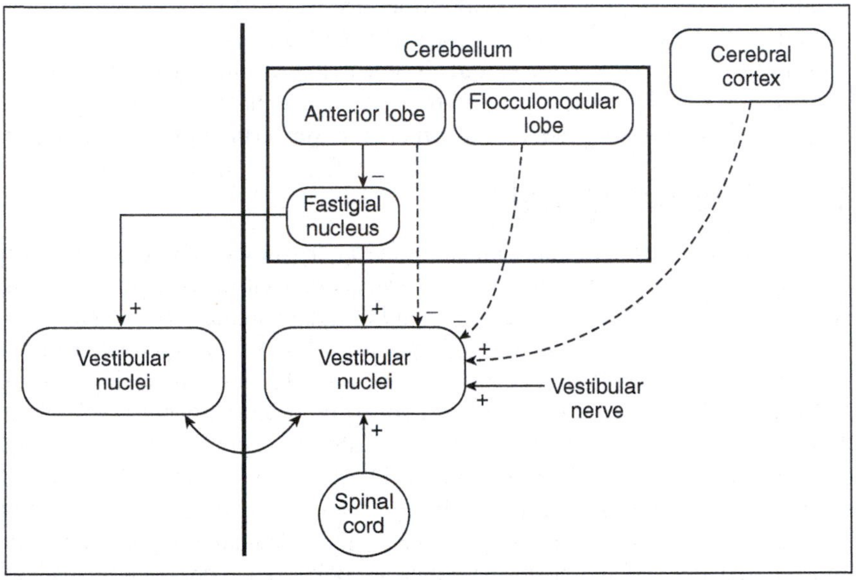

FIG. 9.9. Afferent Projections of the Vestibular Nuclei.

The inferior vestibular nucleus (spinal or descending nucleus) has a salt-and-pepper appearance in myelin-stained sections.

dorsal column nuclei. In transverse sections, the inferior vestibular nucleus has a distinctive "salt and pepper" appearance caused by descending fibers of the lateral vestibulospinal tract and the uncinate fasciculus. The medial vestibular nucleus is located along the medial flank of the inferior and lateral vestibular nuclei. Unlike the other vestibular nuclei, the medial nucleus is composed of small cells and has few myelinated fibers, which gives it a distinctly pale appearance in myelin-stained sections (see Figure 5.10). The superior vestibular nucleus is tucked into the dorsolateral corner of the pontine tegmentum and forms part of the ventrolateral wall of the fourth ventricle.

The semicircular canals project to the vestibular nuclei that influence eye movements.

At the risk of oversimplification, the vestibular complex can be divided on a functional basis into rostral and caudal parts. The rostral component coordinates head and eye movement, and the caudal part modulates posture and muscle tone. The rostral division includes the superior vestibular nucleus, the ventral part of the lateral nucleus, and the rostral portions of the medial and inferior nuclei—all areas that receive projections from the semicircular canals. The caudal part of the vestibular complex consists of the caudal aspects of the medial and inferior vestibular nuclei and receives projections from the saccule and utricle.

The vestibular nuclei that modulate posture and muscle tone receive projections from the otolith organs.

A small contingent of primary vestibular fibers bypasses the vestibular complex and projects directly to the cerebellum. Even though the cerebellum receives projections from almost every sensory system, this is the only instance involving first-order afferent fibers. These fibers join axons of second-order neurons located in the vestibular nuclei and enter the cerebellum through the juxtarestiform body located lateral to the superior vestibular nucleus and medial to the inferior cerebellar peduncle. These afferent vestibulocerebellar fibers terminate in the deep cerebellar nuclei and the vestibulocerebellum (nodulus, uvula, flocculus; see Chapter 12).

Afferent Projections of the Vestibular Nuclei

The vestibular nuclei receive afferent projections from the cerebellum and the cerebral cortex, as well as the contralateral vestibular nuclei and the reticular formation (see Figure 9.9).

Cerebellovestibular Projections. The cerebellum is the largest source of input to the vestibular nuclei. Purkinje cells in the vestibulocerebellum send inhibitory projections to the vestibular nuclei via the juxtarestiform body. Other neurons located in the fastigial nucleus, the most medial of the four deep cerebellar nuclei, project bilaterally to the vestibular nuclei and the adjacent reticular formation. The ipsilateral fibers descend within the juxtarestiform body, and the contralateral axons form the uncinate fasciculus. The uncinate fasciculus is a small tract that crosses within the cerebellum and then courses to the contralateral brainstem along the dorsal surface of the superior cerebellar peduncle. Neurons in the fastigial nucleus, like those in the other deep cerebellar nuclei, use glutamate, aspartate, or both as their neurotransmitters and thus are presumed to facilitate the activity of the vestibular nuclei. Postural and vestibular feedback relayed through the cerebellum enable the vestibular nuclei to continually adjust their output to the axial musculature.

The cerebellum is the single largest source of input to the vestibular nuclei.

Purkinje cells are GABAergic.

The **uncinate fasciculus** (the hooked tract) crosses within the cerebellum and exits along the dorsal surface of the superior cerebellar peduncle.

Corticovestibular Projections. Descending projections from the cerebral cortex normally inhibit the activity of the vestibular nuclei. Damage to this corticovestibular projection disinhibits the vestibular nuclei, which causes either decerebrate or decorticate rigidity, also known as extensor posturing (see below).

Efferent Projections of the Vestibular Nuclei

Thalamocortical Projections. Ascending projections from the medial and inferior vestibular nuclei terminate in the ventral posterolateral, ventral lateral, and posterior thalamic nuclei before projecting to the vestibular cortex (Figure 9.10). Several regions of the cerebral cortex have been implicated in vestibular function, but most of the evidence supports a circumscribed area on the postcentral gyrus close to the face representation. Vestibular sensation may enter the conscious sphere, but this seldom happens in healthy individuals.

Vestibular sensations reach consciousness at the cortical level.

Vestibulocerebellar Projections. The cerebellum uses sensory input to refine movements of the axial and appendicular musculature. The small contingent of primary vestibular fibers that projects to the cerebellum is supplemented by a larger group of second-order projections from the vestibular nuclei. All of the vestibular nuclei except the lateral nucleus project to the

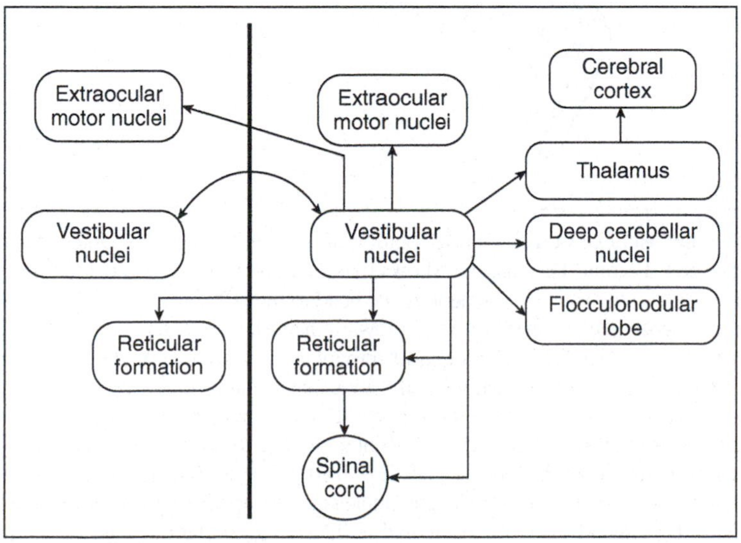

FIG. 9.10. Efferent Projections of the Vestibular Nuclei.

cerebellum, but the heaviest projections originate in the caudal portions of the medial and inferior vestibular nuclei. These projections to the cerebellar cortex and the deep cerebellar nuclei relay information from the otolith organs about head tilt and linear acceleration.

Projections to the Extraocular Motor Nuclei. Extensive projections from the vestibular nuclei to the abducens, trochlear, and oculomotor nuclei enable a moving observer to maintain visual fixation on a stationary object. These projections form the basis of the vestibulo-ocular reflex (VOR).

The VOR mediates compensatory eye movements that stabilize visual images on the retina during head and body movements. As with other reflexes, the VOR is executed by a three-neuron pathway. The sensory limb of the VOR consists of the primary afferent neurons of the vestibulocochlear nerve that signal rotation of the head. Neurons in the medial and superior vestibular nucleus act as the interneurons that project via the medial longitudinal fasciculus to the efferent limb of the reflex: the motor neurons of the extraocular muscles. In general, vestibular projections to the contralateral extraocular nuclei are excitatory, whereas ipsilateral projections are inhibitory. Motor nuclei that move the eyes to the right receive afferent projections from the vestibular neurons that respond to leftward head rotation and vice versa. The VOR operates in all three planes as well as at intermediate angles, but from a pedagogical standpoint, it is easiest to discuss this reflex in the horizontal plane (Figure 9.11). Because head rotation typically activates more than one semicircular canal, compensatory eye movements usually involve several extraocular muscles.

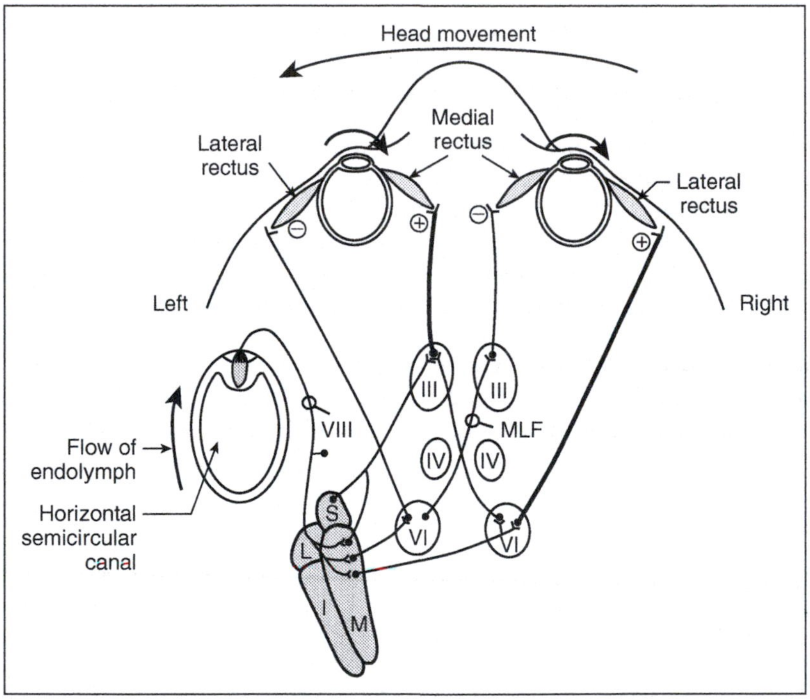

FIG. 9.11. Vestibulo-Ocular Reflex (VOR). During rotation of the head, the VOR counterrotates the eyes to stabilize the image on the retina. This diagram shows that rotation of the head to the left initiates compensatory eye movements to the right. Movement of the head to the left causes inertial flow of endolymph in the left horizontal semicircular canal to the right toward the utricle, which increases neural activity in the vestibular branch of cranial nerve VIII. Increased activity in the vestibular nuclei is relayed to the motor nuclei of the extraocular muscles. Projections to the abducens nucleus initiate contraction of the right lateral rectus muscle, whereas those to the oculomotor nucleus contract the left medial rectus muscle. The corresponding antagonist muscles relax. The VOR interconnects all 12 extraocular muscles with the vestibular apparatus to operate in all three planes. MLF = medial longitudinal fasciculus; III = oculomotor nucleus; IV = trochlear nucleus; VI = abducens nucleus; S = superior vestibular nucleus; M = medial vestibular nucleus; L = lateral vestibular nucleus; I = inferior vestibular nucleus.

The VOR is the basis for the doll's eye maneuver, one of the diagnostic tests used to evaluate brainstem integrity in unconscious patients. The doll's eye maneuver tests most of the vestibulo-ocular circuitry from the periphery to the midbrain as well as the efferent pathways to the extraocular eye muscles. A significant brainstem lesion would likely affect the vestibular pathway in some way. The test is performed with the patient in the supine position. After confirming that the patient has not sustained an injury to the cervical spine, the head is rotated from side to side. If all vestibulo-ocular pathways are intact, both eyes will move together in the direction opposite that of the head movement, as if fixed on a stationary object in the center of the visual field.

Doll's eye maneuver: turn head left, eyes turn right (and vice versa)

Commissural Projections. Commissural projections coordinate vestibular activity derived from the left and right sides. At the synaptic level, this coordination differs for the semicircular canals and the otolith organs. Excitatory connections typically are found between the vestibular nuclei that receive afferent projections from the otolith organs, whereas inhibitory connections are associated with neurons that respond to stimulation of the semicircular canals. The difference in synaptic polarity between the linear and rotatory systems is based on how the receptors on the left and right sides of the head are displaced during head movement. The otolith organs on both sides of the head move as a unit through space during linear acceleration, so excitatory commissural projections reinforce neural activity on the contralateral side. During head rotation, however, one side of the head moves forward while the other side moves backward. For example, turning the head to the left increases the firing rate in the left vestibular nerve and decreases the firing rate of the right vestibular nerve (Figure 9.12). Inhibitory commissural projections between the vestibular nuclei accentuate the signal difference already present on the left and right sides during head rotation. These commissural projections are normally spontaneously active. As illustrated in Figure 9.12, as activity in the left vestibular nucleus increases, the inhibitory commissural pathway suppresses activity in the contralateral

The left and right semicircular canals inhibit one another; left and right otolith organs reinforce each other.

Disinhibition: Dumping a pail of water on a fire will extinguish (inhibit) the flames. Anything that prevents (inhibits) the water from being poured on the fire (e.g., tripping and spilling the pail) will allow the fire to grow (excitation).

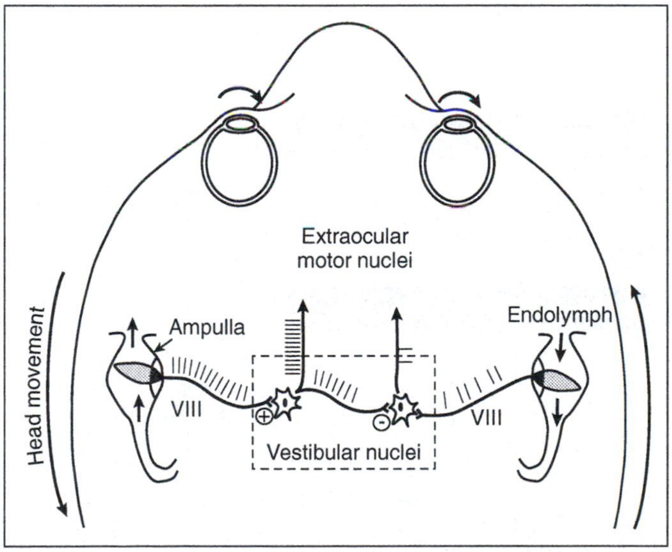

FIG. 9.12. Commissural Vestibular Projections. If the head is turned to the left, the endolymph in the left semicircular canal flows to the right through the ampulla, depolarizes the hair cells in the crista ampullaris, and increases the firing rate of the vestibular nerve on the left side. The left vestibular nuclei, by inhibiting neurons in the contralateral vestibular nuclei, accentuates the left/right difference in the evoked activity. On the right side, the endolymph within the horizontal canal flows away from the utricle, which hyperpolarizes the hair cells and lowers the firing rate of the ipsilateral vestibular nerve and nuclei. The sluggish activity in the right vestibular nuclei reduces the effectiveness of its inhibitory projection to the left side (not shown), which further facilitates neural activity in the left vestibular nuclei.

vestibular nucleus. The influence of the right vestibular nucleus on the contralateral side, although not shown in Figure 9.12, is the mirror image of this circuit. Lower activity in the right nerve/nucleus reduces the inhibition (disinhibits) normally exerted on the left side. These commissural projections, by exaggerating the differences in vestibular activity between the left and right sides, improve response sensitivity and resolution. Commissural connections also assist in vestibular compensation, the restoration of balance between the left and right vestibular nuclei that takes place following unilateral damage to the vestibular nuclei, nerve, or end organ.

Descending Projections. Muscle tone is regulated by several descending pathways, including the lateral and medial vestibulospinal tracts. The lateral vestibulospinal tract modulates muscle tone based on information about the body's equilibrium derived from the maculae of the otolith organs. The medial vestibulospinal tract, by comparison, ensures that movement of the head is coordinated with eye movements triggered by stimulation of the semicircular canals.

The **lateral vestibulospinal tract** descends the full length of the spinal cord and facilitates extensors.

Lateral Vestibulospinal Tract. The lateral vestibulospinal tract originates mainly from the lateral vestibular nucleus and terminates on α-motor and γ-motor neurons in the anterior horn (see Figure 4.23). Although the lateral vestibulospinal tract descends the entire length of the spinal cord, most of its axons terminate at cervical and lumbar levels. Stimulation of the lateral vestibulospinal tract releases glutamate or acetylcholine at its axon terminals, which facilitates extensors and inhibits flexors of the ipsilateral arm and leg.

The actions of the lateral vestibulospinal tract normally are modulated by descending projections from the cerebral and cerebellar cortices and the rubrospinal tract. Extensor posturing, more commonly referred to as decerebrate rigidity, is often observed following brainstem damage at the mid-collicular level (Figure 9.13). Patients

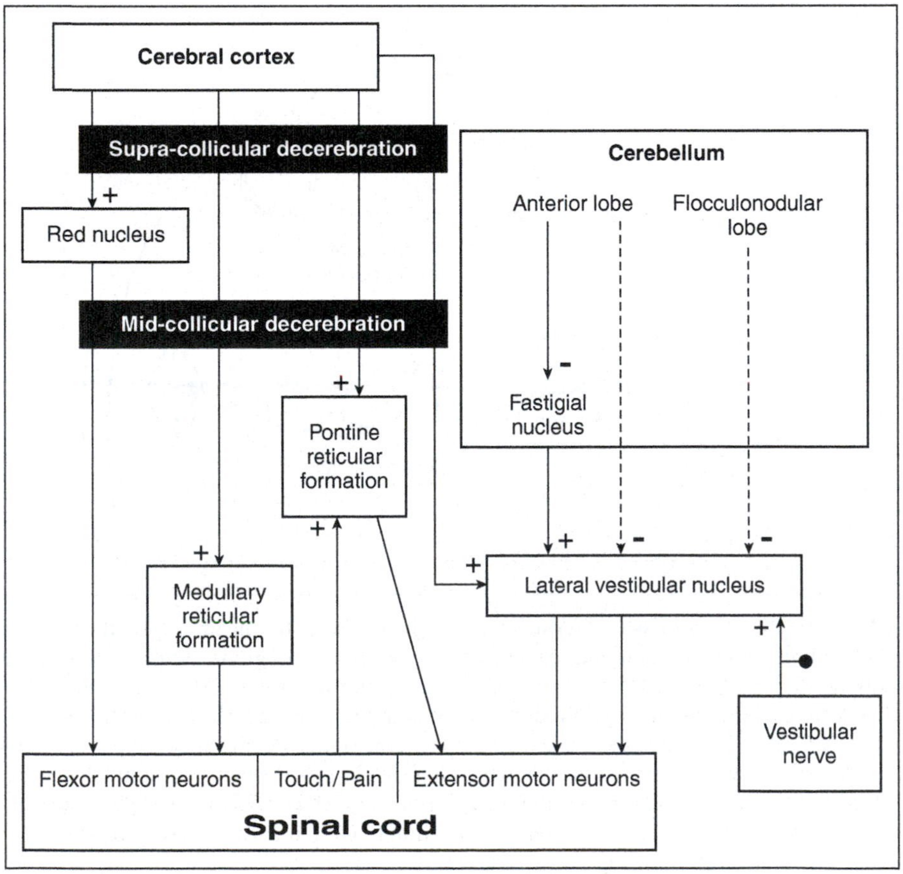

FIG. 9.13. Neural Circuits Underlying Decerebrate Rigidity. Decerebrate rigidity occurs following mid-collicular damage that isolates the spinal cord and caudal brainstem from the forebrain. This damage has four actions. First, the lateral vestibular nucleus and the pontine reticular formation are released from the inhibitory control of the cerebral cortex. Loss of cortical inhibition facilitates the extensor motor neurons that control the arms and legs. Second, output from the pontine reticular formation is increased by excitatory nociceptive input from the anterolateral system. Third, projections from the red nucleus to the spinal cord, which would normally inhibit extensor motor neurons, are severed. Fourth, the medullary reticular formation, which like the red nucleus inhibits extensor motor neurons, remains connected to the spinal cord but is inoperative without excitatory input from the cerebral cortex. The net effect is a profound and unopposed facilitation of the extensor motor neurons of the arms and legs.

with decerebrate rigidity show pronounced extension of the arms and legs, the so-called antigravity muscles. Decerebrate rigidity is caused, in part, by the unopposed actions of the pontine reticulospinal and the lateral vestibulospinal tracts on the α-motor and γ-motor neurons of the ventral horn. Because activity in the pontine reticular formation is driven by excitatory projections of the anterolateral system (ALS), noxious stimulation may cause patients with upper brainstem lesions to show pathologic extension of the arms and legs. Sectioning the dorsal roots or the vestibular nerves reduces the excitatory input to the vestibular nuclei and diminishes the symptoms of decerebrate rigidity. Because descending GABAergic projections from the anterior and flocculonodular lobes of the cerebellum normally restrain the lateral vestibular nucleus, cerebellar damage exacerbates decerebrate rigidity. Loss of inhibitory control over the fastigial nucleus following damage to the anterior cerebellum also augments extensor posturing.

Patients with brainstem damage rostral to the superior colliculus show flexion of the arms and extension of the legs, a presentation called decorticate rigidity. Arm flexion in decorticate rigidity is believed to be mediated by the rubrospinal tract, which remains connected to the spinal cord in patients with supra-collicular damage (see Figure 9.13). Symptom progression from decorticate to decerebrate rigidity typically signals spread of the damage caudally and a poor prognosis for the patient.

> Decerebrate rigidity = mid-collicular damage
> Decorticate rigidity = supra-collicular damage

Medial Vestibulospinal Tract. Stimulation of the labyrinth, in addition to initiating the VOR, triggers the vestibulo-collic reflex, a series of compensatory head movements designed to stabilize the head during movement. The vestibulo-collic reflex is mediated by the medial vestibulospinal tract, which consists of descending projections from the medial vestibular nucleus to cervical α-motor and γ-motor neurons that innervate the neck muscles. The medial vestibulospinal tract descends through the caudal brainstem and cervical cord within the medial longitudinal fasciculus (see Figures 4.23 and 5.10). Whereas the medial vestibulospinal tract terminates bilaterally within the reticular formation of the caudal brainstem, its projections to the spinal cord are strictly ipsilateral.

> The **medial vestibulospinal tract** travels within the medial longitudinal fasciculus, descends only as far as the lower cervical cord, and stabilizes the head during movement.

Central Modulation of Vestibular Transduction. Small groups of neurons located near the lateral border of the abducens nucleus project via the vestibular nerve to the hair cells of the maculae and the cristae (see Figure 9.4). These crossed and uncrossed cholinergic projections are believed to modulate the dynamic range of the vestibular hair cells.

CLINICAL SIGNS AND SYMPTOMS

The vestibular system prevents movement-induced fluctuations in balance, muscle tone, and visual tracking. Under most circumstances, the vestibular system is able to maintain order by making slight adjustments to these systems. Extreme or unfamiliar movements that overwhelm the vestibular system cause sensory, motor, and autonomic symptoms. These symptoms also may arise when the vestibular system is unable to reconcile information derived from different sensory systems, such as vision and balance. Unilateral dysfunction of the vestibular end organ, nerve, or nuclei may produce a neurophysiologic imbalance, which has a similar effect. In summary, vestibular signs and symptoms are caused by failure of the vestibular system to maintain the status quo. These sensory, motor, and autonomic effects range from mildly unpleasant to completely disabling.

Motion Sickness

The combination of visual, kinesthetic, somatosensory, and vestibular information usually presents an unambiguous assessment of how the body is oriented, moving, or both, through the environment. When these sensory systems provide discordant information or even novel sensations, motion sickness may occur. Motion sickness usually starts as malaise but may

> **Motion sickness** is caused by a mismatch of sensory signals.

When I'm seasick, first I'm afraid I'm going to die; then I'm afraid I won't.

progress to nausea and vomiting. The other symptoms of motion sickness such as profuse sweating, chills, pallor, hyperventilation, and vertigo are mediated by the area postrema, the nucleus of the solitary tract, and the dorsal motor nucleus of the vagus. Motion sickness is not considered a pathologic response but rather a normal visceral response to mismatched sensory stimuli. When riding in a car, for example, the stationary image of the dashboard may clash with the vestibular and kinesthetic sensations caused by motion of the car. For this reason, motion sickness may be relieved by looking out the car window or exacerbated by reading a book on your lap. Staring at the horizon helps the motion-sick traveler because the horizon, unlike the dashboard, truly is stationary, and this enables the brain to get a single message from the visual, vestibular, and proprioceptive systems: movement is taking place. Because the vestibular system is so plastic, people gradually adapt to sickness-inducing stimuli, as suggested by the expression to "get your sea legs." After motion sickness starts, however, relief is often hours away. Scuba divers have discovered the secret to a quick fix for motion sickness: jump in and descend. After one is submerged, the mismatch between movement of the ocean and the visual cues disappears and sea sickness resolves within seconds. Pharmacologic prevention of motion sickness utilizes drugs such as the anticholinergic scopolamine or the antihistamine dimenhydrinate (Dramamine®) that inhibit neural activity in the vestibular nuclei.

Vertigo and Dizziness

Vertigo is the illusion that you or your environment is moving. **Dizziness,** unlike vertigo, has no localizing value.

Vertigo is the illusion of movement of either self or environment caused by asymmetric activation of the vestibular system. In addition to the perception of movement, which corresponds to activity in the cerebral cortex, the sufferer may exhibit ocular and postural signs as well as autonomic symptoms. Vertigo typically causes a rhythmic oscillation of the eyes called nystagmus, which is a disturbance of the VOR. Postural imbalance is caused by disturbances in the descending vestibulospinal systems. Autonomic symptoms, such as sweating, nausea, vomiting, and hyperventilation, are due to activation of medullary autonomic areas, including the area postrema, the nucleus of the solitary tract, and the dorsal motor nucleus of the vagus.

Dizziness is a more diffuse phenomenon that includes lightheadedness, sensations of swimming or floating, and giddiness, but not necessarily an illusion of movement. Whereas vertigo and its related signs and symptoms are considered the hallmark of vestibular dysfunction, dizziness has no signs associated with it and usually originates outside the vestibular system. Dizziness has no localizing value.

Meniere's Disease

Tinnitus is a ringing, buzzing, or clicking sound that the patient localizes to the ear.

Meniere's disease, which is caused by excessive accumulation of endolymph, was described in Chapter 8. Patients with Meniere's disease have recurrent, unpredictable attacks of tinnitus, sensorineural hearing loss, and vertigo. Those with severe symptoms experience nausea, may resist moving their heads, and require assistance when standing. The duration of these attacks ranges from minutes to hours, during which time the symptoms of vertigo gradually dissipate. The treatment of choice for patients with severe symptoms is surgical installation of a shunt.

Nystagmus

The **direction of nystagmus** is defined by its quick phase because it is easier to observe.

Nystagmus is a pathologic oscillation of one or both eyes in one or more planes. Nystagmus involves a slow saccade in one direction followed by a quick excursion in the opposite direction. Even though the slow phase is the pathologic component of nystagmus and the quick phase is merely a compensatory adjustment, the quick phase is used to define the direction because it is easier to observe. Spontaneous nystagmus may signal damage to the vestibular apparatus or nerve, the brainstem, or the cerebellum. For patients with suspected lesions in these areas, induction of nystagmus is an important part of the clinical examination because it enables the physician to observe the operation of the vestibular system.

Nystagmus can be induced in healthy individuals by either caloric stimulation of the external auditory meatus or bodily rotation. Caloric stimulation creates convection currents in the semicircular canals that induce endolymphatic flow. The easiest semicircular canal to stimulate is the horizontal canal because it lies closest to the external ear. The patient's head is typically elevated at a 60° angle to put the horizontal canal in the vertical plane. Irrigating the ear with cool (30° C) water creates convection currents in the endolymph, which then flows away from the ampulla. The resultant hyperpolarization of the hair cells causes the patient's eyes to turn slowly toward the stimulated ear; the rapid phase is in the opposite direction (**c**old, **o**pposite). The effect is reversed if warm water is used (**w**arm, **s**ame).

> The mnemonic **COWS** (**c**old, **o**pposite; **w**arm, **s**ame) summarizes the direction of rapid eye movement following caloric stimulation of the ear.

In certain circumstances, rotation of the head induces nystagmus. As described earlier, the VOR is a set of compensatory eye movements that oppose normal head rotation during visual tracking. Unusually large rotations of the head that force the eyes beyond the limits imposed by the orbits initially trigger a normal VOR. When the eyes reach the limit of their excursion, however, they quickly rebound to a central fixation point and then resume their slow tracking movement opposite to the direction of head rotation.

> Hot air (and hot endolymph) rises.

In the clinic, nystagmus can be invoked with the aid of a Bárány chair. The Bárány chair allows a patient to be rotated at a constant speed in one direction for 15–20 seconds before the rotation is suddenly stopped. Prior to stopping, the movement of the endolymph matches that of the labyrinth; after stopping, the inertia of the endolymph carries it through the labyrinth and past the ampulla, stimulating the crista. The abrupt stop causes the patient's eyes to move slowly in the same direction as the prior rotation. These slow excursions are punctuated by quick movements in the direction opposite of the chair's rotation. For example, if the patient were rotated to the left, the slow phase of nystagmus would be to the left, and the quick phase would be to the right. This patient, if asked to point at a stationary target, would past-point—that is, point further to the left. If this patient were to stand up, there would be a tendency to fall in the direction of the prior rotation. The Bárány chair, unlike caloric stimulation, requires specialized equipment and does not permit separate testing of each ear.

> In the Bárány chair:
> Postural disturbances and past-pointing → same direction as the previous rotation
> Vertigo and nystagmus (fast phase) → opposite direction of previous rotation

RESOLUTION OF CLINICAL CASE

The patient was diagnosed with benign paroxysmal positional vertigo (BPPV), the most common type of vertigo. Idiopathic BPPV may strike at any age but is most common in the elderly, and women are more often afflicted than men. Postmortem studies have shown that patients with BPPV have utricular degeneration. It is believed that otoconia liberated from the diseased utricle migrate into the semicircular canals, typically the posterior one. Attacks of vertigo are triggered when angular rotation pushes these "floaters" into the ampulla and against the cupula. In most cases, BPPV resolves spontaneously within 1 month. Physicians often prescribe exercises designed to dislodge the debris from the cupula and disperse them into the endolymph of the utricle and saccule.

REVIEW QUESTIONS

Directions: For each of the following questions, choose the **one** best answer.

1. Which of the following statements best describes the lateral vestibulospinal tract?

A. The caudal continuation of the medial longitudinal fasciculus (MLF)
B. Descends ipsilaterally from its origin in the medial vestibular nucleus
C. Facilitates the extensors of the arms and legs
D. Extends only as far as the cervical spinal cord and plays a role in the postural control of the head
E. Together with the rubrospinal tract, controls posture by facilitating the extensor muscles of the legs

2. An unconscious 23-year-old man was brought into the emergency department after being found lying on the sidewalk outside a tavern. Blood oozed from the deep scalp laceration at the mastoid protuberance and the external auditory meatus. After ruling out injury to the cervical spine, the attending physician performed the doll's eye maneuver. As a diagnostic test, the doll's eye maneuver usually does not pinpoint damage within the brain, but rather rules out damage to particular structures. Which of the following structures can be assessed by the doll's eye maneuver?

A. Medial vestibulospinal tract
B. Lateral vestibulospinal tract
C. Thalamic vestibular relay
D. Vestibular nerve
E. Cerebellum

3. Which of the following areas receives a direct projection from vestibular neurons located in the vestibular ganglion?

A. Cerebellum
B. Nucleus abducens
C. Brainstem reticular formation
D. Medial longitudinal fasciculus (MLF)
E. Spinal cord

4. Which of the following statements about the vestibular nuclei is true?

A. Ascending projections from the vestibular nuclei travel to the oculomotor nuclei within the central tegmental tract.
B. Commissural connections between vestibular nuclei are excitatory for linear acceleration and inhibitory for angular acceleration.
C. Electrical stimulation of the fastigial nucleus decreases extensor muscle tone.
D. The superior vestibular nucleus receives afferent projections from the semicircular canals and modulates muscle tone.
E. Direct projections from the vestibular nuclei to the neostriatum help regulate voluntary motor control.

5. Which of the following events would be caused by turning the head to the left?

A. Neural activity in the vestibulocochlear nerve on the left side of the head increases.
B. The stereocilia of the horizontal semicircular canal on the left side of the head bend away from the utricle.
C. Endolymph flows toward the utricle on the right side of the head.
D. Descending lateral vestibulospinal projections execute compensatory adjustments of the head and neck.
E. The medial rectus muscle of the right eye contracts.

6. Which of the following procedures exacerbates the symptoms of decerebrate rigidity?

A. Sectioning the dorsal roots in the cervical enlargement
B. Lesioning the lateral vestibular nucleus
C. Denervation of the labyrinths
D. Sectioning the ventral roots in the cervical enlargement
E. Electrical stimulation of the vestibular nerve

7. Which of the following two vestibular structures control eye movements in the same direction?

A. Posterior semicircular canal and the saccule
B. Horizontal semicircular canal and the saccule
C. Vertical semicircular canal and the utricle
D. Lateral semicircular canal and the saccule
E. Saccule and utricle

8. You begin to get seasick during a cruise on a small boat. Returning to the dock is not an option. What should you do?

A. Lie down and rest.
B. Crawl into the cabin where it's quiet.
C. Distract yourself by reading a book.
D. Put on your scopolamine patch.
E. Stand on the deck and stare at the horizon.

9. Which of the following statements is true about the stereocilia of the vestibular apparatus?

A. All hair cells within the ampullae of the left ear are oriented in the same direction.
B. Hair cells depolarize when the stereocilia bend away from the kinocilium.
C. Hair cells signal the direction of movement.
D. Bending hair cells toward the striola of the utricle signals dorsoventral motion.
E. Vestibular hair cells, unlike those in the auditory system, are not damaged by streptomycin.

10. After a patient underwent several minutes of clockwise rotation in a Barany chair, the physician abruptly stopped the chair. The physician asked the patient to stand and point to the doorway. Which of the following observations would you expect in a patient with no vestibular pathology?

A. Loss of balance upon standing and a tendency to fall to his left as he pointed to the right of the doorway
B. Left nystagmus while pointing to the left of the doorway
C. Lost of balance upon standing, and a tendency to fall to his left while showing a right nystagmus
D. The patient complaining that the room was spinning to the right, while he was pointing to the left of the doorway
E. Left nystagmus and pointing to the right side of the doorway

ADDITIONAL READING

Classic Literature

Angaut P, Brodal A: The projection of the "vestibulocerebellum" onto the vestibular nuclei in the cat. *Arch Ital Biol* 105:441–479, 1967.

Benson AJ: The vestibular sensory system. In: Barlow HB, Mollon JD, eds. *The Senses*. New York, NY: Cambridge University Press, 1989:333–368.

Brodal A: The vestibular nuclei in the macaque monkey. *J Comp Neurol* 227:252–266, 1984.

Brodal A, Brodal P: Observations on the secondary vestibulocerebellar projections in the macaque monkey. *Exp Brain Res* 58:62–74, 1985.

Carpenter MB: Vestibular nuclei: afferent and efferent projections. *Prog Brain Res* 76:5–15, 1988.

Haines DE: Cerebellar corticonuclear and corticovestibular fibers of flocculonodular lobe in a prosimian primate *(Galago senegalensis)*. *J Comp Neurol* 174:607–630, 1977.

Reviews and Landmark Research Articles

Andrews JC: Intralabyrinthine fluid dynamics: Meniere disease. *Curr Opin Otolaryngol Head Neck Surg* 12:408–412, 2004.

Baloh RW, Halmagyi GM, eds: *Disorders of the Vestibular System*. New York, NY: Oxford University Press, 1996.

Barmac NH: Central vestibular system: vestibular nuclei and posterior cerebellum. *Brain Res Bull* 60:511–541, 2003.

Boyle R: Activity of medial vestibulospinal tract cells during rotation and ocular movement in the alert squirrel monkey. *J Neurophysiol* 70:2176–2180, 1993.

Brandt T: Vertigo. In: Brandt T, Caplan LR, Dighgans J, Diener HC, Kennard C, eds. *Neurological Disorders: Course and Treatment*. New York, NY: Academic Press, 1996.

Buttner-Ennever JA, Gerrits NM: Vestibular System. In: Paxinos G, Mai JK, eds. *The Human Nervous System*. New York, NY: Elsevier, 2004.

Duque-Parra JE: Perspective on the vestibular cortex throughout history. *Anat Rec* 280B:15–19, 2004.

Fernandez C, Goldberg JM, Abend WK: Response to static tilts of peripheral neurons innervating otolith organs of the squirrel monkey. *J Neurophysiol* 35:978–987, 1972.

Fukushima K: Corticovestibular interactions: anatomy, electrophysiology, and functional considerations. *Exp Brain Res* 117:1–16, 1997.

Goldberg JM, Fernandez C: Efferent vestibular system in the squirrel monkey: anatomical location and influence on afferent activity. *J Neurophysiol* 43:986–1025, 1980.

Hamann K-F, Arnold W: Meniere's disease. *Adv Oto-Rhino-Laryngol* 55:137–168, 1999.

Leigh RJ: Human vestibular cortex. *Ann Neurol* 35:383–384, 1994.

Leigh RJ, Brandt T: A re-evaluation of the vestibulo-ocular reflex: new ideas of its purpose, neural substrate, and disorders. *Neurol* 43:1288–1295, 1993.

Nakashima T, Teranishi M, Hibi T, Kobayashi M, Umemura M: Vestibular and cochlear toxicity of aminoglycosides—a review. *Acta Otolaryngol* 120:904–911, 2000.

Parnes LS, Agrawal SK, Atlas J: Diagnosis and management of benign paroxysmal positional vertigo (BPPV). *Canad Med Assoc J* 169:681–693, 2003.

Semont A, Freyss E, Vitte P: Curing the BPPV with liberatory maneuver. *Adv Oto-Rhino-Laryngol* 42:290–293, 1988.

Tran Ba Huy P, Toupet M: Peripheral disorders in the otolith system: a pathophysiological and clinical overview. *Adv Oto-Rhino-Laryngol* 58:110–127.

Wazen JJ: Dizziness and hearing loss. In: Rowland LP, ed. *Merritt's Textbook of Neurology*. Philadelphia, PA: Williams and Wilkins, 1995:30–35.

Zakir M, Dickman JD: Regeneration of vestibular otolith afferents after ototoxic damage. *J Neurosci* 26:2881–2893, 2006.

INTERNET RESOURCES

American Academy of Otolaryngology: Head and Neck Surgery
Dizziness and Motion Sickness
http://www.entnet.org/healthinfo/balance/dizziness.cfm

Canadian Medical Association Journal
Benign Paroxysmal Positional Vertigo (BPPV)
http://www.cmaj.ca/cgi/content/full/169/7/681

Mayo Clinic
Benign Paroxysmal Positional Vertigo (BPPV)
http://www.mayoclinic.com/health/vertigo/DS00534/DSECTION=1

MedicineNet.com
Vertigo, Motion Sickness, and Dizziness
http://www.medicinenet.com/vestibular_balance_disorders/article.htm

National Institutes of Health (MedlinePlus)
Dizziness and Vertigo
http://www.nlm.nih.gov/medlineplus/dizzinessandvertigo.html
National Institute on Deafness and Other Communication Disorders
Balance Disorders
http://www.nidcd.nih.gov/health/balance/balance_disorders.asp
Pennsylvania Neurological Associates, LTD.
Dizziness
http://www.pneuro.com/publications/dizzy/
Benign Paroxysmal Positional Vertigo (BPPV)
http://www.pneuro.com/publications/dizzy/bppv.html
Tulane University
An Inner Ear Primer
http://www.som.tulane.edu/departments/pathology/fermin/InnerEarPrimer.html
University of California at San Diego, Department of Surgery
Dizziness and Benign Positional Vertigo
http://health.ucsd.edu/specialties/Surgery/otolaryngology/Ear/bppv.htm
University of Maryland Medical Center
Motion Sickness
http://www.umm.edu/altmed/ConsConditions/MotionSicknesscc.html
Vestibular Disorders Association
http://www.vestibular.org/vestibular-disorders/diagnostic-tests.php

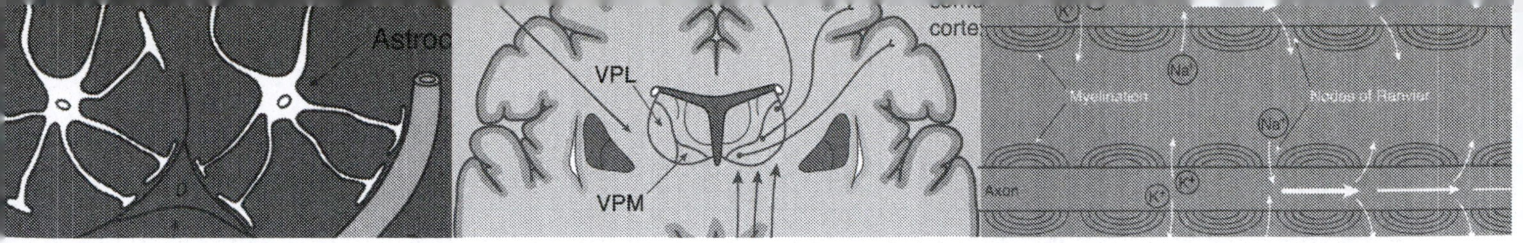

CHAPTER 10

Chemical Senses

INTRODUCTION OF CLINICAL CASE

A 30-year-old female victim of an automobile accident was unconscious when she was brought to the emergency department. The assorted minor cuts and bruises on her forehead were probably caused when her head struck the windshield. The patient regained consciousness shortly after arriving at the hospital, but she was mildly confused. The attending physician ordered computerized tomography (CT) scans of the head, which showed that the patient had a broken nose but no skull fracture or intracranial bleeding. She showed no signs of hemiplegia, aphasia, or cranial nerve palsies, but she had a severe headache. By the time the patient was discharged from the emergency department, her headache had improved considerably. Her nose had stopped bleeding but was now slowly discharging a clear fluid. The physician diagnosed a mild concussion and instructed the patient to rest for a few days. The patient's husband was instructed to awaken her every 3 hours her first night home. One week later during her follow-up examination, the patient mentioned that food seemed tasteless since the accident. The physician tested her sense of taste with sugar and salt, which she was able to correctly identify. The physician completed the neurologic examination; all other tests were unremarkable. To this day, this patient steadfastly insists that she has no sense of taste, but she has not been re-examined.

OVERVIEW OF THE CHEMICAL SENSES

The chemical senses include the so-called common chemical sense as well as smell and taste. The common chemical sense, which is the most primitive of the three, protects us from noxious odors and fluids. Taste and smell guide a variety of motivated behaviors and, in humans, contribute to our quality of life. Unlike other sensory systems, taste and smell often evoke strong emotional reactions that range from delight to disgust.

Flavor: an amalgam of taste, smell, and somesthetic sensations

Smell and taste stand at the threshold between the internal milieu and the outside world. From this ideal vantage point, smell and taste monitor food selection to ensure that our diets are both safe and nutritious. The gustatory system also triggers ingestive and digestive reflexes that modulate oral, gastric, pancreatic, and intestinal secretions. The virtually seamless coordination of smell and taste belies the fact that each is a separate sense with its own receptors, pathways, and sensations. Smell results from chemical stimulation of receptors located in the nasal cavity; taste sensation arises from chemical stimulation of receptors on the tongue and throughout the oral cavity. Flavor is the fusion of gustatory, olfactory, and somatosensory (i.e., touch, pain, and temperature) stimulation that takes place during eating.

COMMON CHEMICAL SENSITIVITY

The common chemical sense detects noxious chemical stimulation of mucous membranes associated with the eyes, nose, mouth, respiratory tract, and anal and genital openings. The pain caused by chemical irritation triggers lacrimal and withdrawal reflexes, which protect vital tissues from prolonged, potentially damaging stimulation. The range of noxious chemical stimuli is virtually limitless and may include substances such as pungent spices (e.g., onion, garlic, chili pepper), lacrimators (e.g., tear gas), sternutators (e.g., black pepper), and skin irritants. High concentrations of some olfactory and gustatory stimuli (e.g., hydrochloric acid [HCl], sodium chloride [NaCl]) have irritant properties as well. The receptors for the common chemical sense are free nerve endings, which lack the specialization and sophistication of the olfactory and gustatory end organs. Stimulation of these free nerve endings evokes pain, which produces both reflexive and protective physiological responses. For example, sneezing, closure of the nares and glottis, respiratory depression, and increased nasal secretion limit exposure to noxious odors.

OVERVIEW OF OLFACTION

Smell serves several important functions in humans, and its loss has serious consequences, especially on the quality of life. Approximately 1% of the population has a complete and permanent olfactory deficit. Olfactory dysfunction is particularly common in the elderly, the most rapidly expanding segment of the population. Because smell loss may be an early warning sign of a chronic degenerative disease, olfaction should be tested during routine neurological examinations.

Olfactory Epithelium

The receptors in the olfactory system are bipolar neurons that cover 1 cm^2 of the posterodorsal roof of the nasal cavities, the medial nasal septum, and part of each superior nasal turbinate. The olfactory receptors are unique because they are the only neurons that are embedded within the sensory epithelium and thus directly exposed to the environment (Figure 10.1). The olfactory epithelium consists of olfactory receptor neurons intermixed with sustentacular cells, basal (stem) cells, and Bowman's glands. Respiratory epithelium,

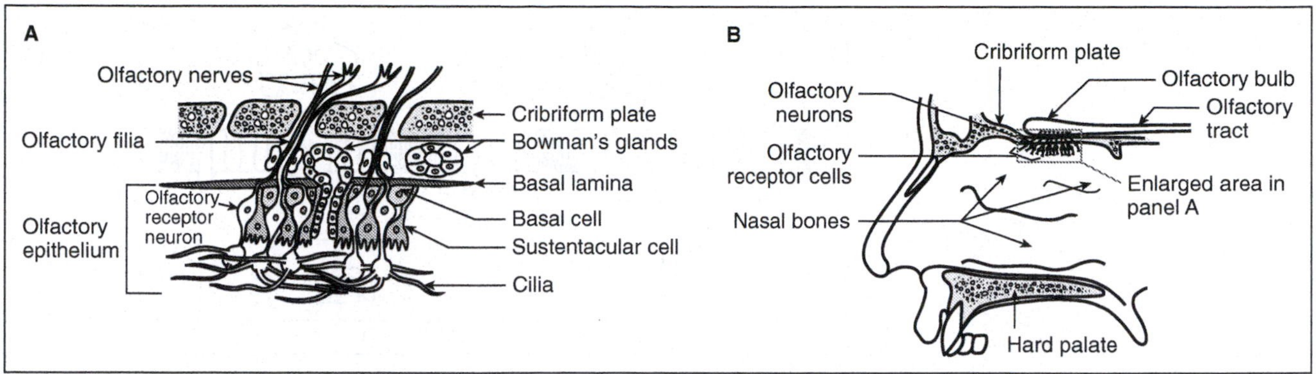

FIG. 10.1. Diagram of the Olfactory Epithelium in situ. (A) The axons of olfactory receptor neurons enter the cranium through small foramina in the cribriform plate of the ethmoid bone. (B) The location of the olfactory epithelium along the roof of the nasal cavity.

which covers the remaining 60 cm^2 of the nasal cavity on each side, lacks olfactory receptors and thus has no direct role in smell.

ORNs have a life span of 30–120 days.

The distal end of each olfactory receptor neuron (ORN) has a knob-like swelling capped with a tuft of 6–12 cilia. The cilia are covered with receptor-binding sites and coated with mucus secreted by the Bowman's glands. The glial-like sustentacular cells secrete various immunoglobulins, antimicrobial proteins, and enzymes that protect the ORNs from the environmental toxins and viruses that invade the nasal cavity with each breath. It is unclear whether ORNs succumb to these external agents or are preprogrammed for death, but they are replaced every 30–120 days. Replacement cells are derived by mitosis of the basal cells. Because radiation and chemotherapy target rapidly dividing cells, ORNs are susceptible to antineoplastic agents. Even in patients who never undergo cancer treatment, ORN replacement does not keep pace with degeneration. As ORNs die, the olfactory epithelium is gradually replaced by respiratory epithelium. Hence, loss of olfactory epithelium is most apparent in the elderly.

Olfactory Transduction

Before molecules can activate the olfactory receptors, they must traverse the mucous layer that covers the olfactory epithelium. Odorant molecules are carried across the mucous layer by odorant-binding proteins that also remove odorants from the olfactory epithelium after sensory transduction has run its course.

Olfactory transduction starts when an odor molecule binds to a subset of the 1000 transmembrane receptors located on the olfactory cilia. Because single receptors respond to multiple odors and all odors bind to numerous receptors, the quality of each smell is represented by the pattern of activity across the population of all olfactory receptors. By using the spectrum of evoked activity across so many olfactory receptors, the olfactory system is able to recognize more than 10,000 different odors. Receptor binding activates local G-proteins, which trigger one of two different second-messenger pathways (Figure 10.2). The first pathway uses a G-protein-mediated increase in adenylate cyclase–cyclic adenosine monophosphate (cAMP) to open sodium (Na^+) channels. The influx of Na^+ depolarizes the ORN, and this generates action potentials at the axon hillock. Pleasant fruity and floral odors may preferentially use the cAMP pathway. The other pathway relies on G-protein-mediated activation of phospholipase C to increase the intracellular concentration of inositol triphosphate (IP_3). Increased concentrations of IP_3 open calcium (Ca^{2+}) channels and depolarize the ORNs. The IP_3 pathway has not been linked to a particular class of odorants. The olfactory epithelium consists of individual zones whose constituent ORNs express a single odorant receptor.

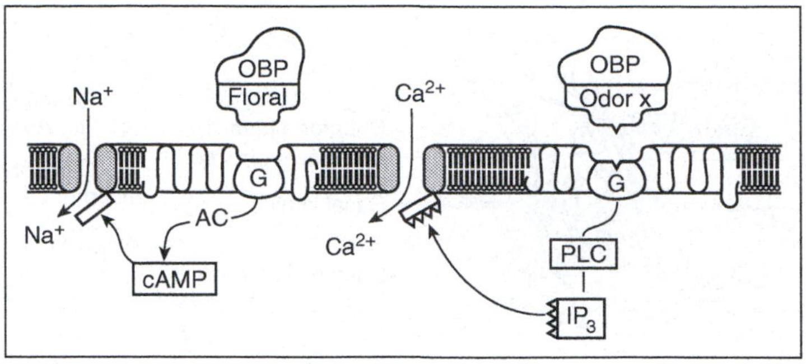

FIG. 10.2. Pathways of Olfactory Transduction. Two separate pathways, one using cyclic adenosine monophosphate (cAMP) and the other inositol triphosphate (IP_3), mediate olfactory transduction. AC = adenylate cyclase; G = G-protein; OBP = olfactory-binding protein; PLC = phospholipase C.

Olfactory Bulb

The olfactory bulb has six layers.

The extremely fine, unmyelinated axons of the ORNs are gathered into small bundles called "filia" that form the olfactory nerve (cranial nerve I) and enter the cranial vault through small perforations in the cribriform plate of the ethmoid bone. Severe head trauma that shifts the brain within the skull may stretch or sever these delicate axons where they pass through the cribriform plate. Because local edema and scar formation usually limits regeneration of the olfactory filia, olfactory deficits caused by head trauma are usually permanent. Interestingly, many patients who have lost their sense of smell are unaware of their olfactory impairment; instead, they report an inability to taste food.

Axons of the olfactory nerve enter the anterior cranial fossa and terminate in the ipsilateral olfactory bulb. The olfactory bulb is a flattened disk sandwiched between the cribriform plate and the ventral surface of the orbital cortex. The olfactory bulb consists of six layers. Starting from the outer surface, these layers are (1) the olfactory nerve layer, (2) the glomerular layer, (3) the external plexiform layer, (4) the mitral cell layer, (5) the granule cell layer, and (6) the anterior olfactory nucleus (Figures 10.3 and 10.4). The elaborate circuitry of the olfactory bulb converts the signals received from the olfactory cilia into highly processed codes before sending them to the forebrain.

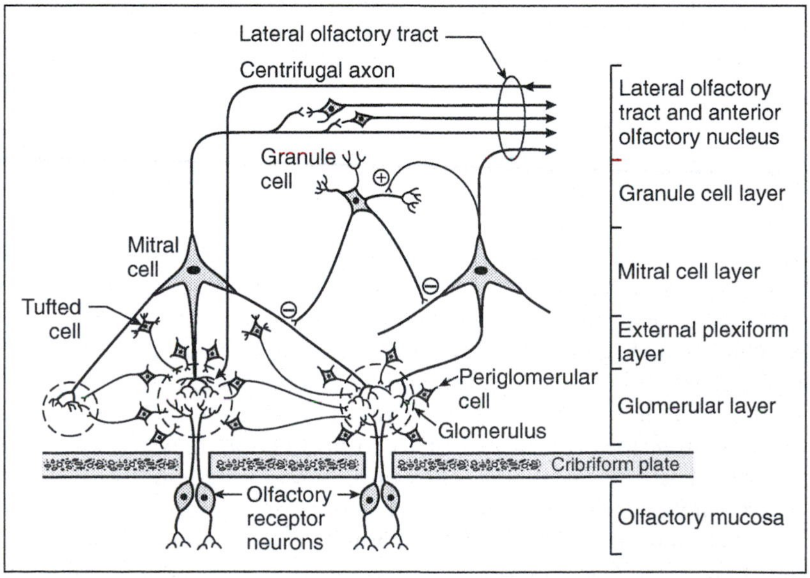

FIG. 10.3. Schematic Diagram Illustrating the Internal Circuits of the Olfactory Bulb.

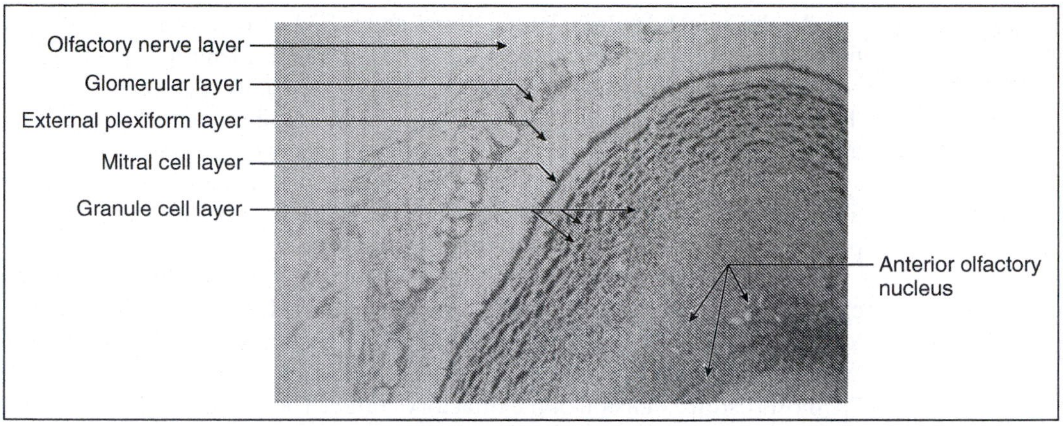

FIG. 10.4. Horizontal Section of the Rat Olfactory Bulb. Although the laminar organization of the olfactory bulb is similar in humans and rats, the layers are easier to distinguish in the rat.

Olfactory bulb glomerulus: an acellular plexus of axonal and dendritic terminals

Olfactory nerve axons line the surface of the rostral olfactory bulb before piercing its surface and terminating in cell-sparse areas called glomeruli. Each glomerulus is an elaborate plexus in which the glutamatergic terminals of the ORNs synapse on the axons and dendrites of periglomerular cells and on the apical dendrites of mitral and tufted cells (Figure 10.5; see also Figure 10.3). The soma of each periglomerular cell forms a cup or calyx around one glomerulus, but its axons and dendrites may infiltrate as many as ten neighboring glomeruli. Periglomerular cells, which use γ-aminobutyric acid (GABA), dopamine, substance P, and enkephalin as neurotransmitters, improve the coding of odor quality by highlighting the activity in a few glomeruli while inhibiting its neighbors. Mitral and tufted cells, whose dendrites invade the glomeruli, are the efferent neurons of the olfactory bulb. Olfactory information carried by the ORNs undergoes tremendous convergence as it passes through the olfactory bulb. For every thousand axons that enter a glomerulus, only one dendrite exits. The glomeruli also receive projections from the contralateral olfactory bulb, as well as noradrenergic, serotonergic, and cholinergic projections from the locus ceruleus, midline raphe, and basal forebrain, respectively.

Because the ORN axons originating within a single zone of the olfactory epithelium converge onto one or two glomeruli, the olfactory bulb has a similar, although more constricted, zonal organization. Although the presence of zones within the olfactory epithelium and the olfactory bulb suggest that the glomerulus is the basic unit of olfactory discrimination and that the olfactory bulb uses spatial organization to represent odor quality, the lack of chemosensory zones at the cortical level suggests that the process is more complicated, at least at its central terminus.

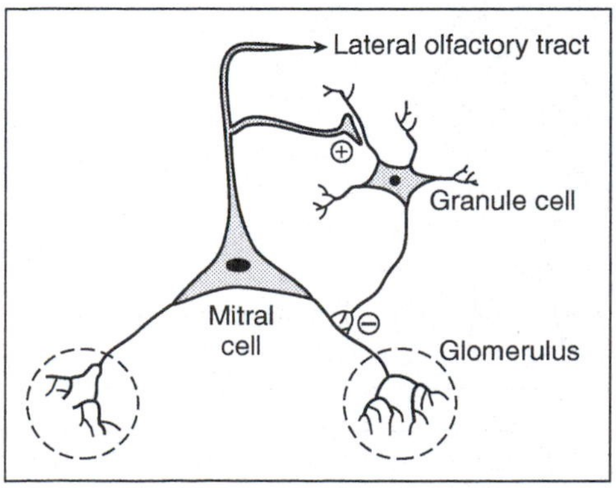

FIG. 10.5. Granule Cell Mediated Recurrent Inhibition of Mitral Cell Activity.

Granule cells have no axons.

As the apical dendrites of the mitral and tufted cells pass through the external plexiform layer, they are inhibited by GABAergic dendrodendritic synapses from granule cells. Because granule cell inhibition is initiated by excitatory axodendritic synapses from the mitral cells (see Figure 10.5), the mitral cells are, in effect, terminating their own signal. This recurrent inhibitory circuit improves the temporal resolution of the olfactory system by limiting the duration of the mitral cell response. Granule cells, like the glomeruli, also receive projections from the anterior olfactory nucleus bilaterally, other parts of the olfactory cortex, and the limbic system.

The core of the olfactory bulb is formed by the axons of mitral and tufted cells, which exit the caudal end of the bulb and form the lateral olfactory tract (see Figure 10.3). Scattered clusters of cells within this medullary core constitute the anterior olfactory nucleus. Although the anterior olfactory nucleus does not have a laminar structure, it is considered the most rostral extension of the olfactory cortex. The left and right olfactory bulbs are interconnected by projections from the anterior olfactory nuclei through the rostral part of the anterior commissure.

Central Projections of the Olfactory Bulb

The central organization of the olfactory system differs from the other sensory systems in several important ways. First, projections to the brain from the olfactory bulb (excluding the anterior olfactory nucleus) are entirely ipsilateral. Second, smell information reaches the primary olfactory cortex without passing through the thalamus. Third, the primary olfactory cortex is three-layered paleocortex instead of six-layered neocortex. Fourth, the olfactory system is more strongly integrated with the limbic system than any other sensory system.

There is a medial olfactory stria, but no medial olfactory tract.

All olfactory information enters the brain through the lateral olfactory tract, which lies within the olfactory sulcus of the orbital cortex (Figure 10.6). As the lateral olfactory tract approaches the anterior perforated substance, it divides into lateral and medial striae. The lateral olfactory stria is the main conduit for cortically bound olfactory information; the medial stria projects to the septal area and the hypothalamus. Smell information that reaches the hypothalamus guides reproduction, feeding, and drinking, as well as maternal and aggressive behaviors.

Axons in the lateral olfactory stria terminate in layer I of the olfactory cortices, which is densely innervated by the apical dendrites of the pyramidal cells located in layers II and III. The pyramidal cells in layers II and III constitute the efferent neurons of the primary olfactory cortex.

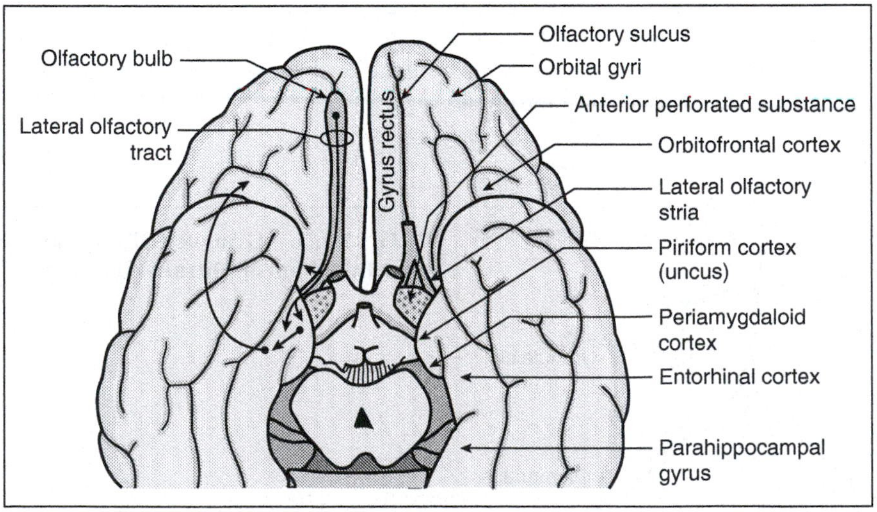

FIG. 10.6. Cortical Olfactory Projections.

Primary olfactory cortex consists of six cytoarchitecturally distinct regions: the anterior olfactory nucleus, the olfactory tubercle, the piriform cortex, the periamygdaloid cortex, the corticomedial amygdaloid nucleus, and the entorhinal cortex.

Anterior Olfactory Nucleus. Commissural projections of the anterior olfactory nucleus may enable interhemispheric transfer of olfactory memories.

Olfactory Tubercle. The olfactory tubercle is located on the ventral surface of the forebrain just medial to the lateral olfactory stria. The three poorly defined layers of the olfactory tubercle are difficult to distinguish from the overlying nucleus accumbens and ventral striatum. Motivated behavior appears to be influenced by the olfactory tubercle.

Piriform Cortex. The largest constituent of primary olfactory cortex, the piriform cortex, forms the dorsomedial surface of the temporal lobe near its attachment to the frontal lobe. Piriform cortex projects to every other part of primary olfactory cortex as well as the hypothalamus, the lateral preoptic area, the mediodorsal nucleus of the thalamus, the diagonal band of Broca, and the taste areas located in the insula and orbitofrontal cortex.

Amygdala. Olfactory projections from the periamygdaloid nucleus to the amygdala proper provide an avenue for odors to affect visceral and emotional responses. The corticomedial amygdaloid nucleus projects to reproduction-related areas in the anterior hypothalamus.

Entorhinal Cortex. Entorhinal cortex, the most caudal part of primary olfactory cortex, is located in Brodmann area 28 in the rostral part of the parahippocampal gyrus. Because the entorhinal cortex resembles both paleocortex and neocortex, its cytoarchitecture is described as transitional. The entorhinal cortex projects to the orbitofrontal cortex, the hippocampus, and the mediodorsal dorsal nucleus of the thalamus. The projections to the hippocampus may form the anatomic link for the strong association between smell and memory. Direct and indirect (via the mediodorsal nucleus) projections from the entorhinal cortex to the orbitofrontal cortex may be part of the anatomical substrate for flavor perception.

Due to the phylogenetic antiquity of the olfactory system, smell information passes directly to the primary olfactory cortex without synapsing in the thalamus. By comparison, the smell projection to the secondary olfactory area in the orbitofrontal cortex follows a more conventional route through the mediodorsal nucleus of the thalamus. Given the small size of the transthalamic pathway to this neocortical site, it is probably less important than the projections from the piriform and the entorhinal cortices.

The mediodorsal nucleus is the thalamic relay for smell.

Neural Coding of Odor Quality

The most persistent controversies in olfaction (and taste) concern the neural mechanisms for coding quality. The problem in olfaction is particularly acute because we can identify thousands of different odors. Attempts to organize the olfactory world on the basis of chemical composition have been largely unsuccessful, but psychophysical studies have shown that most odors fall into one of several qualitative categories (Table 10.1). These

Olfactory stimuli cannot be arranged along a continuum like visual and auditory stimuli.

TABLE 10.1 Prototypical Stimuli of the Primary Odor Qualities

Odor Quality	Prototypical Stimuli
Flowery	Rose
Fruity	Fruit and wine
Ambrosial	Musk and sandalwood
Aromatic	Camphor and spices
Sweaty	Isovaleric acid
Rotten	Rotten eggs and feces
Stinging	Formic acid

qualitative categories typically relate to plant and animal sources that generate odors such as orange, rose, and musk. This insight, unfortunately, has done little to advance our understanding of quality coding in the olfactory system. Unlike primary colors, these qualitative categories cannot be used like building blocks to assemble new odors.

The difficulty in determining how the nervous system codes for stimulus quality in the chemical senses has been attributed, in part, to our lack of understanding of basic olfactory transduction mechanisms. Recent breakthroughs in receptor transduction mechanisms should serve as a framework for future studies on quality coding within the central nervous system. Early speculation that individual smell (and taste) neurons are dedicated lines that respond to a single stimulus quality was refuted by experimental data showing that most chemosensory neurons respond to several stimuli. Broad tuning sacrifices specificity within individual neurons but increases the information-carrying capacity of the system.

Clinical Aspects of Olfaction

Olfactory deficits pose safety and quality-of-life issues.

Olfactory disorders can be caused by upper respiratory infection, nasal and sinus disease, toxic odors (e.g., formaldehyde, paint solvents), radiotherapy and chemotherapy, head trauma, and dozens of prescription and nonprescription drugs. Tables 10.2 and 10.3 list a small sample of the diseases and disorders, and classes of medications that disrupt olfactory perception. It is unclear why only some patients who are treated for these conditions or taking these medications develop olfactory problems. Fortunately, most secondary olfactory symptoms resolve after the disease or disorder has run its course or after the patient has discontinued taking the medicine.

Negative disturbance: reflects lost function

Positive disturbance: reflects the expression of surviving structures

Olfactory deficits may be complete (anosmia), partial (hyposmia), distorted (dysosmia), hallucinatory (phantosmia), and in rare cases an inability to recognize smells (agnosia). Anosmias and hyposmias are negative disturbances, which vary in degree only. Dysosmias and phantosmias, by comparison, are positive disturbances, which have an entirely different etiology. The diagnosis of an olfactory agnosia requires that the patient's olfactory and cognitive skills be intact.

Negative olfactory deficits are caused by transport problems and sensorineural damage. Transport problems impede the flow of odorants to the olfactory epithelium, and, depending on their severity, they can cause either hyposmia or anosmia. Because most transport problems are caused by paranasal disease (e.g., nasal polyps, neoplasms, sinusitis), surgical removal of the nasal obstruction usually restores olfactory function.

Sensorineural problems are associated with neurologic damage or dysfunction of either peripheral or central structures. Sensorineural olfactory deficits can be caused by

TABLE 10.2 Medical Conditions and Exposures That Alter the Sense of Smell

Aging	Huntington's disease
Alcoholism	Hypothyroidism
Alzheimer's disease	Multiple sclerosis
Brain tumors	Parkinson's disease
Diabetes	Rhinitis
Epilepsy	Trauma
Herpes simplex encephalitis	Upper respiratory infection
HIV	

TABLE 10.3 Medications That Alter Olfactory Perception

Anesthetics (topical)	Opiates
Antihypertensive drugs	Sympathomimetic drugs
Anti-inflammatory drugs	

a wide range of factors including viral infections, head trauma, radiation therapy, environmental toxins and pollutants, prescribed medication, and endocrine imbalances. Nearly two-thirds of all chronic anosmia and hyposmia cases are caused by permanent damage to the olfactory epithelium due to upper respiratory disease, head trauma, and nasal sinus disease. Olfactory deficits may also accompany intracranial tumors (e.g., olfactory groove meningiomas, frontal lobe gliomas) that compress the lateral olfactory tract or the medial aspect of the temporal lobe. Hyposmia is an early presenting symptom of Alzheimer's disease and human immunodeficiency virus (HIV) infection and often accompanies idiopathic Parkinson's disease, Korsakoff's psychosis, and Huntington's disease.

Upper respiratory infections are the most common cause of permanent olfactory loss.

Blows to the head, particularly those from the rear, may sever the olfactory filia.

Patients with dysosmias report that normally pleasant smelling odors are unpleasant. Dysosmias and phantosmias are positive disturbances caused by abnormal patterns of neural activity. Some dysosmias develop while the olfactory system is recovering from an insult, but most are idiopathic with an indeterminate locus. Phantosmias typically accompany epileptiform activity within the medial temporal lobe and its limbic neighbors, the amygdala and hippocampus. Schizophrenic and psychotic patients may experience olfactory hallucinations, which are almost always unpleasant.

Seizures involving the temporal lobe are often preceded by olfactory hallucinations or auras.

Olfaction shows a gradual deterioration with age and accelerates rapidly after age 70. For patients in their 80s, hyposmia is the rule rather than the exception, and anosmia is common. Although there may be multiple causes for the age-related decline of smell, erosion of the olfactory epithelium is one known cause. Due to the significant loss of olfactory glomeruli and mitral cells in most seniors, age-related olfactory deficits interfere with flavor perception and have a significant impact on feeding and nutrition in the elderly.

Frequency of smell loss:
Before age 65, <1%
Age 65–80, 50%
Older than 80, 75%

OVERVIEW OF TASTE

Transduction of gustatory information is mediated by specialized receptors whose central projections terminate in neocortex rather than paleocortex. The sense of taste mediates several ingestive reflexes and guides complex behaviors such as foraging for food.

Taste Quality

Taste stimuli are usually grouped into four discrete qualitative categories: salty, sweet, sour, and bitter (Table 10.4). Some data suggest that the beef-like taste of monosodium glutamate may be a fifth primary taste quality called umami (deliciousness), but there is no consensus on this point. Each of these primary taste qualities is related to the nutritional content and safety of food. For example, sweet stimuli are preferred and eagerly ingested because most are sugars, carbohydrates, or other calorie-rich foods. Ingestion of table salt replaces sodium, an essential mineral that is continuously lost through sweating and urination. Sour and bitter stimuli are rejected because they are associated with food spoilage and poisons, respectively. There are exceptions to these "rules," however. Saccharin, which tastes sweet, has no nutritional value, and lead acetate, a sweet-tasting salt, is poisonous. Lithium chloride, a toxic salt, tastes like sodium chloride.

The **four basic taste qualities:** salty, sweet, sour, and bitter

Flavor is a complex percept resulting from the synthesis of gustatory, olfactory, and somatosensory (touch, temperature, pain) information obtained during food and beverage consumption. Odors released in the mouth reach the olfactory receptors through the

TABLE 10.4 Prototypical Stimuli of the Primary Taste Qualities

Taste Quality	Prototypical Stimuli
Salty	Sodium chloride (NaCl)
Sweet	Sucrose
Sour	Hydrochloric acid (HCl)
Bitter	Quinine hydrochloride (QHCl)

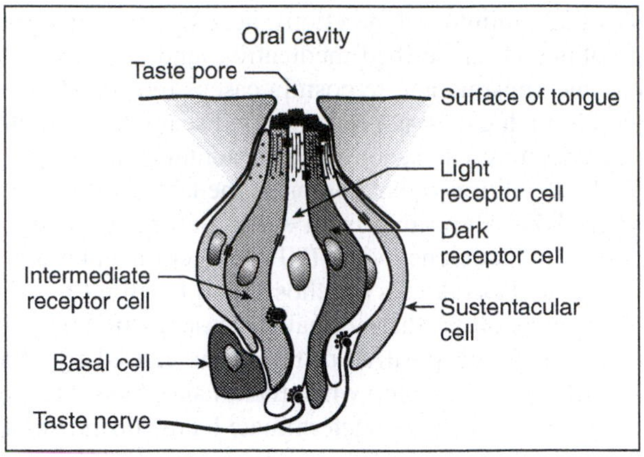

FIG. 10.7. Cross Section of an Individual Taste Bud. Each taste bud has a concentric arrangement of basal, sustentacular, and receptor cells.

nasopharynx, a process known as retronasal stimulation. Few people appreciate the contributions of odors to the flavor of food until a head cold blocks their nasal air flow. The overwhelming tendency to attribute olfactory stimulation to the palate accounts for the fact that most patients who report a loss of taste, in fact, are unable to detect odors.

Taste Buds

Taste buds are microscopic structures embedded within taste papillae.

Taste buds are goblet-shaped clusters of 50–150 receptor, sustentacular, and basal cells arranged concentrically like the segments of an orange (Figure 10.7). The receptor cells are capped by microvilli that protrude into an apical pore that is bathed by the fluids that coat the tongue surface. Fluids in the oral cavity that enter the apical pore contact and bind to the taste receptors located on these microvilli. Taste receptor cells are divided into light, dark, and intermediate types based on the granularity of the cytoplasmic matrix. These cell types may reflect different classes of receptor cells or different developmental stages of a single type, but all of them have synapses located along their basolateral surfaces. The harsh environment of the oral cavity takes its toll on the taste receptor cells, which have a life span of only 10–14 days. As receptor cells degenerate, basal cells located at the perimeter of the taste bud migrate to the center and differentiate into receptor cells. Sustentacular cells provide support for the basal and receptor cells, but they do not play a direct role in taste transduction.

Distribution of Taste Buds

Taste buds are located on the tongue, soft palate, epiglottal folds, uvula, larynx, pharynx, and upper third of the esophagus (Figure 10.8). Taste buds on the tongue are encased within papillae; those on the soft palate, epiglottis, uvula, larynx, and esophagus are embedded in the surface epithelium. There are no taste papillae on the ventral tongue surface and few, if any, along the midline of the dorsal tongue. The taste buds on the epiglottis protect the airway from fluid aspiration. The function of the taste buds within the esophagus is not known, but they are unlikely to play a role in taste perception, per se.

Fungiform, from Latin, means "mushroom-like."

Foliate, from Latin, means "leaf-ike."

There are four different types of papillae within the oral cavity, but only three contain taste buds. Fungiform papillae line the lateral margin and the tip of the anterior tongue. Foliate papillae, which are buried within four to six vertically oriented trenches four to six vertically oriented trenches along the lateral edge of the tongue near the palatoglossal arches near the palatoglossal arches, have limited access to tastants except those released when food is crushed by the molars. Circumvallate papillae, numbering between seven and eleven, form a chevron near the base of the tongue. These bunker-like papillae have

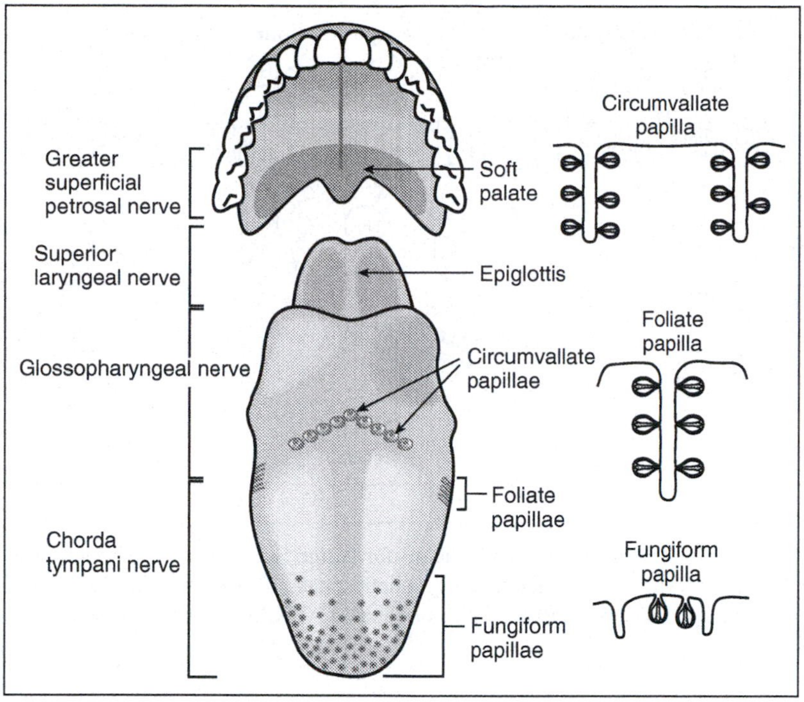

FIG. 10.8. Distribution of Taste Buds. The distributions for the chorda tympani, glossopharyngeal, superior laryngeal, and superior petrosal nerves are shown on the left side. Cross sections of fungiform, foliate, and circumvallate papillae are shown on the right side.

their taste buds in the walls of the trenches of the mucous-filled moats that surround these structures. Filiform papillae, which cover most of the tongue's dorsum, do not contain taste buds. These cone-shaped pillars of cornified epithelium give the tongue its rough texture.

Saliva makes at least four important contributions to taste perception and oral hygiene. First, saliva solubilizies foods and fluids so that they can enter the apical taste pore and bind with the taste receptors. Second, saliva protects the delicate surfaces of the intraoral cavity by diluting, buffering, and cooling hot foods and fluids. Third, saliva rinses tastants from the tongue, which readies the taste receptors for the remainder of the meal. Fourth, saliva's trophic properties help maintain the integrity of the taste buds. Damage to the salivary glands by radiation produces severe and usually permanent dry mouth (xerostomia) which, in turn, leads to halitosis and dental caries.

Saliva contributes to taste transduction and maintains the taste buds and teeth.

Regional Taste Sensitivity

Despite the fact that all parts of the oral cavity populated by taste papillae respond to all four of the basic taste stimuli, there are regional differences in taste thresholds. The lowest thresholds for sweet and salty stimuli are near the front of the tongue, whereas those for sour and bitter stimuli are lowest on the posterior tongue and soft palate. The basis for these regional differences in taste thresholds is not understood.

All four basic taste qualities can be detected by all of the taste buds located on the tongue.

Taste Transduction

Taste transduction begins when sapid stimuli bind to receptors located on the microvilli within the taste pore. Research within the last 5–10 years has shown that the mechanism for taste transduction is different for each of the primary taste qualities, but probably similar across different classes of taste papillae (Figure 10.9). Salty taste depends on the dissociation of NaCl into Na^+ and chloride (Cl^-) ions within the saliva prior to receptor

Salty and sour taste are initiated by Na^+ and Ca^{2+} influx.

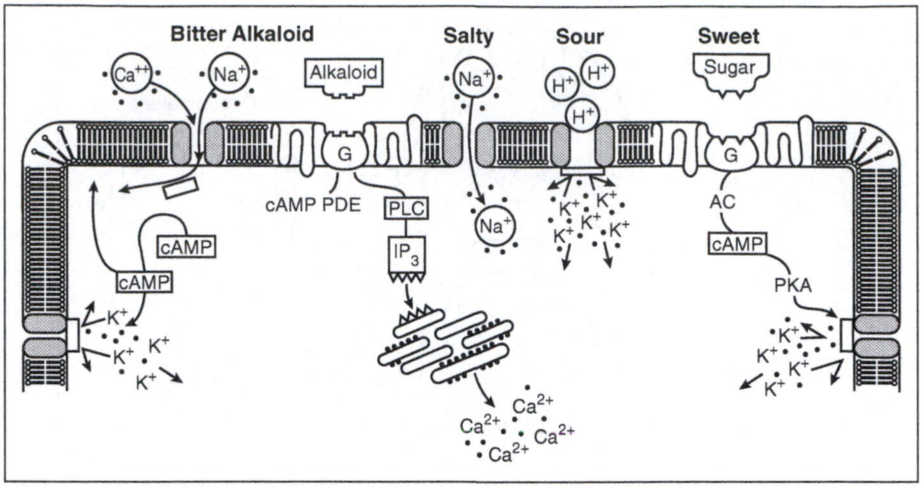

FIG. 10.9. Taste Transduction Mechanisms for Bitter, Salty, Sour, and Sweet Stimuli. AC = adenylate cyclase; cAMP = cyclic adenosine monophosphate; G = G-protein; IP_3 = inositol triphosphate; PDE = phosphodiesterase; PLC = phospholipase C; PKA = protein kinase A.

binding. Transduction of salty taste is initiated by the voltage-independent diffusion of Na^+ ions through amiloride-sensitive pores located along the surface of the microvilli. The influx of positively charged Na^+ ions down its concentration gradient depolarizes the receptor cell directly, which releases neurotransmitter into the synapses at the base of the taste receptor cell. Sour stimuli depolarize taste receptor cells in two ways. First, protons (H^+) donated by stimuli such as hydrochloric acid flow through the amiloride-sensitive sodium channels. Second, protons block the apically located potassium (K^+) channels, which stops the taste cell's resting outward K^+ current.

Sweet transduction depends on specific membrane receptors rather than ion channels. Sweet-tasting stimuli include carbohydrates (e.g., monosaccharides and disaccharides), D-amino acids, dipeptides (e.g., aspartame), artificial sweeteners (e.g., saccharin, cyclamate), certain proteins (e.g., thaumatin, monellin), and some heavy metal salts (e.g., lead acetate). Although the number of different sweet receptors remains unknown, at least two separate sweet transduction pathways have been described. After sugar binds to a membrane-bound G-protein, it triggers an adenylate cyclase–cAMP reaction that depolarizes the cell by closing K^+ channels. Synthetic sweeteners use an alternate IP_3-mediated pathway to release Ca^{2+} from intracellular stores and elicit action potentials.

Bitterness, like sweetness, is associated with a wide range of chemically diverse agents and relies on membrane-resident receptors. Bitter agents include many L-amino acids (e.g., L-phenylalanine, L-tryptophan), alkaloids (e.g., caffeine, quinine), glycosides (e.g., digitalis), divalent cations (e.g., Ca^{2+}, Mg^{2+}), and various peptides. Given the prevalence of bitter stimuli in the wild, bitterness could be described as the default taste quality. Several lines of evidence indicate that there are multiple G-protein-activated bitter transduction pathways. For some receptors, G-proteins activate phospholipase C, which triggers an IP_3-mediated release of Ca^{2+} from intracellular stores and neurotransmitter release. In other cases, phosphodiesterase removes the cAMP block on cation (e.g., Na^+, Ca^{2+}) influx. Quinine hydrochloride and bitter salts such as $CaCl^2$ function like protons and block K^+ efflux from the cell. Each of these transduction pathways depolarizes the taste receptor cell, which triggers action potentials and neurotransmitter release from the base of the cell.

Taste Bud Innervation

Damage to the facial nerve (VII) causes Bell palsy.

From an embryological standpoint, the tongue consists of anterior and posterior parts. Taste buds located on the anterior two-thirds of the tongue are innervated by the

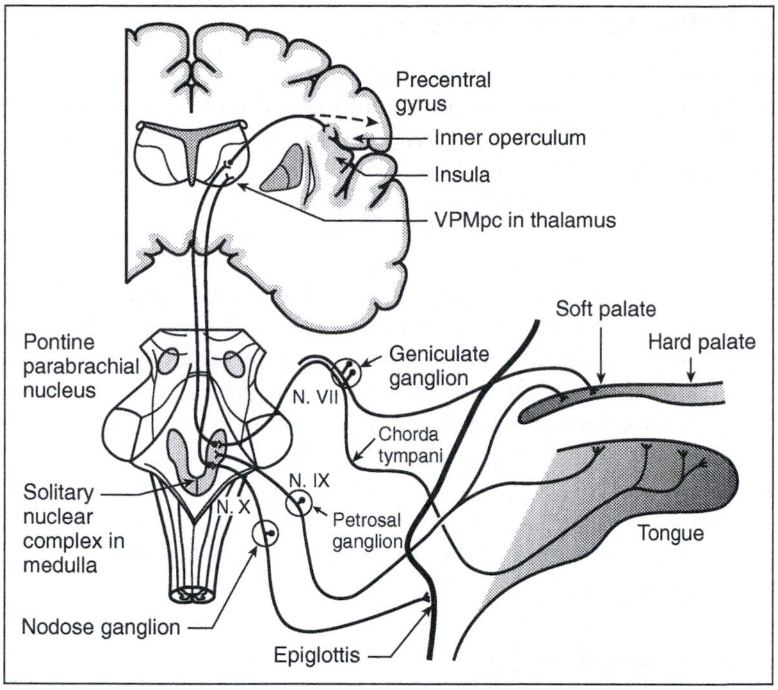

FIG. 10.10. Peripheral and Central Taste Pathways. Taste buds in the oral cavity are innervated by cranial nerves VII, IX, and X. Each of the first-order nerves terminates in the nucleus of the solitary tract (NST) of the medulla; second-order neurons ascend to the parvicellular division of the ventroposteromedial nucleus (VPMpc) of the thalamus. The primary taste cortex is located in the anterior insula. Gustatory information ascends from the oral cavity to cortex along ipsilateral pathways.

chorda tympani branch of the facial nerve (VII) and the lingual branch of the trigeminal nerve (V; Figure 10.10). The chorda tympani nerve conveys gustatory information, and the lingual nerve provides somatosensory innervation. Damage to the facial nerve may cause a variety of symptoms including loss of taste, hyperacusis, impaired salivation and lacrimation, and facial paralysis. The precise combination of symptoms depends on the location of the damage along the facial nerve (see Chapter 5). When the root of the facial nerve is crushed by acoustic neuromas growing within the cerebellopontine angle, all of these symptoms are present (see Chapter 8). Because the chorda tympani nerve crosses the tympanic membrane during its journey to the tongue, it is susceptible to damage during surgical repair of the eardrum (tympanoplasty) as well as during removal and replacement of the stapes in otosclerotic patients. A common but underreported cause of lingual/chorda tympani nerve damage is third molar ("wisdom tooth") extractions. Nerve bruising may cause taste loss and an unpleasantr parathesia/anesthesia of the tongue. If the lingual/chorda tympani nerve is sectioned, anastomosis of the cut ends must be done within several days to avoid permanent disability.

"Wisdom tooth" extraction is one of the most common causes of injury to the facial nerve.

Taste buds within the circumvallate papillae, as well as other stray taste buds on the posterior one-third of the tongue, are supplied by the lingual-tonsillar branch of the glossopharyngeal nerve (IX), which contains both gustatory and somatosensory fibers. The foliate papillae straddle the chorda tympani and glossopharyngeal fields. Taste buds on the soft palate are supplied by the superior petrosal nerve, a branch of the facial nerve, and the glossopharyngeal nerve; those within the esophagus and on the epiglottal surface communicate with the central nervous system via the superior laryngeal nerve, a branch of the vagus nerve. The neurotransmitter used by taste receptor cells has not been identified but is presumed to be glutamate.

The **glossopharyngeal nerve** (IX) innervates the posterior third of the tongue soft palatefoliate papillae.

Innervation of the foliate papillae:

- Chorda tympani nerve (anterior half)
- Glossopharyngeal nerve (posterior half)

Central Gustatory Projections

Taste information ascends ipsilaterally through the central tegmental tract.

The gustatory thalamic relay is VPMpc.

The chorda tympani, glossopharyngeal, and vagus nerves are the distal processes of pseudounipolar neurons whose cell bodies are located within ganglia located near the brainstem. Their central processes enter the rostral medulla and terminate in the nucleus of the solitary tract (NST; see Figure 5.10), which contains a rough topographic map of the tongue. Taste buds innervated by the chorda tympani nerve project to the rostral part of the NST, whereas the glossopharyngeal and vagal nerves project to progressively more caudal regions of the nucleus. Axons of second-order neurons within the NST enter the central tegmental tract and ascend ipsilaterally to the parvicellular division of the ventroposteromedial nucleus (VPMpc) of the thalamus (see Figures 10.10 and 6.3). Third-order neurons in the thalamus project to the primary taste cortex located at the junction of the anterior insula and the inner operculum. A minor projection to the foot of the precentral gyrus exists in monkeys, but its presence in humans and its role in taste perception, if any, has not been determined. Neurons in the primary taste cortex project to the orbitofrontal cortex, which also receives convergent projections from the visual, somatosensory, and olfactory systems. The multimodal nature of the orbitofrontal cortex suggests that it may provide the neural substrate for flavor perception.

Coding of Taste Quality

There is empirical support for both the dedicated line and pattern theories.

As in olfaction, most taste neurons respond to more than one stimulus; hence, they are broadly tuned. The ambiguity associated with broad tuning means that taste quality must be represented by the pattern of activity across many neurons. This view, called the pattern theory, has empirical support. Psychophysical and neurophysiologic experiments have shown that similar tasting chemicals evoke similar patterns of neural activity in the nervous system (Figure 10.11). Alternatively, neurons may act as dedicated lines, in which activity in a specific group of cells represents a specific taste. The theory that the taste system relies on dedicated cells garners support from the fact that people typically use a limited vocabulary to describe taste quality (i.e., salty, sweet, sour, bitter). The mechanisms of taste transduction, although not fully understood, are consistent with the notion that only a limited number of stimulus qualities exists. Because dedicated lines can be tested more easily than the pattern theory, it has received more criticism. At present, both theories have firm empirical support and loyal followings. Future studies are likely to show that the nervous system uses both to encode taste and smell quality.

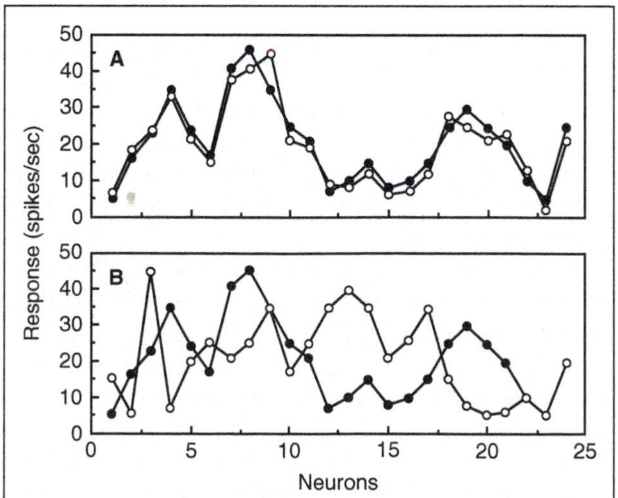

FIG. 10.11. Pattern of Neural Activity Across Neurons. (A) The pattern of neural activity across 24 neurons is very similar when two similar-tasting chemicals are applied to the tongue. (B) When two dissimilar tasting chemicals are applied to the tongue, the pattern of activity across the same 24 neurons is distinctly dissimilar.

Functions of the Gustatory System

Oral Reflexes. Foods with appetitive tastes initiate reflexive swallowing, whereas aversive tastes (e.g., bitter or sour-tasting foods) trigger gapes and other oral motor reflexes that eject food from the mouth. These reflexes are executed by circuits formed by the first-order taste neurons, interneurons within the NST and reticular formation, and output neurons within the facial and hypoglossal motor nuclei.

Stimulation of the epiglottal taste buds triggers the gag reflex, which prevents fluid aspiration into the upper airway. The superior laryngeal branch of the vagus nerve, which constitutes the afferent limb of this reflex, projects to the posterior NST, whose cells act as interneurons for this reflex arc. The efferent limb of the gag reflex is executed by cholinergic neurons within the nucleus ambiguus.

Gustatory-mediated reflexes protect the airway and aid digestion.

The taste of food also triggers salivation, as well as vagally mediated gastric and pancreatic secretions that aid digestion. Salivation is mediated by a four-neuron reflex involving the chorda tympani and glossopharyngeal nerves, neurons in the NST, preganglionic parasympathetic neurons in the superior and inferior salivatory nuclei, and the postganglionic parasympathetic neurons. The efferent projections of the superior salivatory nucleus are contained within the chorda tympani nerve; those of the inferior salivatory nucleus reside within the glossopharyngeal nerve. Food in the oral cavity also triggers gastric acid release, which prepares the stomach for the arrival of food. Oral administration of glucose releases pancreatic insulin. This preabsorptive release of insulin exceeds that following intravenous glucose administration. The efferent limb of these visceral reflexes is mediated by the subdiaphragmatic branch of the vagus nerve.

Taste and Learned Behaviors. Many animals, including humans, form strong associations between taste cues and the consequences of feeding. The clearest demonstration of this phenomenon is a conditioned taste aversion (CTA), the association between the taste of a novel food and subsequent gastrointestinal malaise. Ambient odors and the physical setting may interact with learning and expression of CTAs, but are of secondary importance. Conditioned taste aversions represent a form of classical conditioning in which the taste of the novel food serves as the conditioned stimulus (CS). The illness-inducing agent (e.g., *Salmonella,* radiation, or a toxic chemical) acts as the unconditioned stimulus (UCS), which evokes illness, the unconditioned response (UCR). Sometimes only a single pairing of the CS (taste) and the UCS is sufficient to form a CTA. Radiation and cancer chemotherapy are potent emetics that may act as UCSs by linking food consumed before therapy with subsequent gastrointestinal malaise. Patients sometimes consume a snack just prior to chemotherapy to make it the scapegoat CS for CTA learning, thereby sparing the foods they consumed during the previous meal.

The ability to associate taste with the beneficial consequences of feeding forms the basis for conditioned taste preferences. For example, when an animal depleted of an individual micronutrient is given an opportunity for repletion, a taste preference develops for that micronutrient.

CLINICAL ASPECTS OF TASTE

The innervation of the taste buds by three different cranial nerves makes a total loss of taste sensation (ageusia) unlikely, although not impossible. Regional ageusias, however, are more common following viral infections involving the middle ear and local trauma to primary taste nerves (e.g., Bell's palsy) or central structures. Because the gustatory system emphasizes taste quality rather than the locus of taste stimulation, most people are unaware of regional ageusias. For this reason, detection of an ageusia often requires separate testing of the gustatory fields innervated by chorda tympani and glossopharyngeal nerves on each side of the tongue. Patients who do notice a problem may report a generalized decrease in taste intensity (hypogeusia).

TABLE 10.5 Medical Conditions and Exposures That Alter Taste Perception

Alzheimer's disease	Depression
Acoustic neuromas	Diabetes
Bell's palsy	Middle ear surgery
Brain tumors	Psychiatric disorders
Chemotherapy	Radiation therapy
Cirrhosis of the liver	Renal failure
	Third molar extractions

TABLE 10.6 Medications That Alter Taste Perception

Anticoagulants	Antiviral drugs
Antiepileptic drugs	Bronchodilators
Antihistamines	Diuretics
Antihypertensive drugs	Hypnotics
Antiseptics	Sympathomimetic drugs
Antiulcerative agents	Vasodilators

Dysgeusias are almost always aversive.

Positive taste disturbances such as dysgeusias and phantoms are poorly understood, but they are potentially more serious because they are usually long lasting and almost universally unpleasant. Dysgeusias are errant perceptions triggered by a sapid stimulus in the mouth. Taste phantoms, or hallucinations, appear in the absence of verifiable gustatory stimulation. Some dysgeusias and phantoms have a metallic taste; others assume a bitter or fecal quality. Dysgeusias and phantoms triggered by trauma or disease may respond to sectioning one or more of the remaining taste nerves; those that appear spontaneously are more resistant to treatment. Less common yet are gustatory agnosias, a failure to recognize sensations in patients who have intact cognition and taste apparatus.

Gustatory deficits may be caused by hundreds of medicines; fortunately, few patients are susceptible.

Several studies indicate that taste acuity declines with age, but in general, gustatory perception is more resistant to aging than olfaction. Like olfaction, however, taste disorders may accompany a formidable array of medical conditions as well as dozens of prescription and non-prescription drugs (Tables 10.5 and 10.6). Similarly, not every patient afflicted with the conditions or taking the medications listed in Tables 10.5 and 10.6 experiences gustatory problems. This is fortunate, because gustatory deficits are often difficult to treat. Post-traumatic gustatory loss, which accounts for 18% of all reported taste problems, is virtually untreatable but sometimes resolves spontaneously after several months. Persistent gustatory problems impair the patient's quality of life, which in many cases causes depression and anxiety. Approximately 24% of all patients with intractable taste problems report mild to severe depression; conversely, 35% of all depressed patients experience taste problems. In general, a patient's gustatory symptoms are more likely to improve when the cause is a medical or dental condition that does not directly involve the gustatory system (e.g., allergies, upper respiratory infections, gingivitis, depression). In cases such as these, the taste disorder often improves as the medical or dental condition resolves or the medications are discontinued.

RESOLUTION OF CLINICAL CASE

Taste loss following traumatic closed-head injury is rare and not well understood. Careful testing of patients who report taste loss shows that, in most cases, their sense of smell has been disrupted and taste perception is normal. Most people, including many physicians, appreciate the enormous contribution of olfactory information to flavor perception only when they have clogged nostrils from a head cold. When this patient hit her head on the windshield, her brain surged forward and struck the inner surface of the skull, causing a concussion. Such severe brain movement may sever the delicate olfactory filia where they pass through the cribriform plate. Olfactory function may return if the olfactory nerves are merely stretched or compressed by local edema. In this case, the patient showed a permanent loss, suggesting that her olfactory nerves were severed in the accident. This patient, like most who have sustained olfactory loss, was convinced that she lost her sense of taste. Another issue that should have been addressed in the emergency department was the leakage of clear fluid from the nose (rhinorrhea) of this patient. Rhinorrhea following head trauma may signal cerebrospinal fluid leakage into the nasal cavity through a fracture of the cribriform plate. Fractures of the cribriform plate may enable bacteria in the nasal cavity to infiltrate and infect the meninges, a serious but preventable complication of head trauma.

REVIEW QUESTIONS

Directions: For each of the following questions, choose the **one** best answer.

1. Which area receives a direct projection from the olfactory bulb?
   A. Orbitofrontal cortex
   B. Piriform lobe
   C. Insula
   D. Nucleus of the solitary tract (NST)
   E. Mediodorsal thalamic nucleus

2. What is involved in the taste transduction mechanism for NaCl?
   A. Reversible binding to receptors located on the microvilli of the taste bud, which triggers Ca^{2+} entry into taste cells
   B. Direct entry of Na^+ ions into the cell through ion-sensitive gates, which depolarizes the taste cell
   C. Reversible binding to receptors located on the apical surface of the taste bud, which triggers a G-protein-mediated release of cAMP
   D. A G-protein-initiated cascade that involves the second messenger inositol triphosphate (IP_3)
   E. Binding to a G-protein receptor, which triggers an adenylate cyclase–cAMP-mediated opening of a cation channel that allows Na^+ flow into the cell

3. From the standpoint of perception, which of the following sensory modalities is most closely related to the common chemical sense?
   A. Taste
   B. Smell
   C. Flavor
   D. Touch
   E. Pain

4. What are the source and the destination, respectively, of gustatory information carried by the central tegmental tract?
   A. The parvicellular division of the ventroposteromedial nucleus (VPMpc) of the thalamus and the ipsilateral mediodorsal (MD) nucleus of the thalamus
   B. The nucleus of the solitary tract (NST) and the contralateral primary gustatory cortex
   C. The VPMpc and the ipsilateral primary gustatory cortex
   D. The NST and the contralateral MD nucleus of the thalamus
   E. The NST and the ipsilateral VPMpc of the thalamus

5. Which of the following is true about olfactory receptors?
   A. They are bipolar neurons.
   B. They are located in the olfactory bulb.
   C. They are replaced every 10–14 days.
   D. They are durable and resist chemotoxic but not traumatic injury.
   E. They are free nerve endings.

6. Where is primary taste cortex located?
   A. Foot of the postcentral gyrus
   B. Rostral insula
   C. Uncus
   D. Adjacent to the somatosensory representation of the tongue
   E. Brodmann area 43

7. Where does convergence of taste and smell information take place?
   A. Rostral insula
   B. Primary taste cortex
   C. Orbitofrontal cortex
   D. Entorhinal cortex
   E. VPMpc nucleus of the thalamus

Directions: For the remaining questions, match the lettered option below with statements 8-12. Each lettered option may be used once, more than once, or not at all.

A. Only smell
B. Only taste
C. Both taste and smell
D. Neither taste nor smell

8. Receptor cells regenerate.

9. Transduction involves second messengers.

10. Receptor cells are neurons.

11. The apical end of receptors is capped by microvilli.

12. Central projections are primarily contralateral.

ADDITIONAL READING

Classic Literature

Amoore JE, Hautala E: Odor as an aid to chemical safety: odor thresholds compared with the threshold limit values and volatiles for 214 industrial chemicals in air and water. *J Appl Toxicol* 3:272–290, 1983.

Beidler LM, Smallman RL: Renewal of cells within taste buds. *J Cell Biol* 27:263–272, 1965.

Erickson, RP: Sensory neural patterns and gustation. In: Zotterman Y, ed. *Olfaction and taste*. New York, NY: Pergammon Press, 1963:205–213.

Pfaffmann, C: Gustatory afferent impulses. *J Cell Comp Physiol* 17:243–258, 1941.

Shepherd GM: Synaptic organization of the mammalian olfactory bulb. *Physiol Rev* 52:864–917, 1972.

Reviews and Landmark Research Articles

Beckstead RM, Morse JR, Norgren R: The nucleus of the solitary tract in the monkey: projections to the thalamus and bran stem nuclei. *J Comp Neurol* 190:259–282, 1980.

Buck L, Axel R: A novel multigene family may encode odorant receptors: a molecular basis for odor recognition. *Cell* 65:175–187, 1991.

Buck LB: Information coding in the mammalian olfactory system. *Cold Spring Harb Symp Quant Biol* 61:147–155, 1996.

Carmichael ST, Clugnet MC, Price JL: Central olfactory connections in the macaque monkey. *J Comp Neurol* 346:403–434, 1994.

Deems DA, Doty RL, Settle RG, Moore-Gillon V, Shaman P, Mester AF, Kimmelman CP, Brightman VJ, Snow Jr. JB: Smell and taste disorders, a study of 750 patients from the University of Pennsylvania Smell and Taste Center. *Arch Otolaryngol Head Neck Surg* 117:519–528, 1991.

Doty RL, Deems DA, Stellar S: Olfactory dysfunction in parkinsonism: A general deficit unrelated to neurologic signs, disease stage, or disease duration. *Neurol* 38:1237–1244, 1988.

Doty RL, Shaman P, Applebaum SL, Gibertson R, Siksorski L, Rosenberg L: Smell identification ability: changes with age. *Science* 226:1441–1443, 1984.

Doty RL, Shaman P, Dann M: Development of the University of Pennsylvania Smell Identification Test: a standardized microencapsulated test of olfactory function. *Physiol Behav* 32:489–502, 1984.

Duncan HJ, Smith DV: Clinical disorders of olfaction. In: Doty RL, ed. *Handbook of Olfaction and Gustation*. New York, NY: Marcel Dekker, 1995:345–365.

Firestein S: How the olfactory system makes sense of scents. *Nature* 413:211–218, 2001.

Herness MS, Gilbertson TA: Cellular mechanisms of taste transduction. *Annual Rev Physiol* 61:873–900, 1999.

Margolskee RF: Receptor mechanisms in gustation. In: Doty RL, ed. *Handbook of Olfaction and Gustation*. New York, NY: Marcel Dekker, 1995:575–595.

Miller IJ: Anatomy of the peripheral taste system. In: Doty RL, ed. *Handbook of Olfaction and Gustation*. New York, NY: Marcel Dekker, 1995:521–547.

Mombaerts P: Molecular biology of odorant responses in vertebrates. *Annual Rev Neurosci* 22:487–509, 1999.

Price JL: Olfaction. In: Paxinos G, Mai J, eds. *The Human Nervous System*. 2nd ed. New York, NY: Elsevier, 2004:1197–1211.

Pritchard TC, Eslinger PJ, Wang J, and Yang Q: Smell and taste disorders. In: Rizzo M, Eslinger PJ, eds. *Principles and Practice of Behavioral Neurology and Neuropsychology*. Philadelphia, PA: Saunders, 2004:335–359.

Pritchard TC, Hamilton RB, Morse J, Norgren R: Projections of thalamic gustatory and lingual areas in the monkey, *Macaca fascicularis*. *J Comp Neurol* 244:213–228,1986.

Pritchard TC, Norgren R: Gustatory system. In: Paxinos G, Mai J. *The Human Nervous System*. 2nd ed. New York, NY: Elsevier, 2004:1171–1196.

Ronnett GV: The molecular mechanisms of olfactory signal transduction. In: Doty RL, ed. *Handbook of Olfaction and Gustation*. New York, NY: Marcel Dekker, 1995:127–145.

Travers SP, Norgren R: Organization of orosensory responses in the nucleus of the solitary tract of rat. *J Neurophysiol* 73:2144–2162, 1995.

Vassar R, Chao SK, Sitcheran R, Nunez JM, Vosshall LB, Axel R: Topographic organization of sensory projections to the olfactory bulb. *Cell* 79:981–999, 1994.

Zatorre RJ, Jones-Gottman M, Evans AC, Meyer E: Functional localization and lateralization of human olfactory cortex. *Nature* 360:339–340, 1992.

INTERNET RESOURCES

American Academy of Otolaryngology
Head and Neck Surgery
http://www.entnet.org/healthinfo/topics/smell_taste.cfm

American Rhinologic Society
http://american-rhinologic.org/

Anosmia Foundation
http://www.anosmiafoundation.org/index.shtml

Association for Chemoreception Sciences
http://www.achems.org/

National Institute on Deafness and Other Communication Disorders
http://www.nidcd.nih.gov/

Sense of Smell Institute
http://www.senseofsmell.org/

Yale University School of Medicine
Olfactory Nerve Overview
http://info.med.yale.edu/caim/cnerves/cn1/cn1_1.html

Specific questions about taste and smell can be answered at:

Clinic@monell.org

nidcdinfo@nidcd.nih.gov (800-241-1044)

BellamyT@UPHS.upenn.edu

Taste and Smell Clinics. Proper identification and treatment of taste and smell disorders often requires specialized training that few physicians receive as medical students or residents. Physicians at the three taste and smell clinics in the United States listed below not only treat chemosensory disorders but also perform state-of-the-art research on the chemical senses.

The Smell and Taste Center at the University of Pennsylvania
http://www.med.upenn.edu/stc/

Nasal Dysfunction Clinic at University of California at San Diego
http://health.ucsd.edu/specialties/surgery/otolaryngology/nasal/

Taste and Smell Center at the University of Connecticut Health Center
http://www.uchc.edu/uconntasteandsmell/

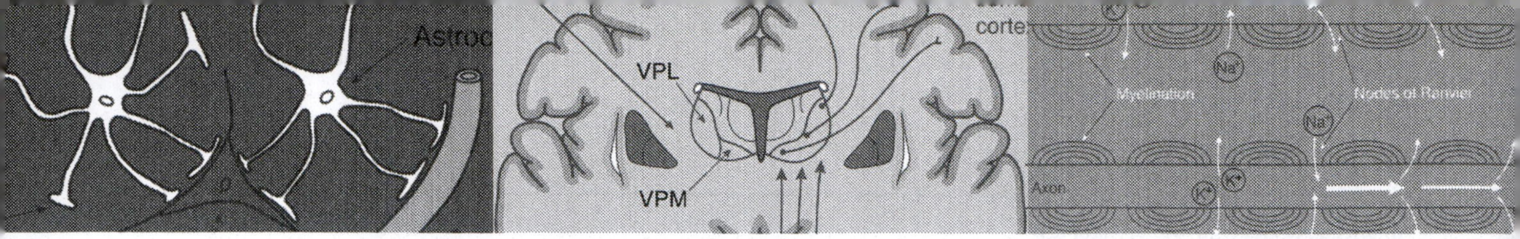

CHAPTER 11

Visual System

INTRODUCTION OF CLINICAL CASE

A 37-year-old woman was seen by her physician because of recurring headaches and blurred vision. The patient reported difficulty driving because cars in adjacent lanes seemed to "pop out from nowhere." Her eye movements appeared normal and she did not complain of double vision. Direct and consensual pupillary light reflexes were normal, and there was no indication of a relative afferent pupillary defect. An ophthalmoscopic examination was also unremarkable; there was no evidence of papilledema or retinopathy, nor were there any signs of hemorrhage, aneurysm, or retinal exudates. The optic cup in each eye had a well-defined margin, and both the lens and vitreous were free of opacities. A visual field test, however, revealed bilateral loss of the temporal fields and complete loss of central vision in the left eye. Although the patient did not exhibit any other physical symptoms, her blood was drawn for an endocrine evaluation, and she was taken to a nearby medical center to obtain a magnetic resonance image (MRI) of her brain.

OVERVIEW OF THE VISUAL SYSTEM

Most people rely on vision more than any other sensory system to acquire information about the external world. Our visual system creates a vivid spatial representation of the world that allows us to determine the size, shape, color, and location of objects in three-dimensional space. When these objects move, our visual system informs us of their direction and relative speed. Furthermore, our motor system receives projections from the visual system to guide eye movements that are associated with visual attention and our interactions with objects in the environment.

The visual system includes the eyes and all of the brain regions that receive information from the eyes. These regions form an extensive neural network that occupies 40% of the cerebral cortex and interconnects the cortex with numerous nuclei in the thalamus and brainstem. Because of this widespread distribution, many diseases and injuries can affect one or more parts of the visual system. The central visual pathways have a precise topographic organization, knowledge of which is clinically useful for determining the location of lesions that impair vision or other central nervous system (CNS) functions.

THE EYE

The eyes are highly specialized structures that allow light to be perceived by the CNS. In the posterior part of each eye lies the retina, a laminated neural structure that transduces light into neural signals. The neuronal circuits of the retina transform light information into a neural code that is used by the brain to construct a visual representation of the external world.

Development of the Eye

The eye is an outgrowth of the brain.

Eye development begins in the prosencephalon during the third week of embryologic growth, as shown in Figure 11.1. On day 22, the optic vesicles begin their extension from both sides of the ventral forebrain but remain connected to the diencephalon by hollow optic stalks. As the optic vesicles grow laterally, their distal ends enlarge and gradually displace the overlying mesenchyme until they appose the surface ectoderm on day 28. By day 34, the ectoderm has thickened and formed the lens placode so that the underlying optic vesicle may induce the lens placode to invaginate and form the lens vesicle. Between days 34 and 38, the cells in the neck of the lens placode fuse together and the lens vesicle separates from the surface ectoderm before it develops into the lens of the eye.

Formation of the lens vesicle is accompanied by invagination of the distal end of the optic vesicle into a two-layered structure called the optic cup. After the lens vesicle separates from the ectoderm, the distal rim of the optic cup bends inward and embraces the lens vesicle to form the iris. The inferior surface of the optic cup is indented by the optic fissure, a small cleft that contains mesenchyme and hyaloid blood vessels that supply the retina and the lens vesicle. The edges along the optic fissure eventually grow around the hyaloid vessels and merge. With further development, the distal tributaries of the hyaloid vessels degenerate, but the proximal branches become the central retinal artery and vein.

The optic cup is composed of two distinct layers. The inner, thicker layer is called the nervous layer because it differentiates into the neuronal layers of the retina. The outer, thinner layer is called the pigment layer because it eventually forms the pigment epithelium. These two layers are separated by the intraretinal space, a slender cavity that originates from the lumen of the optic vesicle and gradually disappears as the pigment and nervous layers grow closer together to form a fully developed retina. The pigment and nervous layers may later separate in response to head trauma, a condition known as a retinal detachment.

The lens vesicle induces cell proliferation in the nervous layer, causing it to form a thick neuroepithelium that differentiates into several layers of neurons. Axons from the retinal ganglion cells grow across the inner surface of the nervous layer and migrate into the lumen of the optic stalk, where they form the optic nerve. The optic nerve fibers from both eyes proceed caudally until they meet at the optic chiasm located at the base of the brain. Those fibers originating from the nasal portion of each retina (approximately 60% of the fibers) cross the midline of the optic chiasm before entering the brain, whereas those from the temporal side enter the brain without crossing the midline.

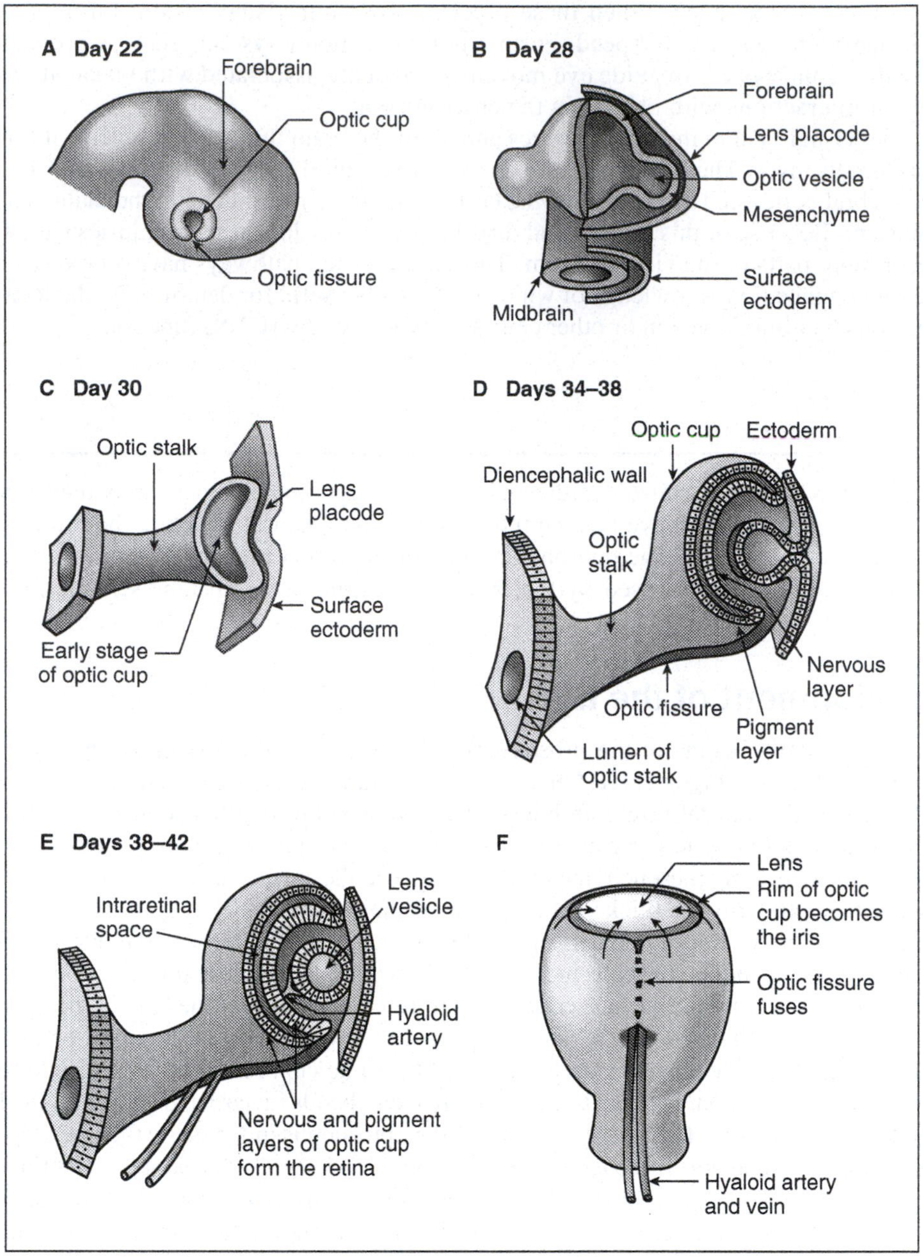

FIG. 11.1. Development of the Eye. (A) Surface view of the optic vesicle evaginating from the ventral surface of the forebrain. (B-E) Sectional views showing the development of the optic stalks and the induction of the lens from the surface ectoderm. (F) The optic fissure closes around the hyaloid artery and vein.

Anatomy of the Eye

The eye is a complex structure that contains many intricate components. The major components of the eye are shown in Figure 11.2.

The **sclera** protects the eye.

Sclera and Choroid. An extremely tough membrane called the sclera, or more commonly the "white of the eye," covers most of the eye. The sclera surrounds the eyeball and is continuous with the cornea on the anterior side and with the dura surrounding the optic nerve on the posterior side. A dense, fibrous connective tissue, the sclera protects the

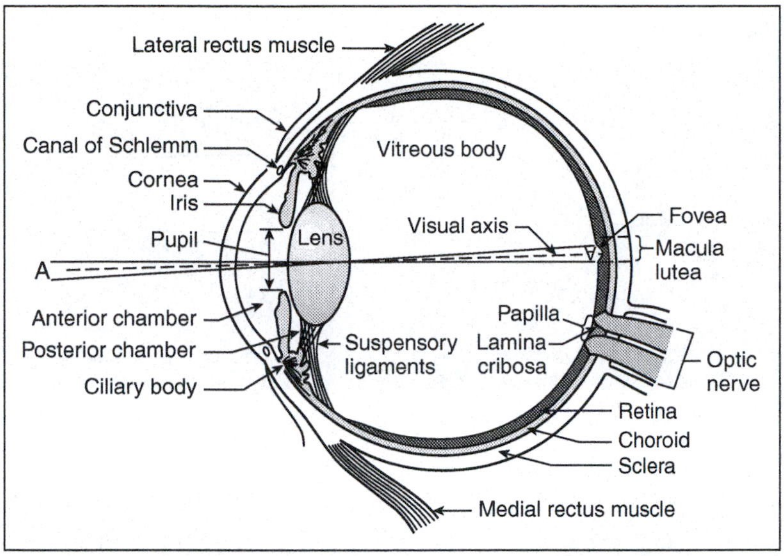

FIG. 11.2. Components of the Eye. Horizontal section through the eye illustrates the visual axis and its relationship to the lens, the macula, and other structures in the eye.

interior of the eye by resisting punctures and other injuries. In addition, the sclera is invested by six extraocular muscles that control the direction of visual fixation.

The choroid is a thin, highly vascularized and pigmented layer that lies between the sclera and the retina. Branches of the ophthalmic artery supply blood to the choroid layer, which in turn supplies nutrients to the photoreceptors of the retina. The sclera and the choroid are both derived from mesenchyme tissue surrounding the optic cup. During development, the distal rim of the choroid differentiates into the ciliary body and the iris.

Cornea. The cornea forms the anterior surface of the eye in front of the iris and pupil. Although the cornea is continuous with the opaque sclera, it is transparent and permits light transmission into the interior of the eye. The cornea has a highly curved surface that refracts light more than any other component in the eye and is essential for focusing images onto the retina.

The **cornea** refracts light more than any other part of the eye.

Due to its exposed location on the anterior aspect of the eye, the cornea is vulnerable to abrasion by small particles. To detect minor irritants, the cornea is densely innervated by a plexus of free nerve endings that originate in the ophthalamic division of the trigeminal ganglion. In fact, the cornea is the most densely innervated part of the body. The central projections of the corneal afferents terminate in the spinal trigeminal nucleus, which projects to the facial nucleus to mediate the corneal blink reflex.

Iris. The iris is an adjustable, pigmented diaphragm that controls the size of the pupil and, hence, modulates the amount of light entering the eye. Pupil diameter can vary from 1 to 8 mm and is controlled by two sets of nonstriated muscles in the iris. Thus, the pupil constricts during contraction of the pupillary sphincter and dilates during contraction of the pupillary dilator. The sphincter is an annular muscle located around the inner rim of the iris; it receives parasympathetic innervation from a small number of postganglionic neurons in the ciliary ganglion, which is located just posterior to the eye. The dilator muscle, by comparison, has a radial organization around the circumference of the pupil and is located along the posterior wall of the iris. The dilator muscle receives sympathetic innervation from the postganglionic neurons of the superior cervical ganglion, which is located in the base of the neck.

The **iris** controls the amount of light entering the eye.

Loss of sympathetic innervation of the eye causes Horner's syndrome, which is characterized by a small pupil (miosis) and a partial drooping of the eyelid (ptosis). The pupil becomes miotic because sympathetic innervation of the dilator muscle is interrupted; ptosis results from the decreased innervation of a small strip of muscle in the upper eyelid

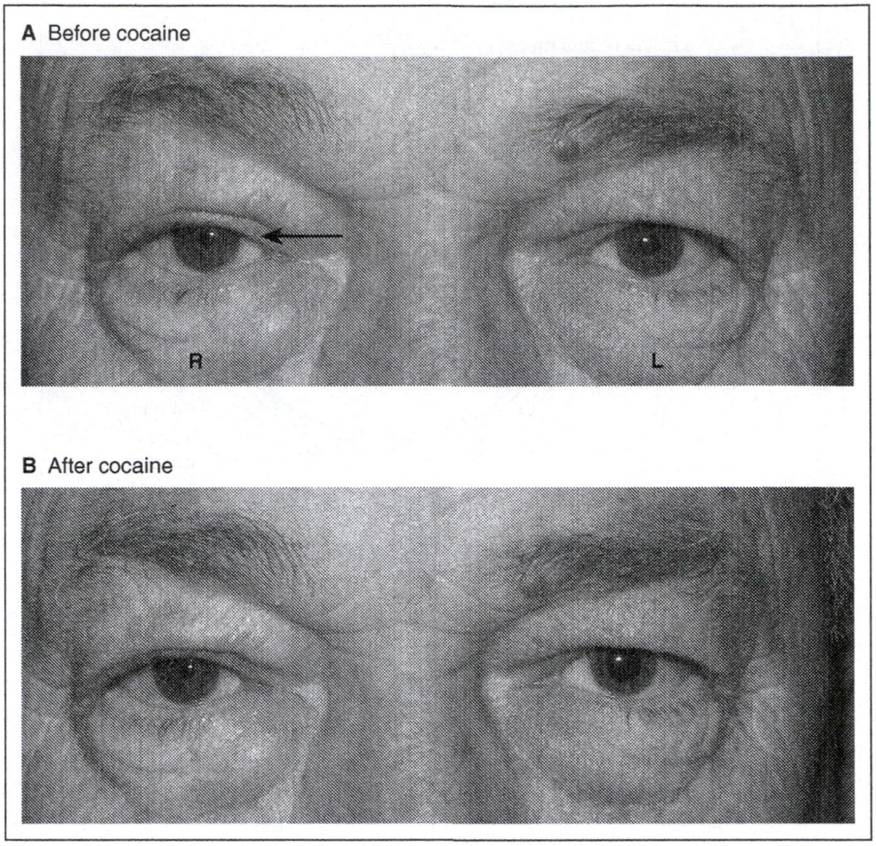

FIG. 11.3. Horner's Syndrome. (A) Horner's syndrome is suspected because the upper eyelid of the right eye is slightly ptotic (arrow). (B) The pupil of the left eye, which is normal, dilates in response to cocaine, which is an indirect sympathomimetic that blocks reuptake of norepinephrine at the postganglionic noradrenergic terminals of the sympathetic nervous system. The pupil of the right eye, however, does not dilate in response to cocaine because its sympathetic innervation is lost. (Photographs provided courtesy of Dr. William Cantore, Pennsylvania State University.)

called Mueller's muscle. Anhidrosis may also accompany a Horner's syndrome if the lesion is preganglionic and involves the fibers that innervate the sweat glands of the face. Clinically, the presence of Horner's syndrome is easily revealed by determining whether the pupil responds to topical application of a sympathomimetic drug such as cocaine (Figure 11.3; see also Chapters 5 and 13).

Ciliary muscles control the shape of the **lens.**

Ciliary Body. The ciliary body, which consists of muscle fibers underneath the ciliary process and ciliary epithelium, has a ring-like structure that follows the outer perimeter of the iris. The ciliary process produces aqueous humor, a clear fluid similar to cerebrospinal fluid. Aqueous humor carries nutrients to the lens and the cornea. Suspensory ligaments, which are sometimes called zonal fibers, connect the ciliary body to the equator of the lens.

The ciliary body develops from mesenchyme tissue and differentiates into three layers of annular, oblique, and longitudinal muscle fibers. These ciliary muscles are innervated by most of the postganglionic neurons in the ciliary ganglion. Contraction of these muscle fibers causes the anterior edge of the ciliary body to move slightly toward the equator of the lens, thereby reducing the tension along the suspensory ligaments. This action allows the lens to bulge, an effect that increases its refractive power (Figure 11.4).

Lens. The lens is a transparent, oval-shaped structure composed of interlocking crystalline fibers enclosed in a basement membrane called the lens capsule. The main function of the lens is to alter light refraction so that the eye may focus on objects located at

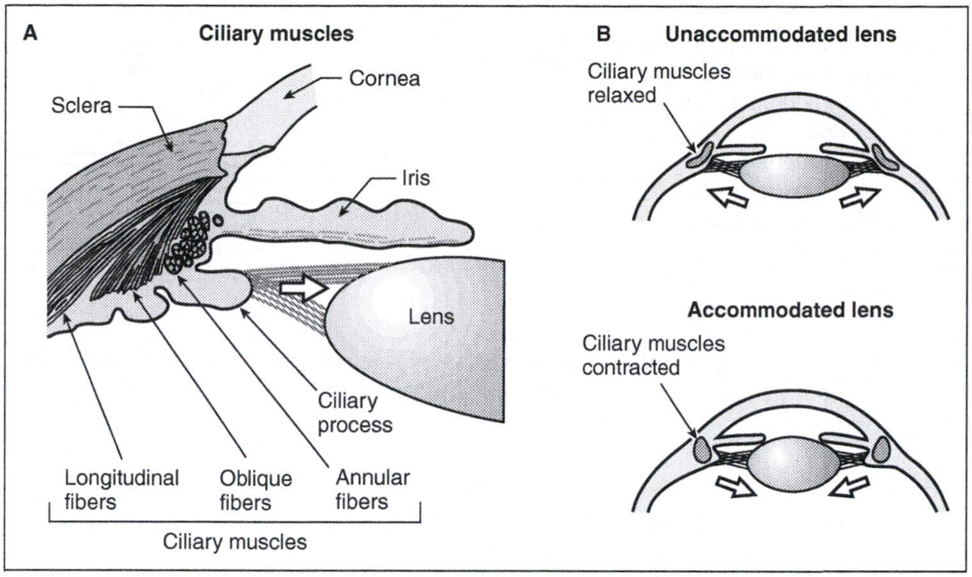

FIG. 11.4. Ciliary Muscles. (A) This diagram shows the structure of the three sets of ciliary muscle fibers after removing the cornea and sclera. The white arrow indicates the direction of movement of the ciliary body during contraction of the ciliary muscles. (B) The ciliary muscles control the shape of the lens. When distant objects are viewed, the ciliary muscles are relaxed and the lens flattens. When nearby objects are viewed, the ciliary muscles contract and the lens bulges because of decreased tension along the suspensory ligaments.

different distances. Because the lens capsule and its enclosed fibers are highly elastic, the shape of the lens varies with changes in the amount of tension along the suspensory ligaments. The curvature of the lens surface determines the degree of light refraction; therefore, lens shape is controlled within narrow limits to bend light rays more or less as the eye focuses on near or distant objects, respectively. Thus, light refraction is greatest when the lens bulges during contraction of the ciliary muscles and is lowest when the lens flattens during relaxation of the ciliary muscles (see Figure 11.4).

The lens focuses light onto the retina.

With age, the lens may gradually become cloudy and interfere with visual acuity. This condition, known as a cataract, is easily corrected by surgically removing the cloudy lens and implanting a plastic lens in the lens capsule.

Retina. During embryologic development, the nervous layer of the optic cup differentiates into several layers of neurons to form the retina. One layer in the retina is composed exclusively of photoreceptors, which transduce photons of light into neural signals that are subsequently processed by neighboring layers of neurons. Ultimately, these signals are sent to the retinal ganglion cells, whose axons converge at the optic disk and project to the brain as the optic nerve. The detailed structure of the photoreceptors and the other layers of the retina are discussed in "The Retina."

Photoreceptors transduce light into neural impulses.

The structure of the retina varies considerably across its surface. The macula lutea, which lies in the center of the retina, represents the central part of the visual field. A small depression in the macula lutea, called the fovea, has the highest density of photoreceptors and, consequently, the highest spatial resolution of the visual field. The optic disk, which lies on the nasal side of the macula lutea, represents the point at which the optic nerve emerges from the retina. There are no photoreceptors at the optic disk, and hence, it is often called the blind spot (Figure 11.5).

Pigment Epithelium. The pigment epithelium develops from the pigment layer of the optic cup and lies between the choroid on its outer surface and the photoreceptors on its inner surface. The proximity of the pigment epithelium and the photoreceptors allows

The **pigment epithelium** supports the cellular functions of the retina.

FIG. 11.5. Blind Spot. To demonstrate the blind spot, close your left eye and view the plus sign with your right eye while holding the page 6 inches away. The filled circle "disappears" when its image is projected onto the optic disk. The blind spot is usually not noticed because the visual system "fills in" the missing portion of the visual scene. This is demonstrated by viewing the lower portion of the figure as described above; all the lines appear continuous despite the presence of a gap.

interactions that are vital to visual functions. The pigment epithelium also contains a high concentration of melanin, which absorbs light and reduces the reflection of light onto the photoreceptors.

Optic Nerve. The optic nerve is composed of myelinated axons that convey visual information from the retina to the brain. The central retinal artery and vein travel through the center of the optic nerve and supply blood to the inner layers of the retina. At the posterior surface of the optic disk, the optic nerve and retinal blood vessels perforate the sclera and choroid at the lamina cribrosa (Figure 11.6). The three meningeal layers (i.e., dura mater, arachnoid, and pia mater) lining the optic nerve are continuous with the meninges surrounding the brain. As the optic nerve enters the eye, the dura mater merges with the sclera.

Fluid-Filled Chambers in the Eye. The chambers lying immediately anterior and posterior to the lens are filled with aqueous humor, a clear watery fluid that is secreted by the ciliary process into the posterior chamber lying between the iris and lens (see Figure 11.2). The aqueous humor in the posterior chamber passes through the pupil and into the anterior chamber, which lies between the iris and the cornea. Aqueous humor supplies nutrients to the lens and cornea before it leaves the anterior chamber via the canal of Schlemm, a portal into the venous system that is located near the junction of the iris and cornea. When the outflow of aqueous humor is impeded, the intraocular pressure increases and may produce glaucoma, a leading cause of blindness.

The vitreous body, the large spherical chamber between the lens and the retina, is filled with a thick, gelatinous fluid called vitreous humor (see Figure 11.2). The vitreous

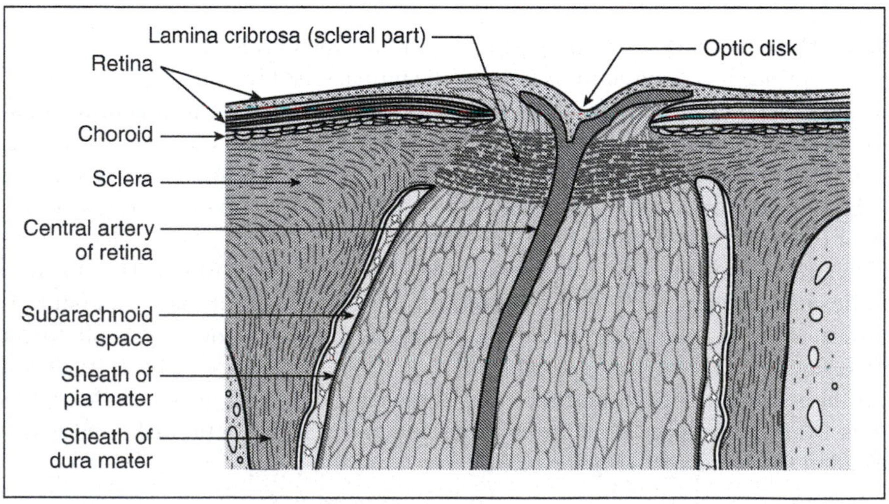

FIG. 11.6. Optic Nerve. Horizontal section through the optic nerve shows the nerve fibers perforating the sclera to form the lamina cribrosa.

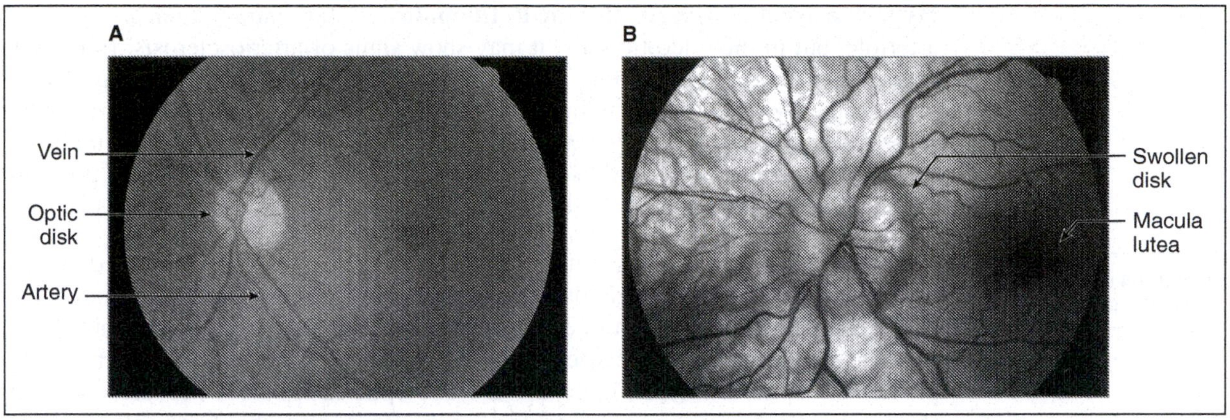

FIG. 11.7. Ophthalmoscopic Views of the Eye. (A) Optic disk in a normal left eye. The margins of the optic disk are well defined, and the central retinal artery and vein are seen emerging from the optic cup before bifurcating into branches that radiate along the surface of the retina. (B) Fundus with papilledema. The margins of the optic disk are blurred because the optic disk is swollen. (Photographs provided by Dr. William Cantore (photo A) and Dr. Thomas Gardner and Mr. Timothy Bennett (photo B), Pennsylvania State University.)

humor maintains the shape of the eyeball and contains phagocytic cells that remove blood and other cellular debris that might interfere with light transmission.

Ophthalmoscopic Examination of the Eye

Macula lutea is the region in the retina that represents the central part of the visual field.

An ophthalmoscope is used to look through a patient's pupil to inspect the retina, the optic disk, and the blood vessels on the inner surface of the retina (Figure 11.7). The macula lutea ("yellow spot") is the general area in the center of the retina that lies within a ring of vascular arcades. The fovea appears as a small bright spot in the center of the macula, and it contains a small depression, the foveola. The foveola and the surrounding part of the macula are devoid of surface blood vessels; this effectively increases the chance that light reaches the photoreceptors located in the fovea. The macula has a darkly stained appearance because it contains the highest density of photoreceptors and, thus, has a high concentration of melanin and other pigments. The macular region, especially the fovea and foveola, consists mainly of cone photoreceptors, which subserve color vision and the perception of fine details. The optic disk, or papilla, is located approximately 3 mm medial to the macula lutea and appears as a bright pinkish disk. The central part of the disk, which is lighter in color, is characterized by a depression or cup in the optic disk. The central retinal artery and vein enter the eye by passing through the optic disk, where they radiate into several branches across the surface of the retina.

Ophthalmoscopic (or funduscopic) examination is an important part of every neurologic exam because the appearance of the retina is often altered by head trauma or systemic disease. Furthermore, the central retinal artery and vein lie on the surface of the retina, and inspection of their "nude" state provides an opportunity to detect signs of vascular disease produced by diabetes mellitus, hypertension, or arteriosclerosis.

Diabetic Retinopathy. The most serious ocular complication of chronic diabetes mellitus is retinopathy. Although insulin administration may control blood sugar levels, vascular pathology may continue to progress in this disease. Diabetes mellitus produces morphologic changes in the endothelial cells and basement membranes of blood vessels throughout the body, including the eye, where occlusion or leakage of the retinal capillaries may take place. The ophthalmoscopic hallmarks of diabetic retinopathy are a scattering of microaneurysms and blot-like hemorrhages where the capillary walls are weakened. These clinical signs are visualized more easily following injection of a fluorescent dye into the circulation, a technique known as fluorescein angiography.

Hypertensive and Arteriosclerotic Retinopathy. The central retinal artery is really an arteriole, but in the sclerotic state, it may show signs of arteriosclerosis. In the sclerotic state, the normally red arteriole appears lighter in color due to thickening of its vessel wall. In the hypertensive state, increased vascular pressure allows the arterioles to compress the veins wherever they cross each other in the retina. If blood pressure is not controlled, hemorrhages and hard exudates (cellular debris) accumulate in the posterior part of the fundus. Chronic hypertension is often an underlying cause of arteriosclerosis.

Papilledema is a swollen or "choked" optic disk.

Papilledema. Any increase in intracranial pressure, whether produced by a brain tumor, a cerebral hemorrhage, or an infection of the CNS, causes swelling of the optic disks. Although papilledema does not normally affect vision, it is recognized during a funduscopic examination because the swelling obliterates the optic cup and blurs the margins of the optic disk (see Figure 11.7B). The optic disk bulges because continuity between the meninges surrounding the optic nerve and the brain allows increased intracranial pressure to be transmitted through the subdural space. Papilledema may also follow obstruction of venous outflow that occurs secondary to increased pressure in the cavernous sinus that, in turn, elevates the pressure of the ophthalmic vein. In both cases, the optic disk is compliant where the sclera is perforated at the lamina cribrosa by the departing optic nerve fibers.

An increase in intracranial pressure is not the only cause of papilledema, but it is the most common. Papilledema can also be produced by decreases in intraocular pressure or by a marked elevation in blood pressure. As papilledema becomes more advanced, there is an increase in venous engorgement, vascular hemorrhages, and retinal exudates. If papilledema is not treated, vision may become impaired due to secondary atrophy of the optic nerve.

Image Formation on the Retina

Although the cornea refracts light more than any other component of the eye, the ability to focus on objects at varying distances is accomplished mainly by changes in the shape of the lens (Figure 11.8). When we focus on distant objects, the lens becomes flatter. For nearby objects, the lens thickens in order to bend light rays to a greater degree.

The shape of the lens and the size of the pupil are adjustable to focus images on the retina.

The shape of the lens is controlled by two opposing forces: the innate elasticity of the lens and the tension along the suspensory ligaments. When the ciliary muscle relaxes, the ciliary body retracts, and the suspensory ligaments pull on the equator of the lens to flatten it. By contrast, contraction of the ciliary muscle causes the ciliary body to move toward the lens, which decreases tension along the suspensory ligament and allows the elastic lens to assume a more convex shape.

The clarity of images on the retina is partly determined by the size of the pupil. As with microscopes and other optical instruments, light rays passing through the edge of the lens are subjected to chromatic and spherical aberrations. With a small pupil, most light entering the eye is transmitted through the center of the lens, and this reduces optical

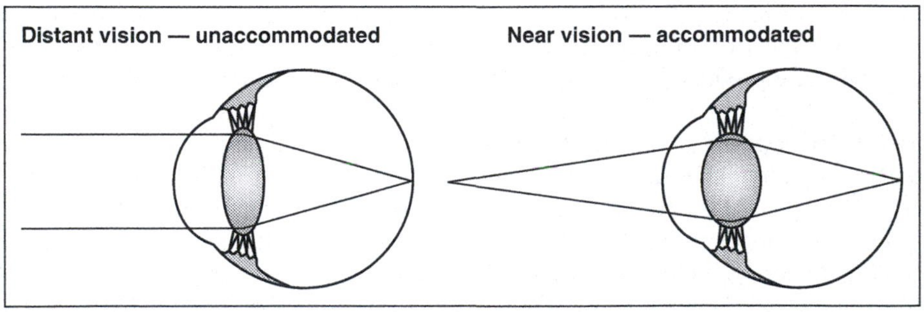

FIG. 11.8. Accommodation. When viewing nearby objects, the lens thickens to increase the angle of refraction.

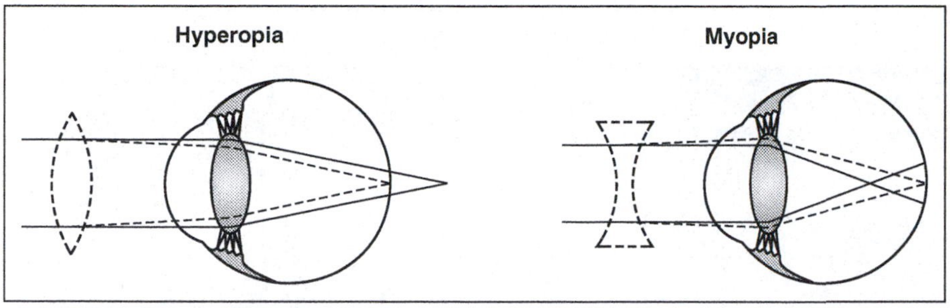

FIG. 11.9. Hyperopia and Myopia. Hyperopic (farsighted) individuals focus light behind the retina because the eyeball is too short. Myopic (nearsighted) individuals focus light in front of the retina because the eyeball is too long. The dashed lines indicate how these refractive errors are corrected by the appropriate lenses.

distortion. Photographers employ the same principle when they reduce the aperture of a camera to improve the depth of field so that objects located at varying distances from the camera are brought into focus. A small pupil, however, interferes with visual acuity by reducing the amount of light entering the eye. For this reason, the visual system adjusts the size of the pupil to limit optical distortion and maximize the depth of field according to the ambient illumination.

Accommodation-Convergence Reaction. The ability to focus on objects near the face is accomplished by coordinating the activities of several muscles, a response called the accommodation-convergence reaction. This ocular reflex is demonstrated by having a patient fixate on the examiner's finger as it is moved toward the nose. As the patient watches the approaching finger, the eyes converge toward the midline. This convergence response is mediated by contraction of the medial recti muscles of both eyes. Furthermore, as the eyes converge, the lens in each eye becomes more spherical, and both pupils constrict. This accommodation response is mediated by simultaneous contraction of the ciliary muscle and the pupillary sphincter, both of which receive parasympathetic innervation from postganglionic neurons in the ciliary ganglion.

Myopia and Hyperopia. Myopia and hyperopia represent refractive errors in which light rays are not properly focused on the retina because the focal plane of the lens and the shape of the eye are mismatched (Figure 11.9). Myopia, or nearsightedness, results when distant objects are focused in front of the retina either because the cornea is too curved or the eyeball is too long. Hyperopia, or farsightedness, results when nearby objects are focused behind the retina either because the cornea is not curved enough or because the eyeball is too short. Both types of refractive errors can be corrected with an appropriate set of concave (for myopia) or convex (for hyperopia) lenses.

> **Myopic** individuals are "nearsighted"; images from distant objects are focused in front of the retina.
>
> **Hyperopic** individuals are "farsighted"; images from near objects are focused behind the retina.

Presbyopia. In nearly all persons, aging causes the lens to lose elasticity and limits the degree of curvature that can be achieved by the lens when the ciliary muscles contract (see Figure 11.4B). As the accommodative power of the lens decreases with age, the closest point that can be brought into focus gradually recedes. This condition, known as presbyopia, is usually present by age 45 and may interfere with reading or other near-vision tasks. Presbyopia can be corrected by an appropriate set of convex lenses.

> **Presbyopia** occurs during normal aging; the lens loses elasticity and is unable to accommodate to nearby objects.

THE RETINA

The retina originates from the neural tube during embryologic development and is, therefore, considered part of the CNS. Consistent with its origin, the retina contains a variety of neurons that are organized into circuits for processing visual information.

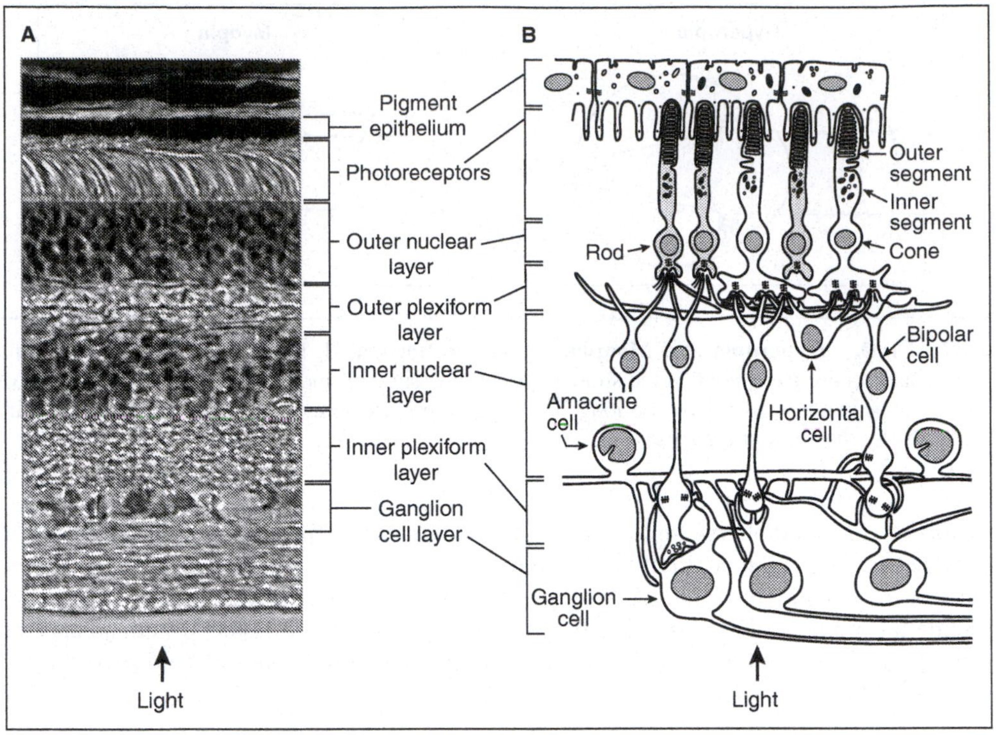

FIG. 11.10. Organization of the Retina. (A) Photomicrograph of the human retina. (B) Diagram of the neuronal components in the retina. Vertical transfer of information from photoreceptors to bipolar cells and then to ganglion cells provides the most direct route into the brain. Horizontal cells and amacrine cells mediate lateral interactions between neighboring parts of the retina.

Laminar Organization of the Retina

The retina contains five types of neurons: photoreceptors, bipolar cells, ganglion cells, horizontal cells, and amacrine cells. These neurons and their processes are organized into several layers that are identified with respect to the vitreous body (Figure 11.10). The outer nuclear layer, which is adjacent to the pigment epithelium and is most distant from the vitreous body, contains two types of photoreceptors: rods and cones. The outer plexiform layer lies closer to the vitreous body and contains the presynaptic terminals of rods and cones as well as the postsynaptic processes associated with bipolar and horizontal cells. The inner nuclear layer contains the cell bodies of bipolar, horizontal, and amacrine cells. Progressing toward the vitreous humor, the inner plexiform layer contains the synaptic connections between the bipolar, amacrine, and ganglion cells. Finally, the cell bodies of the ganglion cell layer give rise to a layer of nerve fibers that converge in the optic disk and exit the retina as the optic nerve.

The retinal neurons form specific circuits that process visual information before conveying it to the brain. Serial connections between the photoreceptors, bipolar neurons, and ganglion neurons represent the most direct route for sending visual information to the brain. By contrast, the horizontal and amacrine cells have lateral processes that interconnect adjacent groups of photoreceptors, bipolar cells, and ganglion cells. These lateral connections provide a mechanism for modulating the neural output that represents neighboring portions of the visual field. Because of these lateral interactions, spatial changes in illumination that indicate the edge of an object are perceived more easily.

Photoreceptors

Rods and cones are the only cells in the visual system that are directly activated by light. Characterized by similar structures, both types of photoreceptors contain outer and inner

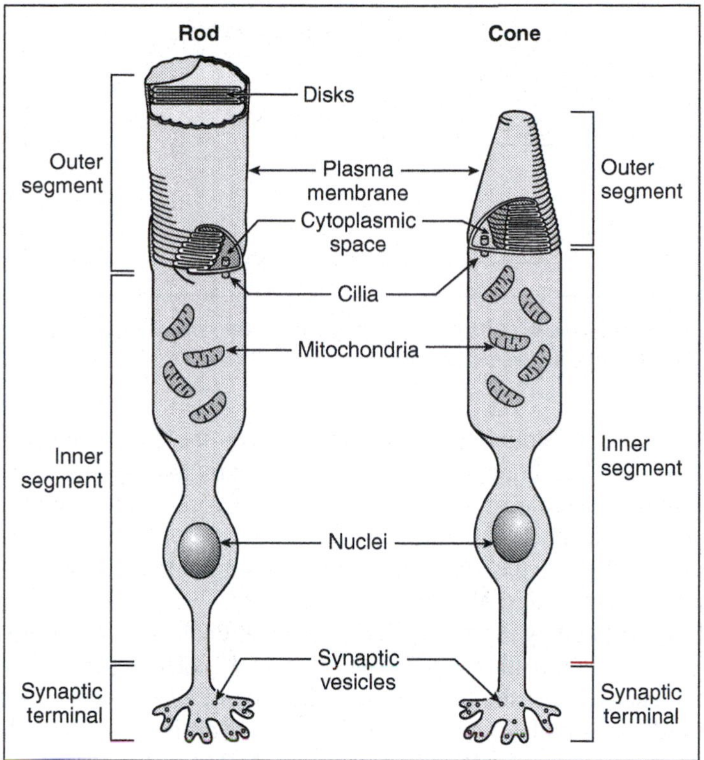

FIG. 11.11. Photoreceptors. Although similar in structure, cones have short outer segments and contain fewer disks than rods. The outer segments contain photopigments and other proteins needed for transducing light into electrophysiologic signals; the inner segments contain organelles that synthesize the components of the outer segments. The synaptic terminals contain vesicles and neurotransmitter molecules.

segments that are connected by a cilium (Figure 11.11). The outer segments contain stacks of membranous disks that are loaded with photopigments and other proteins needed to transduce light into neural signals. The inner segments contain a nucleus, mitochondria, and organelles needed for biosynthesis of the disks and other molecules used in phototransduction. The inner segments also synthesize synaptic vesicles and maintain the synaptic terminals for neurotransmission in the outer plexiform layer.

Most students are initially surprised to learn that photoreceptors are in the outermost layer of the retina because this indicates that light must pass through several layers of cells and their processes before reaching the rods and cones. Fortunately, the inner layers of the retina are virtually transparent and absorb only a small fraction of the incoming light. The location of photoreceptors in the outer layer of the retina reflects their physiologic dependence on the pigment epithelium. As new disks are formed at the base of the outer segment, the oldest disks at the tip are shed into the intraretinal space. In fact, the life span of a disk is about 12 days as it proceeds from the base of the outer segment to its distal tip. To accommodate this turnover rate, detached disk fragments are removed from the intraretinal space by the phagocytic activity of the pigment epithelium. The pigment epithelium also recycles bleached photopigment molecules after they participate in phototransduction. Retinal detachments, which occur in response to head trauma or disease, interfere with these critical functions and cause the photoreceptors to degenerate.

Photopigments are the combination of a protein and 11-*cis* retinal.

Phototransduction. Phototransduction is the process by which photoreceptors convert light energy into neural signals. This process involves one light-sensitive step followed by a cascade of biochemical reactions that alter the membrane potential of the photoreceptor. The only light-dependent step in the transduction process involves the absorption of a photon of light by a photopigment molecule. Four types of photopigments are present in the human eye, and all of them consist of a protein covalently linked to 11-*cis* retinal, an aldehyde derivative of the carotenoid alcohol known as vitamin A. In rods, for example, the protein coupled to 11-*cis* retinal is opsin, and the combination of opsin and 11-*cis* retinal is called rhodopsin. Cones have one of three different proteins that combine with 11-*cis* retinal, and each is sensitive to a different range of wavelengths in the visible spectrum. In fact, this differential wavelength sensitivity of the cone photopigments is due to their protein components.

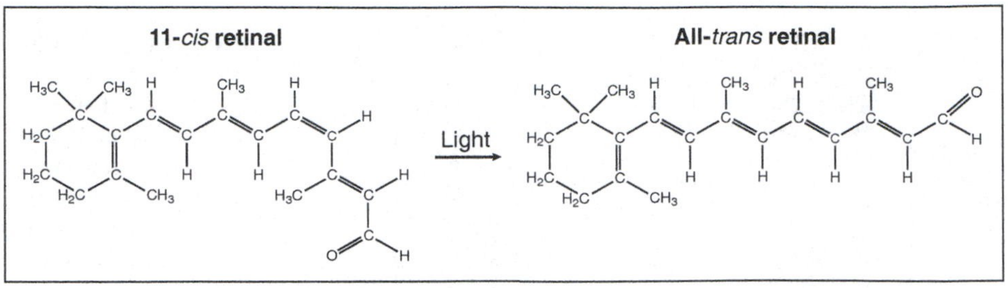

FIG. 11.12. **Photoactivation of Retinal.** Absorption of light alters the conformational structure of retinal from the 11-*cis* form to the all-*trans* configuration.

Each opsin molecule contains 348 amino acid residues that span the disk membrane seven times. The hydrophobic transmembrane regions are connected by hydrophilic loops of amino acids that extend into the cytoplasm of the outer segment. Cross-links within the transmembrane regions form a tight pocket around a bound molecule of 11-*cis* retinal. Hence, the conformational structure of the opsin molecule resembles the structure of metabotropic neurotransmitter receptors described in Chapter 2.

The absorption of light by a photoreceptor causes a cascade of biochemical events.

When a photon of light is captured by rhodopsin, the conformational structure of retinal is altered from the 11-*cis* form to the all-*trans* form (Figure 11.12). The all-*trans* isomer causes a conformational change in opsin that induces activation of a G protein called transducin. In response, transducin stimulates phosphodiesterase to hydrolyze a nucleotide called cyclic guanosine monophosphate (cGMP). Removal of cGMP from the cytoplasm leads to closure of the sodium (Na^+) channels in the outer segment (Figure 11.13). Thus, activation of a single rhodopsin molecule stimulates hundreds of transducin molecules, each of which hydrolyzes hundreds of cGMP molecules. It has been estimated that a single photoactivated rhodopsin molecule may close 300 Na^+ channels, or nearly 3% of the Na^+ channels that are normally open in a dark-adapted rod.

After all-*trans* retin*al* detaches from the protein component, it is reduced to all-*trans* retin*ol*, which enters the pigment epithelium where it is recycled back into 11-*cis* retinal. Subsequently, 11-*cis* retinal is transported from the pigment epithelium to the photoreceptor outer segments where it combines with a protein to form a new photopigment molecule.

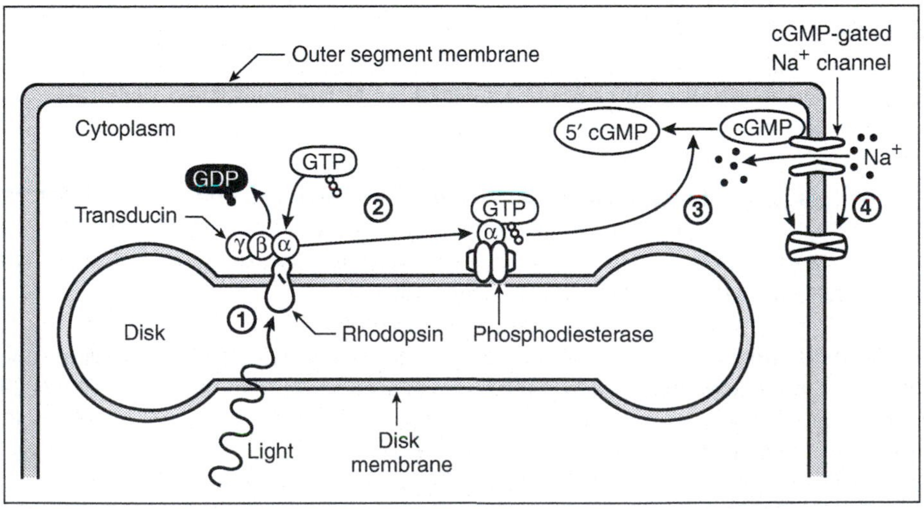

FIG. 11.13. **Phototransduction.** Phototransduction in rods involves four steps: (1) light stimulates rhodopsin to activate the G protein transducin; (2) transducin activates phosphodiesterase; (3) phosphodiesterase hydrolyzes cGMP to convert it to 5′ cGMP; (4) the removal of cGMP from the cytoplasm closes the cGMP-gated Na^+ channels. cGMP = cyclic guanosine monophosphate; GTP = guanosine triphosphate; GDP = guanosine diphosphate.

Photoreceptor Membrane Potentials. In darkness, cGMP maintains Na^+ channels in the open state and permits a passive flow of Na^+ into the cytoplasm of the photoreceptor outer segment. The steady influx of Na^+ in the dark depolarizes the photoreceptor and maintains the membrane potential at −40 mV. In this partially depolarized state, the photoreceptor's inner segments allow potassium (K^+) to leak out of the cell through K^+ channels. Thus, the steady influx of Na^+ into the outer segment is balanced by an efflux of K^+ from the inner segment; together these ionic movements establish a circular flux of current known as dark current (Figure 11.14). The concentration gradients for K^+ and Na^+ are maintained at physiologic concentrations by ion pumps in the inner segment that uses metabolic energy to pump Na^+ out and K^+ in (see Chapter 1).

During illumination of the retina, the Na^+ channels close. The decrease in Na^+ influx hyperpolarizes the membrane potential because K^+ continues to leak out of the inner segment. Although the membrane potential never shifts completely to the equilibrium potential for K^+ (−80 mV), illumination may hyperpolarize the photoreceptor to −65 mV. Like other neurons, the vesicular release of neurotransmitter from a photoreceptor requires depolarization of the membrane potential; hence, photoreceptors release more neurotransmitter when illumination is reduced. In moderate levels of illumination, the amount of neurotransmitter release fluctuates continuously in response to changes in brightness. Thus, transmitter release decreases with a gain in luminance and increases when luminance declines.

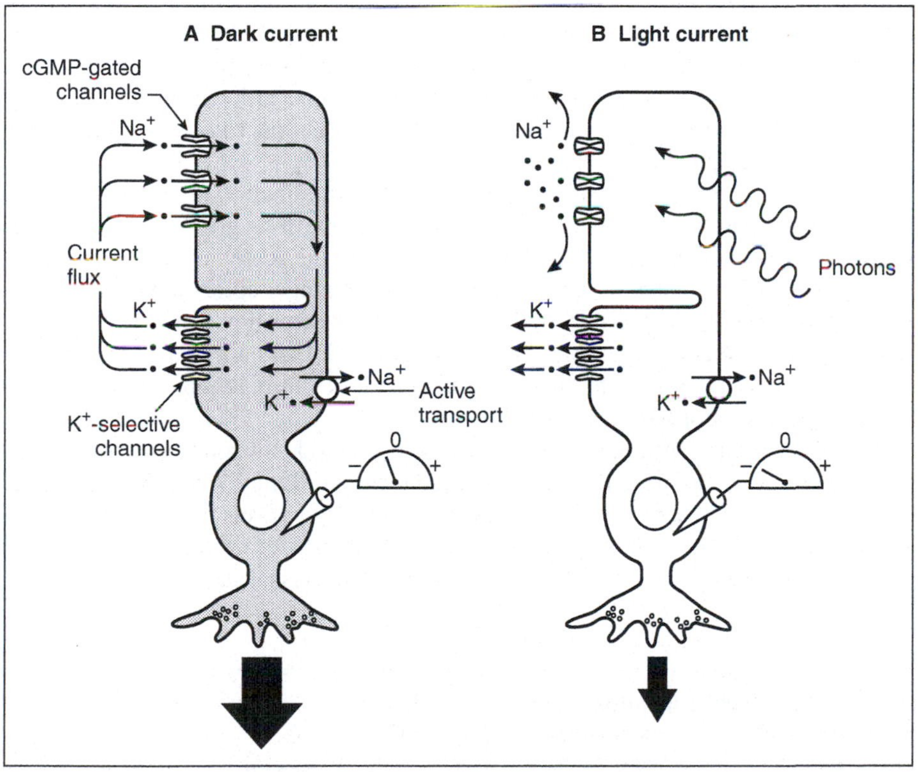

FIG. 11.14. Photoreceptor Membrane Potentials. (A) In the dark, cGMP-gated Na^+ channels are open, thereby allowing a passive influx of Na^+ current, which depolarizes the photoreceptor to −40 mV. Further depolarization is prevented by leakage of K^+ current from the inner segment. Concentration gradients of Na^+ and K^+ are maintained by ion pumps in the inner segment. (B) During light stimulation, removal of cGMP causes Na^+ channels to close, and the photoreceptor hyperpolarizes because K^+ continues to leak out of the inner segment. Shading indicates depolarization, and arrow size indicates the magnitude of neurotransmitter release cGMP = cyclic guanosine; Na^+ = sodium ion; K^+ = potassium ion.

TABLE 11.1 Structural and Functional Differences between Rods and Cones

Properties of Rods	Properties of Cones
High sensitivity to light	Low sensitivity to light
Large quantity of photopigment	Small quantity of photopigment
Scotopic (night) vision	Photopic (day) vision
Low spatial acuity	High spatial acuity
Highly convergent retinal circuits	Retinal circuits less convergent
Located outside fovea	Concentrated in fovea
Achromatic	Chromatic
One photopigment (rhodopsin)	Three color-sensitive photopigments

Rod and Cone Comparisons. Although rods and cones are both sensitive to light, important distinctions between these cells allow them to serve different visual functions. Rods and cones differ in size, shape, photopigment, retinal distribution, and their synaptic connections with other neurons (Table 11.1). The rod system is specialized to detect low levels of illumination and stimulus motion. By comparison, the cone system needs higher levels of illumination to resolve spatial detail with greater acuity than the rod system.

Scotopic: rod vision
Photopic: cone vision

Sensitivity to Illumination. The most striking structural difference between rods and cones concerns the size and shape of their outer segments. Rods have longer outer segments that contain many more disks than cones and, consequently, contain more photopigment than cones. Furthermore, rod rhodopsin is more efficient at transducing light than the cone photopigments. Collectively, these factors endow rods with greater sensitivity to low levels of illumination than cones.

Human vision occurs over a much wider range of illumination than would be possible if rods and cones had the same sensitivity to light. Because of its greater sensitivity, the rod system allows vision during low light levels that occur in the scotopic range (e.g., starlight). At higher levels of illumination, known as the mesopic range, colors are detected because both rods and cones are responsive. In daylight, vision is determined almost exclusively by cones because the rods have reached their saturation point and are unable to exhibit additional responses to increased illumination. This range of illumination, known as photopic vision, mediates most of our visual perception.

Differences in the sensitivity and time course of the rod and cone systems are apparent when leaving a well-illuminated area to enter a dark room. Initially, it is difficult to see because neither the cones nor the rods are sensitive to low light levels immediately after being exposed to intense light. In a few minutes, however, rhodopsin levels in the rods become more concentrated, and this process of dark adaptation improves visual sensitivity (Figure 11.15).

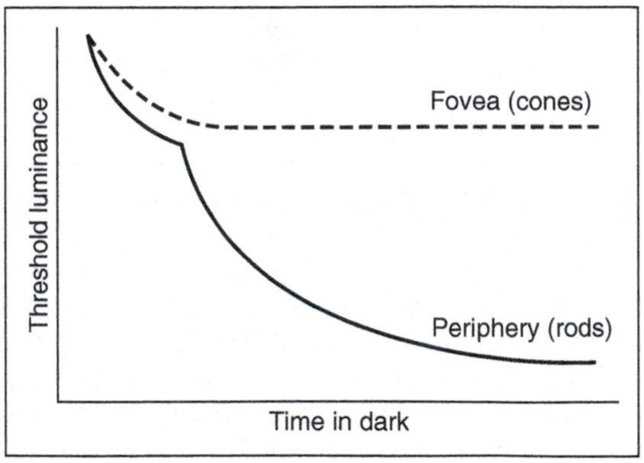

FIG. 11.15. Dark Adaptation. This figure illustrates changes in threshold sensitivity as a function of elapsed time in the dark. The light intensity of a small target was constantly adjusted to a level that was barely detectable. The threshold sensitivity of the fovea depends mainly on cones, whereas sensitivity in the peripheral retina depends on rods.

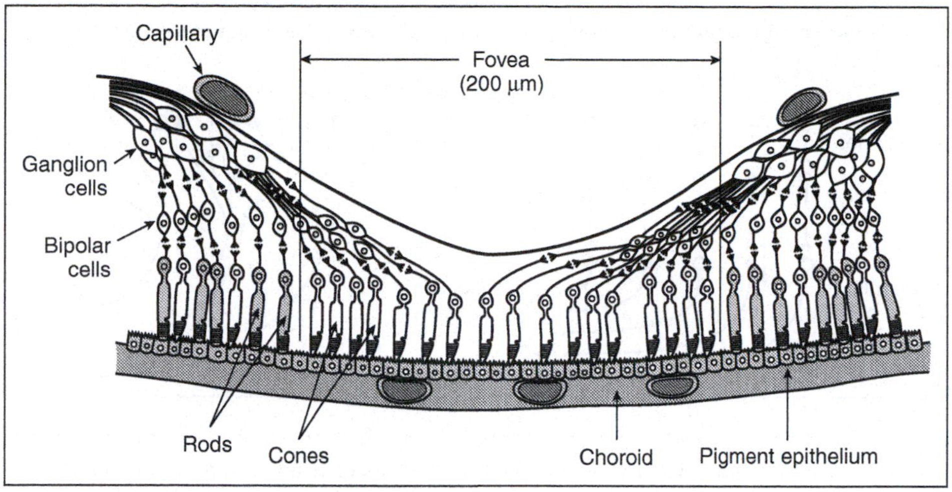

FIG. 11.16. Macula Lutea. A cross section through the macula lutea shows how bipolar and ganglion cells are displaced from the central part of the fovea. Only cones are present in the center of the fovea, and each cone communicates with one bipolar and one ganglion cell.

Distribution of Rods and Cones. Each eye contains approximately 110 million rods and 6 million cones. Although the cones are scattered throughout the retina, they are most densely concentrated in the macula lutea, which represents the central 5 degrees of the visual field. In fact, the fovea, which lies in the center of the macula, contains only cones. By comparison, rods are densest in the regions surrounding the macula lutea.

These regional variations reflect the distinct functions of the macula lutea and the surrounding retina. Whereas the macula lutea has high spatial acuity, the surrounding regions are specialized for detecting visual motion. Thus, reading and other tasks that require high spatial resolution are dependent on visual signals received from the macula. By comparison, signals originating from the outer part of the retina initiate the head and eye movements that occur when visual attention shifts to objects moving in the peripheral visual field.

The fovea and the rest of the macula have better spatial resolution than the surrounding retina for several reasons. First, the fovea is devoid of any overlying blood vessels that might interfere with light transmission. Second, the inner layers of the retina are displaced laterally so that light can interact directly with photoreceptors without having to pass through multiple layers of neurons (Figure 11.16). Finally, the fovea only contains cones that are much narrower than those in the rest of the retina; this permits the fovea to have a much higher density of photoreceptors than the surrounding retina.

The regional variation in visual acuity is also related to the degree of synaptic convergence in the rod and cone systems. A tremendous amount of convergence exists in the retina, a fact that is apparent from comparing the different cell layers of the retina. As Figure 11.10 indicates, a large number of photoreceptors send information to a small number of ganglion cells. In regions surrounding the macula, many rods project onto a few bipolar cells, which in turn project to even fewer ganglion cells. In the fovea, however, there is much less convergence from the cones to the bipolar cells, and from the bipolar cells to the ganglion cells. Hence, cones in the fovea essentially have a private channel into the brain that enables the fovea to provide a high degree of spatial resolution (Figure 11.17). By comparison, the rod system cannot signal precise stimulus positions because this system is characterized by a high degree of convergence. Although convergent circuits interfere with spatial acuity, they enable the rod system to excel at spatial and temporal summation, which increases the likelihood of detecting a moving stimulus (Figure 11.17). Because of the convergent circuits of the rod system, our attention is drawn to objects that move in the peripheral part of our visual field.

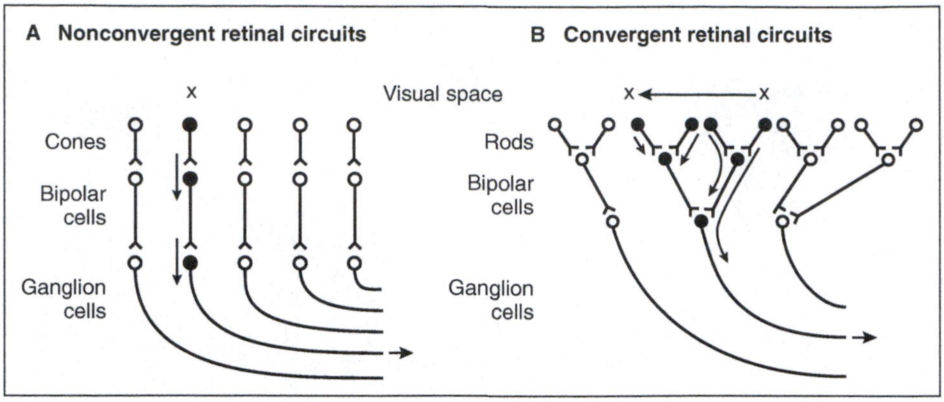

FIG. 11.17. Retinal Circuits. (A) In the fovea, cones have one-to-one communication with bipolar and ganglion cells, which allows the cone system to determine the exact location of a stimulus (x) in the visual field. Arrows indicate the flow of information in the retina. (B) In the periphery, many rods project to a few bipolar cells, which project to even fewer ganglion cells. Because of spatial and temporal summation, the convergent circuits of the rod system enhance sensitivity to moving stimuli but at the expense of spatial resolution. From the vantage point of the retinal ganglion cell, the stimulus could be located anywhere along the arrow.

Macular degeneration is the leading cause of blindness in the elderly.

Macular Degeneration. The importance of the macula for resolving spatial detail is underscored by the degree of visual impairment that accompanies macular degeneration. In many adults, the choroid undergoes age-related degenerative changes that allow blood and other fluids to leak into the retina at the posterior fundus. As the intraretinal space slowly fills with fluid, the macula detaches from the pigment epithelium and eventually forms a scarred region. Patients with macular degeneration usually have normal peripheral vision, but the loss of vision in the central visual field is often disabling because reading is difficult and the patient is unable to drive a car. Although macular degeneration is the leading cause of blindness in persons older than 75, there is no cure for this disease and its etiology remains unknown.

Functions of the Retina

The main task of the visual system is to identify objects in the external world. To accomplish this, the brain must extract information about form and shape from variations in light intensity. Abrupt changes in light intensity, or luminance contrast, provide important cues about the shape of an object. The amount of light reflected from an object is usually constant along its flat surfaces but varies significantly at its edges and corners. In addition, the luminance and color of an object differ significantly from the light originating from the background. Thus, the contrast in light reflected from the corners and edges of an object are used by the visual system to recognize shape and form.

The neural circuits in the retina are organized to enhance the detection of contrast. Unlike most sensory systems that transmit peripheral signals directly to the CNS with little modification, the retina performs a significant amount of processing before sending visual information to the brain. Although photoreceptor output is proportional to the intensity of light reflected from a stimulus, the output of the neurons in the inner layers of the retina is converted into information about luminance contrast. Thus, signals conveyed by the optic nerve fibers do not simply represent the absolute amount of light coming from a particular point in the visual field but, instead, signal spatial locations that contain abrupt changes in light intensity. By transforming light intensity into information about contrast, the retina enhances the perception of stimulus edges.

Visual Receptive Fields. When the eyes are fixated on a point in the center of the visual world, light coming from that fixation point interacts with cones located in the fovea. Similarly, light coming from points in the visual field that are located away from the fixation point interact with different photoreceptors. In fact, because light travels in a straight line, each point in the visual field is represented by a corresponding point on the retina. The area in the visual field in which illumination causes a change in a photoreceptor's membrane potential is called the receptive field for that photoreceptor. All neurons in the retina, including bipolar and ganglion cells, have well-defined receptive fields that are described in terms of the angle, in degrees, away from the fixation point. More generally, the receptive field for any photoreceptor, bipolar cell, or ganglion cell is defined as that region in the visual field that causes a change in the cell's membrane potential when that region is illuminated.

Center-Surround Receptive Fields. Much of our knowledge about the retina comes from physiology studies in which neuronal discharges were recorded from ganglion cells while stimulating the visual field with small spots of light. Experiments performed by Stephen Kuffler in the 1950s showed that retinal ganglion cells have circular receptive fields and respond best to light that stimulates either the center or the circumference of their receptive fields. These studies led to the characterization of two classes of retinal neurons: "on-center" and "off-center" ganglion cells (Figure 11.18). An on-center ganglion cell discharges when light strikes the center of its receptive field but is inhibited by light in the surrounding perimeter. An off-center ganglion cell has an opposite receptive field organization: it discharges in response to light in the perimeter of its receptive field but is inhibited by light in the center.

The population of retinal ganglion cells consists of equal numbers of on-center and off-center cells. Both cell types are distributed uniformly across the retina to signal changes in light intensity that occur in any part of the visual field. Both types of ganglion cells may

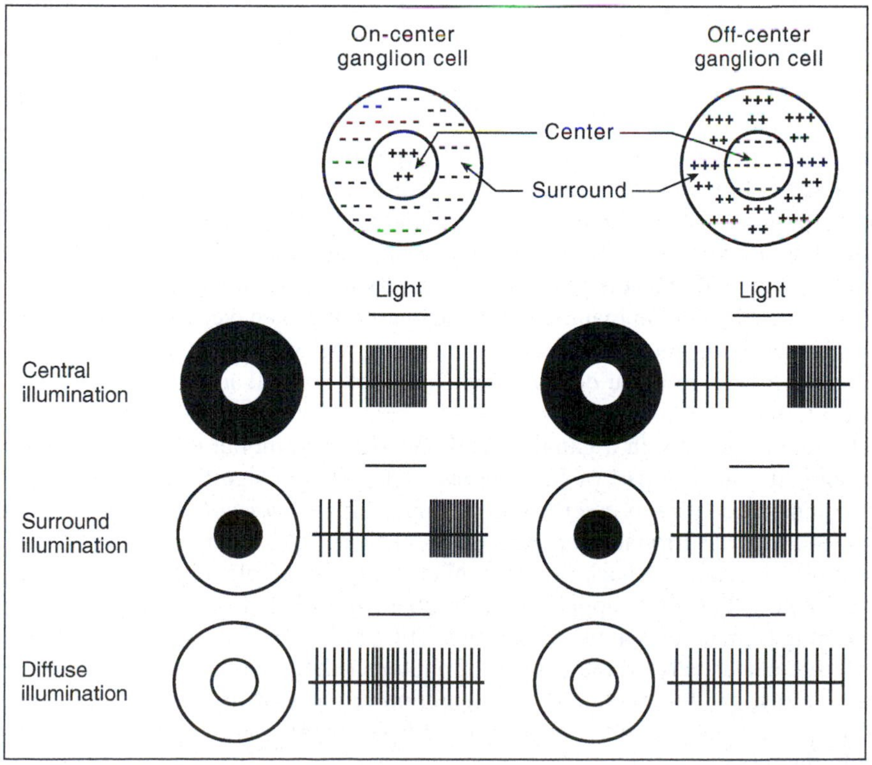

FIG. 11.18. Center-Surround Receptive Fields. On-center and off-center ganglion cells respond differentially to light stimulating the center or perimeter of their receptive fields.

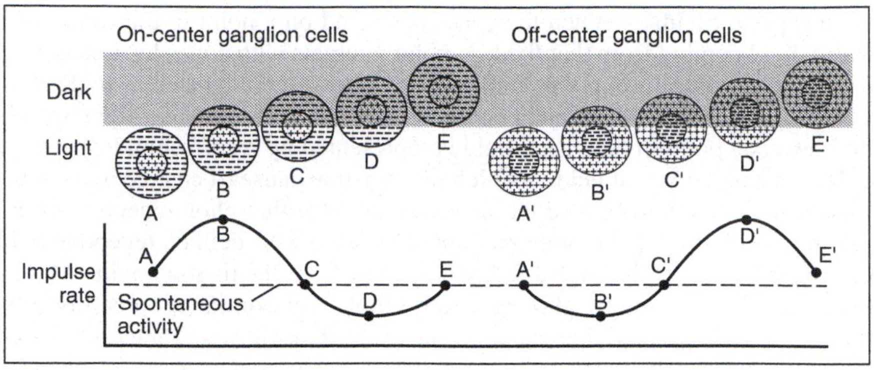

FIG. 11.19. Ganglion Cell Responses to Light-Dark Edges. This figure illustrates the responses of matching sets of on-center and off-center ganglion cells to a light-dark edge. Both types of cells respond best when their receptive fields subtend the light-dark edge. The two sets of cells show different response patterns that distinguish the light and dark sides.

detect a change in luminance; bright light on one side of an edge is signaled by an increase in the firing rate of on-center cells, whereas the darker side of the edge is signaled by an increase in the firing rate of off-center cells. Off-center ganglion cells are necessary because the spontaneous activity of an on-center cell is low and a decrease in illumination would not be signaled by a decline in their firing rate.

Ganglion cells respond best when a light-dark edge falls on their receptive field.

How do cells with circular receptive fields signal the presence of a linear edge of light and dark? The answer to this question is clear from an analysis of ganglion cell responses during different stimulus conditions. The best stimulus for exciting an on-center ganglion cell is a small spot of light that stimulates only the center of the receptive field, whereas the best stimulus for exciting an off-center ganglion cell is a ring of light (an annulus) that illuminates only the perimeter of the receptive field. In both cells, these responses are suppressed by shining light onto the antagonistic part of the receptive field. Thus, illumination of the receptive field perimeter inhibits on-center cells, whereas light on the receptive field center suppresses discharges in off-center cells. Consequently, retinal ganglion cells respond best to stimuli that differentially illuminate the center and surrounding parts of the receptive field (see Figure 11.18). Few visual stimuli, however, consist of small circular lights that stimulate only the center or surround of a ganglion cell's receptive field. Most objects are defined by corners or linear edges characterized by a distinct change in luminance. Although ganglion cells have circular receptive fields, the configuration of antagonistic center-surround regions allows groups of cells to respond differentially to linear edges of light and dark that fall across their receptive fields (Figure 11.19).

The rate of activity in a ganglion cell encodes the amount of contrast between the center and surrounding part of its receptive field. This is significant for perception because luminance contrast is essential for distinguishing an object from its background. The antagonistic center-surround properties of ganglion cells also explain why the perception of brightness is related to background luminance. For example, objects that reflect a uniform amount of light may appear to be brighter or darker depending on the amount of light coming from objects in the background (Figure 11.20). Our perception of brightness is not based exclusively on the density of photons reflected from an object, but depends on the contrast in illumination across neighboring parts of the visual field. The neural basis for perceiving brightness is derived, at least in part, on the encoding mechanisms found in the retina.

Circuit Mechanisms. The antagonistic center-surround properties of on-center and off-center ganglion cells are determined mainly by the afferent connections of the bipolar

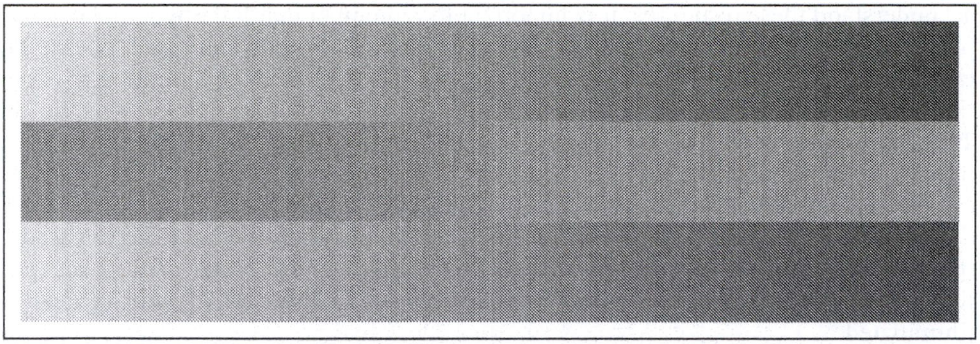

FIG. 11.20. Perceptual Contrast. The center panel reflects a constant amount of light throughout its extent but appears brighter or darker depending on the background illumination. The uniform shading of the center panel can be confirmed by covering the upper and lower panels.

cells. Like ganglion cells, bipolar cells have antagonistic center-surround receptive fields and are classified as on-center or off-center. The primary difference is that bipolar cells do not discharge action potentials because they do not contain voltage-gated Na^+ channels. Because bipolar cells have very short processes, their graded potentials spread passively to the synaptic terminals without a significant reduction in amplitude.

In response to small spots of light stimulating the center of their receptive fields, on-center bipolar cells depolarize and off-center bipolar cells hyperpolarize (Figure 11.21).

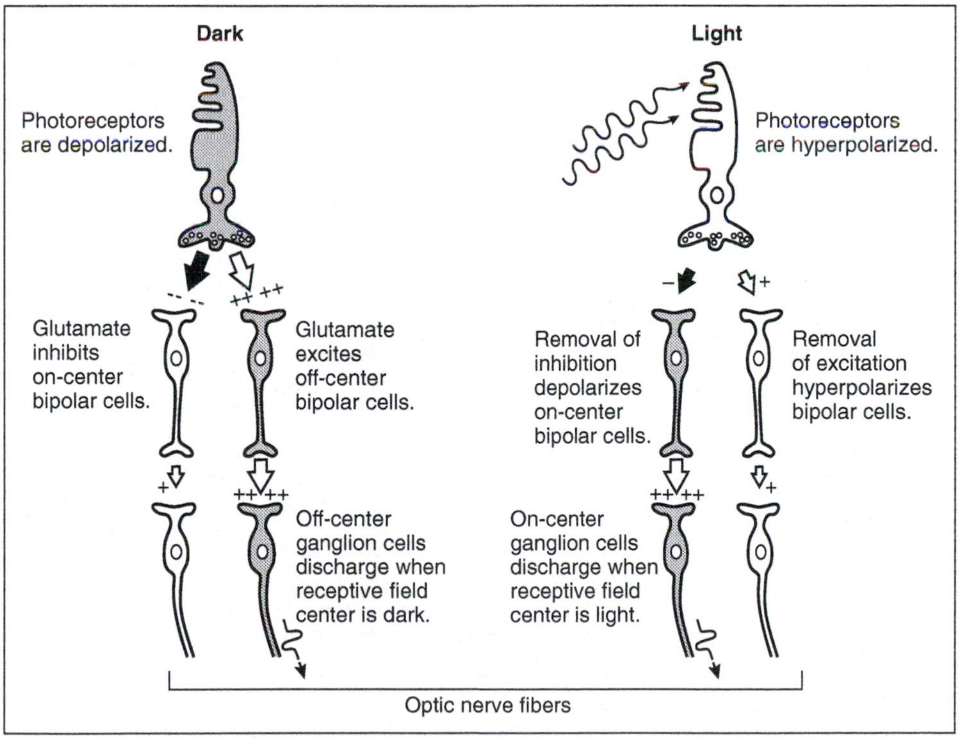

FIG. 11.21. On-Center and Off-Center Responses. Photoreceptors in the dark or light are depolarized (shaded) or hyperpolarized (unshaded) and release more or less glutamate from their synaptic terminals. Glutamate is inhibitory (dark arrows) or excitatory (light arrows), depending on the postsynaptic receptors on the bipolar cells. Arrow size indicates the magnitude of neurotransmitter release.

Glutamate has opposite effects on off-center (excitatory) and on-center (inhibitory) bipolar cells.

Horizontal cells cause neighboring photoreceptors to release more glutamate.

To understand these responses, it is important to remember that light hyperpolarizes the photoreceptors and reduces neurotransmitter release. Both rods and cones release glutamate, which is excitatory in most brain regions, but may produce inhibition or excitation in the retina depending on the type of glutamate receptor on the postsynaptic cell. Thus, glutamate opens the Na^+ channels in off-center bipolar cells, and the resulting influx of Na^+ depolarizes these cells. In the case of on-center bipolar cells, glutamate closes the Na^+ channels but opens their K^+ channels, and the cell is hyperpolarized by the ensuing efflux of K^+. Because light reduces the amount of glutamate released by the photoreceptors, on-center cells are excited by light in the center of their receptive fields, whereas off-center cells are inhibited when their receptive field centers are illuminated.

Light produces opposite effects on bipolar cell activity, depending on whether it stimulates the center or the surrounding part of the cell's receptive field. This antagonistic property is mediated by a lateral network of horizontal cells interconnecting neighboring groups of photoreceptors (Figure 11.22). Bipolar cells do not receive direct synaptic contacts from horizontal cells; instead, horizontal cells synapse directly on the terminals of photoreceptors. This configuration allows horizontal cells to regulate one group of photoreceptors in response to membrane potential changes in a neighboring group of photoreceptors. When a photoreceptor is hyperpolarized by light, the horizontal cells cause adjacent photoreceptors to become depolarized. Thus, on-center bipolar cells are hyperpolarized by light in the peripheral part of their receptive field because the horizontal cells mediate an increase in glutamate release from the photoreceptors representing the receptive field center. Hence, horizontal cells provide a mechanism for mediating opposite responses in adjacent groups of photoreceptors, and this mechanism is used to enhance luminance contrast.

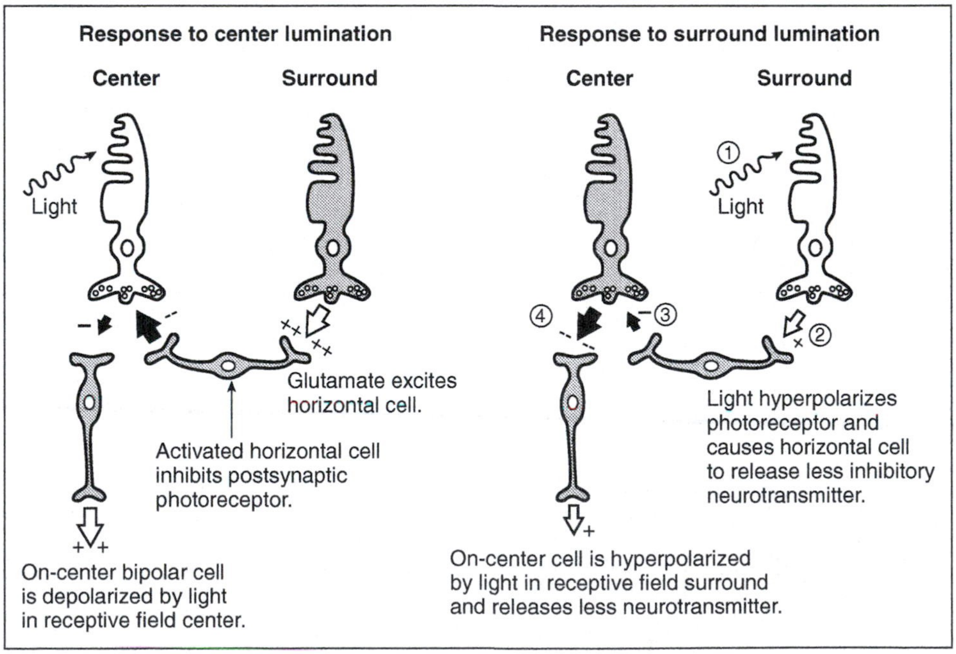

FIG. 11.22. Horizontal Interactions. This diagram shows how horizontal cells alter the responses of an on-center bipolar cell. (1) Light hyperpolarizes photoreceptors in the surround region. (2) As the photoreceptors release less excitatory neurotransmitter, this hyperpolarizes postsynaptic horizontal cells. (3) As the horizontal cells release less inhibitory neurotransmitter, nearby photoreceptors are depolarized. (4) The depolarized photoreceptors release more inhibitory neurotransmitter onto the on-center bipolar cell.

CENTRAL VISUAL PATHWAYS

The visual system consists of a large number of interconnected brain regions that analyze information received from the retina. Visual perception of form, color, motion, and depth is mediated by multiple cortical areas in the occipital, temporal, and parietal lobes. Other brain regions, such as the superior colliculus and specific parts of the motor system, use visual information to guide eye movements and to direct changes in visual attention. Finally, retinal projections to the brainstem mediate pupillary reflexes, whereas projections to the hypothalamus regulate circadian rhythms.

Retinal Projections

Each retina contains 1 million ganglion cells whose axons converge at the optic disk and exit the eye as the optic nerve. The optic nerve proceeds toward the optic chiasm, which lies between the diencephalon and the pituitary gland. At that point, nearly 60% of the optic nerve fibers cross the midline and continue centrally as the optic tract. Individual fibers of the optic tract may terminate in the thalamus, the hypothalamus, or the midbrain.

Primary Visual Pathway. Most retinal ganglion cells project to the lateral geniculate nucleus, which resides in the caudal part of the ventral thalamus (see Chapter 6). Axons from the lateral geniculate nucleus enter the optic radiation and terminate in the primary visual cortex, which occupies the superior and inferior banks of the calcarine sulcus in the occipital lobe (Figure 11.23). The primary visual cortex (Brodmann area 17) is called the striate cortex because freshly cut sections of this area reveal prominent horizontal striations that represent the myelinated fibers passing horizontally within certain cortical layers. The disynaptic retinogeniculostriate pathway is the primary route for conveying visual information to the cerebral cortex. A lesion in any part of this pathway causes partial or total blindness.

Retina → lateral geniculate nucleus → striate cortex

Secondary Visual Pathways. Some projections from the retina terminate in the midbrain to mediate pupillary light reflexes. The afferent circuitry for the pupillary light reflex consists of ganglion cell axons that project to the pretectal olivary nucleus, which lies rostral and lateral to the superior colliculus. Neurons in the pretectal olivary nucleus project

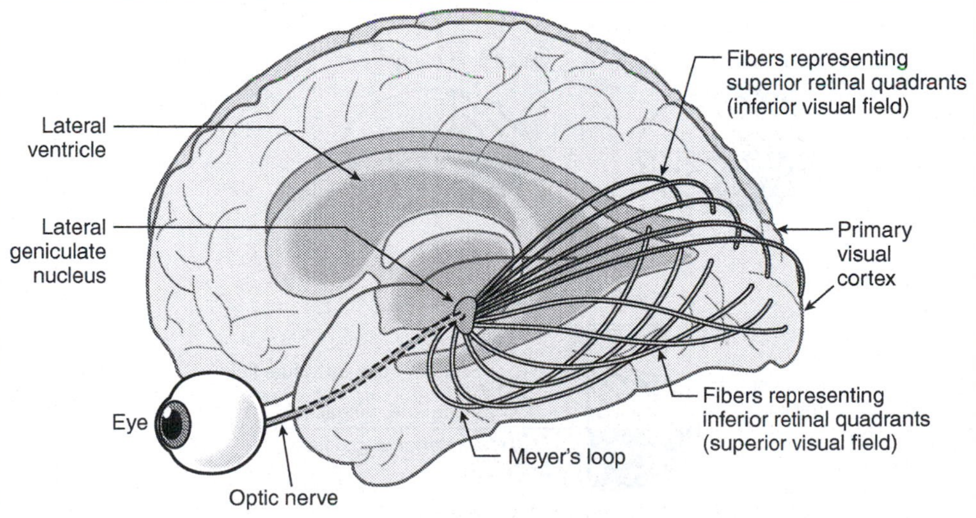

FIG. 11.23. Primary Visual Pathways. Lateral diagram of the brain showing the disynaptic retinogeniculostriate pathway. Geniculostriate projections (or optic radiations) course along the lateral margin of the lateral ventricle. The fibers conveying information from the inferior retina course through the temporal lobe (Meyer's loop) before terminating in the inferior bank of the calcarine sulcus.

bilaterally to preganglionic parasympathetic neurons in the Edinger-Westphal nucleus (see Figure 5.31), which innervate the ciliary ganglion. Postganglionic parasympathetic neurons in the ciliary ganglion innervate the ciliary muscle and the pupillary sphincter of the iris. Thus, in response to shining a light in either eye, the bilateral projections from the pretectal olivary nucleus mediate both direct and consensual pupillary constriction.

If a shadow is cast over either eye, both pupils dilate. Although the pathway mediating this sympathetic response is somewhat uncertain, retinal projections to the midbrain reticular formation comprise the afferent part of this reflex. The midbrain reticular formation sends descending projections to the intermediolateral cell column of the thoracic spinal cord, which contains preganglionic cholinergic cells that project to the superior cervical ganglion. Postganglionic neurons in the superior cervical ganglion ascend in association with blood vessels and innervate the dilator muscle of the iris.

Other retinal ganglion cells project to the superior colliculus, which lies in the tectum of the midbrain. The superior colliculus uses visual, auditory, and somatosensory information to coordinate head and eye movements while tracking a moving object in the visual field or to redirect visual attention in response to a new stimulus (see "Oculomotor Mechanisms" in this chapter).

Finally, a few retinal ganglion cells project to the suprachiasmatic nucleus of the hypothalamus. This brain region uses variations in light intensity to control a broad range of physiologic processes that follow a circadian rhythm.

Visual Fields

The visual space seen by each eye is called the visual field for that eye (Figure 11.24). For descriptive reasons, each visual field is subdivided by vertical and horizontal lines that

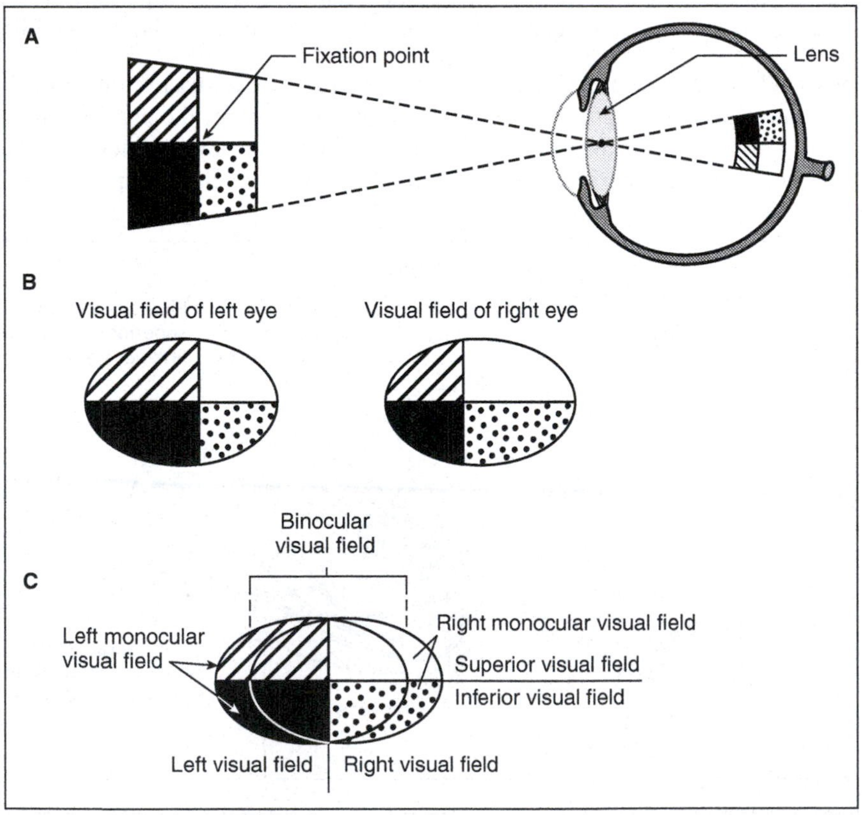

FIG. 11.24. Visual Fields. (A) Fixated images are projected onto the retina upside down and reversed from left to right. (B) Visual fields for each eye are asymmetric because the nasal retina (which views the temporal field) is larger than the temporal retina. (C) The brain fuses the information from each eye into a single image centered around the fixation point. The visual field can be subdivided into left, right, inferior, and superior hemifields.

intersect the point fixated by the fovea. Each visual field is composed of left, right, superior, and inferior hemifields that are "observed" by corresponding portions of the retina. Visual images are inverted by the lens, however, so the visual fields are reversed from left to right and from top to bottom on the retina. Hence, the inferior retina responds to the superior visual field, whereas the superior retina responds to the inferior visual field. The retinal representations for the left and right visual fields are more complicated. The left visual field projects onto the temporal retina of the right eye and the nasal retina of the left eye, and the right visual field is seen by the temporal retina of the left eye and the nasal retina of the right eye.

Both eyes focus on the same fixation point and, consequently, most of their visual fields have substantial overlap. The overlapping region is called the binocular visual field because every point in this area is seen by both eyes; the nonoverlapping regions are called monocular visual fields because they are seen by only one eye (Figure 11.25). The monocular visual fields are crescent-shaped areas that surround the peripheral edge of each side of the binocular visual field and are seen only by the extreme medial portion of the ipsilateral nasal retina. You can demonstrate the existence of monocular visual fields

The nasal retina is more extensive than the temporal retina.

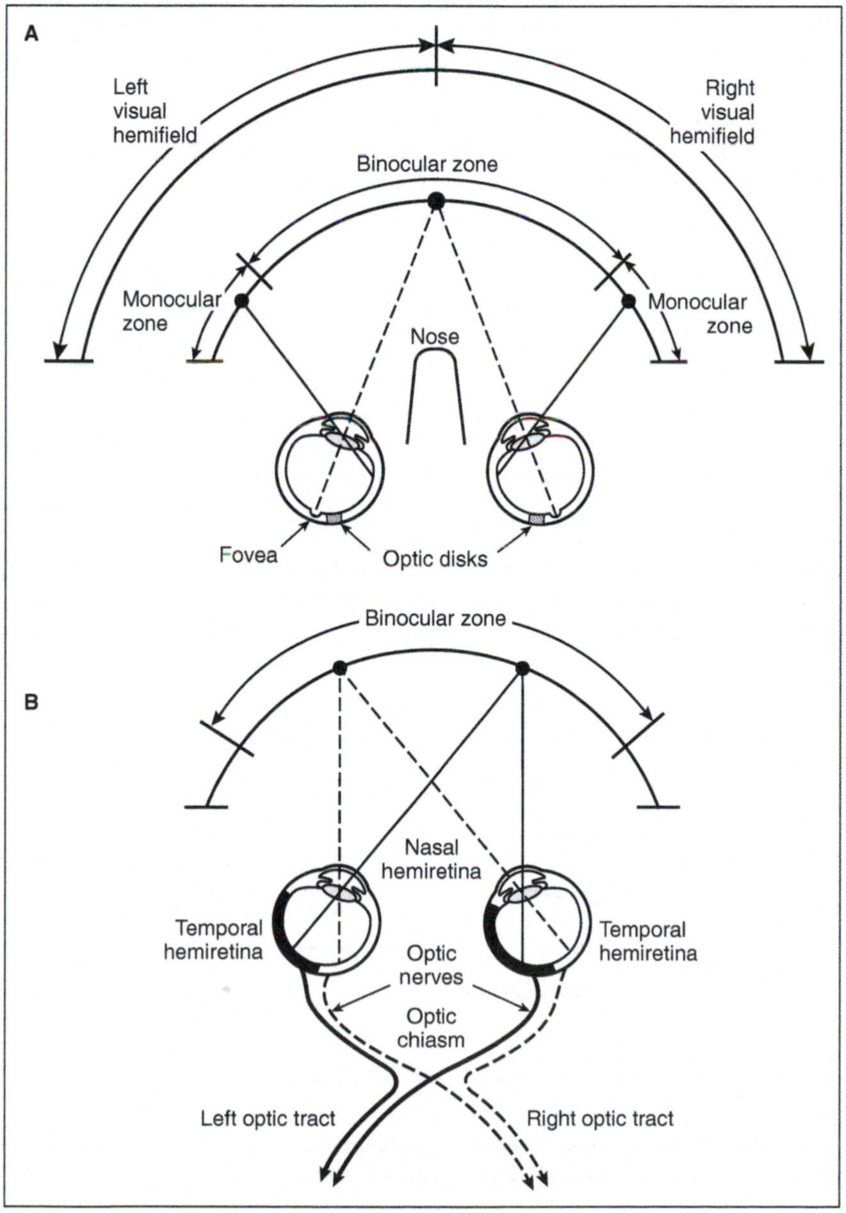

FIG. 11.25. Visual Field Projections onto the Retina. (A) Different parts of the visual field are shown relative to the fixation point. The binocular visual field is seen by both eyes; monocular visual fields are seen only by the extreme medial portion of the nasal retina. (B) Each point in the binocular visual field projects onto a corresponding point in the temporal and nasal retina of both eyes. The partial decussation in the optic chiasm allows information from each side of the visual field to be sent only to the contralateral hemisphere.

by rapidly closing and opening each eye in an alternating sequence. As your field of view switches from one eye to the other, you should notice that objects in the extreme lateral part of one eye's visual field (viewed by the nasal retina) are not seen by the other eye, in part because the latter view is blocked by the nose. In fact, the temporal retina is less extensive than the nasal retina and contributes only 40% of the fibers that comprise the optic nerve; the other 60% of the fibers originate from the nasal retina.

Each cortical hemisphere receives all of its visual information from the contralateral visual field. All ganglion cell axons originating from the nasal retina decussate in the optic chiasm; those fibers coming from the temporal retina remain ipsilateral (see Figure 11.25B). Hence, the optic nerve contains fibers representing both visual fields, but the optic tract conveys information from only the contralateral visual field. Thus, the function of the optic chiasm is analogous to the internal arcuate fibers in the somatosensory system and to the pyramidal decussation in the motor system: each tract ensures that information concerned with one side of the body is processed by the opposite side of the brain.

Topography of the Visual Pathways

The **lateral geniculate nucleus** and **striate cortex** contain retinotopic maps of the contralateral visual field.

The multisynaptic projections from the retina to the cortex are topographically organized. Thus, neighboring ganglion cells in the retina project to neighboring neurons in the lateral geniculate nucleus, which project to neighboring neurons in the striate cortex. By virtue of this point-to-point projection system, the visual system can use the spatial location of neural activity to encode the position of objects in the visual field.

Visual field defects are highly correlated with the location of damage in the visual system, and for this reason it is important for physicians to understand the topographic organization of the visual system. The macular part of the retina, which represents the central 5 degrees of the visual field, is represented in the posterior parts of the lateral geniculate nucleus and the striate cortex. The superior half of the retina projects to the medial half of the lateral geniculate nucleus, which in turn projects through the optic radiations to the superior bank of the calcarine sulcus. By comparison, the inferior half of the retina projects to the lateral half of the lateral geniculate nucleus, which projects anterolaterally into the temporal lobe to form Meyer's loop before coursing posteriorly to terminate in the lower bank of the calcarine sulcus (see Figure 11.23). Due to these projection patterns, the superior visual field is represented in the lower bank of the calcarine sulcus, whereas the inferior visual field is represented in the upper bank (Figure 11.26).

Although the visual system is retinotopically organized, the visual maps in the lateral geniculate nucleus and striate cortex are highly distorted. Nearly half of the neurons in both regions respond to macular stimulation, even though the macula represents only the central 5 degrees of the visual field. The distorted representation of the central visual area reflects the large numbers and high density of ganglion cells in the macula. Furthermore,

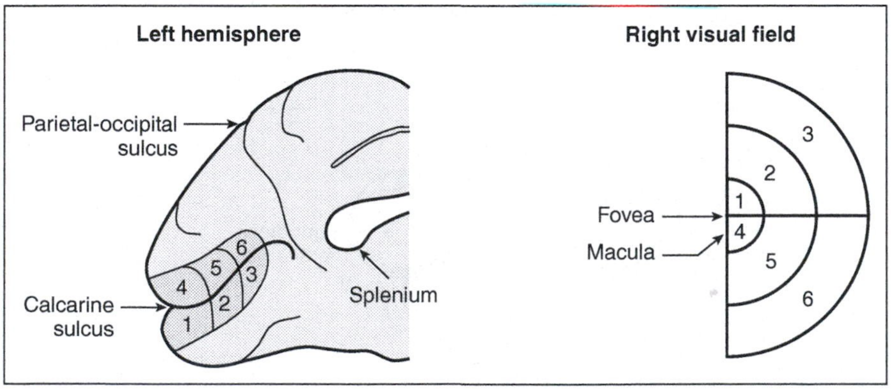

FIG. 11.26. Primary Visual Cortex. This diagram shows how one-half of the visual field is mapped onto the primary visual cortex of the contralateral hemisphere.

because cones in the fovea have a one-to-one relationship with the axons of the optic nerve, this part of the visual field provides a disproportionate share of the visual input to the brain. This disproportionate representation underscores its importance for visual perception and activities such as reading, which require discrimination of fine details.

Visual Field Deficits

Patients suffering from a cerebral vascular accident (or stroke) in the visual system usually experience a loss of vision, or anopsia, in one part of the visual field. Because of its retinotopic organization, focal lesions in one part of the visual system produce a specific visual field deficit. Hence, mapping the visual field of each eye and noting where vision is impaired enables an ophthalmologist to deduce the precise location of a CNS lesion.

Visual field defects provide important clues about the location of lesions in the CNS.

The relationship between lesions in the visual system and specific visual field deficits is illustrated in Figure 11.27. Obviously, damage to one retina or to one optic nerve affects vision for the corresponding eye only. Lesions located more posteriorly in the visual, however, involve the visual fields of both eyes. When the crossing fibers of the optic chiasm are damaged, for example, the visual field deficit is called heteronymous because the visual loss occurs in nonoverlapping parts of the visual fields of the two eyes. In fact, pituitary gland tumors frequently compress the decussating fibers in the optic chiasm and produce heteronymous bitemporal hemianopsia.

Lesions located posterior to the optic chiasm always affect the same part of the visual field in each eye and, therefore, are called homonymous visual field deficits. A complete lesion of the right optic tract, for example, produces left homonymous hemianopsia. More caudal lesions are unlikely to produce complete hemianopsia, however, because the optic radiations occupy extensive brain regions that are almost never destroyed by a single lesion. Damage to Meyer's loop on the right side produces a quadrantic anopsia in the left superior visual field without affecting vision in the inferior quadrant. A vascular accident restricted to the upper or lower cortical bank of the calcarine sulcus produces a quadrantic

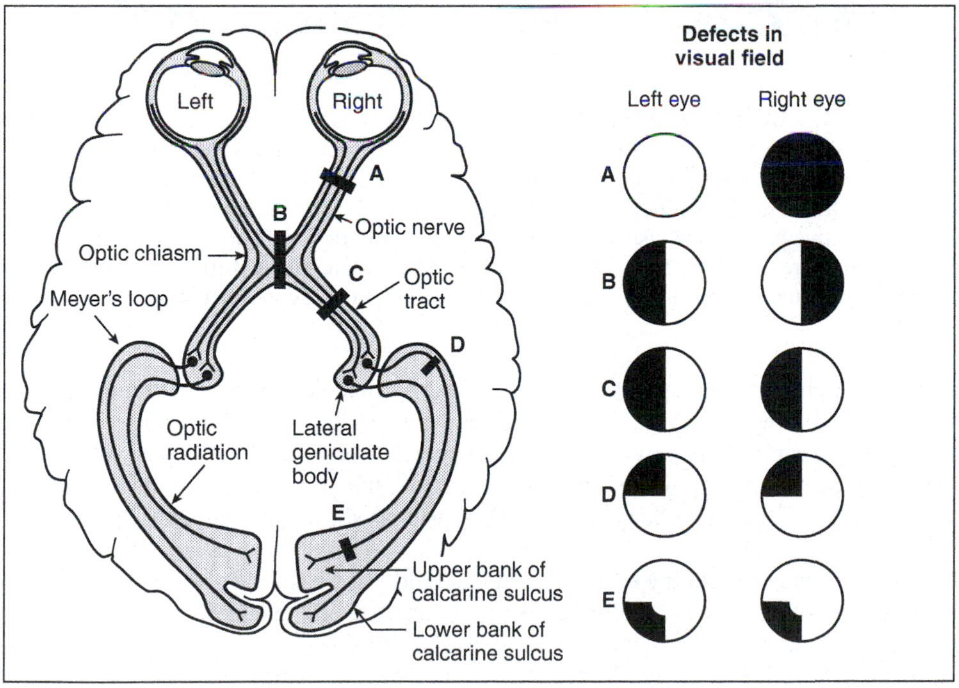

FIG. 11.27. Visual Field Deficits. Lesions in the visual system are correlated with specific visual field deficits. (A) Blindness in the right eye. (B) Bitemporal heteronymous hemianopsia. (C) Left homonymous hemianopsia. (D) Superior quadrantic anopsia. (E) Inferior quadrantic anopsia with macular sparing.

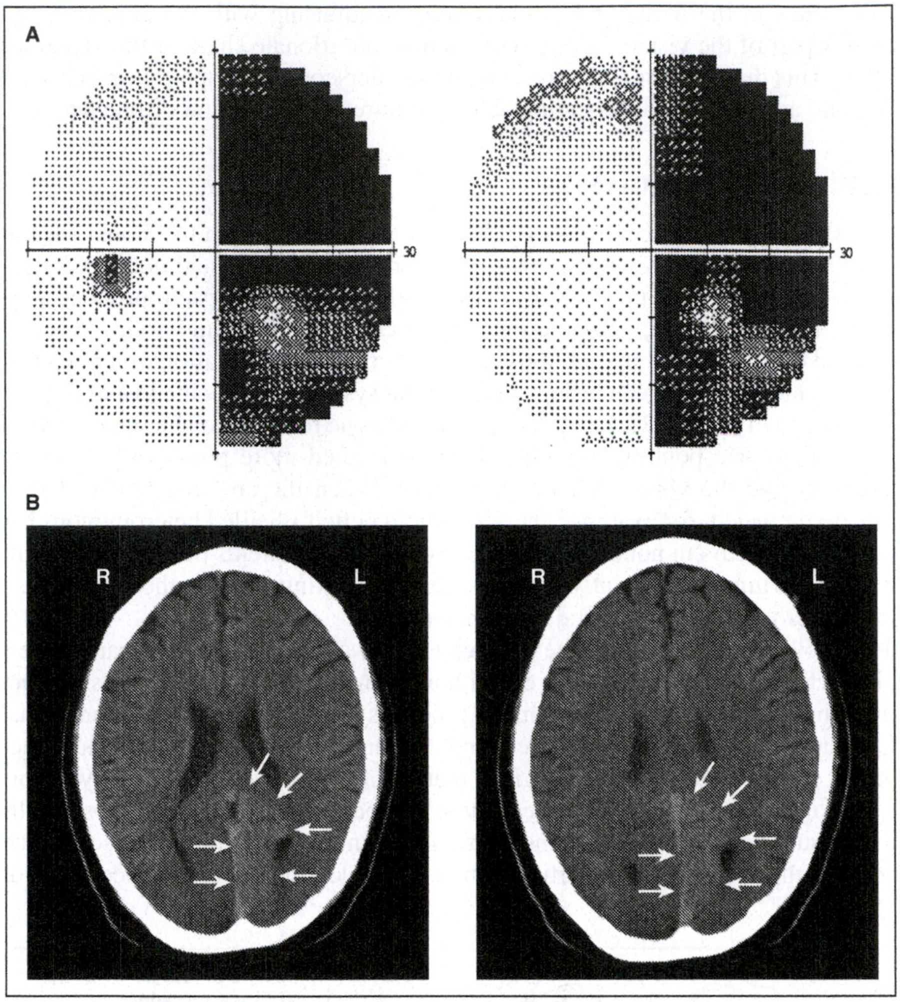

FIG. 11.28. Homonymous hemianopsia. (A) A 24-year-old man underwent cardiac transplantation. When he awoke from surgery, he noticed trouble seeing to his right. Formal visual field testing demonstrated a right homonymous hemianopsia. These diagrams represent the patient's sensitivity to different levels of illumination in the visual field of each eye. As shown, black regions indicate insensitive parts of the visual field; white or light gray regions indicate locations where dim spots of light were detected. (B) An MRI scan revealed an infarct in the distribution of the left posterior cerebral artery (arrows). (Courtesy of Dr. William Cantore, Pennsylvania State University.)

anopsia, which may or may not be accompanied by macular sparing. Although the basis for macular sparing is uncertain, anastomoses between the middle and posterior cerebral arteries may permit blood flow to the occipital pole following a stroke in the posterior cerebral artery. Strokes affecting the blood supply to both the upper and lower banks of the calcarine sulcus produce a homonymous hemianopsia, as shown in Figure 11.28.

Relative Afferent Pupillary Defects. Visual field testing should always be used in conjunction with other tests to determine the likely location of a visual system defect. If a defect in one optic nerve is suspected, the swinging light test can be used to compare the pupillary light reflexes elicited from each eye. In this test, a bright flashlight is directed to one eye and then to the other while the patient stares ahead in a dimly lit room. Dysfunction in one optic nerve causes the pupils to respond more slowly and less completely when compared to the response evoked by the intact optic nerve. In left optic neuritis, for example, both pupils exhibit rapid constrictions in response to shining a light in the right eye. When the light is moved to the left eye, however, the speed and amplitude of the pupillary responses are noticeably decreased. A partial optic nerve lesion may also cause the pupils to constrict only transiently during sustained illumination on the affected side. The clinical value of the swinging light test relies on the fact that the speed and amplitude of the pupillary reflexes are proportional to the number of intact fibers in the optic nerve. In contrast to efferent defects produced by an oculomotor nerve lesion, both pupils are always equal in size in an afferent defect.

A relative pupillary defect may also occur if the optic tract has a lesion or is compressed by a tumor. Even though the optic tract contains fibers from both eyes, a slower pupillary reflex is more likely to be elicited when light is shone into the eye with temporal hemianopsia because the fibers from the nasal retina, which are more numerous than those from the temporal retina, have been damaged. The eye located ipsilateral to the optic tract lesion has nasal hemianopsia, but at least 60% of its nerve fibers are intact, and it can mediate a quicker pupillary light reflex.

Lateral Geniculate Nucleus

The lateral geniculate nucleus is a small, laminated structure in the caudal thalamus that relays information from the retina to the striate cortex. As shown in Figure 11.29, the lateral geniculate nucleus contains six layers that vary in neuronal composition. The two most ventral are called magnocellular layers 1 and 2 because they are composed of large multipolar neurons with large dendritic fields. More dorsally, layers 3 through 6 are called parvocellular layers because they contain smaller neurons.

Each layer of the lateral geniculate nucleus represents the contralateral visual field and receives visual input from only one eye. Layers 1, 4, and 6 receive crossed projections from ganglion cells in the contralateral nasal retina, and layers 2, 3, and 5 receive uncrossed projections from the ipsilateral temporal retina. This pattern of retinal projections

Layers 2, 3, and 5 receive inputs from the eye on the same (ipsilateral) side. (2 + 3 is the same as 5.)

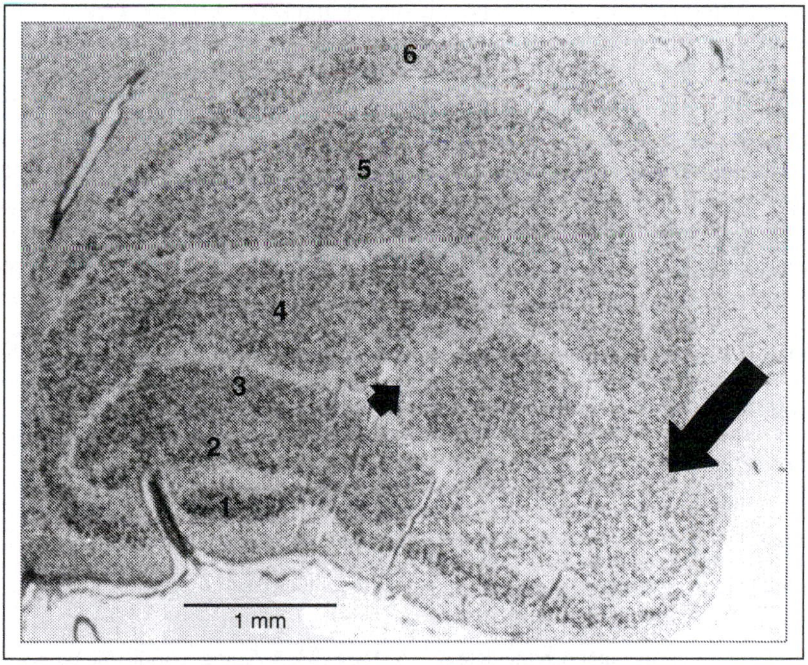

FIG. 11.29. Lateral Geniculate Nucleus. A coronal section illustrates the six layers of the lateral geniculate nucleus. Layers 1 and 2 are the magnocellular layers; layers 3, 4, 5, and 6 are the parvocellular layers. The small arrow indicates the representation of the blind spot in layer 4; the large arrow indicates where layers 4 and 6 have merged together to represent the monocular segment. (Source: Reprinted with permission from Hickey TL, et al: Variability of laminar patterns in the human lateral geniculate nucleus. *Comp Neurol* 183:221–246, 1979.)

explains two morphologic features of the lateral geniculate nucleus (see Figure 11.29). First, the monocular visual field is represented only within layers 1, 4, and 6; layers 2, 3, and 5 are absent because no part of the temporal retina views this part of the visual field. Second, a cell-sparse region appears in layers 4 and 6, but not in layers 3 and 5, because this area corresponds to the blind spot located in the nasal retina of the contralateral eye. Lateral geniculate neurons in the blind spot representation disappear during embryologic development because they never receive functional inputs from the contralateral retina.

The contralateral visual field is represented multiple times among the different layers of the lateral geniculate nucleus. Thus, neurons located directly above or below each other in the different layers of the lateral geniculate nucleus represent the same point in the visual field even though they receive projections from different eyes.

Magnocellular and Parvocellular Comparisons. All neurons in the lateral geniculate nucleus have concentric center-surround receptive fields with "on" and "off" antagonistic regions that are similar to the receptive fields of the retinal ganglion cells. However, the parvocellular neurons differ from the magnocellular neurons in several important respects. Parvocellular neurons have smaller receptive fields and are color selective, whereas magnocellular neurons have larger receptive fields and respond equally to all colors. Magnocellular neurons display transient responses to a flash of light; parvocellular neurons, by comparison, exhibit sustained responses. These functional differences are directly related to the types of retinal ganglion cells that project to the magnocellular and parvocellular layers.

Several structural and functional criteria have been used to classify retinal ganglion cells into two different subtypes (Table 11.2). Retinal ganglion cells that project to the magnocellular layers of the lateral geniculate nucleus are called M cells; those that project to the parvocellular layers are called P cells. The M cells have large cell bodies and large dendritic fields that integrate visual information from a wide expanse of the retina; P cells are smaller and respond only to a small part of the retina. The P ganglion cells tend to be concentrated near the fovea, whereas the M ganglion cells are scattered throughout the retina. Finally, the terminal arborizations of the P ganglion cells are smaller and more densely packed than those of the M ganglion cells.

The functions of the M and P cell types have been studied by analyzing the effects of focal lesions in the lateral geniculate nucleus. Lesions restricted to the parvocellular layers impair color vision and reduce visual acuity. Removal of the magnocellular layers, however, does not affect color vision or visual acuity but interferes with motion perception. These results suggest that the parvocellular layers are critical for detailed visual discrimination, whereas the magnocellular layers detect and analyze moving objects.

TABLE 11.2 Structural and Functional Properties of Retinal Ganglion Cells

M Ganglion Cells	P Ganglion Cells
Large receptive fields	Small receptive fields
Large dendritic arbors	Small dendritic arbors
Large soma	Small soma
Magnocellular projections	Parvocellular projections
Broad terminal arbors	Narrow terminal arbors
Layers 1 and 2 of the lateral geniculate	Layers 3, 4, 5, and 6 of the lateral geniculate
Function: motion processing	Function: visual acuity
Cells scattered throughout retina	Cells concentrated in fovea
Brief, transient responses	Sustained responses
Insensitive to color	Sensitive to color

Note. M = magnocellular; P = parvocellular.

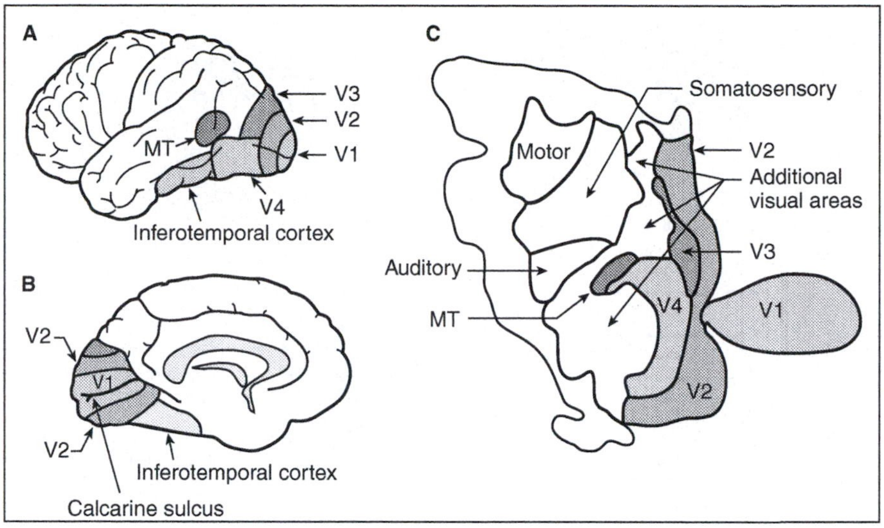

FIG. 11.30. Visual Cortex. (A) Diagram of the left cerebral hemisphere showing the location of the striate cortex (V1) and other major visual areas including V2, V3, and V4. (B) View of the medial surface. (C) A flattened view of the cortex, which reveals the comparative area devoted to motor and sensory functions. More than 25 distinct cortical regions mediate specific aspects of visual function; collectively, they occupy approximately 40% of the total cortical area. MT = medial temporal area.

Visual Cortex

One of the most striking aspects of the brain is the enormous amount of cortex that is devoted to processing visual information. The visual cortex includes all of the occipital lobe and a substantial portion of the temporal and parietal lobes (Figure 11.30). The cerebral cortex contains at least 25 distinct regions that are concerned exclusively with visual function and another 10–15 areas that play a limited role in visual processing. Collectively, approximately 40% of the cerebral cortex is involved in visual perception.

Striate Cortex. The striate cortex is often called the primary visual cortex (or V1) because it is the primary target of the lateral geniculate nucleus. The striate cortex occupies both banks of the calcarine sulcus and contains a complete topographic map of the contralateral visual field.

> Neurons in the striate cortex detect specific features in the visual world.

Unlike neurons in the retina or the lateral geniculate nucleus, neurons in striate cortex do not respond very well to circular spots of light shone on the retina. In the 1960s, David Hubel and Torsten Wiesel showed that striate cortical neurons respond much more to rectangular stimuli that have a light-dark edge. The responses of these neurons vary as a function of the orientation of the light-dark edge, and each neuron has a preferred orientation (Figure 11.31). Cortical neurons that respond to stationary bars of light at a preferred orientation are called simple cells. Simple-cell response properties are a product of convergent inputs from lateral geniculate neurons whose circular receptive fields occupy adjacent, linear parts of the visual field. The dependence of simple cells on convergent inputs from the lateral geniculate nucleus is evident from the fact that simple cells reside near layer IV, which receives geniculocortical projections.

> **Simple cells** detect specific **orientations.**

Other neurons in the striate cortex have receptive field properties that are more complicated. Neurons classified as complex cells, for example, have much larger receptive fields and do not respond well to stationary bars of light. Instead, complex cells respond optimally to bars of light with a preferred orientation that move in a specific direction. Neurons known as hypercomplex cells also have a preferred orientation but become inhibited if the bar exceeds a specific length. These response properties suggest that complex and hypercomplex cells receive convergent inputs from populations of simple cells

> **Complex cells** are orientation and **direction selective.**

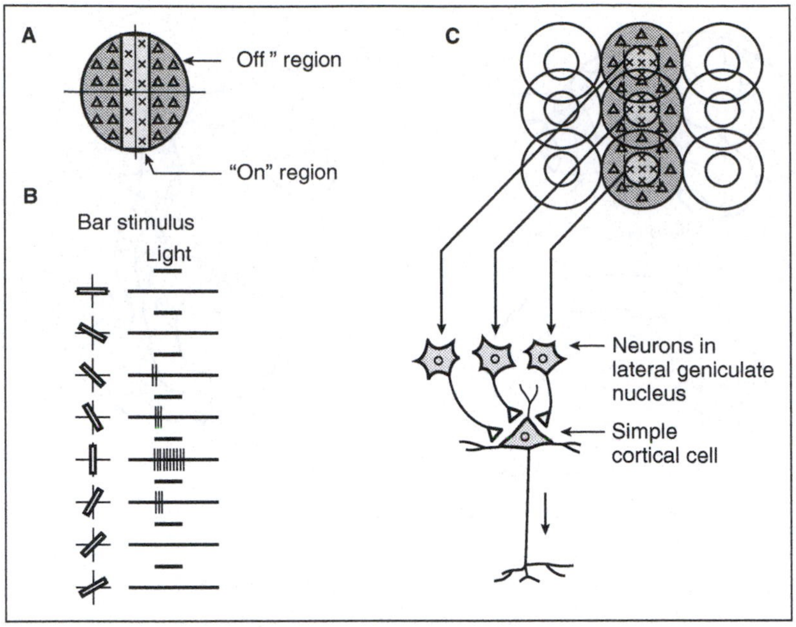

FIG. 11.31. Simple Cell Receptive Fields. (A) Simple cells in the striate cortex have rectangular receptive fields with excitatory (on) and inhibitory (off) regions. (B) Simple cells are orientation sensitive. (C) The rectangular receptive field of a simple cell results from convergent inputs from lateral geniculate neurons with aligned receptive fields.

that respond to adjacent parts of the visual field. Complex and hypercomplex cells are most prevalent in layers II, III, V, and VI, and these layers receive much of their input from the simple cells located near layer IV.

The fact that simple and complex cells respond to specific stimulus features suggests that the striate cortex is organized to detect particular aspects of a visual scene. Furthermore, striate cortex is several times larger than the lateral geniculate nucleus, probably because many more neurons are required to construct the circuits that detect all possible orientations that might appear in any part of the visual field. With these built-in circuits, the specific shape and orientation of objects in the visual field are automatically encoded when specific populations of cortical neurons become active.

Columnar Organization of the Striate Cortex. The striate cortex is organized into repeating modules or columns of cells that respond to specific stimulus features in one part of the visual field. The columnar organization of striate cortex was discovered by comparing the response properties of neurons that were sequentially encountered during orthogonal and tangential electrode penetrations (Figure 11.32). If the electrode traveled orthogonal to the cortical surface, it encountered neurons with similar receptive fields and orientation preferences. If the electrode traveled parallel to the cortical surface, however, the orientation preferences gradually shifted until a complete range of orientations was encountered.

Each neuron in layer IV of the striate cortex responds to photic stimulation of one eye or the other but not to both eyes (see Figure 11.32). Left and right eye dominance occurs in alternating columns of neurons that are 800 μm wide. Neurons located above and below layer IV may respond to both eyes but are more responsive to the eye that activates the neurons in layer IV. Hence, the similarity in ocular dominance represents a functional column. The columnar basis for ocular dominance is determined primarily by the pattern of projections from the lateral geniculate nucleus. Each 800 μm-wide band in layer IV receives its visual information either from layers 2, 3, and 5, which represent the ipsilateral eye, or from layers 1, 4, and 6, which represent the contralateral eye. Vertical projections

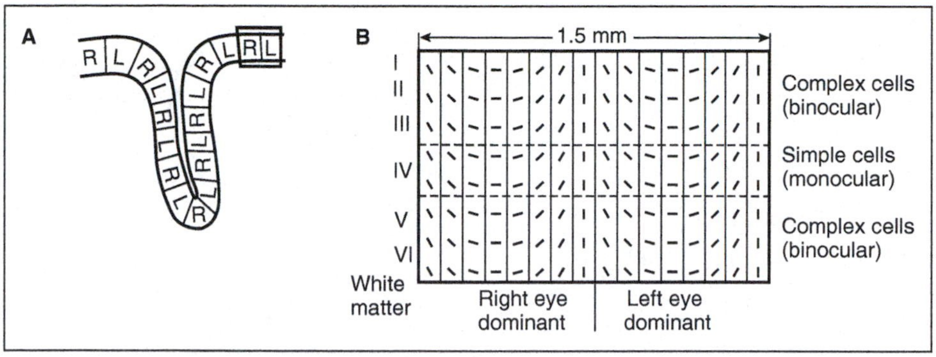

FIG. 11.32. Columnar Organization. (A) Diagram of the striate cortex with an inset of two adjacent ocular dominance columns. (B) Each ocular dominance column contains a series of smaller orientation columns arranged systematically to represent orientations spanning 180 degrees. Simple cells respond to one eye and reside near layer IV. Complex cells may respond to both eyes and usually reside above and below layer IV. R = right; L = left.

from layer IV cause neurons in the supragranular and infragranular layers to have responses characterized by a similar ocular dominance (see Figure 6.9).

Electrophysiologic studies have shown that orientation and ocular dominance columns are superimposed on one another in the striate cortex. Each ocular dominance column (800 μm) contains an orderly representation of all possible orientation preferences. Thus, within two adjacent ocular dominance columns, all possible orientations are represented twice, once for each eye. Other stimulus attributes such as color sensitivity, motion sensitivity, and spatial frequency are also organized into columns or modules that repeat at regular intervals throughout the striate cortex. Neurons sensitive to color, for example, are clustered into segregated regions called "blobs" that contain high concentrations of cytochrome oxidase.

Stereopsis. Neurons located above or below layer IV of striate cortex may respond to visual inputs from both eyes. For some of these neurons, the information received from each eye represents adjacent parts of the visual field, and these binocular responses are used for encoding depth perception. Stereopsis, or vision with two eyes, is critical for depth perception because objects outside the plane of fixation evoke images with some degree of retinal disparity (Figure 11.33). To understand how retinal disparity contributes to depth perception, use only one eye to look at the tip of your finger as you position it in front of an object located a few yards away. As you continue to fixate on your fingertip, open the other eye and you will notice that you perceive two images of the distant object. Fortunately, your visual system interprets the duplicated image as an indication of depth and does not conclude that the object magically replicated itself!

Although the neuronal circuits that mediate stereopsis are not entirely understood, it is well established that binocular responses in the striate cortex depend on normal inputs from both eyes during early postnatal development. Binocular responses do not develop if the cortex is deprived of images from one eye because of uncorrected refractive errors, if the lens is cloudy (congenital cataract), or if images from both eyes cannot be fused because the extraocular muscles fail to align the eyes properly (amblyopia or "lazy eye"). If binocular responses do not develop during childhood, retinal disparity is an ineffective cue for depth perception, and this interferes with certain visual-motor tasks. Therefore, children should be screened for visual problems at an early age so that corrective actions can be taken as soon as possible.

> Binocular vision leads to **retinal disparity,** an important cue for **depth.**

Extrastriate Cortex. Experimental studies have identified numerous cortical areas around the striate cortex that process visual information. Areas located close to V1 are named according to their functional proximity to the striate cortex (i.e., V2, V3, or V4);

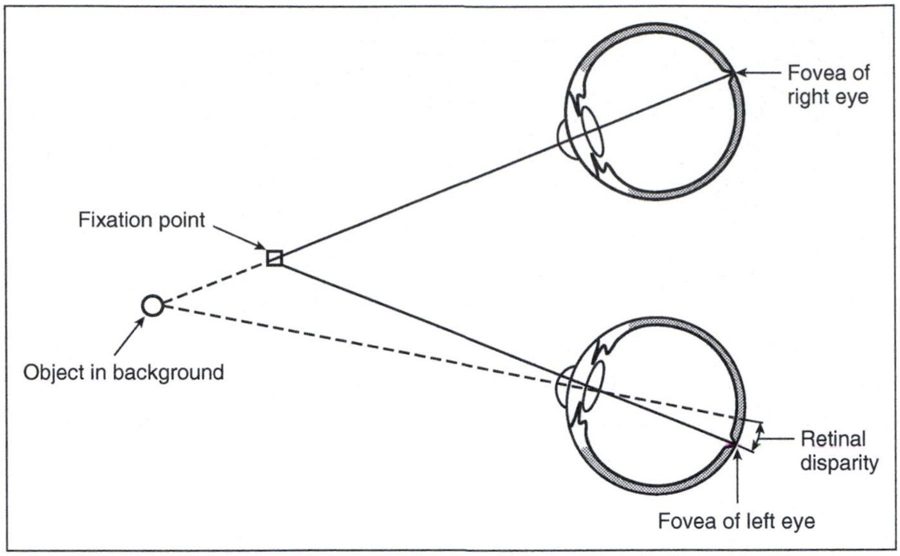

FIG. 11.33. Retinal Disparity. Binocular vision results in retinal disparity for objects that lie outside the fixation plane. In this diagram, two objects are aligned so that their images fall on the fovea of the right eye. The images fall on different parts of the left retina because the background object is located further away.

other extrastriate visual areas are named according to their anatomic location (e.g., middle temporal cortex). Extrastriate cortex includes all of the occipital lobe that lies outside of Brodmann area 17 as well the posterior parietal lobe and the ventral temporal lobe. The striate cortex communicates with these regions through short corticocortical association fibers.

Processing Streams. Stimulus features such as form, color, and motion are analyzed by separate areas within the extrastriate cortex. There are at least two major processing streams in extrastriate cortex that originate largely from the magnocellular and parvocellular layers of the lateral geniculate nucleus (Figure 11.34). The parvocellular and magnocellular layers of

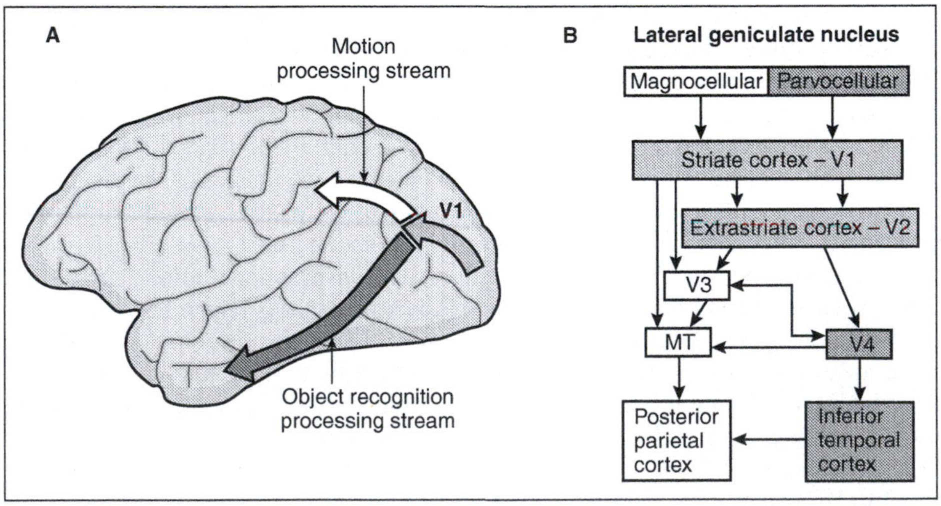

FIG. 11.34. Visual Processing Streams. (A) Lateral view of the brain showing the location of visual processing streams for object recognition and motion perception. (B) Information from the parvocellular and magnocellular layers of the lateral geniculate nucleus is sent through a hierarchical network of cortical areas. Although separate pathways may process specific attributes of a stimulus, lateral connections (reciprocal arrows) probably unify different stimulus features into a single percept. MT = medial temporal area.

the lateral geniculate nucleus project to distinct subdivisions of layer IV in the striate cortex, which in turn project to separate parts of V2 cortex. The magnocellular and parvocellular subregions in V2 form the origin of two separate and divergent processing streams that extend across the remaining extrastriate cortical areas.

The processing stream derived from the parvocellular layers of the lateral geniculate nucleus uses high-resolution information from the macula for pattern perception and object recognition. Regions in V1 and V2 that analyze form and pattern information project to parts of the extrastriate cortex such as area V4 and the inferior part of the temporal lobe. By comparison, the processing stream derived from the magnocellular pathway analyzes stimulus motion and the spatial relationships of objects. The magnocellular pathway receives most of its visual input from the retina surrounding the macula. The parts of V1 and V2 that analyze motion and spatial position project to the medial parts of the extrastriate cortex, including V3, the medial temporal (MT) area, and the posterior part of the parietal lobe. Some evidence suggests the presence of another processing stream for analyzing color information, but this pathway is largely a subset of the parvocellular processing stream.

Parvocellular stream: form and pattern perception
Magnocellular stream: motion perception

The segregation of visual functions into distinct anatomic pathways is reflected by the specificity of symptoms produced by focal lesions in extrastriate cortex. Patients who sustain damage to area MT area, for example, cannot interpret moving objects in a meaningful way. Patients with this disorder, called akinetopsia, recognize objects at rest, but they perceive rapidly moving objects as appearing suddenly at one position and then at another. In another example, patients with bilateral damage to area V4 (on the medial surface of the occipital lobe) have difficulty perceiving color even though their cones function normally. These achromatopsic individuals recognize objects and perceive motion, but their visual world is composed entirely of shades of gray.

There is strong evidence for divergent processing streams in the extrastriate cortex, but it is not clear how segregated pathways might bind different parts of a visual stimulus into a single percept. For example, when students see Dr. Pritchard drive his flashy red sports car along the highway, their visual system automatically links the separate features of this stimulus (i.e., movement, red, car) to form a unified perception. Lateral connections between separate parts of extrastriate cortex (e.g., V4, MT) provide an anatomic substrate for unifying these attributes into a single perception (see Figure 11.34). Recent evidence suggests that these lateral connections are responsible for synchronizing neuronal discharges in the connected regions. Thus, when separate visual features of the same object are analyzed independently by separate cortical areas, synchronous discharges in both regions may provide a perceptual mechanism for binding these stimulus features into a unified percept.

Lateral connections between the processing streams unify separate features into the perception of a single object.

OCULOMOTOR MECHANISMS

To acquire a vivid spatial representation of the world, the visual system constantly directs the motor system to move the eyes so that different points of visual interest are sequentially fixated by the fovea. Signals received from the visual system are used by the motor system to control the precise direction and amplitude of specific eye movements.

Saccadic Eye Movements

We acquire most visual information by making a series of brief, ballistic eye movements called saccades. We emit high rates of saccadic eye movements but usually are unaware of them because the visual system uses only the information acquired during the fixation periods to create a stable representation of the world. Otherwise, the external world would appear to be moving around us because the visual fields are constantly changing with each successive eye movement.

Saccadic eye movements have two motor components: an initial pulse phase followed by a tonic step phase. The pulse phase, which represents the actual ballistic movement of the eyes, is initiated by a burst of activity in the extraocular motor nuclei. The

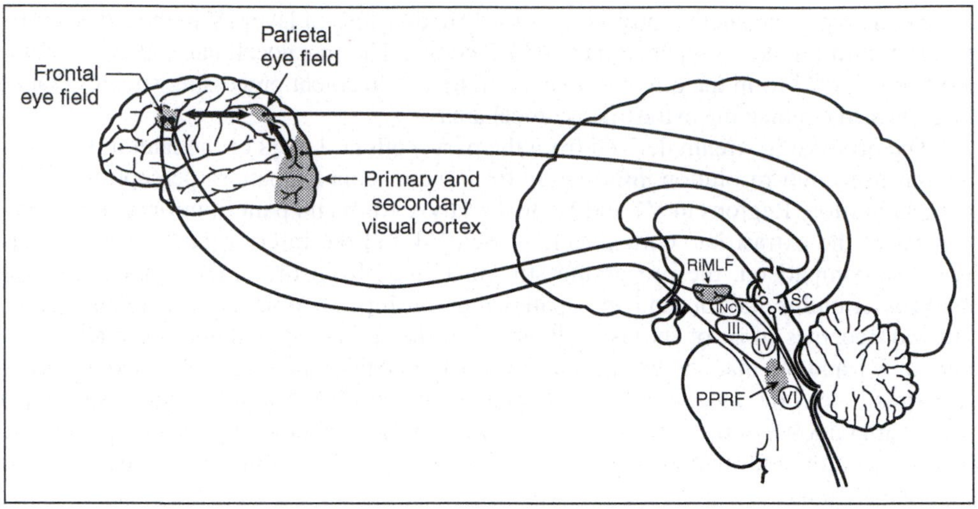

FIG. 11.35. Oculomotor Pathways. Lateral and medial views of the brain depicting the location of the oculomotor structures and their interconnections that mediate saccadic eye movements. RiMLF = rostral interstitial nucleus of the medial longitudinal fasciculus; INC = interstitial nucleus of Cajal; SC = superior colliculus; PPRF = paramedian pontine reticular formation; III, IV, and VI = cranial nerve nuclei.

velocity and amplitude of the pulse phase are determined by the number of active motor neurons and their firing rates. After the pulse phase has been completed, the eyes remain fixated on the target during the step phase because the extraocular muscles remain tonically active. The exact position of the eyes during the step phase is determined by the rate of activity in the neurons innervating each pair of extraocular muscles.

Neural Control of Saccadic Eye Movements. The frontal eye fields and the superior colliculus are responsible for issuing the motor commands that initiate saccadic eye movements. Both of these brain regions receive afferent signals from the visual system and send descending projections to the brainstem nuclei that control horizontal and vertical eye movements (Figure 11.35).

Horizontal and Vertical Gaze Centers. Saccadic eye movements in most directions are composed of distinct movement vectors in the horizontal and vertical directions. Rather than relying on a single brain region to calculate the muscle contractions for a particular saccade, the brainstem contains two separate nuclear regions, known as gaze centers, that independently calculate the motor output needed to produce movement vectors in the vertical and horizontal directions. Thus, all saccadic eye movements represent the combined output of activity from the separate horizontal and vertical gaze centers.

Horizontal gaze movements are controlled by the paramedian pontine reticular formation (PPRF). The PPRF is an elongated region near the midline of the rostral and caudal pontine reticular formation. The PPRF sends excitatory projections to the ipsilateral abducens nucleus and inhibitory projections to the contralateral abducens nucleus. Each abducens nucleus innervates the lateral rectus muscle of the ipsilateral eye and sends crossed projections to the part of the oculomotor complex that controls the medial rectus muscle of the contralateral eye. Hence, the PPRF on each side coordinates the contractions of the lateral rectus and medial rectus muscles of both eyes to execute conjugate horizontal eye movements.

Vertical saccades are controlled by two regions located in the rostral part of the midbrain. The rostral interstitial nucleus of the medial longitudinal fasciculus (RiMLF) controls the pulse phase of vertical saccades, and a nearby region, the interstitial nucleus of Cajal, controls the step phase. Both of these midbrain nuclei project bilaterally to the oculomotor complex, which executes vertical eye movements by activating the superior and inferior rectus muscles.

Superior Colliculus. The superior colliculus is a laminated structure that receives direct projections from some of the retinal ganglion cells, especially M cells, that respond to stimuli moving in the peripheral part of the visual field. Thus, one function of the superior colliculus is to shift visual attention by sending commands to the motor system so that the eyes track specific targets moving through the visual field.

The upper layer of the superior colliculus receives topographical projections from both the retina and the ipsilateral striate cortex. These afferent projections form a detailed map of the contralateral visual field, and each site in this map represents a potential target for visual fixation. In addition, the superior colliculus receives excitatory inputs from the frontal and parietal cortices that direct the superior colliculus to perform eye movements that are consistent with cognitive demands and shifts in visual attention. Electrical stimulation of one point in the superior colliculus elicits saccadic eye movements to the corresponding part of the contralateral visual field. Physiologic recordings have also shown that saccadic eye movements to a visual target are preceded by increased neuronal activity at the corresponding site in the superior colliculus.

The deep layers of the superior colliculus receive visual inputs from the upper layers of the superior colliculus, as well as auditory inputs from the inferior colliculus and somatosensory inputs from the nucleus gracilis and nucleus cuneatus. Hence, the superior colliculus plays a key role in visual fixation by using a variety of sensory modalities to guide eye and head movements to external stimuli.

Projections from the deep layers of the superior colliculus initiate saccadic eye movements and maintain tracking movements of the eyes and head on a moving stimulus. The ventral part of the superior colliculus contains a precise motor map that specifies the direction of eye movements to any point in the contralateral visual field. The oculomotor responses are mediated by ipsilateral tectofugal projections to the RiMLF, the interstitial nucleus of Cajal, and the PPRF. In addition, the superior colliculus sends descending projections to the spinal cord (tectospinal tract) to control head and neck movements.

Reflexive eye movements to objects moving in the peripheral part of the visual field are mediated by the **superior colliculus.**

Frontal Eye Fields. Each frontal lobe contains a small, specialized region that controls voluntary eye movements. Known as Brodmann area 8, the frontal eye fields are located in the posterior part of the middle frontal gyrus and, like other parts of the motor system, receive projections from the cerebellum and basal ganglia. The frontal eye fields also receive massive projections from the extrastriate cortex via the superior longitudinal fasciculus. This visual information is used by the frontal eye fields to direct the eyes toward objects that have visual interest.

Voluntary eye movements are mediated by the **frontal eye fields.**

Efferent projections from the frontal eye fields descend through the internal capsule and crus cerebri to terminate in the ipsilateral superior colliculus, the RiMLF, and the interstitial nucleus of Cajal. Additional fibers proceed further caudally and decussate in the rostral pons to terminate in the PPRF. Hence, unlike the parietal cortex, which projects to the superior colliculus, the frontal eye fields project directly to the eye movement control circuits in the pons. Consistent with these projections, unilateral activation of the frontal eye field produces saccadic eye movements to the contralateral visual field. Unilateral damage of the frontal eye field in one hemisphere may briefly impair saccadic eye movements to the contralateral side, but it does not usually produce a permanent deficit because projections from the superior colliculus provide another route for controlling the pontine eye movement circuits. Similarly, patients may also recover from superior colliculus damage because the frontal eye fields are intact.

RESOLUTION OF CLINICAL CASE

The clinical case in this chapter illustrates signs of pituitary adenoma. Most pituitary tumors are benign and may go undetected if they are asymptomatic. Pituitary adenomas are classified as secretory or nonsecretory. Secretory tumors, which are less common, release anterior pituitary hormones such as prolactin, growth hormone, adrenocorticotropic hormone, follicle-stimulating hormone, and luteinizing hormone. Nonsecretory tumors may cause headaches or produce visual field deficits if the tumor extends superiorly and compresses the fibers of the optic chiasm. Due to the retinotopic arrangement of the optic chiasm, visual loss initially occurs in the superior temporal quadrants and then spreads into the inferior temporal quadrants. Although bitemporal hemianopsia is a classic sign of pituitary adenoma, any pattern of visual loss can occur, including unilateral or homonymous hemianopsia, because the tumor may grow asymmetrically and affect only one side of the optic chiasm. Pituitary tumors may also invade the cavernous sinus and compromise the third, fourth, or sixth cranial nerves to produce diplopia. The best diagnostic procedure for evaluating pituitary adenoma is an MRI scan, because it provides an image of soft tissue without interference from the surrounding bone. Pituitary adenomas can be surgically excised; the mortality rate for this procedure is less than 1%.

REVIEW QUESTIONS

Directions: For each of the following questions, choose the **one best** answer.

1. Which of the following structures participates in the accommodation-convergence reflex?
A. Edinger-Westphal nucleus
B. Pigment epithelium
C. Pupillary dilator
D. Superior colliculus
E. Lateral rectus muscle

2. Which of the following conditions is unlikely to be detected by ophthalmoscopic examination?
A. Diabetic retinopathy
B. Bitemporal hemianopsia
C. Papilledema
D. Hypertension
E. An increase in intracranial pressure

3. What is a likely cause of a bitemporal visual field deficit?
A. Occlusion of the posterior cerebral artery
B. An increase in intracranial pressure
C. Compression of the optic chiasm by a pituitary adenoma
D. Compression of the oculomotor nerve by an aneurysm of the superior cerebellar artery
E. Lesion in one optic nerve

4. Retinal disparity is important for what visual function?
A. Color vision
B. Visual acuity
C. Motion detection
D. Depth perception
E. Saccadic eye movements

5. What ocular function would be impaired by a retinal detachment?
A. Phototransduction
B. Pupillary constriction
C. Accommodation of the lens
D. Conjugate eye movements
E. Blood flow through the central retinal artery

6. A patient has a left homonymous superior quadrantic anopsia without macular sparing. What structure is most likely to be damaged?
A. Right lateral geniculate nucleus
B. Left optic tract
C. Optic radiations in Meyer's loop on the right side
D. Optic radiations in Meyer's loop on the left side
E. Striate cortex in the lower bank of the right calcarine sulcus

7. What part of the eye has neither afferent nor efferent innervation?
A. Lens
B. Cornea
C. Retina
D. Iris
E. Pupillary sphincter

8. What response is produced by parasympathetic activation of the ciliary body?
A. Pupillary dilation
B. An increase in the refractive index of the cornea
C. A decrease in the size of the iris
D. An increase in tension of the zonal fibers
E. An increase in the convexity of the lens

9. Shining light in the left eye produces a consensual pupillary light reflex but not a direct reflex. What is the most likely location of the lesion?
A. Posterior commissure
B. Right oculomotor nerve
C. Left oculomotor nerve
D. Right optic nerve
E. Left optic nerve

10. Which of the following conditions is produced by loss of sympathetic innervation?
A. Pituitary adenoma
B. Horner's syndrome
C. Macular degeneration
D. Crocodile tears
E. Homonymous hemianopsia

ADDITIONAL READING

Classic Literature

Hartline HK, Ratliff F: Inhibitory interaction of receptor units in the eye of *Limulus*. *J Gen Physiol* 40:357–376, 1957.

Hubel DH, Wiesel TN: Receptive fields and functional architecture of monkey striate cortex. *J Physiol (Lond)* 195:215–243, 1968.

——: Receptive fields, binocular interaction and functional architecture in the cat's visual cortex. *J Physiol (Lond)* 160:106–154, 1962.

Kuffler, SW: Discharge patterns and functional organization of the mammalian retina. *J Neurophysiol* 16:35–68.

Reviews and Landmark Research Articles

Behrens MM: Impaired vision. In: Rowland LP. *Merritt's Textbook of Neurology*. 9th ed. Baltimore, MD: Williams & Wilkins, 1995:35–42.

Cheung SH, Legge GE: Functional and cortical adaptations to central vision loss. *Vis Neurosci* 22:187–201, 2005.

Felleman DJ, Van Essen DC: Distributed hierarchical processing in primate cerebral cortex. *Cerebral Cortex* 1:1–47, 1991.

Grill-Spector K, Malach R: The human visual cortex. *Ann Rev Neurosci* 27:649–677, 2004.

Hart WMJ: *Adler's Physiology of the Eye: Clinical Application*, 9th ed. St. Louis, MO: Mosby Year Book, 1992.

Hubel DH: *Eye, Brain and Vision*. New York, NY: W. H. Freeman, 1988.

Klein R, Peto T, Bird A, Vannewkirk MR: The epidemiology of age-related macular degeneration. *Am J Ophthalmol* 137:486–495, 2004.

Koretz JF, Handelman GH: How the human eye focuses. *Sci Am* 259:92–99, 1988.

Nathans J, Thomas D, Hogness DS: Molecular genetics of human color vision: the genes encoding blue, green and red pigments. *Science* 232:193–202, 1986.

Schiller PH, Sandel JH, Maunsell JHR: Functions of the "on" and "off" channels of the visual system. *Nature* 322:824–825, 1986.

Schnape JL, Baylor DA: How photoreceptor cells respond to light. *Sci Amer* 256:40–47, 1987.

Sereno MI, Dale AM, Reppas JB, Kwong KK, Belliveau JW, Brady TJ, Rosen BR, Tootell RB: Borders of multiple visual areas in humans revealed by functional magnetic resonance imaging. *Science* 268:889–893, 1995.

Slakter JS, Stur M: Quality of life in patients with age-related macular degeneration: impact of the condition and benefits of treatment. *Surv Ophthalmol* 50:263–273, 2005.

Sterling P: Retina. In: Shepard GM. *The Synaptic Organization of the Brain*. New York, NY: Oxford University Press, 1990:170–213.

INTERNET RESOURCES

American Macular Degeneration Foundation
http://www.macular.org/

Low Vision Online
http://www.lowvisiononline.unimelb.edu.au/index.htm

National Eye Institute
http://www.nei.nih.gov/

National Institutes of Health
Age-Related Macular Degeneration
http://health.nih.gov/result.asp/416/8

National Institutes of Health
Diabetic Retinopathy
http://www.nei.nih.gov/health/diabetic/retinopathy.asp

Prevent Blindness in America
http://www.preventblindness.org/vpus/vp.html

University of Utah
Primary Visual Cortex
http://webvision.med.utah.edu/VisualCortex.html

Visual Illusions Gallery
http://dragon.uml.edu/psych/illusion.html

Washington University Neuroscience Tutorial
http://thalamus.wustl.edu/course/

William F. Hoyt Neuro-Ophthalmology Collection
http://www.healcentral.org/healapp/searchResults?publicationId=250&page=1

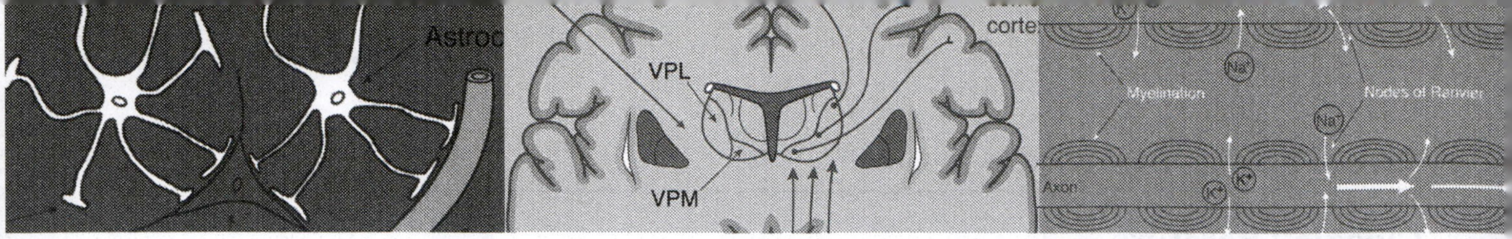

CHAPTER 12

Motor System

INTRODUCTION OF CLINICAL CASE

A 53-year-old man scheduled an appointment with his physician after enduring a litany of seemingly unrelated symptoms for several months. The patient was nervous and jittery most of the time, and he had multiple jerky involuntary movements of the arms. He also noted that his piano playing had deteriorated recently. Perhaps coincidentally, the patient's father had developed similar motor problems when he was about 50 years old, but he died in an automobile accident before seeing a physician. Although the patient dismissed his wife's concerns that business woes were pushing him toward a nervous breakdown, he admitted being depressed and had suicidal thoughts periodically. Among the noteworthy observations during the neurological examination, muscle tone and strength appeared normal, but the patient was unable to sustain a tight handgrip because of constant involuntary movements. In addition, he was unable to visually track the physician's moving pen unless it moved very slowly. The physician prescribed a mild antidepressant and asked the patient to submit a blood sample for genetic testing.

OVERVIEW

Movement is a fundamental activity. The motor system enables us to eat, walk, run, work, and play. When the ability to move is lost, the consequences are catastrophic. Paralysis in the advanced stages of amyotrophic lateral sclerosis (ALS) is so profound that patients are described as "locked in" because the only voluntary movement they retain is the ability to move their eyes.

Amyotrophic lateral sclerosis is known as **Lou Gehrig's disease** in the United States and **Charcot's disease** in the rest of the world.

The central organization of the motor system is complex and involves all levels of the nervous system. The spinal cord and brainstem contain the motor neurons that constitute the final common pathway for motor execution (see Chapters 4 and 5). Subcortical nuclei and the cerebellum refine the temporal and spatial precision of movements. Volitional control of movement is vested in the cerebral cortex. This multi-tiered system is tightly interwoven with the visual, auditory, vestibular, and somatosensory systems, which provide the spatial and temporal contexts within which movement takes place.

The motor system uses elaborate neural loops to plan, execute, and confirm that its actions are being performed properly. As described below, movement is the last step in a multisynaptic loop involving sensory, cognitive, and motor areas of the cerebral cortex. This sensory/cognitive/motor loop is modulated by other loops through the brainstem, the basal ganglia, the cerebellum, and the thalamus that provide the timing and coordination necessary for discrete, efficient, and accurate movement.

CORTICAL CONTROL OF MOVEMENT

The motor cortex consists of three major contiguous areas located in the posterior part of the frontal lobe: primary motor cortex, premotor cortex, and the supplementary motor area. Although there is literature supporting further division of these areas into ten separate motor territories, we limit our discussion to the three major areas. These three divisions of motor cortex differ not only in their histological and connectional properties, but also in their functional characteristics. The cooperative action of these areas is essential for voluntary execution of skilled movements.

Primary Motor Cortex

Movement can be evoked by electrical stimulation of many areas of the cerebral cortex, but the excitation thresholds vary considerably. Charles Sherrington designated the precentral gyrus as the primary motor (MI) cortex because it had the lowest threshold for excitation. The MI cortex (Brodmann area 4) covers the precentral gyrus from the depths of the midsagittal sulcus to the lateral sulcus (see Figure 6.7). Histologically, the MI cortex consists almost exclusively of pyramidal cells with a prominent layer V and an almost nonexistent granular layer IV. Because the MI cortex lacks granule cells, it is referred to as agranular cortex. Betz cells, the largest of the pyramidal cells (70-90 μm), are the histological hallmark of Brodmann area 4, but other than their size, they have no special significance.

In both neurosurgical patients and animals, brief pulses of electric current applied to the MI cortex contract individual muscles of the body on the contralateral side. Most of the projections to the facial and trigeminal motor nuclei, the nucleus ambiguus, and the spinal accessory nucleus are bilateral. Experiments that examined widespread areas of the MI cortex have demonstrated that the entire body is represented along the precentral gyrus in a fashion similar to that of the primary somatosensory cortex on the postcentral gyrus (Figure 12.1; see also Figure 7.10). Based upon experiments using brief electrical stimulation, the organization of the motor homunculus is related to the degree of fine motor control, rather than the size of the peripheral muscle or limb. Thus, the large representations of the face and fingers in the MI cortex provide the basis for the exquisite control we have over those parts of the body. Focal stimulation of the MI cortex has shown that neurons related to particular muscles or muscle groups have a columnar organization, an obvious homolog to the primary

Electrical stimulation of the MI cortex contracts individual muscles.

Homunculus, from Latin, means "small person."

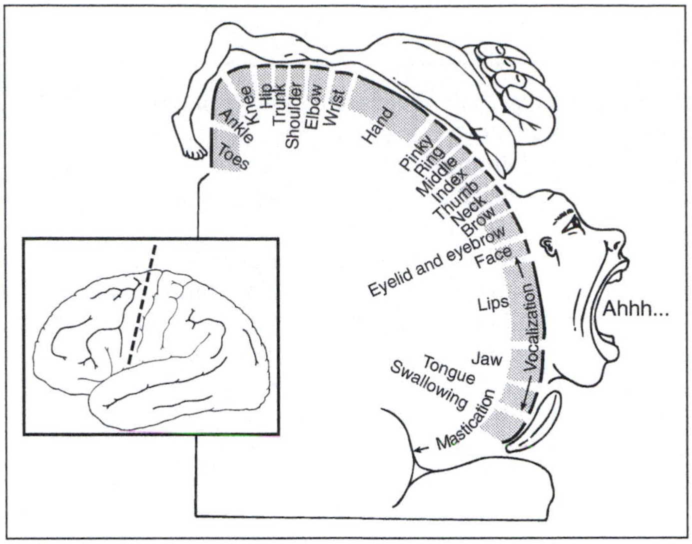

FIG. 12.1. Somatotopic Map of Primary Motor Cortex. The distorted body map represents differences in fine motor control.

somatosensory, auditory, and visual cortices described previously. Individual muscles, especially those related to the digits and the perioral area, are represented at multiple loci within circumscribed areas of cortex. It is believed that muscles with a multiple representation participate in more complex movements than muscles represented only at a single site.

Neuron pools are the basis for motor precision.

Electrophysiological recordings from animals trained to aim a joystick at a target have shown that the activity of individual neurons in the MI cortex is correlated with the direction and force of arm movement. This correlation, however, is too variable to account for the high degree of motor precision shown by the animals. In fact, precise movements are not controlled by individual cortical neurons, but rather by the combined output of many motor neurons. Because each site in MI cortex controls relatively small groups of muscles, complex multimuscle and multijoint movements require coordinated activity across distributed parts of MI cortex.

Some motor coordination may originate within the MI cortex. When long-duration focal stimulation of the MI cortex is used, coordinated and behaviorally relevant movements are evoked. For example, stimulation within the forearm/finger representation of MI cortex evokes a grasping movement by the wrist and fingers followed by a sweeping motion toward the chest or face. Stimulation at other sites moves the arm into defensive or guarding positions. It is noteworthy that the trajectory of these movements varies as a function of the limb's initial position in order to bring the limb to the same final posture (e.g., in front of the face). These data are relatively new, but they are well supported and likely to push the field of neuroscience to reconsider how complex movements are coordinated by the forebrain.

Coordinated movement is imposed upon primary motor cortex by the premotor and supplementary motor cortices.

The more traditional and also well-supported view is that motor coordination is imposed upon MI cortex by the premotor and supplementary motor areas. Both areas have direct projections to the spinal cord but also plan and coordinate complex movements through their projections to the MI cortex. The MI cortex also receives direct projections from the primary somatosensory cortex, as well as indirect projections from the basal ganglia and cerebellum. Collectively, these areas provide MI cortex with the instruction set required to execute skilled movements (Figure 12.2).

Premotor Cortex

Electrical stimulation of the premotor cortex produces complex movements.

Premotor cortex (Brodmann area 6) is located immediately rostral to MI cortex and contains several motor homunculi; none, however, are as well defined as the motor map in the MI cortex (see Figure 6.7). Compared to MI cortex, movements evoked by electrical stimulation of premotor cortex are more complex (e.g., simultaneous turning of the

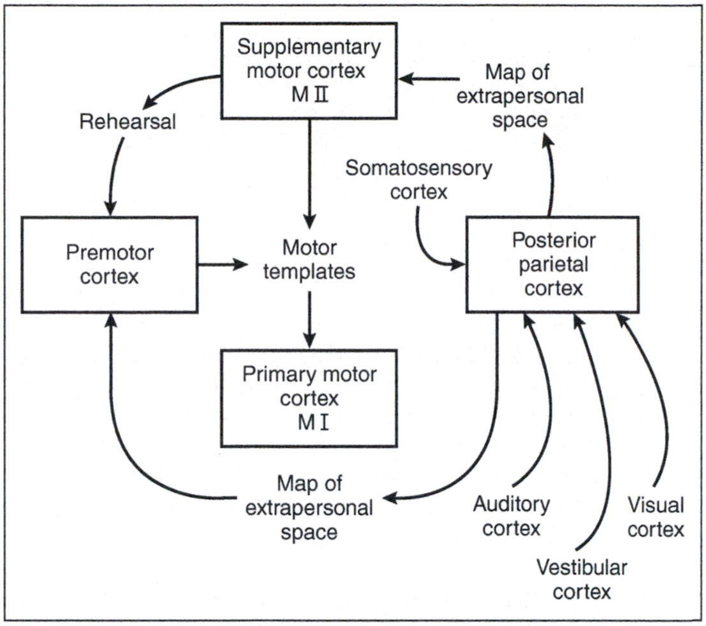

FIG. 12.2. Corticocortical Projections Guide Movement. Movement takes place in the context of our extrapersonal space. Sensory information gathered from the visual, auditory, vestibular, and somatosensory systems is assembled by the posterior parietal cortex into a map of our extrapersonal space. The premotor and supplementary motor cortices create templates for movement within this space. All of the motor cortices, including MI, execute these motor templates.

Premotor cortex creates motor templates for MI.

torso and head) and require stronger electric currents. Premotor cortex exerts direct control over the axial (trunk) and proximal (limb) musculature through its projections to MI cortex, the reticular formation, and the spinal cord. The corticocortical projections to primary motor cortex provide templates or recipes for complex movement that involve not only the trunk and limb muscles, but also the distal musculature (i.e., digits). Control of the digits is the province of the primary motor cortex. The combined action of these corticocortical, corticoreticular, and corticospinal projections enables the premotor cortex to generate complex and coordinated movements of the torso, arms, and fingers.

The motor templates generated by the premotor cortex are reminiscent of those used by Broca's area to orchestrate the oral, perioral, laryngeal, and respiratory movements executed by primary motor cortex during speech. In order to generate these motor templates, premotor cortex must take into account the context in which the planned movement will take place. Contextual information is provided by the posterior parietal cortex, which constructs and maintains a map of the body's extrapersonal space (see Figure 12.2). The role of the posterior parietal cortex in volitional movement is discussed later in this chapter.

Because the premotor cortex provides the spatial and temporal recipe or template for movement, the neural activity there increases prior to that in MI cortex and the spinal cord. These data, as well as the clinical literature, suggest that the premotor cortex is a form of higher-order motor cortex.

Supplementary Motor Area

MII rehearses internally generated movements.

The supplementary motor area (MII) forms the medial part of Brodmann area 6 that is buried within the midsagittal sulcus (see Figure 6.6). Like the premotor cortex, the supplementary motor cortex provides the MI cortex with the motor templates it requires to perform voluntary movement. The MII cortex has a homunculus, but it is not as well defined as the map in the primary motor cortex. Electrical stimulation of the MII cortex produces complex movements of the trunk muscles contralaterally or the limb muscles bilaterally. Like the premotor cortex, neuronal activity in the MII cortex increases prior to the onset of

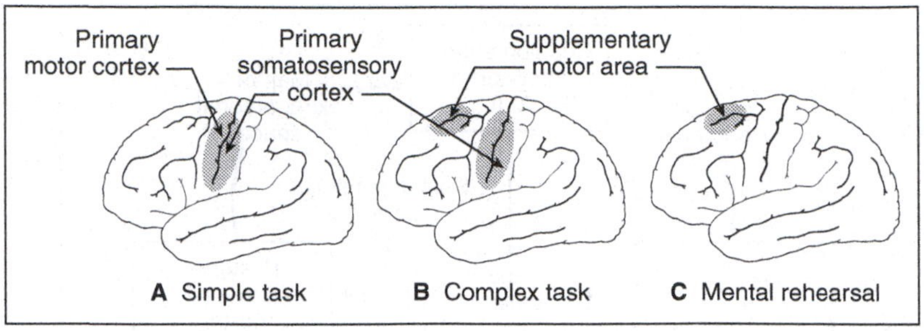

FIG. 12.3. Blood Flow in the Motor Cortices during Three Different Types of Movement. (A) Simple task: Repeated apposition of the index finger and the thumb activates the finger areas of the primary motor and sensory cortices along the central sulcus. (B) Complex task: Apposition of several fingers to the thumb, one at a time in a specified order, activates the same motor and sensory areas as the first task as well as circumscribed areas in the premotor and MII cortices. (C) Mental rehearsal: The subject remains motionless and rehearses the complex task; only the MII cortex is active during mental rehearsal.

movement, which suggests that it also rehearses and organizes complex movements as a service to primary motor cortex (Figure 12.3). Unlike the premotor cortex, the movements driven by the MII cortex are internally generated rather than triggered by sensory stimuli.

Posterior Parietal Cortex

Posterior parietal cortex creates the internal representation of our immediate extrapersonal space.

Brodmann areas 5 and 7 in the superior parietal lobule are sensory association areas that are critical to generating volitional movement (see Figure 6.6). In order for movement to occur, the motor areas in the frontal lobe must have a spatial context in which to operate. The posterior parietal lobe uses visual, auditory, somatosensory, vestibular, and proprioceptive information to construct a map of the body's immediate extrapersonal space.

Projections from the posterior parietal cortex to the premotor and supplemental (MII) motor areas provide the spatial context necessary for reaching, grasping, and tracking objects as well as walking through a crowded a room. Patients with damage to the posterior parietal cortex neglect the contralateral visual and tactile fields and thus are unable to interact with half of their world (see Chapter 6). Although sensory neglect is not a motor deficit per se, the extrapersonal space generated by the posterior parietal cortex is essential for creating motor templates in the premotor and supplementary motor areas, and by extension, for initiating volitional movement (see Figure 12.2).

Descending Projections from Motor Cortex

Seven major descending pathways originate in the motor cortex. The corticobulbar projections that control face and mouth movements were discussed in Chapter 5. The corticothalamic, corticostriatal, and corticopontine projections are the first legs of the multisynaptic neural loops through the thalamus, basal ganglia, and cerebellum that modulate motor performance; each is discussed later in this chapter. The corticospinal, corticorubral, and corticoreticular pathways have a more direct impact on body movements.

Control of the digits is the province of primary motor cortex.

The corticospinal tract controls the axial, proximal, and distal musculature, but its most important responsibility is fine motor control of the digits (see Figures 4.27 and 4.28). For this reason, more than half of its axons terminate in the lateral part of the anterior horn of the cervical enlargement. Despite its close association with precision movements, only 30% of the corticospinal tract originates in MI cortex; the remaining axons derive from Brodmann area 6 (30%) and the parietal lobe (40%). The descending projections from the postcentral gyrus terminate in the posterior horn and modulate sensory information derived from the dorsal roots.

The corticorubral tract originates in the MI, the MII, and the premotor cortices. Neurons in MI cortex terminate in a somatotopic fashion within the red nucleus. The neurons in the

MI cortex that control the fingers terminate in the part of the red nucleus that projects to the lateral half of the anterior horn, which primarily affects the distal musculature. The corticoreticular/reticulospinal and the corticorubral/rubrospinal pathways originate in the MII and premotor cortices, project to the medial half of the anterior horn, and control the trunk and limb muscles (see Figure 4.23). The rubrospinal and reticulospinal tracts coordinate complex, cooperative movements of the trunk and limb muscles such as turning the head and torso while moving the arms and hands.

The **reticulospinal pathways** originate in the pons and medulla.

Lesions of Motor Cortex

Motor deficits caused by cortical lesions vary according to the size and location of the damage. Unlike lower motor neuron damage, which usually causes paralysis, lesions of the motor areas in the frontal lobe produce severe weakness, known as paresis. In addition, patients with cortical lesions rarely show the degree of spastic paralysis that accompanies damage to lower levels of the corticospinal system. Additional symptoms related to upper and lower motor neuron damage are described in Chapter 4.

Cortical lesions are more likely to produce paresis than paralysis.

Patients with primary motor cortex damage initially exhibit a flaccid paralysis followed by slow and incomplete recovery that begins in the axial and proximal musculature and gradually moves toward the digits. Movement of the trunk and arms survives damage restricted to the MI cortex because many descending projections to the axial and proximal musculature originate in the premotor and supplementary motor cortices. Patients with damage to the MI cortex may show some recovery in the digits but are unlikely to recover independent control of their fingers. The inability to fractionate motor control of the fingers interferes with manual dexterity. Thus, damage to the MI cortex interferes with motor proficiency rather than the ability to comprehend, learn, or remember a motor sequence.

Patients with cortical damage rarely show extensor rigidity, but they will show a positive Babinski sign.

Recovery of function: proximal to distal spread

Damage to premotor cortex causes paresis of the trunk and limb muscles and interferes with the choreography of complex movements. Neurological conditions that affect the premotor cortex also produce defects in motor planning and in learning new motor sequences. Complex motor sequences are still possible following damage to the premotor cortex, but they are slow and poorly executed and, by analogy, they are reminiscent of the speech pathology following damage to Broca's area. Because movements generated by premotor cortex are heavily dependent on the map of the extrapersonal space generated by the posterior parietal cortex, visually guided movements are severely affected by damage to the premotor cortex.

Damage to premotor cortex affects choreography of complex movements.

Patients suspected of having premotor cortical damage can be tested at the bedside with the Luria test, in which the examiner demonstrates a repeating sequence of hand gestures in a specific pattern (e.g., fist, chop slap; fist chop, slap). Patients with premotor cortex damage struggle to reproduce the sequence of hand gestures. After the examiner changes the sequence (e.g., chop, slap, fist; chop, slap, fist), these patients may be unable to shift to the novel motor pattern. Prefrontal motor cortex is essential for acquisition, execution, and modification of complex motor tasks. Such motor deficits are seen in patients with Huntington's disease and Pick's frontotemporal dementia.

Whereas lesions in the premotor cortex interfere with visually guided movements, damage to MII cortex hinders internally generated movement sequences. Lesions in MII cortex have their greatest impact on complex motor sequences and goal-directed behaviors that require planning. For example, monkeys with lesions in MII and premotor cortices attempt to obtain food treats by reaching through a transparent screen rather than reaching around it. Lesions in MII cortex also produce motor apraxia, an inability to perform skilled movements that cannot be attributed to paralysis, per se. These patients can use each hand independently, but not cooperatively (e.g., holding a lid open with one hand while removing the contents with the other hand).

Modulation of the Motor System

The MI cortex is responsible for executing voluntary movement, but it depends heavily on input from other brain areas through elaborate, multineuronal loops. As discussed above, the visual, auditory, and somatosensory systems provide the motor system with information about the local environment within which the next movement will take place. Two other parts of the brain, the basal ganglia and the cerebellum, support volitional movement in other ways. The basal ganglia improve the quality and modulate the amplitude of movements, in part by suppressing competing movements. The cerebellum increases the precision of skilled, complex movements. Whereas damage to the motor cortex, its descending pathways, or the lower-order neurons that innervate muscles produces either paresis or paralysis, lesions within the basal ganglia or cerebellum merely degrade motor performance. Nevertheless, both the basal ganglia and the cerebellum play vital roles in motor control.

BASAL GANGLIA

Gross Anatomy

The four parts of the basal ganglia: caudate, putamen, globus pallidus, subthalamic nucleus

Caudate + putamen = **neostriatum**

The basal ganglia include the caudate nucleus, the putamen, the globus pallidus, and the subthalamic nucleus. Other nuclei closely affiliated with the basal ganglia include the substantia nigra, the ventral tegmental area, and the nucleus accumbens (Figure 12.4).

The caudate nucleus and the putamen have the same cytoarchitecture, contain the same neurochemicals, and have similar afferent and efferent connections, so they are grouped into a single entity called the neostriatum. Both parts of the neostriatum are embryologic derivatives of the same cells, but during development they become almost completely separated by the ingrowing fibers of the internal capsule. Rostrally, the putamen is continuous with the head of the caudate nucleus in two places, along the medial edge of the internal capsule and through perforations in the internal capsule called striatal bridges (Figures 12.5 and 12.6).

The caudate nucleus consists of three parts: a large head, a body that tapers posteriorly, and a long, C-shaped tail; all have a close spatial relationship with the lateral ventricle. The head of the caudate nucleus forms the lateral wall of the anterior horn of the lateral ventricle and, for this reason, is an important radiologic landmark (see Figure 12.5). Between the interventricular foramen and the collateral trigone, the body of the caudate nucleus lies on the dorsolateral surface of the thalamus. The tail of the caudate nucleus descends into the inferior horn of the lateral ventricle and ends immediately posterior to the amygdala.

GPi = medial pallidal segment; GPe = lateral pallidal segment

The **subthalamic nucleus** contains glutamatergic neurons.

The putamen, the largest component of the basal ganglia, is located lateral to the internal capsule and the globus pallidus. Together, the putamen and its medial neighbor, the globus pallidus, form a wedge-shaped region called the lenticular nucleus (see Figure 6.1A). A thin layer of myelinated fibers called the external medullary lamina separates the putamen from the globus pallidus; the thinner internal medullary lamina divides the globus pallidus into internal (GPi) and external (GPe) pallidal segments. Some authors refer to the GPi and GPe as the medial and lateral pallidal segments, respectively. The globus pallidus is closely associated with the subthalamic nucleus, a lens-shaped nucleus sandwiched between the zona incerta and the internal capsule in the caudal diencephalon (Figure 12.7; see also

- Basal ganglia
  - Striatum
    - Caudate nucleus
    - Putamen
  - Globus pallidus
  - Nucleus accumbens
  - Subthalamic nucleus
  - Substantia nigra/ventral tegmental area

Putamen + Globus pallidus = Lentiform nucleus

Caudate nucleus + Putamen + Globus pallidus = Corpus striatum

FIG. 12.4. The Basal Ganglia and Their Affiliated Nuclei.

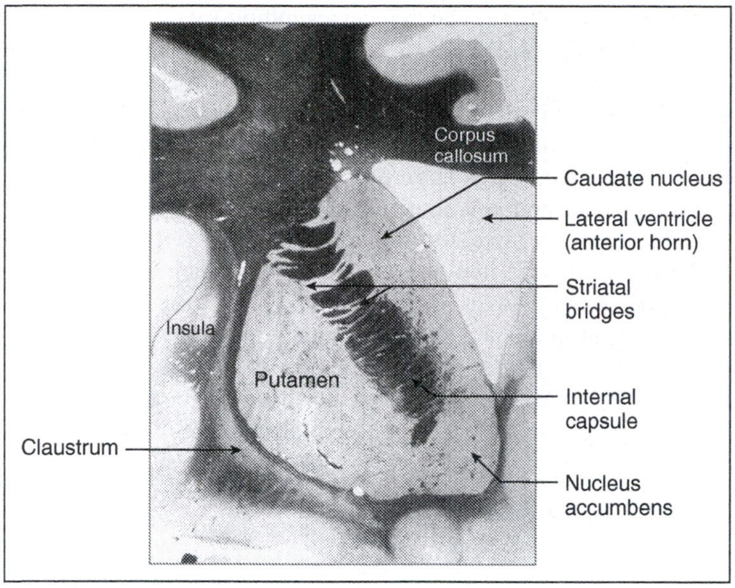

FIG. 12.5. Photomicrograph of the Rostral Neostriatum in the Coronal Plane (Weigert Stain). (Reprinted with permission from the late Dr. Malcolm B. Carpenter.)

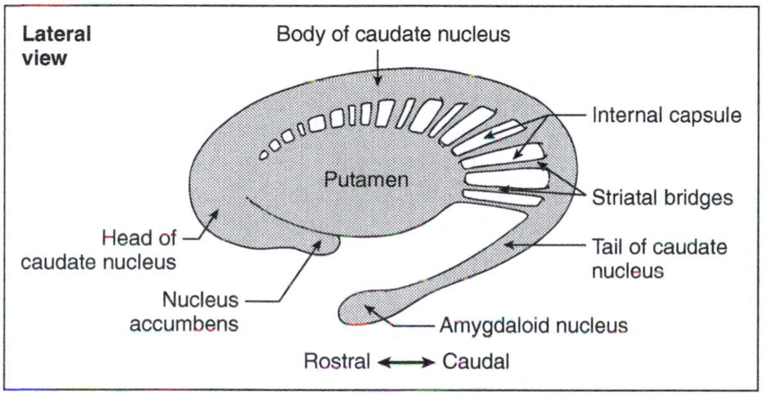

FIG. 12.6. Lateral View of the Caudate and Putamen. This drawing illustrates the continuity of the putamen with the head and body of the caudate nucleus. Rostrally, the head of the caudate nucleus and the putamen are continuous with each other. Further caudally, the caudate nucleus and putamen become separated as the developing fibers of the internal capsule grow between the two nuclei; thin webs of tissue between the putamen and the caudate nucleus are called striatal bridges.

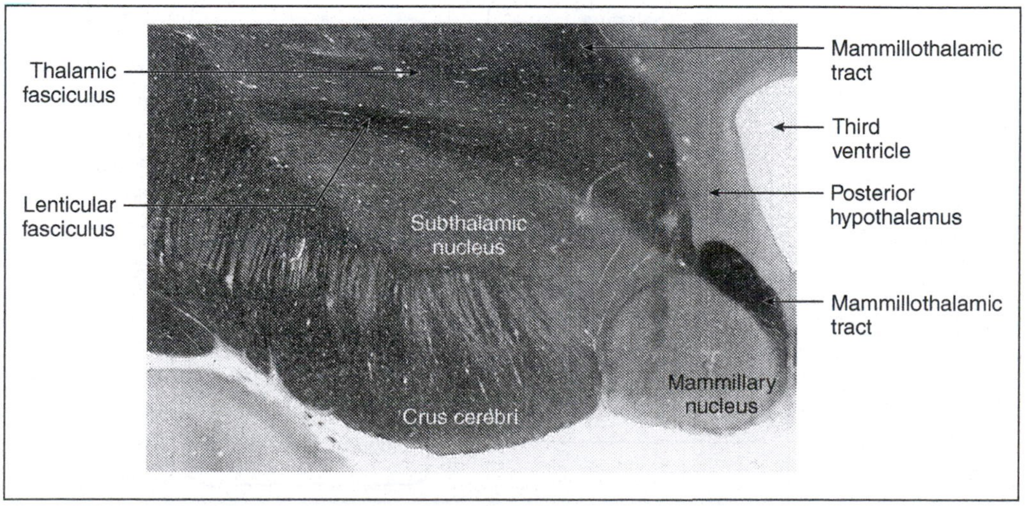

FIG. 12.7. Photomicrograph of the Subthalamic Nucleus, Lenticular Fasciculus, and Thalamic Fasciculus (Weigert Stain).

SNpc and dopamine; SNpr and GABA

GPi and SNpr: similar in many ways

Figures 6.1C, 6.1D). The subthalamic nucleus, which receives inhibitory projections from GPe and excitatory projections from the cerebral cortex, contains the only excitatory neurons in the basal ganglia.

The substantia nigra (see Figure 5.25) and the ventral tegmental area (see Figure 6.1E) are located immediately caudal to the subthalamic nucleus. The substantia nigra consists of a dorsal pars compacta (SNpc) that contains large pigmented, dopaminergic neurons, and a ventral pars reticulata (SNpr) that contains small GABAergic neurons. Although the SNpc and SNpr interact extensively, they are distinctly different nuclei with unique connections and functions. The dopaminergic neurons of the SNpc, which project to the neostriatum, degenerate in Parkinson's disease. Immediately medial to the SNpc is another dopaminergic nucleus, the ventral tegmental area, whose projections to the nucleus accumbens play an important role in limbic functions such as emotion, reward, and motivation. The SNpr and the GPi are usually discussed together because they both contain GABAergic neurons with functionally similar afferent and efferent projections.

Internal Circuitry of the Basal Ganglia

The components of the basal ganglia are classified as input nuclei, output nuclei, and intrinsic nuclei; connections between these nuclei form the direct and indirect pathways (Figure 12.8). Direct projections from the input nuclei (caudate nucleus and putamen) to the output nuclei (GPi/SNpr) comprise the direct pathway. The indirect pathway takes a detour through the intrinsic nuclei (GPe/SNpr; subthalamic nucleus). The direct circuit promotes movement, and the indirect circuit suppresses movement (Figure 12.9).

Input nuclei: caudate nucleus, putamen, nucleus accumbens

Input Nuclei. Almost all afferent projections to the basal ganglia enter through the caudate nucleus, the putamen, and the nucleus accumbens (see Figures 12.8 and 12.9). Cortical association areas in the frontal, parietal, and temporal lobes project primarily to the caudate nucleus; the putamen receives most of its input from the primary sensory and motor cortices, and the nucleus accumbens receives input from limbic cortex. Neurons

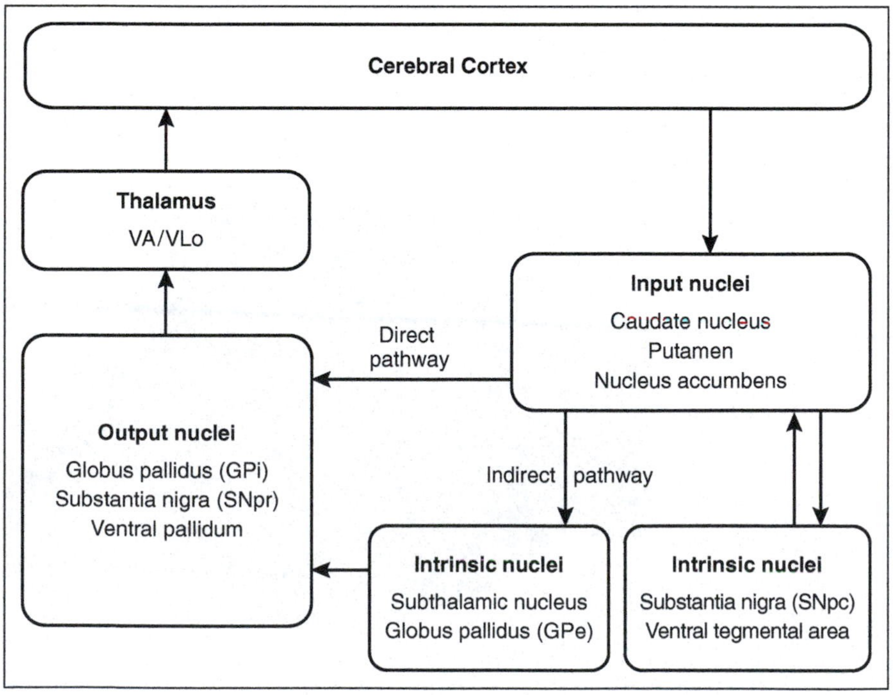

FIG. 12.8. Flow Diagram Showing the Input, Output, and Intrinsic Nuclei of the Basal Ganglia.

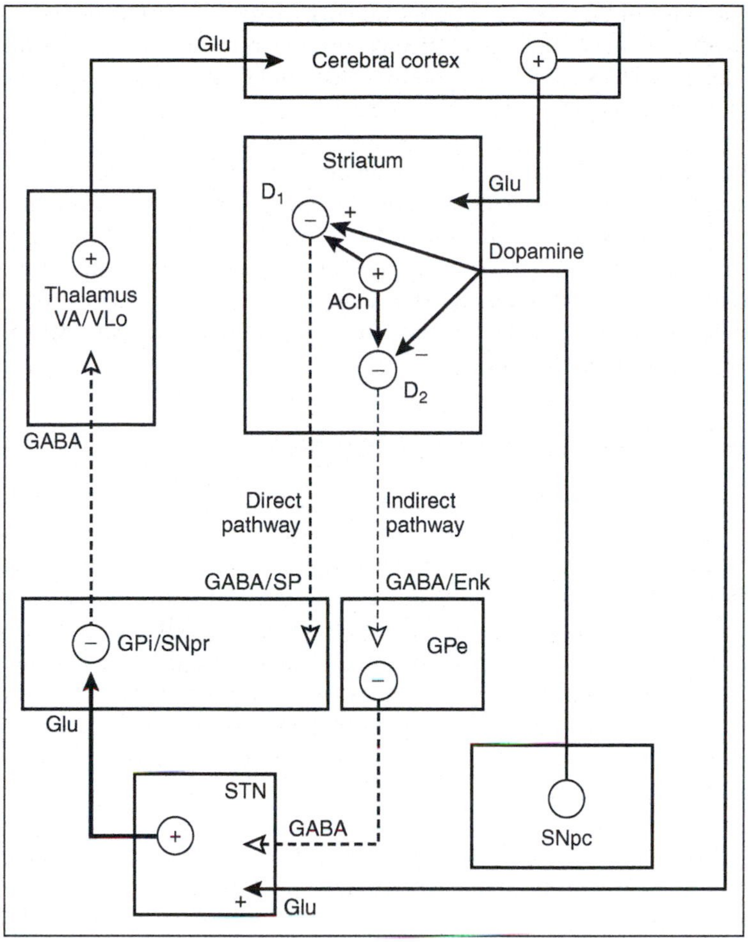

FIG. 12.9. Model of Normal Basal Ganglia Function. Direct and indirect pathways through the basal ganglia modulate the output to the motor thalamus. In the normal individual, dopamine activates the direct pathway, which facilitates movement, and inhibits the indirect pathway, which suppresses movement. ACh = acetylcholine; D_1 and D_2 = spiny striatal neurons with D_1 and D_2 dopamine receptors; GABA = γ-aminobutyric acid; Glu = glutamate; SNpc = substantia nigra, pars compacts; SNpr = substantia nigra, pars reticulata; STN = subthalamic nucleus; VA = ventral anterior nucleus of the thalamus; VLo = the oral part of the ventral lateral nucleus of the thalamus. Adapted from Alexander et al. (1990).

within the putamen form clusters; each neuron within an individual cluster receives corticofugal projections from motor and sensory areas related to the same part of the body (e.g., the same joint or the same limb). In general, these glutamatergic, corticostriatal projections overlap the dopaminergic projections from the SNpc. Evidence that specific regions of the cerebral cortex project to different parts of the neostriatum supports the assertion that the basal ganglia consist of separate, functional channels or processing streams. Five channels have been identified: motor, oculomotor, limbic, dorsolateral prefrontal, and lateral orbitofrontal.

Corticostriatal projections use glutamate and are excitatory.

The complexity of the neostriatum derives primarily from its chemical diversity. More than 90% of the neurons in the neostriatum are GABAergic medium spiny neurons that project to the GPe, GPi, and SNpr. Medium spiny neurons that project to the GPi and the SNpr contain GABA as well as substance P and dynorphin; those that project to the GPe have GABA colocalized with enkephalin. Both D_1 and D_2 spiny striatal neurons receive excitatory projections from the cerebral cortex. Cortical activation of the D_1 receptor containing striatal spiny neurons facilitates movement through the direct pathway. GABAergic aspiny striatal neurons, which also use acetylcholine as a neurotransmitter, synapse on D_2 spiny neurons and suppress movement by activating the indirect pathway (see "Direct and Indirect Pathways").

D_1 spiny neurons: GABA + substance P + dynorphin

D_2 spiny neurons: GABA + enkephalin

Output Nuclei. Basal ganglia output to the thalamus arises from GABAergic neurons located in the GPi and SNpr (see Figures 12.8 and 12.9). Inhibitory projections from the GPi and SNpr to the ventral anterior (VA) and ventral lateral (VLo) thalamic nuclei adjust the level of activity within the premotor and supplementary motor cortices (see Figures 6.1A, 6.1B, and 6.2). Other projections from the SNpr to the superior colliculus modulate eye movements. As neural activity in the thalamus increases, the motor cortices are more likely

Output nuclei: GPi, SNpr

to initiate movement; unfortunately, excessive thalamic activity triggers hyperkinetic movements. Insufficient thalamic activity reduces cortically driven movements and, in the extreme, produces hypokinesis. The key to motor control is to maintain neural activity in the thalamic motor nuclei at an intermediate level.

Intrinsic nuclei: GPe, SNpc, subthalamic nucleus

Intrinsic Nuclei. The afferent and efferent projections of the intrinsic nuclei remain within the basal ganglia. Four nuclei constitute the intrinsic nuclei: the GPe, the subthalamic nucleus, the SNpc, and the ventral tegmental area (see Figures 12.8 and 12.9). The GPe and the subthalamic nucleus form the core of the indirect pathway. Dopaminergic projections from the SNpc and the ventral tegmental area modulate the excitatory effects of the corticostriatal projections. Equilibrium between the direct and indirect pathways is essential for proper function of the motor system.

Efferent Projections of the Basal Ganglia

Thalamic fasciculus: ansa lenticularis, lenticular fasciculus, and cerebellothalamic fibers

Zona incerta: the ventromedial continuation of the reticular nucleus

The intrinsic pathways of the basal ganglia are difficult to identify in histological material, but the output pathways to the thalamus can be readily seen. The efferent projections from the GPi to the thalamus form two separate pathways, the lenticular fasciculus and the ansa lenticularis; both enter the thalamus by joining the crossed cerebellothalamic fibers of the thalamic fasciculus (Figure 12.10; see also Figures 6.1A, 6.1B, 12.8). Axons of the lenticular fasciculus exit the dorsal surface of the GPi, perforate the internal capsule, and then course medially along the ventral border of the zona incerta until they merge with the thalamic fasciculus (see Figures 12.10 and 6.1B). Axons forming the ansa lenticularis exit the GPi from its ventral surface, wrap around the medial tip of the internal capsule, and join the thalamic fasciculus.

Direct and Indirect Pathways. The direct and indirect pathways originate from separate populations of medium spiny neurons in the neostriatum (see Figure 12.9). Both populations receive ascending dopaminergic projections from the SNpc, but one group has D_1 receptors and other has D_2 receptors. Neurons with D_1 receptors are facilitated by nigrostriatal dopaminergic projections; those with D_2 receptors are inhibited. Spiny striatal neurons with D_1 receptors project to GPi and SNpr and form the direct pathway. The spiny striatal neurons with D_2 receptors project to GPe, the first leg in the indirect pathway.

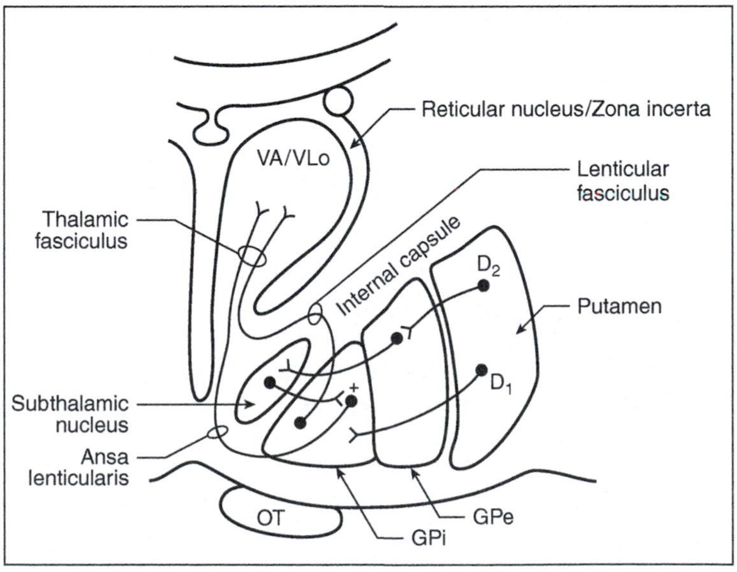

FIG. 12.10. Schematic Diagram of the Intrinsic and Output Pathways of the Basal Ganglia. OT = optic tract. (See Figure 12.9 for definitions of other abbreviations.)

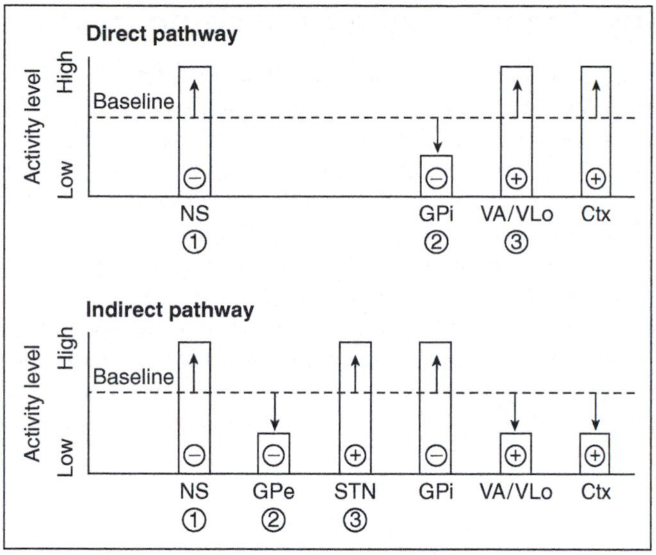

FIG. 12.11. Disinhibition in the Basal Ganglia. Direct pathway (top): As cortically driven activity in the neostriatum (NS) increases, the inhibitory neurons in the GPi are suppressed, which disinhibits the excitatory neurons in the VA/VLo nuclei of the thalamus. Thalamocortical activation promotes movement. Indirect pathway (bottom): Increased neostriatal activity suppresses the inhibitory neurons of the GPe. Reduced activity in the GPe disinhibits the subthalamic nucleus (STN), which contains excitatory neurons. Additional activation of the GPi suppresses the thalamus, which in turn reduces cortically driven movement. Note that the first (1) and second (2) neuron in each circuit are inhibitory, whereas the third (3) is excitatory, and that neurons 1 and 2 move in tandem. Plus and minus signs indicate that the nucleus contains excitatory and inhibitory neurons, respectively Ctx = motor cortex.

Direct Pathway. The direct pathway gets it name because of its direct neostriatal projections to the output nuclei, which, in turn, project to the thalamus. The direct pathway uses a three-neuron, disinhibitory circuit to modulate activity in the motor cortices. In this three-neuron circuit, the first two neurons (in the neostriatum and GPi/SNpr, respectively) are inhibitory, whereas the third neuron (in VA/VLo) is excitatory. Inhibition of the second neuron by the first releases the brake on the third neuron, which increases its activity (Figure 12.11). In the direct pathway, thalamic activity increases as the inhibitory output from GPi/SNpr is suppressed by the neostriatum. Increased activity in the thalamus activates the motor cortices, which promotes movement.

In a disinhibitory circuit, the activity of the first and third elements changes in tandem.

Disinhibition: when a cell is released from inhibition

The direct pathway facilitates movement.

Indirect Pathway. As the name implies, output from the neostriatum to the GPi/SNpr takes a detour to motor cortex. Disinhibition also plays a role in the indirect pathway, but unlike in the direct pathway, the third neuron in the circuit is in the subthalamic nucleus rather than the thalamus. The subthalamic nucleus is the key to understanding how the indirect pathway suppresses movement. In the indirect pathway, the second inhibitory neuron is located in the GPe (see Figure 12.11). Inhibition of the GABAergic neurons in GPe by the neostriatum releases the glutamatergic neurons of the subthalamic nucleus, which, in turn, activates the GABAergic neurons in the GPi/SNpr. As GPi/SNpr activity increases, neural activity in the thalamic VA/VLo nuclei decreases, which reduces cortical activity, making it more difficult to move (see Figure 12.9).

The indirect pathway inhibits movement.

The inhibitory projections from GPe to the subthalamic nucleus are countered by direct excitatory glutamatergic projections from the motor cortices. As dopamine reduces the output of D_2 spiny neurons, the inhibitory influence of GPe on the subthalamus increases. Thus, there is a fine balance between the cortical excitatory input to the subthalamic nucleus and the inhibitory input from the GPe. Because the cortico-subthalamic circuit typically prevails, the indirect circuit opposes the facilitatory action of the direct circuit.

What Do the Basal Ganglia Contribute to Movement?

The once widely held view that basal ganglia dysfunction interferes with the patient's ability to either initiate movement (e.g., Parkinson's disease) or terminate movement (e.g., Huntington's disease, hemiballismus) has been largely discredited. Laboratory studies have shown that lesions of the basal ganglia do not delay movement initiation and that neural activity in other movement-related areas typically precedes that of the basal ganglia. The current view is that the basal ganglia act as a brake that releases desired movements while suppressing competing movements. For example, it would be counterproductive to shuffle your feet or change your posture while trying to press a button on an elevator. In this example, once the motor plan to press the elevator button is conveyed to the basal ganglia by corticostriatal projections, the direct and indirect pathways promote the cortical agenda while suppressing competing oculomotor and postural movements. When basal ganglia disorders upset this balance, either competing movements are expressed or the desired movements are suppressed.

Basal Ganglia Channels

The basal ganglia contain five separate channels or thalamocortical loops. Each loop or channel serves a different function, and like the motor circuit described above, each begins and ends in the cerebral cortex. The circuits are named according the area of the cerebral cortex with which they are most closely associated: motor, oculomotor, limbic, dorsolateral prefrontal, and lateral orbitofrontal. Each circuit not only utilizes a different area of cortex, but also takes a slightly different route through the basal ganglia. For example, most cortical projections in the motor circuit originate in the precentral and postcentral gyri and terminate in the putamen; the corticofugal axons in the oculomotor circuit, by comparison, connect the frontal eye fields with the caudate nucleus. The motor and oculomotor circuits modulate body and extraocular eye movement, respectively.

Mesolimbic dopaminergic system: the dopaminergic projections from ventral tegmental area to the nucleus accumbens, ventral striatum, and medial frontal cortex

Emotional and visceral functions are managed by the limbic loop, which connects the limbic lobe, the hippocampus, and the amygdala with the nucleus accumbens and the ventral striatum. Unlike the other circuits, dopaminergic projections to the nucleus accumbens originate in the ventral tegmental area rather than the SNpc. Basal ganglia output from the nucleus accumbens and the ventral striatum is directed to the mediodorsal nucleus of the thalamus, which has extensive projections to the prefrontal cortex.

The dorsolateral prefrontal and the lateral orbitofrontal loops originate in different parts of the prefrontal cortex, but both circuits contribute to higher-order processing of cognitive and emotional behavior. Executive functions such as problem solving are mediated by the dorsolateral prefrontal circuit. The circuit originating in the lateral orbitofrontal cortex controls our ability to act in a socially responsible manner and show empathy.

Although the nuclei of the basal ganglia are typically discussed as if they were a single entity, most contain areas dedicated to only one of the five loops.

Clinical Aspects

Extrapyramidal disorders relate to the basal ganglia.

Symptoms are experienced by the patient; **signs** are observed by others.

Negative symptoms are deficiencies caused by the loss of specific structures.

For many years, motor symptoms related to dysfunction of the basal ganglia were called extrapyramidal, to distinguish them from deficits mediated by motor cortex and the pyramidal tract. There has been growing awareness over the last few decades that the pyramidal and extrapyramidal systems work as a unit rather than as autonomous systems, and with this realization, the word "extrapyramidal" has gradually fallen into disfavor from a mechanistic standpoint. However, the word is still useful clinically to distinguish between disorders affecting the pyramidal tract from those that involve both the pyramidal tract and the basal ganglia.

Basal ganglia disorders are classified as hypokinetic or hyperkinetic. Hypokinetic disorders cause diminished quality and quantity of movements (e.g., Parkinson's disease). Patients with hyperkinetic disorders have the opposite problem: they display excessive, involuntary movements. Although this classification of movement disorders helps us

TABLE 12.1 Basal Ganglia Deficits

Disorder	Deficit
Akinesia	Absence of movements
Athetosis	Slow, twisting movements
Ballismus	Ballistic, flinging motion of a limb
Bradykinesia	Slowed movements
Chorea	Involuntary, arrhythmic, jerky movements
Cogwheel phenomenon	Ratchet-like resistance during joint flexion
Dyskinesia	Abnormal, involuntary movements
Dystonia	Sustained, abnormal postures
	Contraction of agonist and antagonist muscles
Hypokinesia	Fewer movements
Myoclonus	Shock-like, rapid muscular jerk
Rigidity	Increased resistance to passive movement (e.g., lead pipe rigidity)
Tics	A sudden urge to move or vocalize
Tremor	Rhythmic, oscillating movements of agonist and antagonist muscles
Essential tremor	Mild, benign tremor of adult onset
Intention tremor	Occurs during movement—typically cerebellar
Resting tremor	Occurs at rest—hallmark of Parkinson's disease
Postural tremor	Occurs while limbs are actively held in a fixed position

understand basal ganglia pathophysiology, patients often exhibit both hyperkinetic and hypokinetic symptoms. Table 12.1 lists the more common symptoms associated with diseases of the basal ganglia.

Positive symptoms are caused by the remaining structures.

Parkinson's Disease. Parkinson's disease is a chronic, progressive disorder of unknown origin that primarily affects the motor system. The onset of Parkinson's is slow and insidious, but it typically starts between the ages of 40 and 70. The onset of Parkinson's disease is usually signaled by resting tremor in one hand (pill-rolling) that disappears during volitional movement and increases during stress or emotional turmoil. Rest tremor is typically most obvious when the patient is walking or resting his or her hands on the steering wheel. Although rest tremor brings attention to the disease, it is usually not the disabling feature of the disease. The most significant problems of Parkinson's disease occur 2–5 years after the initial diagnosis when bradykinesia (poverty of movement) causes disability. Common bradykinetic symptoms include difficulty in cutting food, buttoning clothes, and lacing shoes. Handwriting quality deteriorates as the size of their script becomes smaller (micrographia).

Parkinson's disease afflicts 1% of those older than 65.

The increased muscle tone observed in patients with Parkinson's disease is called hypertonia of the rigidity type. This is characterized by increased resistance to passive joint movement in all directions, and it is distinguished from hypertonia of the spasticity type in which tone is increased only in the antigravity muscles. Parkinsonian hypertonia has been called lead pipe rigidity based on the notion that if a thin lead pipe is bent, the resistance will be appreciated in all directions that it is bent. Spasticity is often called clasp knife spasticity, because there is a characteristic give or sudden loss of resistance in one direction. Regardless, patients with Parkinson's disease express hypertonia of the rigidity type and do not exhibit spasticity. This is quite useful clinically. When hypertonia of the rigidity type is superimposed with rest tremor, the passive movement of the limb may give the appearance of shifting gears as a cog falling into place in sequence as in a cog wheel. So, occasionally the term "cogwheel rigidity" is also used to describe the hypertonia of the rigidity type in Parkinson's disease.

The cardinal symptoms of Parkinson's disease include resting tremor, hypertonia of the rigidity type, and bradykinesia.

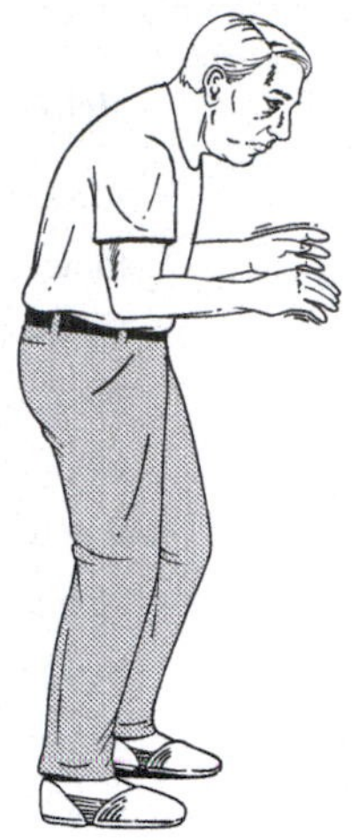

FIG. 12.12. Patient with Parkinson's Disease. The cardinal symptoms of Parkinson's disease include resting tremor of the hands, a slow, shuffling gait, flexion of the trunk, and a mask-like facial expression.

Over time, tremor may appear in the lips, tongue, ipsilateral foot, or hand; eventually the tremor spreads to the axial muscles of the body. Parkinson's patients normally have difficulty initiating movements (akinesia); when movements do occur, they are slow (bradykinesia) and lack normal amplitude. Spontaneous, automatic movements of the face and eyes are replaced by a mask-like expression and an unblinking (reptilian) stare. As the akinesia progresses, speech becomes more difficult, and the patient speaks less often and more softly. Loss of postural reflexes causes bowing of the head and trunk along with flexed elbows, hips, and knees. Walking consists of short steps and a shuffling gait with the hands positioned in front of the body (Figure 12.12). Like the motor system, thinking slows appreciably; approximately 40% of Parkinson's disease patients develop dementia in the late stages of the disease. Because Parkinson's disease usually begins relatively late in life, many patients succumb to other diseases. Although there is no cure for Parkinson's disease, treatment is quite effective and life expectancy is not compromised.

> The symptoms of Parkinson's disease emerge after 70%–80% of the dopaminergic neurons in SNpc degenerate.

Diagnosis is based on the patient's clinical presentation. The symptoms of Parkinson's disease are caused by depletion of striatal dopamine secondary to degeneration of dopaminergic neurons within the SNpc. The first symptoms of parkinsonism appear after approximately 70%–80% of the SNpc cells die; as cell death within the SNpc continues, the number of symptoms and their severity increase.

Nigral degeneration is evident during postmortem examination of the brain by the absence of the dark, neuromelanin-containing neurons in the SNpc. Surviving, but not necessarily healthy, neurons contain Lewy bodies, which are eosinophillic cytoplasmic inclusions. Lewy bodies stain positive for neurofilament proteins, ubiquitin and α-synuclein. Although Lewy bodies are not pathanomonic to Parkinson's disease, their presence in the SNpc is characteristic of idiopathic Parkinson's disease. In the early 1980s, nigral degeneration and Parkinson's disease–like symptoms (parkinsonism) were discovered in a group of young adults who abused a synthetic heroine-like analog of meperidine. Unfortunately, their home brew was contaminated with MPTP (1-methyl-4-phenyl-1,2,5,6-tetrahydropyridine) and its metabolite MPP+, a potent neurotoxin that destroys SNpc neurons. Scientists have capitalized on the selectivity of MPTP for dopaminergic neurons of the SNpc and ventral tegmental area to develop the first truly viable animal model of Parkinson's disease.

> **Hypokinesis** is caused by dysfunction of the direct and indirect pathways.

The hypokinetic symptoms of Parkinson's disease are caused by suppression of the thalamic motor nuclei by the output nuclei of the basal ganglia, GPi and SNpr. As Figure 12.13 shows, loss of nigrostriatal dopamine alters the balance of activity in the direct and indirect pathways. The GABAergic striatal neurons of the indirect circuit respond to the loss of dopamine by increasing their activity, which disinhibits the subthalamic nucleus. Increased activity in the subthalamic nucleus increases the inhibitory output of the GPi/SNpr, which, in

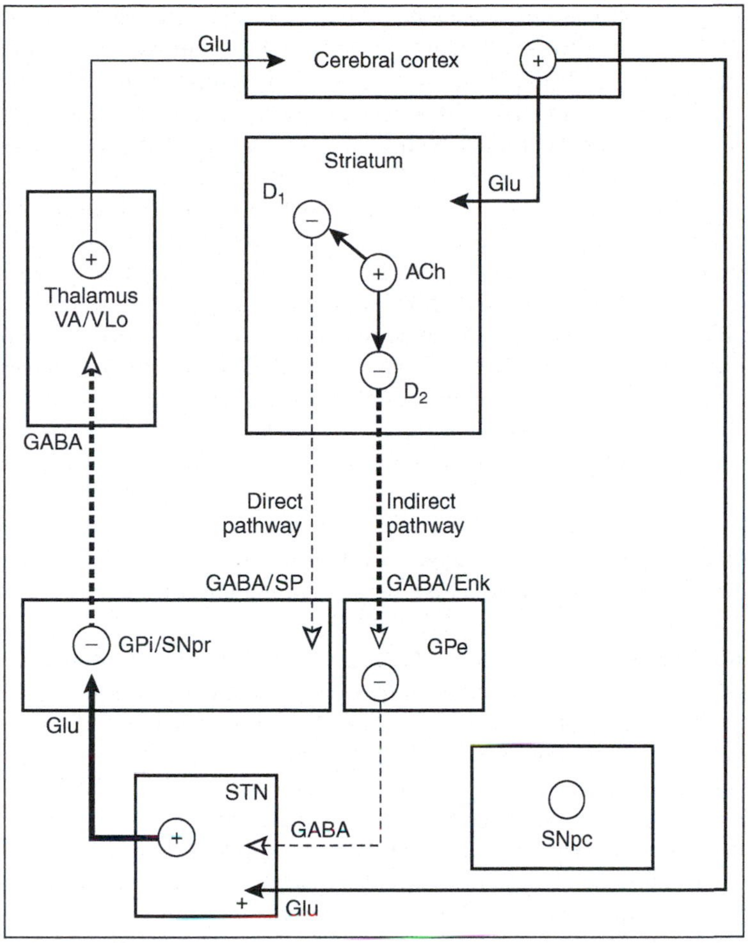

FIG. 12.13. Hypokinetic Model of Basal Ganglia Function. According to this model, the hypokinetic symptoms of Parkinson's disease are caused by a diminution of cortical activation by the thalamic motor nuclei. Loss of nigrostriatal dopamine impairs the direct pathway movement facilitation but promotes the indirect pathway, which suppresses movement. Less activation of the thalamic motor nuclei by the basal ganglia reduces activation of the motor cortex. See Figure 12.9 for abbreviations. Adapted from DeLong (1990).

turn, reduces activity of the VA/VLo nuclei. Loss of dopamine at the striatal D_1 receptors also increases GPi/SNpr inhibition of the thalamic motor nuclei, which ultimately reduces activation of the motor cortex. Ultimately, the hypokinetic symptoms associated with Parkinson's disease are due to inadequate activation of motor cortex (compare Figures 12.9 and 12.13).

Although Parkinson's disease is considered a hypokinetic disorder, these patients exhibit two classic hyperkinetic symptoms: resting tremor and, in patients treated with medications, drug-induced dyskinesia. The origin of resting tremor is believed to be thalamic oscillatory neurons whose firing rate (3-6 Hz) is synchronized with the tremor. Lesioning one of the cerebellar relay nuclei in the thalamus, the ventral intermediate nucleus, destroys these oscillatory neurons and eliminates rest tremor. It is not clear why this works, however, because the ventral intermediate nucleus does not receive projections from the GPi and the SNpr.

Drug-induced dyskinesias typically begin after 3–4 years of treatment with antiparkinsonian medications. The pathophysiology of drug-induced dyskinesias is unclear, but it may be due to the intermittent nature of dopamine replacement that these patients receive. Intermittent stimulation may hypersensitize the striatal dopamine receptors and provoke excessive and abnormal inhibition of subthalamic and pallidal activity. Lesions of the GPi are highly effective in ameliorating drug-induced dyskinesias.

Dopamine does not cross the blood-brain barrier, but its precursor, L-dopa, does.

Management of Parkinson's disease emphasizes dopamine repletion. Replacement therapy is designed to increase dopamine levels in the brain by administering either a dopamine precursor (e.g., L-dopa) or a dopamine agonist (e.g., ropinirole). To ensure that most of the peripherally administered L-dopa reaches the brain, systemic conversion of L-dopa into dopamine must be limited with a decarboxylase inhibitor such as carbidopa. Dopamine levels can also be increased with drugs that suppress dopamine breakdown such as entacapone, which inhibits carboxy-O-methyltransferase, and selegiline, which inhibits monoaminoxidase-B. Amantadine, which blocks the NMDA glutamate receptors, ameliorates resting tremor and drug-induced dyskinesias. Anticholinergic drugs also provide relief by suppressing the aspiny striatal cholinergic neurons.

Surgical intervention may be attempted in Parkinson's disease patients who no longer respond to pharmacologic treatments or in patients with drug-induced dyskinesias. The procedure of choice involves high-frequency electrical stimulation of the subthalamic nucleus via surgically implanted fine wire electrodes. Another surgical intervention involves the GPi, which can be either lesioned (pallidotomy) or electrically stimulated with implanted fine-wire electrodes. Due to the proximity of the GPi to the internal capsule and optic tract (see Figure 12.10), hemiparesis and homonymous hemianopsia are risk factors associated with pallidotomies. Experimental therapies for Parkinson's disease include replacement of dopaminergic cells with stem cells, retinal pigment epithelial cells, or trophic factors.

Huntington's Disease. Huntington's disease is a progressive, autosomal dominant disease typically of adult onset characterized by motor, cognitive, emotional, and behavioral deterioration. In Huntington's disease, the medium spiny projection neurons degenerate, first in the caudate nucleus and eventually in the putamen and globus pallidus. The hallmark of Huntington's disease is the involuntary, dance-like or choreiform movements of the limbs. Early in the disease, these choreic movements and dyskinesias may be incorporated into ongoing voluntary movements of the arms and legs, but eventually these pathologic movements increase in amplitude and overshadow normal motor behavior. Although the dopamine antagonist haloperidol suppresses choreiform movements, it is seldom prescribed because it produces parkinsonian-like symptoms. Because choreiform movements are more embarrassing than disabling to the patient, the benefits of haloperidol are rarely justified. As Huntington's disease progresses, the choreiform movements abate as rigidity and bradykinesia ensue; these symptoms partially respond to dopaminergic therapy.

Huntington's disease is marked by a loss of striatal neurons.

The cognitive impairments that eventually progress to global dementia are the most debilitating symptoms of Huntington's disease. Patients with Huntington's disease also show deficits in executive function, sequencing, motor learning, and complex motor tasks. Depression, alcohol abuse, and suicide, which are very common in young patients, are attributed to caudate atrophy and the loss of frontostriatal circuits. Shrinkage of the caudate nucleus caused by cellular degeneration is visible with neuroimaging.

The cause of Huntington's disease is a mutation of chromosome 4 that produces a proliferation of a normal trinucleotide (CAG). Genetic tests can measure the length of this trinucleotide repeat to confirm Huntington's chorea in symptomatic patients and predict which asymptomatic members of an affected family will likely be stricken with the disease. People whose trinucleotide pattern exceeds 37 will likely develop Huntington's disease. Longer repeats are positively correlated with early onset and more severe symptoms, and if the disease is passed to offspring, even earlier onset—a phenomenon known as anticipation. Huntington's disease is particularly insidious because onset is usually during the third or fourth decade, by which time most patients have started families. Patients with advanced Huntington's disease are bedridden, mute, demented, and require full-time nursing care. Death, which is often caused by respiratory complications, occurs 15–20 years after disease onset.

Hemiballismus: ballistic movements of the ipsilateral limbs

Hemiballismus. Hemiballismus is a hyperkinetic disorder of the basal ganglia marked by a series of involuntary, large-amplitude, ballistic movements of the contralateral extremities. The most common cause of hemiballismus, a focal stroke involving the subthalamic nucleus, decreases the inhibitory output from the GPi, which allows VA and

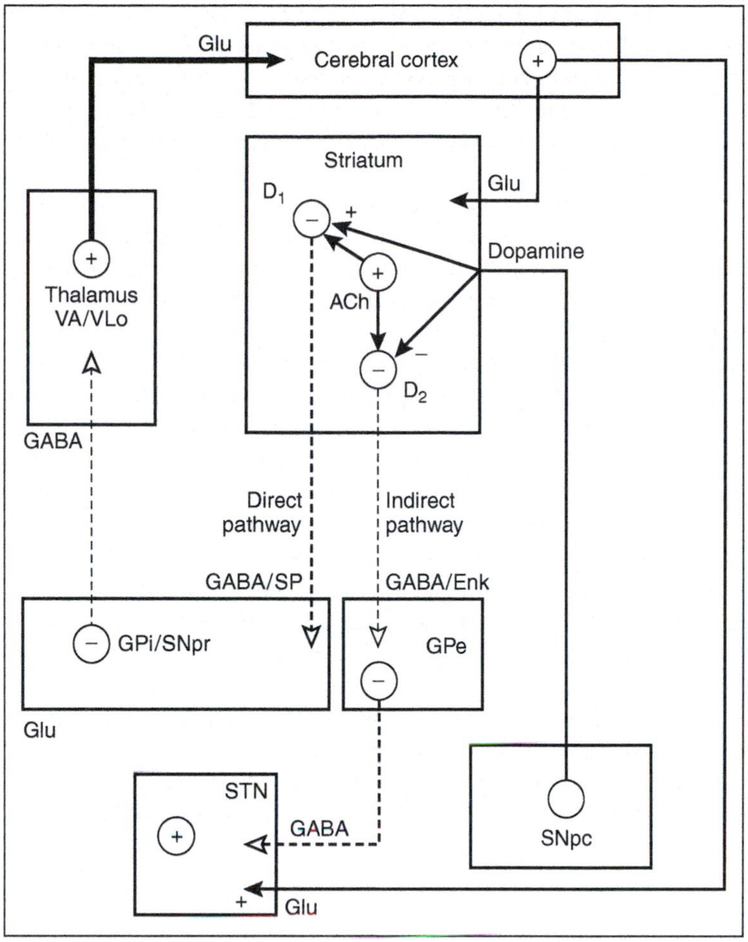

FIG. 12.14. Hyperkinetic Model of Basal Ganglia Function. The hyperkinetic symptoms of hemiballismus are caused by focal damage to the subthalamic nucleus. Damage to the subthalamic nucleus reduces the inhibitory brake on the thalamic motor nuclei by the GPi nucleus. Excessive activation of the thalamus causes over-facilitation of movement by the motor cortices. (See Figure 12.9 for definitions of abbreviations.) Adapted from DeLong (1990).

VLo thalamic activity to rise above normal levels (Figure 12.14). Dopamine-blocking (e.g., haloperidol) or dopamine-depleting (e.g., reserpine) drugs alleviate the symptoms of hemiballismus. Both treatments, by reducing dopamine availability, may create a parkinsonian-like enhancement of the residual subthalamic nucleus activity.

Tourette's Syndrome and Obsessive-Compulsive Disorder (OCD). Tourette's syndrome is a complex and poorly understood disorder characterized by recurrent motor, sensory, and vocal tics. Motor tics are abrupt, brief movements usually confined to one or two joints of a limb. These movements may involve any part of the body, but they usually enlist the upper torso and head. Blinking, shrugging, facial grimacing, and coughing are among the more common tics, which are usually fast and brief rather than slow and sustained. Movements may be simple twitches, or complex, sequential gestures that resemble normal behavior such as hair brushing, jumping, and making obscene gestures. Vocal tics show similar variety and may include grunts, sniffs, coughs, barks, and screams. More complex verbal tics, such as shouting obscenities or repetition of speech, are well publicized but less common. Tic suppression is possible, but it creates unbearable frustration that is immediately relieved when the tic is finally expressed.

Most patients develop Tourette's syndrome before the age of 10, but onset as late as 21 has been reported. Symptoms typically improve by late adolescence and often resolve entirely, but for some patients Tourette's syndrome has a lifelong course. The prevalence of Tourette's syndrome in the population is actively debated, but a mean of 5 cases per 10,000 seems to be generally accepted. There is general agreement that the incidence of Tourette's syndrome is higher in children with special education needs and is strongly linked to obsessive-compulsive disorder (OCD) and possibly attention deficit hyperactivity disorder (ADHD).

80% of Tourette's patients may also have OCD.

The hallmark symptoms of OCD are persistent, intrusive thoughts or compulsive actions that the patient performs in a stereotyped manner, often for such prolonged periods that it interferes with social, family, and work responsibilities. The prevalence of OCD in the general population is about 3%; in the patients with Tourette's syndrome, the incidence may be as high as 80%.

Because the signature symptoms of Tourette's syndrome and OCD—motor and verbal tics, intrusive thoughts, and compulsive actions—represent different types of involuntary behavior, the search for a neural basis has centered on the basal ganglia. Modern imaging studies have confirmed that the basal ganglia play some role in Tourette's syndrome and OCD, but a clear anatomical basis has yet to emerge. The symptoms of Tourette's are relieved by dopamine antagonists and depletors, which is consistent with the assertion that excessive activity in the basal ganglia is responsible for these involuntary behaviors. The role of the basal ganglia in OCD is less clear because selective serotonin reuptake inhibitors (SSRIs), rather than dopamine antagonists, are the preferred pharmacological treatment.

Athetosis. Athetosis is an involuntary, slow, writhing movement of the hands and fingers. In general, the movements in athetosis are slower than those observed in chorea, but all gradations are possible, making the distinction between the two disorders impossible in some instances. Postmortem studies have implicated damage to the globus pallidus and thalamus.

CEREBELLUM

Overview

Feedback is reactive control; **feedforward** is proactive control.

The cerebellum does not initiate movement or directly control the musculature, but it nevertheless plays a vital role in voluntary movement, posture, muscle tone, and balance. The cerebellum guides volitional movement using feedback and feedforward control. Feedback uses sensory information to guide ongoing behavior in a moment-to-moment fashion. An example of feedback control is the process of threading a needle: movements are guided in real time by tactile, proprioceptive, and visual information sent to the cerebellum. Feedforward control relies on the person's experience to anticipate the needs of the motor system and begin movement before feedback is available. For example, ballistic movements too fast to benefit from sensory guidance (e.g., swatting a mosquito) are coordinated by the cerebellum using feedforward control. Cerebellar damage, by affecting the accuracy and timing of movements, disrupts gait, balance, and the execution of precision movements. Other data suggest that the cerebellum contributes to motor learning and language; for clinicians, however, these functions are usually of secondary importance.

Gross Anatomy

The cerebellum, the largest structure in the posterior cranial fossa, is connected to the brainstem by three stout fiber bundles: the inferior, middle, and superior cerebellar peduncles. The tentorium covers the dorsal surface of the cerebellum and secures it to the inner surface of the skull. The cerebellar cortex consists of small, unnamed gyri called folia and two large fissures, the primary and posterolateral, that divide the cerebellum into the anterior, posterior, and flocculonodular lobes, respectively (Figure 12.15; see

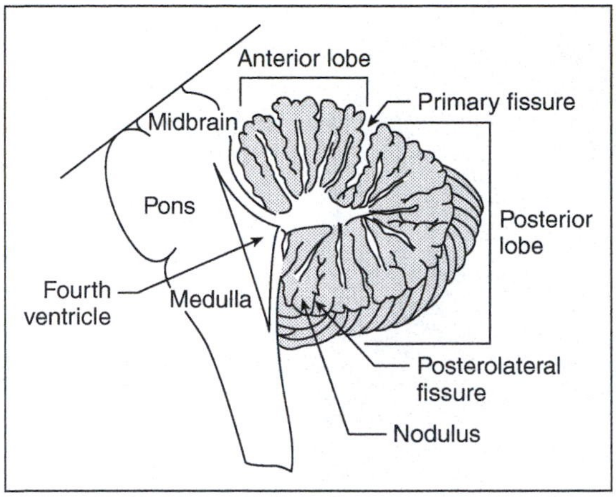

FIG. 12.15. Midsagittal Section of the Cerebellum.

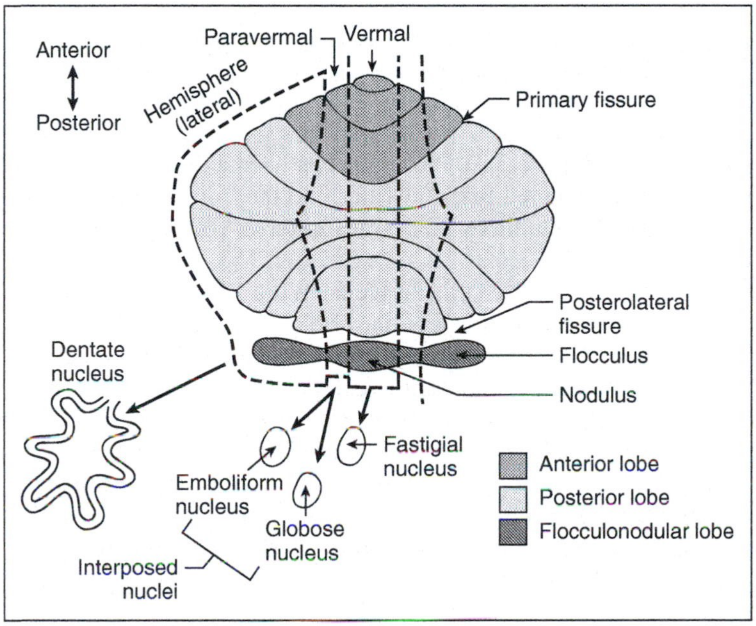

FIG. 12.16. Sagittal Zones of the Cerebellum. The cerebellum consists of three sagittally oriented zones that maintain their topographical relationship with the three sets of underlying deep cerebellar nuclei. Purkinje cells in the vermal zone project to the fastigial nucleus, whereas those in the more lateral paravermal region project to the emboliform and globose (interposed) nuclei. Purkinje cells in the cerebellar hemispheres project to the dentate nuclei.

also Figure 3.10). The cerebellar cortex consists of two hemispheres, a vermal region that straddles the midline, and an intermediate paravermal region (Figure 12.16).

The cortical mantle rests upon the arbor vitae, a dense bundle of myelinated fibers that reciprocally connects the cerebellar cortex with the deep cerebellar nuclei and various brainstem nuclei (see Figure 3.10). The four deep cerebellar nuclei, listed from medial to lateral, are the fastigial, the globose and emboliform (known as the interposed nuclei), and the dentate nucleus (Figure 12.17; see also Figure 12.16). Almost all cerebellar efferent projections originate in the deep cerebellar nuclei. Although the deep cerebellar nuclei receive some afferent projections from extracerebellar sources, most of their afferent projections originate in the cerebellar cortex.

Arbor vitae, from Latin, means "tree of life."

Cortical Cytoarchitecture

Five different types of neurons are found in the cerebellar cortex: Purkinje, stellate, basket, and Golgi neurons, which are inhibitory, and the excitatory granule cells. The most prominent of these neural elements are the large (40-75 μm diameter), flask-shaped

Purkinje cells speak for the cerebellar cortex.

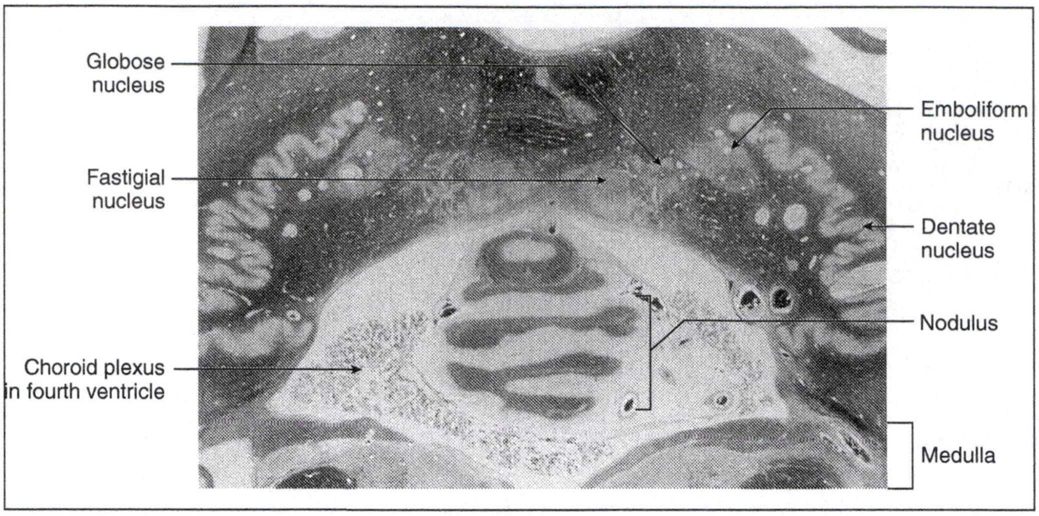

FIG. 12.17. Photomicrograph of the Deep Cerebellar Nuclei. Coronal section of the base of the cerebellum showing the four deep cerebellar nuclei. (Reprinted with permission from the late Dr. Malcolm B. Carpenter.)

Purkinje neurons (Table 12.2; see Figure 1.3). Purkinje cells have a distinctive fan-like dendritic tree whose flat surface is oriented perpendicularly to the long axis of the folia (Figure 12.18). Purkinje cells use the inhibitory neurotransmitter GABA and are the sole efferent neurons of the cerebellar cortex.

Granule cells are the only excitatory neuron of the cerebellar cortex.

Most afferent projections to the Purkinje cells derive from the small (5-8 μm diameter), densely packed granule cells located in cerebellar cortex (Figure 12.19). Granule cells have multiple, short dendrites with claw-like endings that terminate in the cerebellar glomeruli (described in "Cortical Circuitry"). Granule cells use glutamate to excite the apical dendrites of the Purkinje cells. Purkinje cells also receive inhibitory projections from basket cells and stellate cells. The basket cell is the more effective inhibitory neuron because its axon encircles each Purkinje cell's soma; stellate cells, by comparison, synapse on the distal dendrites of the Purkinje cells.

The cerebellar cortex consists of three layers that, unlike in the cerebral cortex, show no regional variation. The deepest layer of the cerebellar cortex is the granule cell layer,

TABLE 12.2 Cerebellar Cortical Neurons

Cell Type	Location	Afferent Source	Efferent Targets	Neurotransmitters	Action
Purkinje	Purkinje layer	Granule cells Basket cells Stellate cells Climbing fibers	Deep cerebellar nuclei Lateral vestibular nuclei	GABA	Inhibition
Granule	Granule layer	Mossy fibers Golgi cells	Purkinje cell dendrites Basket cells Stellate cells Golgi cells	Glutamate	Excitation
Basket	Molecular layer	Granule cells	Purkinje cell somas	GABA Nitric oxide (?)	Inhibition
Stellate	Molecular layer	Granule cells	Purkinje cell dendrites	Taurine (?)	Inhibition
Golgi	Granule layer	Mossy fibers	Granule cell dendrites	GABA	Inhibition

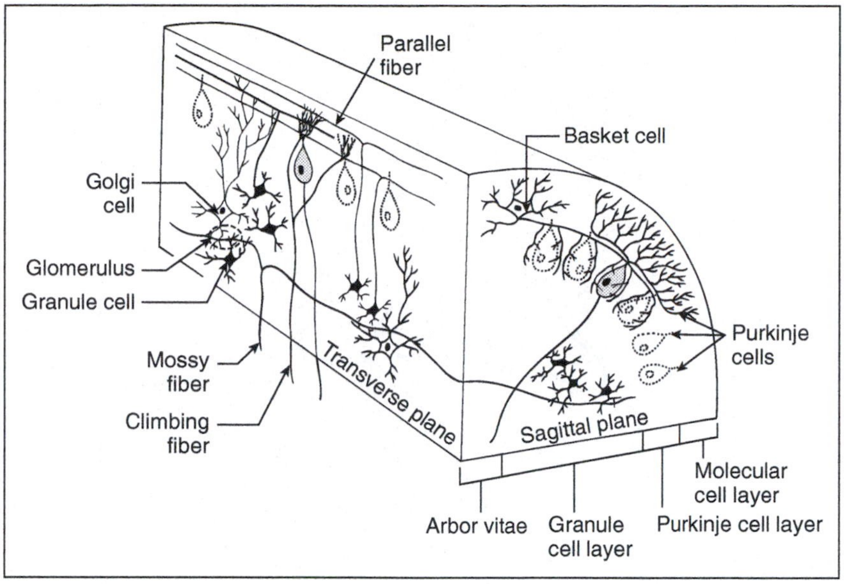

FIG. 12.18. Cerebellar Cortex. The cellular elements of cerebellar cortex are shown in the sagittal and transverse planes. The large, goblet-shaped Purkinje cells form a single layer along the ventral border of the molecular layer. Purkinje cell dendrites have a fan-like appearance when viewed sagittally, but not in the transverse plane. The molecular layer contains few cells but many fibers, including the apical dendrites of Golgi cells and the parallel fibers. Parallel fibers are granule cell axons that enter the molecular layer, bifurcate, and synapse on the apical dendrites of the successive Purkinje cells as they run through the long axis of the folium. Basket cell axons form a pericellular nest that embraces the Purkinje cell somas. The granule cell layer contains cerebellar glomeruli as well as their cellular constituents, the granule and Golgi cells. Input to the cerebellar cortex is provided by mossy fibers and climbing fibers.

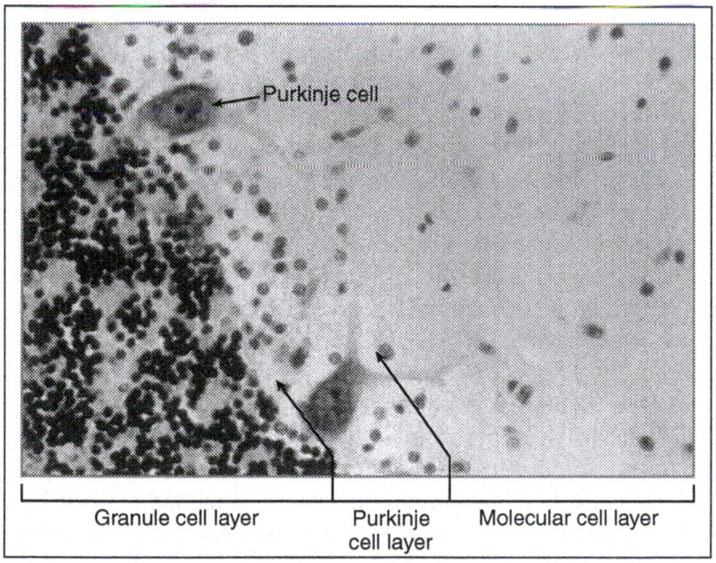

FIG. 12.19. Photomicrograph of Cerebellar Cortex. This section, stained for both cell bodies and myelin, shows the molecular, Purkinje, and granule cell layers. (Reprinted with permission from the late Dr. Malcolm B. Carpenter)

whose constituent neurons are packed so tightly that adjacent neurons seem to touch one another. Purkinje cells form a one-cell-thick layer between the granule cell layer and the overlying molecular cell layer. The molecular layer, which lies closest to the pia mater, consists primarily of granule cell axons (parallel fibers), a few stellate cells, and the dendritic trees of the underlying Purkinje and Golgi cells.

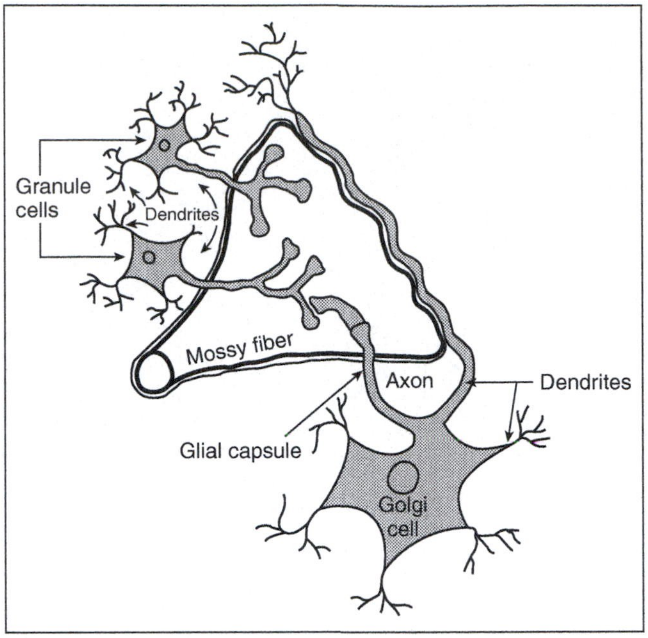

FIG. 12.20. Cerebellar Glomerulus. Mossy fibers terminate in a series of convoluted and lobulated processes called mossy fiber rosettes. The mossy fiber rosette forms the core of the cerebellar glomerulus, a glial encapsulated synaptic ensemble that also contains the claw-like dendrites of several local granule cells and axons and dendrites of local Golgi cells. The inhibitory Golgi axons terminate presynaptically on granule cell dendrites. The mossy fiber provides the excitatory input to the glomerulus, whereas the granule cells serve as the efferent component.

Cortical Circuitry

Most cerebellar afferent projections end as mossy fibers.

Glomerulus (*pl.* glomeruli), from Latin, means "ball."

Afferent projections to cerebellar cortex terminate as either mossy fibers or climbing fibers. Mossy fibers, which originate in the spinal cord, medulla (except the olivary nuclei), and pons, terminate within glial encapsulated structures called glomeruli that are scattered throughout the granule cell layer (Figure 12.20). The mossy fiber designation derives from the moss-like appearance of the lobulated enlargements of the afferent terminals. The large synaptic surface of these lobules provides high-fidelity integration of the mossy fiber signal with the granule cell dendrites, and Golgi cell axons and dendrites. The mossy fiber is the only excitatory component of the rosette. Glomerular output is conveyed by the granule cells whose axons ascend to the superficial part of the molecular layer, bifurcate, and run the length of the folia parallel to the cortical surface and perpendicular to the dendritic fans of the Purkinje cells (see Figure 12.18). Parallel fibers pass through the outstretched dendrites of the Purkinje cells like electrical wires passing through the upper limbs of trees. The lengthy course of each parallel fiber enables individual granule cells to influence a widespread area of the cerebellar cortex.

Climbing fibers originate in the inferior olivary nucleus.

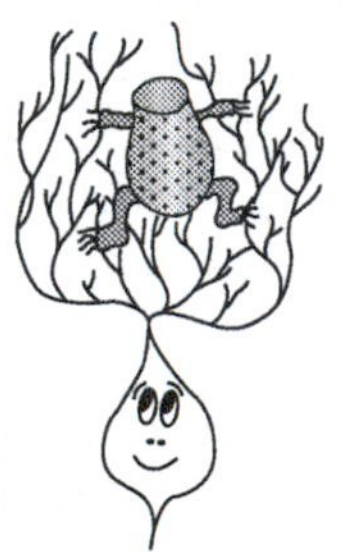
an olive climbing a trellis

Climbing fibers originate in the inferior olivary nuclei and terminate on the apical dendrites of the Purkinje cells (Figure 12.21). Climbing fibers are so named because they climb the dendritic tree of the Purkinje cells like vines on a trellis. Although one climbing fiber may target several Purkinje cells, each Purkinje cell receives only one climbing fiber. Through its multiple excitatory synapses, the climbing fiber exerts a powerful excitatory effect on each Purkinje cell.

The action potentials of a Purkinje cell vary as a function of the type of excitatory input it receives. Simple spikes, similar to those seen throughout the nervous system, are triggered by excitation of the distal dendrites by the parallel fibers. Complex spikes, which have a prolonged and elaborate multiphasic waveform, are evoked by the multiple excitatory synapses of the climbing fibers on the Purkinje cell. It is possible that the

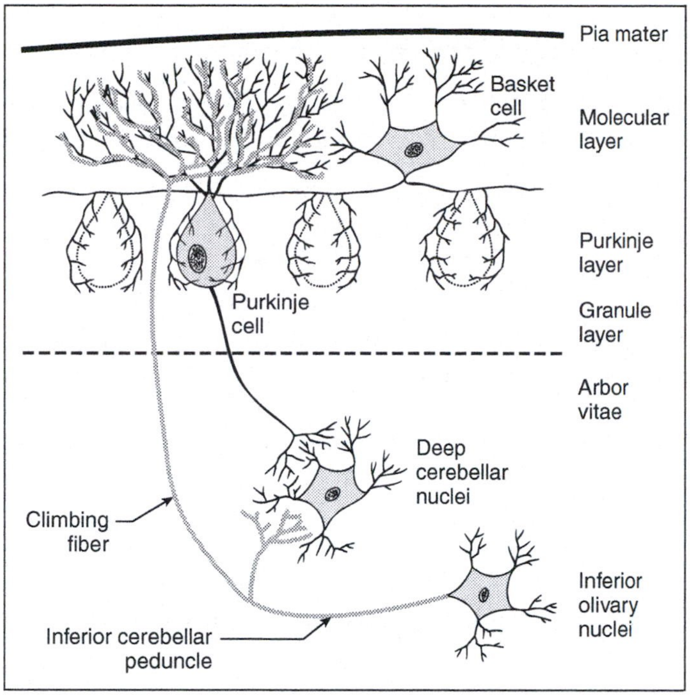

FIG. 12.21. Purkinje Cell Circuitry. A transverse section through a folium shows the fan-like profile of four cerebellar Purkinje cells. Climbing fibers, which originate in the inferior olivary nucleus, climb and repeatedly synapse on the apical dendrites of one Purkinje cell. The Purkinje cell axon, shown leaving the ventral surface of the soma, terminates in one of the deep cerebellar nuclei. The basket cell is named for its basket-like termination around Purkinje cell soma.

changes in calcium conductance produced by complex spikes triggers a cascade of intracellular second messenger–mediated events related to motor learning.

If Purkinje cells and climbing fibers were married to one another, the Purkinje cells would be monogamous and the climbing fibers would be polygamous.

The cerebellar cortex also receives noradrenergic projections from the locus ceruleus, dopaminergic projections from the substantia nigra and the ventral tegmental area, and serotonergic projections from the raphe nuclei. These projections are distributed throughout all layers of the cerebellar cortex and, to a lesser degree, the deep cerebellar nuclei. Like similar projections to the cerebral cortex, these neurotransmitters modulate ongoing activity at their targets.

The cerebellar cortex contains several topographical maps of the body, but none are as well organized as those of the primary somatosensory cortex. In the cerebellar cortex, the orderly representation of one body part (e.g., arm) may be juxtaposed to a detailed map of an unrelated area (e.g., leg). This so-called fractured somatotopy may be the basis for coordinating multiple parts of the body during complex movements. The head and trunk representations are located within the vermal and paravermal zones; receptive fields of the limbs are located laterally.

Deep Cerebellar Nuclei

The fastigial, globose, emboliform, and dentate nuclei contain the primary efferent neurons of the cerebellum (see Figure 12.17). The deep cerebellar nuclei receive collateral projections from brainstem and spinal cord neurons that project to the cerebellar cortex, but most of their afferent projections derive from the cerebellar cortex. Their output is exclusively excitatory and is mediated by the neurotransmitter glutamate.

Fastigial, Globose, Emboliform, Dentate (**F**at **G**uys **E**njoy **D**onuts)

Three sagittal planes:
- Vermal/fastigial
- Paravermal/interposed
- Lateral/dentate

The projections to the deep cerebellar nuclei from the cerebellar cortex form three sagittally oriented zones (see Figure 12.16). The medially located fastigial nucleus receives most of its projections from the midline vermal zone of the cerebellar cortex. The more laterally located interposed and dentate nuclei receive most of their projections from

TABLE 12.3 Cerebellar Circuitry

Functional Modules	Location	Afferent Projections	Efferent Pathway	Efferent Targets	Deep Cerebellar Nuclei	Function
Vestibulocerebellum	Flocculonodular lobe	Scarpa's ganglion Vestibular nuclei Inferior olive	Uncinate fasciculus Juxtarestiform body	Vestibular nuclei Reticular formation	Fastigial nucleus	Balance Posture VOR
Cerebrocerebellum	Lateral hemisphere	Pontine nuclei Inferior olive	Superior cerebellar peduncle	Red nucleus VLc and VPLo nuclei	Dentate nucleus	Motor timing Motor precision
Spinocerebellum	Vermis Paravermal hemisphere	Spinocerebellar tracts	Uncinate fasciculus Juxtarestiform body	Red nucleus	Fastigial nucleus Globose nucleus Emboliform nucleus	Balance Precision movements Movement termination

Note. VOR = vestibulo-ocular reflex; VCc = ventral lateral numleus, pars caudalis; VPLo = ventroposterolateral nucleus, pars oralis.

the paravermal and lateral zones of the cerebellar cortex, respectively. These sagittally oriented zones correspond to the functional organization of the cerebellum.

Functional Organization of the Cerebellum

The cerebellum provides the sensory information that the motor system requires for precise operation. As an embryologic derivative of the alar plate, the cerebellum receives significant projections from the somatosensory, vestibular, visual, and auditory systems. The pattern of afferent projections divides the cerebellum into three functional modules: the vestibulocerebellum, the cerebrocerebellum, and the spinocerebellum (Table 12.3).

Vestibulocerebellum: balance, posture, and VOR

Juxtarestiform body contains reciprocal connections between the cerebellum and the brainstem, and first-order vestibulocerebellar fibers.

Direct projections from the Purkinje cells to the vestibular nuclei are GABAergic.

Nystagmus: an involuntary, rapid movement of the eyeball in any plane

Vestibulocerebellum. The vestibulocerebellum consists of the flocculonodular lobe as well as parts of the vermis and fastigial nuclei. As its name implies, the vestibulocerebellum contributes to balance, posture, and visual fixation through its close relationship to the vestibular system. Primary projections from the vestibular ganglion and secondary projections from the vestibular nuclei enter the cerebellum through the juxtarestiform body located along the medial aspect of the inferior cerebellar peduncle. The vestibulocerebellum also receives significant visual and somatosensory projections from the contralateral inferior olivary nuclei. These olivocerebellar projections enable the cerebellum to adjust the sensitivity of the vestibulo-ocular reflex (VOR) to correct perturbations in peripheral or central vestibular sensitivity caused by age, disease, or trauma.

The vestibulocerebellum adjusts posture and maintains balance through its efferent projections to the vestibular nuclei and the reticular formation (Figure 12.22). Unlike most of the remaining cerebellar cortex, efferent projections from the flocculonodular lobe project to the ipsilateral vestibular nuclei and reticular formation without first synapsing in the deep cerebellar nuclei. These inhibitory projections contribute to balance, control of the extraocular eye muscles, and coordination of head and eye movements. The fastigial nucleus, which facilitates neural activity in the vestibular nuclei and reticular formation, is inhibited by descending projections from the nodulus. These fastigiobulbar projections, like the direct corticobulbar projections, traverse the juxtarestiform body and the uncinate fasciculus, a small fiber bundle that exits the cerebellum along the dorsal surface of the superior cerebellar peduncle. Clinical signs related to damage of the vestibulocerebellum include disorders of balance, gait, posture, and eye movement (e.g., nystagmus). Patients with vestibulocerebellar damage often assume a broad-based gait to compensate for their poor balance and may not show a normal VOR.

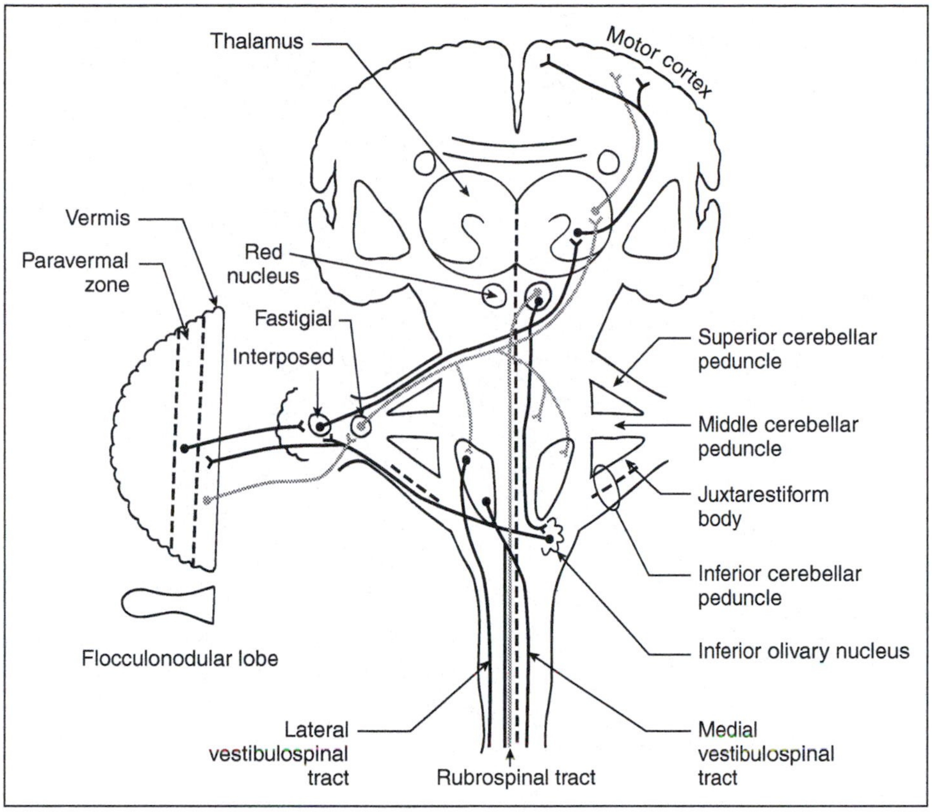

FIG. 12.22. Projections of the Vestibulocerebellum. The efferent projections of the vestibulocerebellum originate in the vermis and the fastigial nuclei.

Cerebrocerebellum. The cerebrocerebellum improves the timing and accuracy of movements through its projections to the premotor and primary motor cortices. This complicated process is carried out by a multisynaptic motor loop that begins and ends in the cerebral cortex (Figure 12.23). Neurons in both cortical sensory and motor areas project to the ipsilateral pontine nuclei, whose neurons project to the contralateral cerebellum through the middle cerebellar peduncle. The deep cerebellar nuclei receive some collateral projections, but most of these axons terminate as mossy fibers in the cerebellar cortex. By comparison, olivocerebellar projections conveying visual and somatosensory information terminate as climbing fibers on Purkinje cells in the lateral zone. As the recipient of both motor output and sensory feedback, the cerebrocerebellum is able to compare intended and actual movements. Purkinje cell axons originating in the cerebrocerebellum terminate in a topographical manner within the dentate nuclei. Efferent projections of the dentate nucleus form the superior cerebellar peduncle, which exits the cerebellum rostrally, decussates in the caudal mesencephalon, and finally terminates in the VLc and VPLo nuclei of the thalamus. These thalamic nuclei project to the premotor and primary motor cortices, thereby closing the cortical-pontocerebellar-thalamocortical loop that improves motor precision by reducing the disparity between intended and actual movements (see Figure 12.2).

Cerebrocerebellum: the lateral zones of the anterior and posterior lobes

The cerebrocerebellum improves motor precision.

The subscript "c" in VLc stands for "caudal," not cerebellar.

Spinocerebellum. The spinocerebellum consists of the vermal and paravermal zones of the anterior and posterior lobes, and their corresponding deep cerebellar nuclei. The vermal and paravermal zones adjust torso and limb position based on feedback from muscle spindles (la fibers) and Golgi tendon organs (lb fibers). Proprioceptive information from the upper limbs is conveyed by the cuneocerebellar tract, whereas the lower limbs are innervated by the dorsal and ventral spinocerebellar tracts. The trajectories of these ascending pathways differ substantially, but all three convey information from the periphery to the ipsilateral cerebellum. Of the three cerebellar lobes, only the spinocerebellum receives somatosensory information directly from the spinal cord.

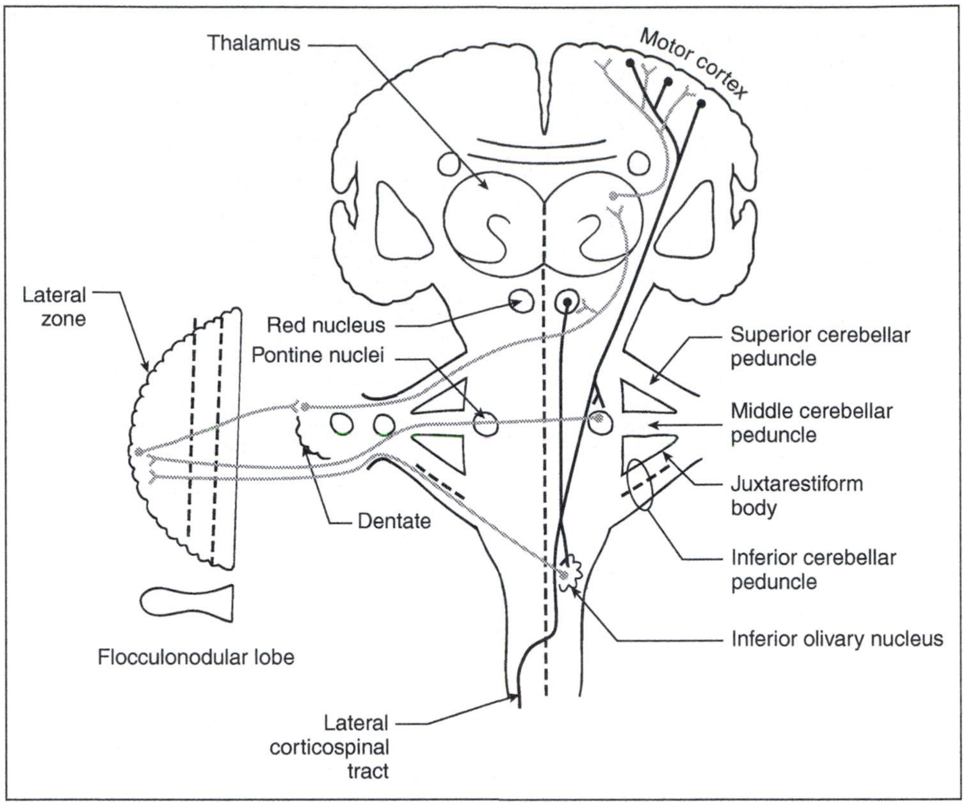

FIG. 12.23. Cerebrocerebellar Circuitry. The ascending projections from the cerebellum cross to the contralateral side of the brain. Because descending corticospinal projections cross back, cerebellar damage causes ipsilateral motor deficits.

Extracerebellar projections from the vermal and paravermal zones originate in the fastigial and interposed nuclei (Figure 12.24). Projections from the fastigial nuclei to the vestibular nuclei and reticular formation, like those of the vestibulocerebellum described above, enable the vermal zone to adjust the trunk muscles of the body. Most fastigial efferents exit the cerebellum within the uncinate fasciculus and terminate in the contralateral vestibular nuclei and the reticular formation. Another contingent of fastigial efferents exits the cerebellum through the ipsilateral juxtarestiform body. Both sets of excitatory fastigiobulbar projections use glutamate as their neurotransmitter.

The projections from the paravermal zone to the interposed nuclei, by comparison, modulate muscle tone and affect movement of the limb muscles. Most of the axons originating in the interposed nuclei exit the cerebellum through the superior cerebellar peduncle, decussate in the caudal mesencephalon, and terminate in the red nucleus. These cerebellorubral projections terminate in the caudal, magnocellular region from which the rubrospinal tract originates. The rubrospinal tract, working in concert with the corticospinal tract, facilitates the flexors of the distal musculature. A small contingent of fibers from the globose and emboliform nuclei terminate in the VLc and VPLo nuclei of the thalamus, which project to the MI cortex.

As would be predicted from the efferent projections of the spinocerebellum, damage to the vermal and paravermal areas upsets balance and the precision of movements executed by the trunk and limb musculature. As with the cerebrocerebellum, spinocerebellar damage also disrupts velocity and force of individual movements as well as the timing of complex movements. It is unusual, however, for patients to have damage restricted to the spinocerebellum.

Feedforward Modulation

Feedback control by the cerebrocerebellum is a cumbersome process best suited for finetuning relatively slow or deliberate movements. For rapid movements that cannot be guided in real

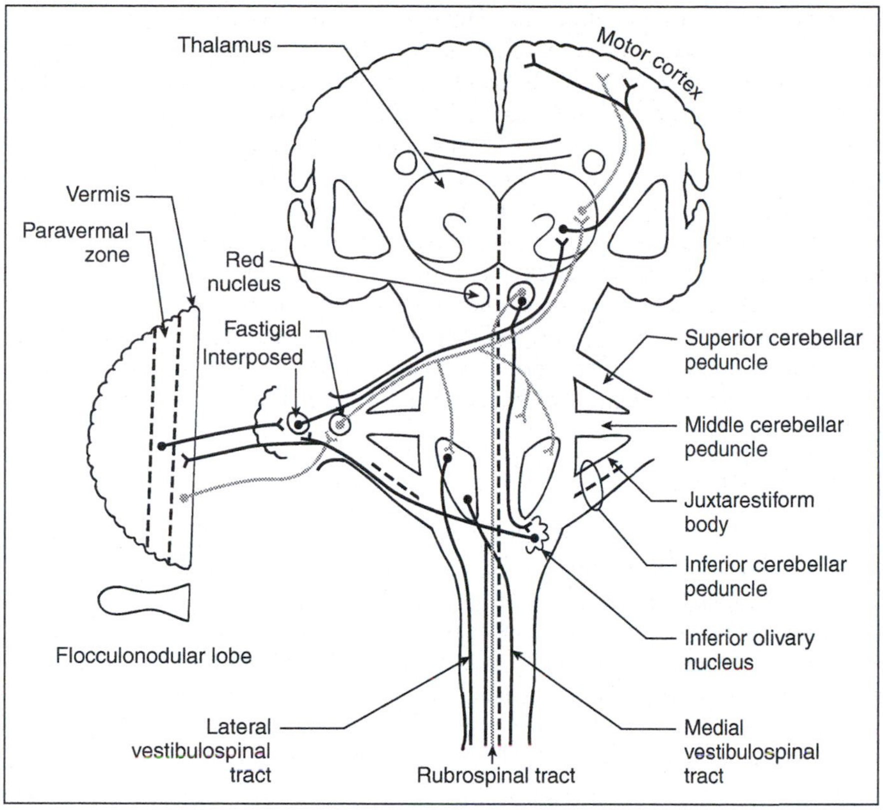

FIG. 12.24. Projections of the Spinocerebellum. Efferent projections of the spinocerebellum resemble those of the vestibulocerebellum and the cerebrocerebellum.

time by feedback, a feedforward or proactive system must be used. Feedforward control is a predictive system capable of executing ballistic and seldom-performed movements, as well as terminating movements smoothly.

In feedback mode, the cerebellum uses sensory information to make real-time adjustments to a motor sequence.

In feedforward mode, the cerebellum uses previous experience to generate a motor sequence.

To play golf, it's more important to have an excellent cerebellum than an expensive set of clubs.

Ballistic Movement. In feedforward mode, the cerebellum guides movements that are too quick to benefit from feedback (e.g., a golf swing). Swinging a golf club requires only a fraction of a second to complete, which is too brief a period to be guided by real-time sensory feedback. Ballistic movements are preprogrammed based on past experience. For an experienced golfer, the mechanics of a golf swing are performed automatically by the cerebellum; conscious adjustment of the swing by the cerebral cortex is usually counterproductive. When a new golf swing is adopted, it is under the voluntary control of primary motor cortex. With practice, the cerebellum assumes control of the timing, balance, and flow of the golf swing and executes it automatically.

Seldom-Performed Movement. By predicting the speed, force, and direction of a movement, the cerebellum provides a good first approximation for how that movement should be executed. For example, even the occasional bowler knows before picking up a bowling ball that it will be heavy and should be cradled from the bottom. A different strategy is used to pick up a fragile item like a wedge of cake. Our past experience with bowling balls and cake is sufficient to create motor templates appropriate for other heavy/bulky or light/fragile objects. When we encounter an object that is heavier than expected and the initial motor strategy fails, we abort the grasp, reposition our grip or stance, and use a different motor strategy to address the object.

Movement Termination. Feedforward control is used to terminate limb movement smoothly. Consider when a paperweight is dropped into someone's outstretched hand. The arm extends briefly before contraction of the biceps muscle returns the arm to its original position. In this example, extension of the arm by the weight stretches the biceps muscle, which triggers the stretch reflex–mediated rebound of the arm. The triceps muscle must provide the brake that prevents the arm from rebounding past its original position. If the braking action of the triceps muscle were entrusted to the stretch reflex, however, it would begin too late to prevent excessive rebound flexion of the arm. The arm would assume a pendular motion as additional cycles of extension and flexion steadied the arm. In healthy individuals, feedforward contraction of the triceps muscle begins during the initial extension of the arm—that is, before the stretch reflex in the triceps muscle is activated. Early activation of the triceps muscle terminates arm rebound near the arm's original position without excessive or repeated oscillation. Lacking feedforward control, patients with cerebellar damage rely on the stretch reflex to terminate limb movement. Movement termination in patients with cerebellar damage is marked by excessive limb oscillation (pendular reflexes).

Clinical Aspects

Despite the importance of the cerebellum to movement, its removal does not cause paralysis or paresis. Patients with cerebellar damage can do almost everything that a healthy person does, but the quality of performance is poor. The core deficit underlying all cerebellar symptomology appears to be poor temporal coordination because cerebellar damage disrupts the timing sequences that synchronize complex, multi-joint/multi-muscle movements related to balance, posture, walking, reaching, speaking, and visual fixation. Cerebellar lesions affect the ipsilateral side of the body because most of the efferent projections of the cerebellum decussate in the midbrain before terminating in the red nucleus and the thalamus. The rubrospinal tract, by recrossing in the ventral tegmental decussation, returns to the original side of the body. The motor nuclei of the thalamus project to primary motor cortex, the origin of the corticospinal tract, which recrosses at the pyramidal decussation.

Cerebellar ataxia resembles drunkenness.

Ataxia. Ataxia is irregular, uncoordinated movement and the cardinal symptom of cerebellar damage. Vermal damage of the anterior and posterior lobes, by disrupting control of the axial musculature, produces an unsteady, broad-based gait called truncal ataxia. Falls are common, usually after staggering toward the side of the lesion. Damage of the paravermal and lateral cerebellum produces limb or appendicular ataxia. Impaired balance and ataxia are caused by damage further posterior in the flocculonodular lobe, but these signs are likely to be accompanied by abnormal eye movements, vertigo, nausea, and vomiting. The staggering of ataxic patients resembles that of drunkenness; similarly, one diagnostic test for cerebellar ataxia is heel-toe walking.

Patients with vestibulospinal damage are unable to close their eyes without falling (positive Romberg sign).

The Romberg test is used to determine whether an ataxic gait is of sensory or cerebellar origin. Standing is a postural reflex that depends on visual, vestibular, and proprioceptive information; at least two of the three systems must be intact for a person to stand unsupported. Patients with mild to moderate vestibular damage or loss of proprioceptive input due to injury of the posterior roots or columns rely on visual cues to stand alone. Following damage to the posterior column, patients are unable to stand with their eyes closed. This is a positive Romberg sign. Patients with mild to moderate cerebellar damage are able to stand with their feet together and eyes closed. Patients with severe vestibular or midline cerebellar damage may be unable to stand, even with their eyes open.

Dysmetria describes movements that overshoot or undershoot their target.

Dysmetria. Patients with dysmetria are unable to gauge the distance to a target accurately. Reaching motions overshoot the object and may be accompanied by tremor and oscillating movements until the patient eventually homes in on the target. Patients with saccadic dysmetria show a similar pattern of overshoot and oscillation during visual fixation. Dysmetria is caused by loss of feedforward control.

Cerebellar tremor is movement-induced; **Parkinson's tremor** occurs at rest.

Intention Tremor. Patients may show marked tremor and erroneous corrections during the final moments before touching an object. Intention tremors reflect a loss of feedforward control.

Cerebellar Hypotonia. The cerebellum does not project to the spinal cord, but it projects to many areas of the brain that do. Cerebellar damage produces hypotonia because decreased output from the deep cerebellar nuclei reduces cortical activation of the α-motor and γ-motor systems. Loss of muscle tone can be observed by direct inspection or by testing for motor rebound. Testing for rebound involves pulling against the patient's flexed arm and then suddenly letting go. Normal patients are able to prevent the arm from striking them in the face. Hypotonia may also contribute to pendular reflexes.

Dysdiadochokinesia. One of the hallmark symptoms of lateral cerebellar damage is dysdiadochokinesia, an inability to perform rapid, alternating movements. Patients with cerebellar damage are unable to alternately pronate and supinate their hands while patting their thighs rapidly. Dysdiadochokinesia is caused by a combination of timing and synchronization deficits, and the difficulty these patients have initiating movements.

Decomposition of Movement. Patients with lateral cerebellar damage often have trouble initiating movements, especially those that involve either multiple muscle groups or coordination of the axial and distal musculature. To compensate, patients may decompose complex movements into their component parts. For example, swinging a tennis racket, which normally involves a sweeping arm motion combined with rotation of the torso, would be performed as sequential rather than simultaneous motions. Decomposition of movement is caused by a breakdown in timing between agonist and antagonist muscle groups and gives movement a robotic appearance.

RESOLUTION OF CLINICAL CASE

The patient was showing early signs of Huntington's chorea. He showed minor choreiform movements of the arms and minor impairment of manual dexterity. These problems will progress until the diagnosis of Huntington's chorea is unmistakable. Although it is too soon to tell if his business problems reflect cognitive impairment, eventually the patient will not be able to manage either his business or his family affairs. Most patients require antidepressant therapy. The physician will be able to make a more certain diagnosis after receiving the results from the genetic testing.

REVIEW QUESTIONS

Directions: For each of the following questions, choose the **one** best answer.

1. Which of the following is a hyperkinetic symptom of Parkinson's disease?
A. Bradykinesia
B. Tremor
C. Reptilian stare
D. Lead pipe rigidity
E. Micrographia

2. Which of the following is the only excitatory neuron in the cerebellar cortex?
A. Basket cell
B. Purkinje cell
C. Granule cell
D. Golgi cell
E. Stellate cell

3. If a patient experiences a seizure in the shoulder and the epileptiform activity spreads laterally across cortex, how would the seizure progress across the body?
A. Shoulder, elbow, wrist, fingers, face, mouth
B. Shoulder, face, mouth, fingers, wrist
C. Shoulder, trunk, leg, foot
D. Shoulder, elbow, wrist, fingers, maxillary face, ophthalmic face
E. It would not spread.

4. Glutamatergic neurons are located in which nucleus of the basal ganglia?
A. Neostriatum
B. Subthalamic nucleus
C. Substantia nigra, pars compacta (SNpc)
D. Internal segment of the globus pallidus (GPi)
E. External segment of the globus pallidus (GPe)

5. A 62-year-old woman presented with an 8-month history of gradually progressive incoordination of the right arm and leg. Examination revealed hypotonia and ataxia of the limbs on the right side. What is the most likely diagnosis?
   A. Stroke involving the anterior spinal artery on the left side above the pyramidal decussation
   B. Tumor within the right cerebellar hemisphere
   C. Tumor within the left subthalamic nucleus
   D. Stroke involving the crus cerebri on the right side
   E. Tumor at the C5 level of the spinal cord affecting most of the lateral funiculus on the right side

6. Why does cerebellar damage produce symptoms on the ipsilateral side of the body?
   A. Because it projects to the ipsilateral red nucleus
   B. Because it projects to the ipsilateral thalamus
   C. Because it has contralateral thalamocortical projections
   D. Because it receives sensory information from the contralateral side of the body
   E. Because it projects to the ipsilateral basal ganglia

7. Which area or areas of the cerebral cortex are active during complicated multifinger movements, but not during the simple movements involving only two fingers?
   A. Primary motor cortex and primary sensory cortex
   B. Supplementary motor cortex(MII)
   C. Posterior parietal cortex (Brodmann areas 5 and 7)
   D. Brodmann areas 4, 6, 3, 1, 2, and 5
   E. Premotor cortex

Damage to the basal ganglia may cause hypokinetic or hyperkinetic symptoms. Match one of the lettered options below with statements 8–13.
   A. Increased movement
   B. Decreased movement

8. An infarct of the subthalamic nucleus

9. Surgical placement of a lesion in GPi (pallidotomy)

10. Administration of an anticholinergic drug

11. A thalamic infarct

12. Administration of a dopamine precursor, L-dopa

13. Administration of a dopamine antagonist

ADDITIONAL READING

Classic Literature

Alexander GE, Crutcher MD: Functional architecture of the basal ganglia circuits: neural substrates of parallel processing. *Trends Neurosci* 13:266–271, 1990.

Alexander GE, DeLong MR, Strick PL: Parallel organization of functionally segregated circuits linking basal ganglia and cortex. *Ann Rev Neurosci* 9:357–381, 1986.

Roland PE, Larsen B, Lassen NA, Skinhoj E: Supplementary motor area and other cortical areas in organization of voluntary movements in man. *J Neurophysiol* 43:118–136, 1980.

Reviews and Landmark Research Articles

Bastien AJ, Thach WT: Cerebellar outflow lesions: a comparison of movement deficits resulting from lesions at the levels of the cerebellum and thalamus. *Ann Neurol* 38:881–892, 1995.

Bergman H, Wichmann T, DeLong MR: Reversal of experimental parkinsonism by lesions of the subthalamic nucleus. *Science* 249:1436–1438, 1990.

Bingaman KD, Bakay RA: The primate model of Parkinson's disease: its usefulness, limitations, and importance in directing future studies. *Prog Brain Res* 127:267–297, 2000.

Comings DE: Tourette's syndrome: a behavioral spectrum disorder. *Adv Neurol* 65:293–303, 1995.

DeLong MR: Primate models of movement disorders of basal ganglia origin. *Trends Neurosci* 13:281–285, 1990.

DeLong MR, Wichman T: Basal ganglia—thalamocortical circuits in parkinsonian signs. *Clin Neurosci* 1:18–26, 1993.

Deogaonkar MS, Subramanian T: Pathophysiological basis of treatment strategies for drug-induced dyskinesias in Parkinson's disease. *Brain Research Reviews* 50:156–168, 2005.

Georgopoulos AP, Kalaska JF, Caminiti R, Massey JT: On the relations between the direction of two-dimensional arm movements and cell discharge in primate motor cortex. *J Neurosci* 2:1527–1537, 1982.

Gerfen CR: Dopamine receptor function in the basal ganglia. *Clin Neurophramacol* 18:S162–S177, 1995.

Goetz CG, DeLong MR, Penn RD, Bakay RAE: Neurosurgical horizons in Parkinson's disease. *Neurology* 43:1–7, 1993.

Graziano, MSA, Taylor CSR, Moore T, Cooke DF: The cortical control of movement revisited. *Neuron* 36:349–362, 2002.

Hague SM, Klaffke S, Bandmann O: Neurodegenerative disorders: Parkinson's disease and Huntington's disease. *J Neurol Neurosurg Psychiatry* 76:1058–1063, 2006.

Parent A, Cicchetti F: The current model of basal ganglia organization under scrutiny. *Mov Disorders* 13:199–202, 1998.

Pereira EAC, Aziz TZ: Parkinson's disease and primate research: past, present, and future. *Postgrad Med J* 82:293–299, 2006.

Tanji J: The supplementary motor area in the cerebral cortex. *Neurosci Res* 19:251–268, 1994.

Tanji J, Shima K: Role for supplementary motor area cells in planning several movements ahead. *Nature* 371:413–416, 1994.

Thach WT, Goodkin HP, Keating JG: The cerebellum and the adaptive coordination of movement. *Ann Rev Neurosci* 15:403–442, 1992.

Tolosa E: The diagnosis of Parkinson's disease. *Lancet* 5:75–86, 2006.

Walter BL, Vitek JL: Surgical treatment for Parkinson's disease. *Lancet Neurol* 3:719–728, 2004.

INTERNET RESOURCES

American Academy of Family Physicians
Update on Parkinson's Disease
http://www.aafp.org/afp/990415ap/2155.html

American Speech-Language-Hearing Association
Huntington's Disease
http://www.asha.org/public/speech/disorders/Huntington-Disease.htm
Amyotrophic Lateral Sclerosis (ALS)
http://www.asha.org/public/speech/disorders/Amyotrophic-lateral-sclerosis.htm

Baltimore Huntington's Disease Center of the Johns Hopkins University
Huntington's Disease
http://www.hopkinsmedicine.org/bhdc/about/

California State University, Chico
Cerebellum
http://www.csuchico.edu/~pmccaff/syllabi/CMSD%20320/362unit7.html
Neuroanatomy of Speech, Swallowing and Language
http://www.csuchico.edu/~pmccaff/syllabi/CMSD%20320/362%20index.html

The Mayo Clinic
Huntington's Disease
http://www.mayoclinic.com/health/huntingtons-disease/DS00401

National Institute of Neurological Disorders and Stroke (NINDS)
Huntington's Disease
http://www.ninds.nih.gov/disorders/huntington/detail_huntington.htm
Parkinson's Disease
http://www.ninds.nih.gov/disorders/parkinsons_disease/parkinsons_disease.htm

Leslie E. Packer, PhD.
Tourette Syndrome
http://www.tourettesyndrome.net/

Tourette Syndrome Association, Inc.
http://www.tsa-usa.org/

University of Western Ontario
Motor Cortex, Cerebellum, et al.
http://www.physpharm.fmd.uwo.ca/undergrad/medsweb/

University of Wisconsin Medical School
Parkinson's Disease
http://www.neuroanatomy.wisc.edu/selflearn/Parkinson%27spesticides.htm

The Global Cerebellum' 97
http://www.neuroanatomy.wisc.edu/cere/text/cere/contents.htm

Washington University School of Medicine
Basal Ganglia and Cerebellum
http://thalamus.wustl.edu/course/cerebell.html
Thalamus
http://thalamus.wustl.edu/course/basmot.html

We Move.org
Parkinson's Disease, Huntington's Disease, Dystonia, Tourette's Syndrome
www.wemove.org

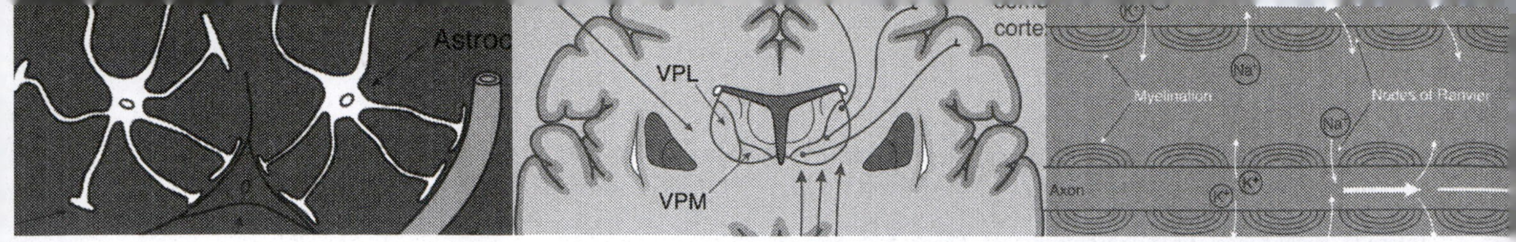

CHAPTER 13

Neural and Neuroendocrine Control of Autonomic Function

INTRODUCTION OF CLINICAL CASE

After months of gradually deteriorating health, a 47-year-old man finally scheduled an appointment with his physician following a recent bout of unrelenting headaches. The patient reported unusual fatigue and an almost unquenchable thirst. For him, the thirst was not as much of a problem as the frequent urination, which interfered with sleep, work, shopping, and travel. Testing was performed over a 3-day period. Reflexes were normal, and there was no evidence of papilledema. The patient's vision, which had been corrected to 20/20 with his recent eyeglass prescription, was only 20/40 now. His urine had a low specific gravity (1.003), but glucose was within normal limits. A subcutaneous injection of vasopressin reduced the volume of urinary output and increased its osmolarity. A magnetic resonance imaging (MRI) scan of the head was scheduled, and additional blood was taken. After reviewing the results of the MRI, the physician requested that the patient have his visual fields measured in the ophthalmology clinic; a bitemporal hemianopsia was detected.

OVERVIEW

The afferent and efferent innervation of the cardiovascular, pulmonary, gastrointestinal, renal, hepatic, endocrine, and reproductive systems, as well as the skin and musculature, is collectively known as the autonomic nervous system (ANS) because it functions almost exclusively outside our sphere of consciousness. The pervasiveness of the ANS enables it to meet the body's changing needs for oxygen, nutrients, and electrolytes as well as maintain proper serum osmolarity and core body temperature. During stressful situations or exercise, the ANS releases glycogen from the liver and increases cardiopulmonary output while diverting energy from the skin and digestive tract. At rest, the process is reversed as energy stores are increased. In short, the ANS adjusts visceral activity to meet the ever-changing demands placed on the body, a process called homeostasis.

Autonomic function is under both neural and hormonal control. Neural control ensures quick and timely activation, but the effects are often short lived. Hormonal effects are more persistent, but they develop more slowly. Homeostasis requires the coordinated action of both systems. Neural control of autonomic function originates from multiple areas in the brain and spinal cord, whereas hormonal control derives from both central (e.g., hypothalamus, hypophysis) and peripheral (e.g., adrenal gland, gonads) sites.

Neural = quick action
Hormonal = prolonged action

Although the ANS is predominantly a motor system, it differs significantly from the somatic motor system. The most obvious difference between the somatic and visceral motor systems is the relative lack of volitional control over autonomic function. In addition, their degree of reliance on central innervation differs. Denervation of somatic muscles causes paralysis, but denervated viscera and glands continue functioning, although they are unable to respond to a physiologic challenge such as exertion. Activation of the ANS often affects multiple systems in the body, unlike the somatic motor system, which is capable of more discrete action. Not surprisingly, there are a host of anatomic differences between the somatic and visceral motor systems.

Autonomic Nervous System

The ANS consists of three divisions: the sympathetic nervous system (SNS), the parasympathetic nervous system (PNS), and the enteric nervous system (ENS). The SNS and PNS control smooth muscle, cardiac muscle, and glandular secretory cells. Although most smooth muscle lines the viscera of the thoracic and abdominal cavities, other sites under autonomic control include the iris, the vasculature of the skin and muscles, the sweat glands, and the muscles of piloerection. Many, but not all, targets of the ANS receive complementary innervation from both the SNS and the PNS. Several notable exceptions include white and brown adipose tissue, sweat glands, and peripheral blood vessels, which are supplied exclusively by the SNS. The ENS is an elaborate neural network that controls intestinal motility and digestive secretions. Mechanical and chemosensory feedback from receptors in the walls of the thoracic, abdominal, and pelvic viscera, as well as the upper gastrointestinal tract, reaches the central nervous system (CNS) along multiple pathways (see below).

SNS + PNS + ENS = ANS

Partition of the ANS into three discrete parts, with the SNS and PNS typically having complementary actions, is a gross oversimplification of homeostatic control. As each component of the ANS is described in turn, bear in mind that there is an extensive autonomic hierarchy linking the visceral afferent and efferent networks of both the SNS and the PNS. Other central circuits link the SNS and PNS to each other, to the somatic musculature, and to the neuroendocrine system. Collectively, this integrative system is known as the central autonomic network (CAN). Although the hypothalamus, known historically as the "chief autonomic ganglion," plays a key role in the CAN, widespread areas of the limbic system including the amygdala, the bed nucleus of the stria terminalis, the septal nuclei, the hippocampus, and the cerebral cortex (cingulate, orbital, insular) are also active participants.

Sympathetic Nervous System

The SNS mobilizes the body's resources for fight or flight behaviors. Sympathetic effects include widespread changes in cardiac, pulmonary, hepatic, and gastrointestinal activity, all of which ready the body for some type of emergency. Sympathetic activation takes place quickly, but its effects are transient. The organization of the SNS is ideally suited for these purposes.

The **SNS:** flight or fight behaviors

Ganglion (*pl.* ganglia): a collection of neurons located outside the CNS

Sympathetic preganglionic neurons are located in the lateral horn of the spinal cord (intermediolateral nucleus; Rexed lamina VII) between segments T1 and L2-L3 (Figure 13.1;

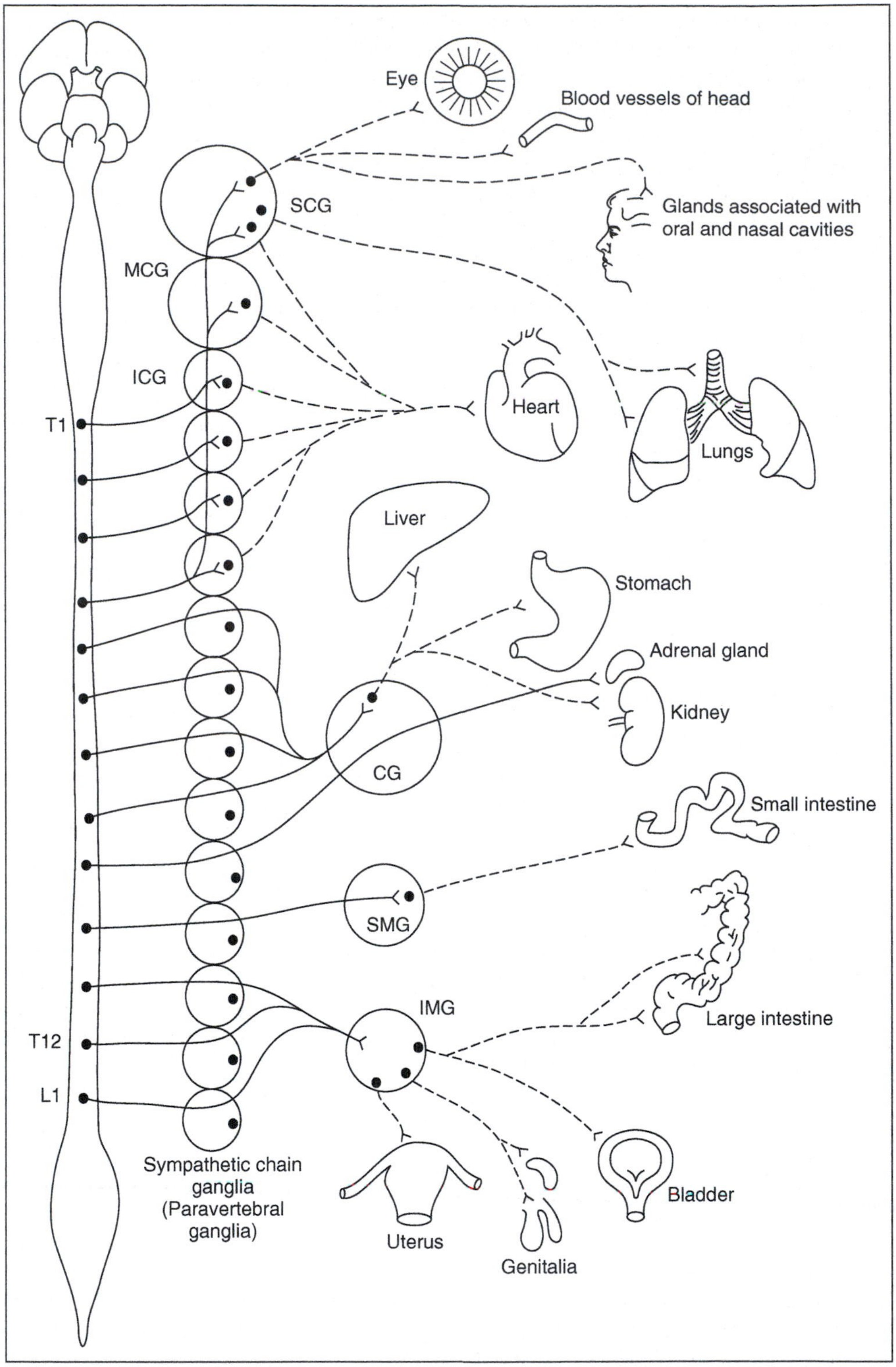

FIG. 13.1. Sympathetic Division of the Autonomic Nervous System. Solid lines are presynaptic fibers; dashed lines are postsynaptic fibers. CG = celiac ganglion; ICG = inferior cervical ganglion; MCG = middle cervical ganglion; IMG = inferior mesenteric ganglion; SCG = superior cervical ganglion; SMG = superior mesenteric ganglion.

see also Figure 4.8D). All preganglionic axons exit the spinal cord through the ventral roots and synapse in the paravertebral ganglia, the prevertebral ganglia, or the adrenal medulla. The paravertebral ganglia, also called the sympathetic chain ganglia, form a continuous column of postganglionic neurons along the lateral margin of the vertebral column from the

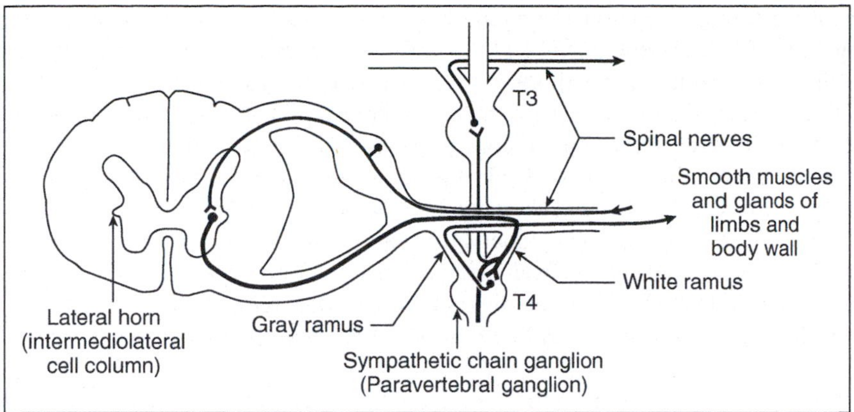

FIG. 13.2. Sympathetic Efferent Pathways. Sympathetic preganglionic neurons exit the spinal cord through the ventral roots, join the spinal nerves briefly, and finally enter the sympathetic chain (paravertebral) ganglia as the white rami where they synapse on the postganglionic neurons. Postganglionic neurons exit the chain ganglia within the gray rami, rejoin the spinal nerves, and synapse on sebaceous glands and piloerector muscles of the skin, and blood vessels of the limbs.

base of the skull to the coccyx. The postganglionic neurons in the more distant prevertebral ganglia are adjacent to the abdominal aorta or its major branches.

Sympathetic Paravertebral Ganglia. The preganglionic axons bound for the paravertebral ganglia leave the spinal cord within the ventral root and form a white communicating ramus that enters the chain ganglia (Figure 13.2). Repeated branching of the preganglionic axons within the ganglia enables each preganglionic neuron to synapse on multiple postganglionic cells. Because each postganglionic neuron is a synaptic target of multiple preganglionic neurons, substantial convergence takes place as well. This divergence and convergence within the sympathetic chain ganglia explains how the SNS is able to command such widespread, coordinated, and nearly simultaneous actions.

As axons of postganglionic neurons exit the paravertebral ganglia, they follow two routes. Some fibers leave the chain ganglia within the gray (unmyelinated) communicating ramus, rejoin their respective spinal nerves, and distribute to blood vessels, sweat glands, and hair follicles in the extremities (see Figure 13.2). These structures are unique in that they do not receive complementary innervation from the PNS. Other postganglionic axons, upon leaving the chain ganglia, form the cervical and thoracic cardiac nerves and pulmonary nerves, as shown in Figure 13.3. These axons course directly to the smooth muscle of the heart and esophagus, the vascular smooth muscle of the heart, and the glandular respiratory epithelium.

This complex pattern of divergence and convergence obscures but does not eliminate the segmental organization and innervation of the body by the SNS. At mid-thoracic, lumbar,

Ramus (*pl.* rami): a small branch or offshoot of a larger structure (e.g. nerve, blood vessel)

The white communicating ramus consists of thinly myelinated preganglionic fibers.

The **final common pathway:** in the somatomotor system, one neuron; in the visceromotor system, two neurons

The gray communicating rami consist of unmyelinated, postganglionic fibers.

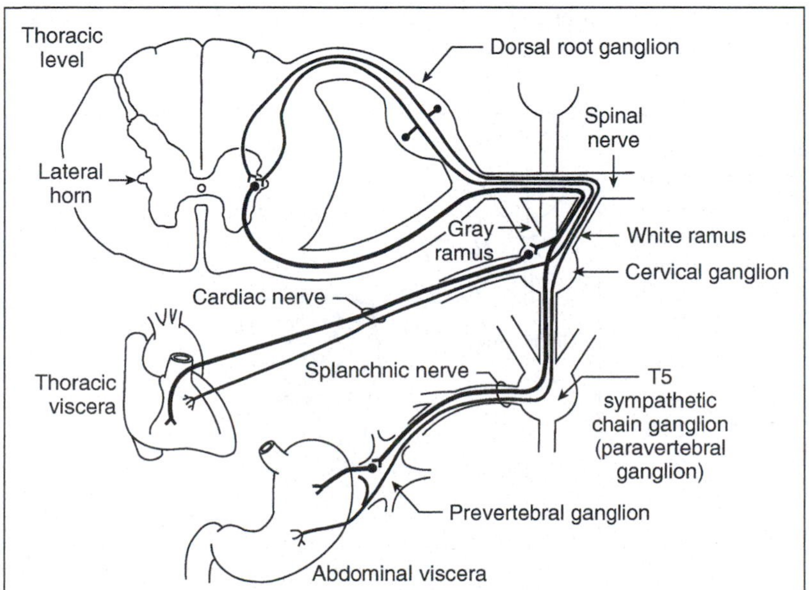

FIG. 13.3. Pathways of the Cardiac and Splanchnic Nerves. The splanchnic nerves are preganglionic axons that pass through the sympathetic chain ganglia without synapsing and terminate on postganglionic neurons in the prevertebral ganglia. The cardiac nerves are the six postganglionic branches of the sympathetic nervous system that run from the superior, middle, and inferior cervical ganglia to the cardiac plexus.

and sacral levels, the sympathetic chain ganglia have a one-to-one relationship with their corresponding spinal nerves (see Figure 13.1). Rostrally, however, the sympathetic preganglionic fibers derived from the upper thoracic cord coalesce and funnel into the superior, middle, and inferior cervical ganglia. The superior cervical ganglia, the largest and most important of the three, innervates visceral targets within the head such as the salivary, sweat, and lacrimal glands, the pupillary dilator muscle, the blood vessels of the brain, as well as the vasculature of the skin of the head and neck, whose somatosensory innervation derives from the C2-C4 segments. Loss of sympathetic innervation caused by damage to the superior cervical ganglion or its afferent projections from the hypothalamus or solitary nucleus produces pupillary constriction (miosis), loss of sweating (anhidrosis), drooping of the eyelid (ptosis), and flushing of the face—a constellation of symptoms known as Horner's syndrome (see Chapter 5).

Postganglionic sympathetic neurons in the mid and lower thoracic chain ganglia receive projections from preganglionic neurons at corresponding levels of the spinal cord and innervate the abdominal viscera. The pelvic viscera and the lower trunk and legs are innervated by preganglionic and postganglionic neurons located at lower thoracic and upper sacral levels.

The **splanchnic nerves** are preganglionic axons that terminate in the prevertebral ganglia.

Sympathetic Prevertebral Ganglia. Some preganglionic fibers pass through the paravertebral ganglia without synapsing and coalesce into the splanchnic nerves that terminate in the prevertebral ganglia (see Figure 13.3). Postganglionic neurons located in the celiac, aorticorenal, superior mesenteric, inferior mesenteric prevertebral ganglia innervate the abdominal and pelvic viscera.

Functionally, the chromaffin cells of the adrenal medulla are analogous to the postganglionic neurons of the sympathetic ganglion.

Chromaffin Cells of the Adrenal Medulla. Other preganglionic sympathetic fibers bypass both the paravertebral and prevertebral ganglia and terminate on chromaffin cells of the adrenal medulla. Chromaffin cells are neural crest derivatives that act like the postganglionic neurons located in the sympathetic ganglia. Unlike the postganglionic neurons that release norepinephrine at synapses within a target organ, however, chromaffin cells release epinephrine (and some norepinephrine as well) into the systemic circulation. Although the vasculature is a slow delivery system, it provides sustained and widespread activation of the viscera and somatic musculature that complements the quick-acting but transient responses elicited by the preganglionic/postganglionic SNS projections at specific targets.

Exception: Postganglionic sympathetic neurons that innervate sweat glands are cholinergic.

Neurotransmitters in the Sympathetic Nervous System. Preganglionic neurons in the SNS use acetylcholine as their neurotransmitter; postganglionic neurons are adrenergic, using either epinephrine or norepinephrine (Figure 13.4). The effects of adrenergic transmission depend on which subclass of alpha-adrenergic or beta-adrenergic receptors are found in the target organ. Stimulation of α_1 receptors causes vasoconstriction, pupillary dilation, and relaxation of the gut. Adrenergic stimulation of β_2 receptors relaxes smooth muscle, which causes bronchodilation, vasodilation in skeletal muscles, and decreased

FIG. 13.4. Efferent Limb of the Sympathetic Nervous System. The widespread effects of the sympathetic nervous system are due, in part, to the synapsing of individual preganglionic neurons onto many postganglionic neurons.

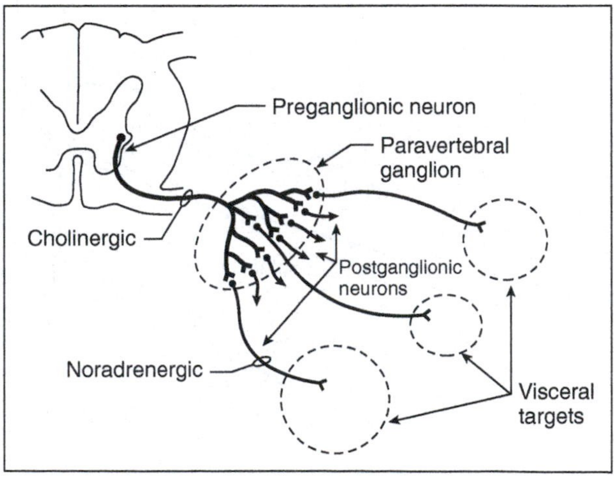

intestinal peristalsis. Activation of β_2 receptors located in cardiac muscle increases heart rate and cardiac output. Epinephrine, a more effective agonist than norepinephrine at both alpha-adrenergic and beta-adrenergic receptors, is used as a bronchodilator for asthma attacks and a cardiac stimulant following arrest of the heart.

Neuropeptides co-localized in autonomic postganglionic neurons may serve as neuromodulators that enable individual neurons to have customized effects at the end organ. Somatostatin and neuropeptide Y are expressed in many sympathetic postganglionic neurons, whereas vasoactive intestinal peptide (VIP) and calcitonin gene-related peptide (CGRP) are found in parasympathetic neurons. The neuropeptide cocktail that is released by each postganglionic neuron appears to be determined by that cell's firing rate and pattern of discharge.

Visceral Sensation. Ischemia, pressure, physical trauma, and cramping of the abdominal and pelvic viscera produce pain, which enters the CNS through the sympathetic nerves. The cell bodies of these visceral afferent neurons are located in the dorsal root ganglia, and their central processes enter the spinal cord through the dorsal root. Although the central projections of these visceral afferent neurons have not been completely elucidated, some ascend with the anterolateral system to the ventral posterior nucleus of the thalamus. Unlike the somatosensory system, visceral afferent sensations are poorly localized; indeed, sensations from the viscera often refer to skin, muscles, or limbs, as discussed in Chapter 7. Other nociceptive sensations that ascend through the spinoreticular tract eventually reach the hypothalamus, which plays a central role in autonomic regulation.

Parasympathetic Nervous System

The PNS is most active when the time for flight or fight has passed and the body is ready to rest, digest, and conserve energy. The PNS conserves energy by slowing cardiopulmonary function and attending to digestion (salivation, gastrointestinal peristalsis, secretion), urination, defecation, and reproduction. The differences between the SNS and the PNS are listed in Table 13.1.

The **PNS** saves energy; the **SNS** spends energy.

Parasympathetic preganglionic neurons, like their sympathetic counterparts, have their embryologic origin in the general visceral efferent (GVE) cell column (see Figure 5.1). Unlike the sympathetic preganglionic neurons distributed throughout the thoracic-lumbar

SNS = thoracic-lumbar
PNS = craniosacral

TABLE 13.1 Comparison of the Sympathetic and Parasympathetic Divisions of the Autonomic Nervous System

Trait	Sympathetic Division	Parasympathetic Division
Preganglionic cell location	T1-L2 (intermediolateral cell column)	S2-S4 Cranial nerve nuclei III, VII, IX, and X
Course of preganglionic fibers	White rami (T1-L2), sympathetic trunks, and splanchnic nerves	Pelvic nerves and cranial nerves III, VII, IX, and X
Postganglionic cell location	Paravertebral ganglia Prevertebral ganglia Adrenal cortex	Walls of viscera Cranial nerve autonomic ganglia (III = ciliary; VII = pterygopalatine and submandibular; IX = otic)
Course of postganglionic fibers	Long course Travel to target organs and tissues Nerve plexuses that run along arteries supplying the head and body	Short course Travel within target organ
Target	Smooth and cardiac muscle Secretory cells	Primarily viscera of the head, thoracic, abdominal, and pelvic cavities
Preganglionic neurotransmitter	Acetylcholine	Acetylcholine
Postganglionic neurotransmitter	Norepinephrine	Acetylcholine
Action	Energy mobilization (flight or fight)	Energy conservation (rest and digest)

spinal cord, the parasympathetic preganglionic neurons are located in the brainstem and in sacral segments S2-S4 (Figure 13.5). The parasympathetic preganglionic neurons in the sacral spinal cord occupy the lateral edge of the central gray, despite the fact that there is no lateral horn, per se, at sacral levels.

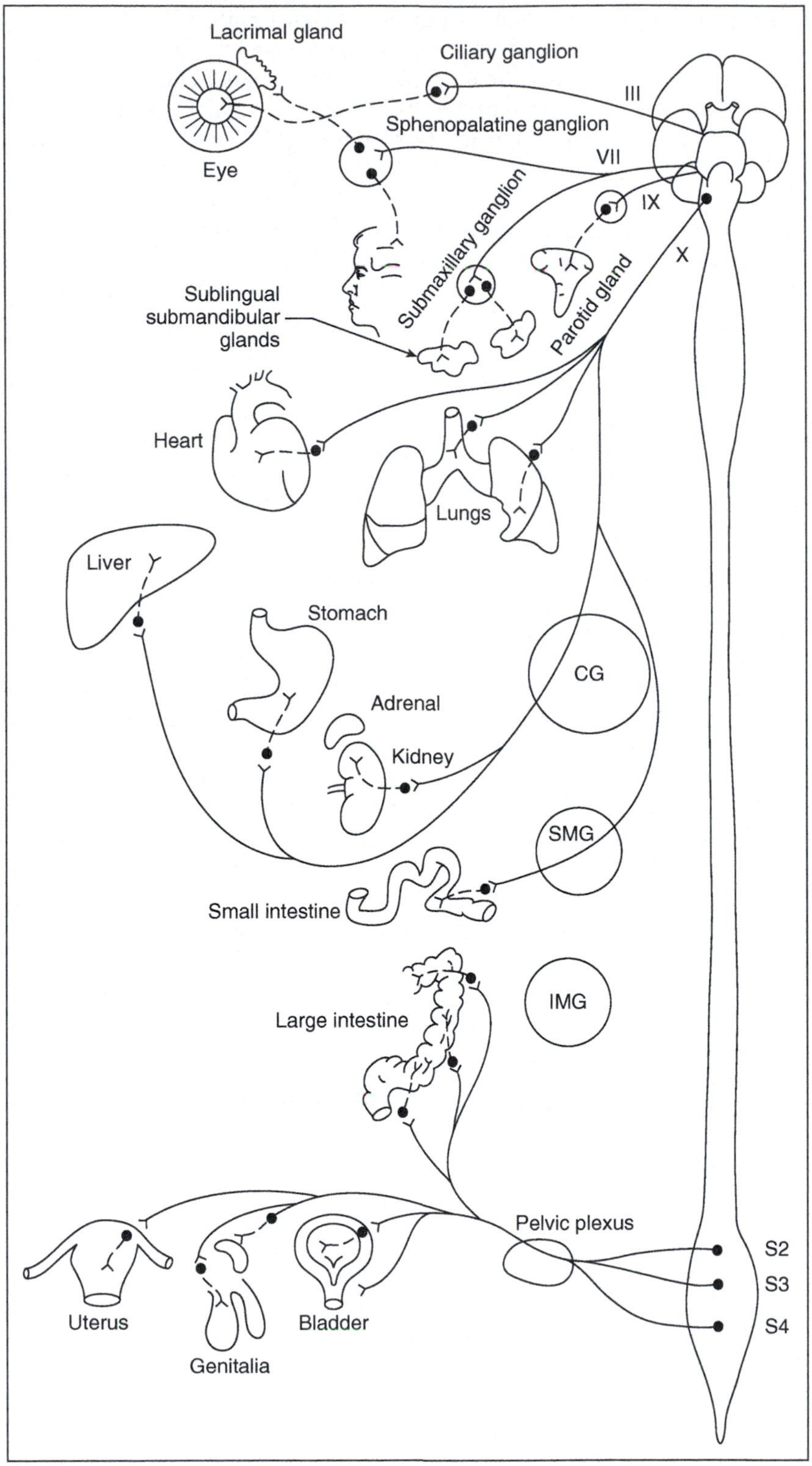

FIG. 13.5. Parasympathetic Division of the Autonomic Nervous System. Solid lines are presynaptic fibers; dotted lines are postsynaptic fibers. CG = celiac ganglion; IMG = inferior mesenteric ganglion; SMG = superior mesenteric ganglion.

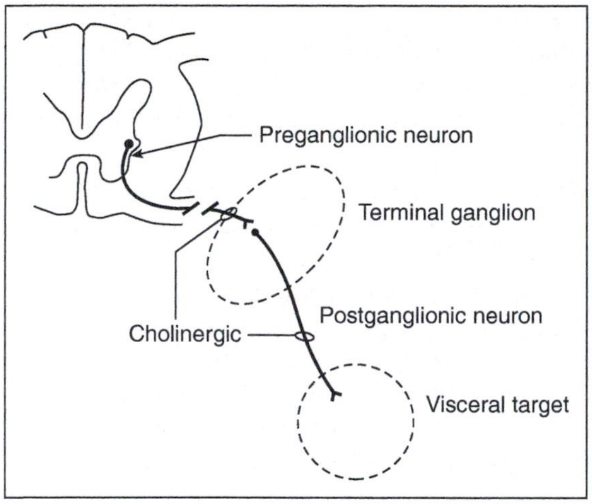

FIG. 13.6. Efferent Limb of the Parasympathetic Nervous System. The relatively discrete actions of the parasympathetic nervous system are due to the near one-to-one relationship between individual preganglionic and postganglionic neurons.

Like the SNS, the final common pathway of the PNS consists of preganglionic and postganglionic neurons. In contrast to the chain ganglia of the SNS, however, the parasympathetic postganglionic neurons are located in discrete ganglia close to or even within the walls of their visceral targets. For example, the postganglionic neurons that innervate the iris and the ciliary muscle are located in the ciliary ganglion, which is located in the posterior part of the orbit. Because the parasympathetic postganglionic neurons are adjacent to their visceral targets, their preganglionic axons are much longer than their postganglionic axons. This contrasts with the SNS in which preganglionic axons are shorter than the postganglionic fibers (see Table 13.1).

The proximity of the autonomic ganglia to their respective target organs enables the actions of the PNS to be more focused than those of the SNS. The specificity of the PNS is also reflected in the synaptic organization of the parasympathetic ganglia where preganglionic axons typically synapse on relatively few postganglionic neurons (Figure 13.6). Both preganglionic and postganglionic neurons in the PNS are cholinergic.

The organ specificity of the PNS derives, in part, from the use of a long preganglionic axon and a short postganglionic axon.

Afferent projections from non-nociceptive receptors in the pharynx, larynx, trachea, lungs, esophagus, heart, stomach, and liver form the sensory limbs of several visceromotor, vasomotor, and secretory reflexes (see below and Chapter 5). These projections, which enter the CNS through the glossopharyngeal and vagus nerves, terminate in the caudal half of the nucleus of the solitary tract (NST).

Ascending projections originating in the solitary nucleus send this visceral afferent information further rostrally to the pontine parabrachial nucleus and the paraventricular nucleus (PVN) of the hypothalamus. The parabrachial nucleus is an important gateway to the limbic system, which is heavily invested in emotion, motivation, and learning (see Chapter 14). The PVN influences cardiovascular function directly via descending sympathetic projections to the neurons in the lateral horn of the thoracic spinal cord, and indirectly through vasopressin release by the neurohypophysis.

Cranial Division. The cranial division of the PNS consists of the preganglionic parasympathetic fibers within the oculomotor (III), facial (VII), glossopharyngeal (IX), and vagus (X) nerves. These nerves participate in a variety of autonomic reflexes, which, like their somatomotor counterparts, consist of both afferent and efferent limbs. This section describes the autonomic reflexes associated with cranial nerves III, VII, IX, and X; these functions and others are described in more detail in Chapter 5.

The cranial division of the PNS: cranial nerves III, VII, IX, and X

Oculomotor Nerve (CN III). The oculomotor nerve contains the general somatic efferent (GSE) fibers that innervate four of the six extraocular muscles and the general visceral efferent (GVE) fibers that mediate the accommodation and pupillary reflexes. These GVE fibers are the axons of the preganglionic neurons located in the Edinger-Westphal nucleus of the oculomotor complex. The postganglionic targets of these GVE neurons, located in the ciliary ganglion, innervate the ciliary muscles that focus the lens and the sphincter pupillae muscles that constrict the pupil. The parasympathetic actions on the pupillary sphincter muscles are opposed by sympathetic projections to the dilator pupillae muscle. The postganglionic axons that innervate the dilator muscle originate in the superior cervical ganglion. Chapter 5 contains a more detailed description of the oculomotor system.

The superior salivatory nucleus is located near the medial edge of the NST.

Patients with **"crocodile tears"** report that foods or beverages trigger tearing instead of salivation.

Facial Nerve (CN VII). Gustatory stimulation of the oral cavity triggers salivatory and secretory reflexes that aid digestion. The facial nerve, which responds to gustatory stimulation of the anterior tongue, projects to the NST whose neurons, in turn, innervate the superior salivatory nucleus. Preganglionic parasympathetic neurons in the superior salivatory nucleus project to the pterygopalatine and submandibular ganglia via the intermediate nerve, a branch of the facial nerve. Postganglionic neurons in the pterygopalatine ganglion innervate the lacrimal glands (tears), and those in the submandibular ganglion supply the submandibular and sublingual glands (saliva). Regrowth of damaged facial nerve fibers sometimes results in crossed innervation of the lacrimal and salivary glands, producing the disorder popularly known as "crocodile tears." Other efferents from the NST to the nearby dorsal motor nucleus of the vagus trigger gastric acid release in the stomach and insulin secretion by the islet cells in the pancreas.

Glossopharyngeal Nerve (CN IX). Salivation mediated by the inferior salivatory nucleus is triggered by gustatory stimulation of taste buds innervated by the glossopharyngeal nerve, which projects to the NST. Neurons in the NST synapse on preganglionic parasympathetic neurons in the inferior salivatory nucleus, which, in turn, terminate in the otic ganglion. Postganglionic neurons in the otic ganglion complete the reflex through their projections to the secretory cells of the parotid gland.

The glossopharyngeal nerve also contains visceral afferent projections from chemoreceptors in the carotid body and baroreceptors in the wall of the carotid sinus. Chemoreceptors located in the carotid *body* sample blood pH and arterial oxygen and carbon dioxide levels through its fenestrated capillaries. Baroreceptors located in the carotid *sinus* respond to rapid changes in blood pressure that require corrective action. This information is transmitted to the caudal NST, which corrects blood pressure through its connections with the dorsal motor nucleus of the vagus (a vasodepressor area), the caudal ventrolateral medulla (CVLM) and the rostral ventrolateral medulla (RVLM, a vasopressor area), and the nucleus ambiguus (Figure 13.7). The baroreceptor reflex is discussed in more detail in the next section. Symptoms associated with lesions of the glossopharyngeal and vagus nerves are discussed in Chapter 5.

Vagus Nerve (CN X). The vagus nerve is a mixed nerve of branchiomeric origin that contains both special visceral afferent (SVA) and general visceral afferent (GVA) fibers. The SVA component innervates taste buds around the epiglottis (see Chapter 10). Several autonomic reflexes are mediated by the GVA fibers that supply the pharynx, larynx,

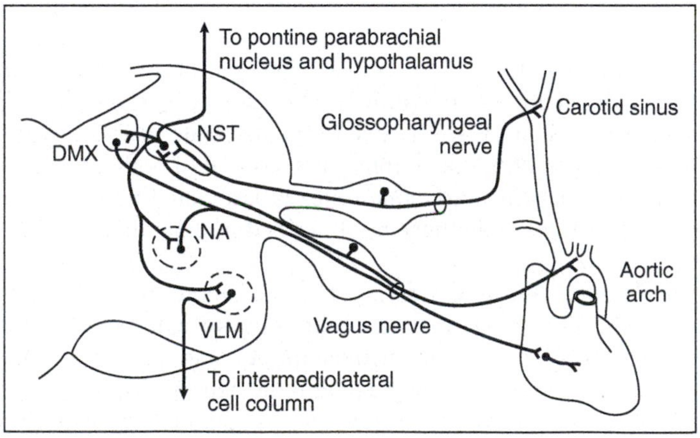

FIG. 13.7. Carotid Sinus Reflex. Afferent projections from receptors located in the carotid sinus and aortic arch terminate in the caudal part of the nucleus of the solitary tract (NST). Ascending projections enter the limbic system through the pontine parabrachial nucleus and hypothalamus. Efferent projections from the dorsal motor nucleus of the vagus (DMX) and the nucleus ambiguus (NA) make compensatory adjustments to the heart. VLM = caudal and rostral ventral lateral medulla.

trachea, lungs, esophagus, heart, liver, pancreas, stomach, and liver. The afferent limb of these SVA- and GVA-mediated reflexes is carried by the vagus nerve to the caudal NST.

Fluid or mechanical stimulation of the larynx and pharynx initiates coughing, gagging, and vomiting reflexes designed to preserve airway patency.

The GVA fibers that innervate baroreceptors and chemoreceptors along the aortic arch, the atria, and the left ventricle are vagal analogs to the pressure and chemical sensors in the carotid sinus and carotid body described above. These afferent vagal pathways mediate the baroreceptor reflex, which counteracts the drop in blood pressure caused by changing from a supine position to a standing position. As Figure 13.8 shows, the decrease in baroreceptor activity caused by a drop in blood pressure triggers both sympathetic and parasympathetic compensatory mechanisms that increase heart rate and cardiac output (stroke volume) as well as vascular resistance in the skeletal muscles and viscera, while preserving blood supply to the heart and brain. The parasympathetic effects are mediated by excitatory projections from the NST to the dorsal motor nucleus of the vagus and the nucleus ambiguus. Increased sympathetic tone is mediated by a reduction of the NST inhibitory influence on the CVLM. The CVLM projects to the vasopressor center located in the RVLM, which contains the sympathetic preganglionic neurons whose axons

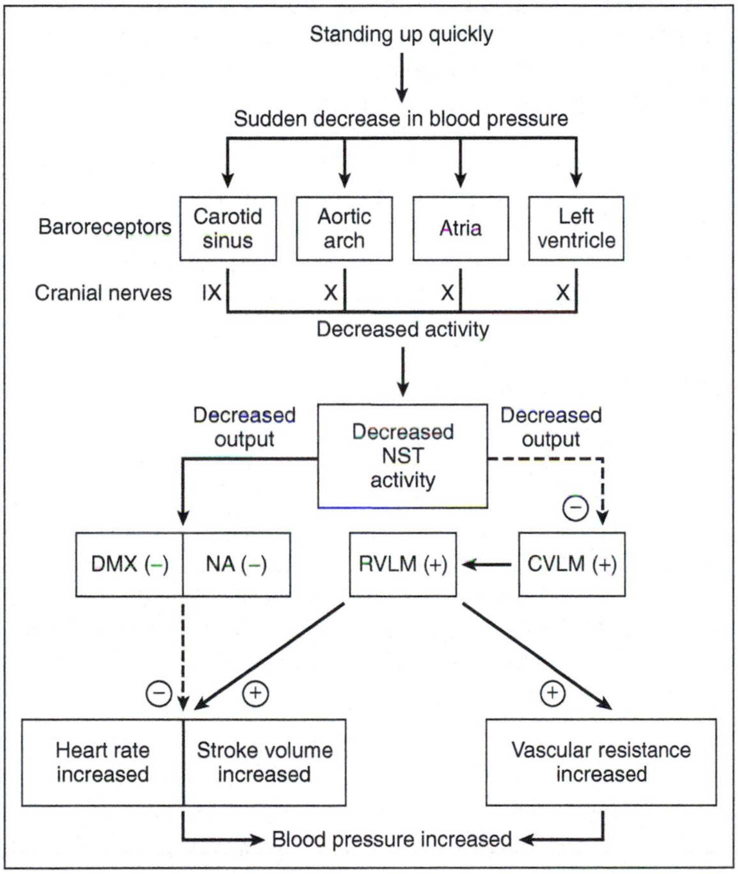

FIG. 13.8. Baroreceptor Reflex. Decreased blood pressure reduces the firing rate of the baroreceptors located in the carotid sinus, the aortic arch, the atria, and the left ventricle, which, in turn, reduces neural activity in the NST. Reduced activation of the NST decreases inhibition of the CVLM/RVLM vasopressor circuit. Increased firing of RVLM neurons improves sympathetic tone, which raises heart rate and cardiac output and increases vascular resistance. These actions are complemented by decreased excitatory output from the NST to the DMX, which disinhibits (i.e., increases) heart rate and cardiac output. The net effect is an increase in blood pressure to counteract the decrease caused by standing. CVLM = caudal ventrolateral medulla; DMX = dorsal motor nucleus of the vagus; NA = nucleus ambiguus; NST = nucleus of the solitary tract; RVLM = rostral ventrolateral medulla. Arrows with dashed lines are inhibitory projections.

descend through the medulla and terminate in the intermediolateral cell column. Stimulating the RVLM increases both heart rate and cardiac output. The same circuitry makes the appropriate (i.e., opposite) compensatory adjustments following an increase in blood pressure.

> The **baroreceptor reflex** has both sympathetic and parasympathetic components.

A sluggish baroreceptor reflex may cause orthostatic hypotension, whose primary symptom of vertigo is usually followed by the groggy exclamation, "Oh, I stood up too fast." The diagnosis of orthostatic hypotension is made if standing causes the systolic blood pressure to decrease by 20 mm Hg or more.

> **Syncope:** a temporary loss of consciousness due to transient generalized cerebral ischemia

Sometimes an unusual set of circumstances conspire to trigger the baroreceptor reflex at an inappropriate time, resulting in vasovagal syncope. For example, an "expectant" father witnessing the birth of his first child is probably flushed with adrenalin, which produces vasodilation of the somatic musculature. Pooling of the blood in the lower body during either standing or sitting reduces venous return to the heart, causing additional sympathetic stimulation. If the normal compensatory response of increasing the rate and force of left ventricular contractions stimulates the pressure receptors located there, the baroreceptor reflex might be triggered, thereby leading to a further reduction in heart rate and cardiac output and, ultimately, fainting.

Preganglionic neurons located in the dorsal motor nucleus of the vagus also project to postganglionic neurons located in terminal ganglia embedded within the walls of the thoracic and abdominal viscera. These descending projections, consistent with the "rest and digest" role of the PNS, constrict bronchioles, decrease heart rate and blood pressure, and increase peristaltic movements and secretions of the gut.

Sacral Division. The sacral division of the PNS consists of preganglionic neurons located in the lateral part of the central gray of spinal segments S2-S4. Preganglionic axons, after exiting the spinal cord in the ventral roots, synapse with the postganglionic neurons located in the walls of the target organs. The short postganglionic axons innervate the bladder, the descending colon, the rectum, and the reproductive organs.

Enteric Nervous System

> The ENS may contain as many neurons as the spinal cord.

The ENS is an elaborate neural network that controls the motility of the gastrointestinal tract as well as secretions of the pancreas and gallbladder. The ENS consists of sensory receptors located throughout the gut that are linked with motor neurons in the spinal cord by interneurons located in the myenteric and submucosal plexuses. Food in the lumen of the gastrointestinal tract initiates secretion of gastric acid and bile into the stomach and small intestine as well as peristaltic movements that propel food through the gastrointestinal tract. Although the ENS usually operates independently of the CNS, both the PNS and SNS are capable of exerting some control. For example, during emergencies the SNS may interrupt peristalsis and secretion.

AUTONOMIC FUNCTIONS

Micturition

> Urination depends upon the cooperation of the SNS, the PNS, and the somatic motor system

Urinary retention and evacuation depend on the cooperation of the SNS, the PNS, and the somatic motor system. Micturition involves volitional control as well as an elaborate hierarchy of segmental and suprasegmental reflexes organized across spinal, brainstem, and cortical levels. In general, urination is controlled by parasympathetic pathways, and urinary retention is maintained by sympathetic and somatomotor circuits (Figure 13.9). Urinary continence is maintained by the internal and external urethral sphincters, which are innervated by neural circuitry located in the spinal cord. Bladder emptying is achieved by relaxing these sphincter muscles and contracting the detrusor muscles located in the walls of the bladder.

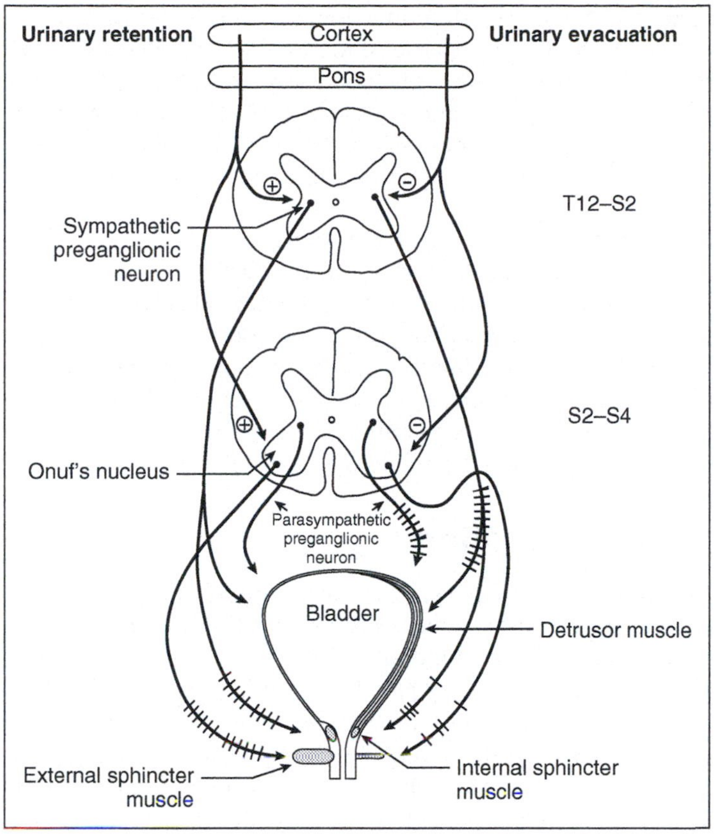

FIG. 13.9. Motor Pathways for Urinary Retention and Evacuation. Control over micturition is exerted by the cerebral cortex, the pons, and the spinal cord. Urinary retention (left) is initiated by neurons in the cerebral cortex and pons that facilitate sympathetic preganglionic neurons in spinal segments T12-S2 and somatic motor neurons at sacral levels. Urinary evacuation (right) is initiated by cortical and pontine neurons that relax the internal and external sphincter muscles by inhibiting the retentive circuits and then contract the detrusor muscle of the bladder.

Bladder distention, detected by stretch receptors and nociceptors in the bladder walls, is transmitted to the spinal cord through spinal nerves whose cell bodies are located in the S2-S4 dorsal root ganglia. Unlike somatosensory projections that enter the cord through the dorsal root, these parasympathetic afferent fibers pass through the ventral root and synapse on neurons in the dorsal and lateral horns. Viscerosensory information terminating in the dorsal horn is conveyed to the thalamus through the anterolateral and lemniscal systems. Third-order neurons in the thalamus project to the parietal operculum near the postcentral sulcus and the insula where conscious perception of a full bladder takes place. Other visceral afferent projections ascend within the spinoreticular tract to the hypothalamus, where various supraspinal autonomic reflexes are initiated. The afferent fibers that terminate in the lateral horn engage preganglionic parasympathetic neurons, which govern spinal automatic reflexes.

When bladder distention is low, somatomotor neurons in the anterior horn of the S2-S4 segments (Onuf's nucleus) reflexively tighten the striated muscles of the external urinary sphincter. Additional security is provided by sympathetic preganglionic neurons in the T12-S2 segments that contract the smooth muscles of the internal urinary sphincter and relax the detrusor muscles that line the walls of the bladder. These guarding reflexes are facilitated by direct and indirect projections from the pons and cerebral cortex, which activate the somatomotor neurons in Onuf's nucleus.

For urination to take place, the somatic and sympathetic retentive reflexes must be inhibited by micturition centers in the pons and cerebral cortex. When bladder distention increases and reaches a threshold level, we become conscious of the need to urinate.

Medial frontal lobe damage produces an **uninhibited bladder.**

Voluntary urination is initiated by the cortical micturition center located along the medial wall of the superior frontal gyrus. Corticospinal projections release the external urethral sphincter that normally retains urine. The pontine micturition center coordinates release of the external sphincter with relaxation of the sympathetic brake on the internal sphincter and contraction of the detrusor muscles by the preganglionic parasympathetic neurons at the S2-S4 levels. After the micturition reflex has begun, it continues until the bladder is virtually empty.

An **automatic bladder** fills to capacity and then voids automatically.

Lower motor neuron damage at the sacral level produces an **atonic bladder.**

The widely distributed circuitry for micturition makes the system vulnerable to injury. Damage to the medial frontal lobes disables the pontine micturition center and produces involuntary urination, also known as an uninhibited bladder. Lesions that interrupt supraspinal micturition pathways produce an automatic bladder, which, as the name implies, voids automatically after filling to capacity. Damage to the sacral cord or the root fibers within the cauda equina produces an atonic bladder, which fills to capacity but, lacking parasympathetic control, cannot be emptied voluntarily. Some patients with an atonic bladder can void by compressing their abdominal muscles; most must be catheterized.

Erection and Ejaculation

Erection is driven by the PNS.

The physiologic mechanisms that operate the male and female sex organs are remarkably similar and, like micturition, reflect the coordinated actions of the SNS, the PNS, and the somatic motor system. Penile and clitoral erection can be initiated by peripheral or psychogenic stimulation and executed by parasympathetic preganglionic neurons located in the S2-S4 segments of the spinal cord. Production of the ejaculate by the seminal vesicles and the prostate gland and secretions from the vaginal walls are controlled by sympathetic neurons in the thoracic and lumbar spinal cord. Following seminal emission into the posterior urethra by the SNS, reflexive somatic motor contractions initiate ejaculation.

Defecation

The stimulus for defecation is distention of the sigmoid colon by feces. Fecal matter is retained by an internal smooth muscle sphincter and an external striated muscle sphincter. The internal sphincter is innervated by sympathetic and parasympathetic fibers exiting the lower lumbar and sacral segments of the spinal cord, respectively. The muscles of the external sphincter are innervated by motor neurons located in the S2-S4 segments but, unlike other striated muscles, they are under both reflexive and voluntary control. Reflexive control of the external sphincter preserves continence during sleep. Distention of the sigmoid colon produces a sense of fullness, mediated by the parasympathetic afferent neurons, accompanied by sympathetic relaxation of the internal sphincter and reflexive tightening of the external sphincter. Defecation takes place following simultaneous parasympathetic contraction of the distal rectum and voluntary relaxation of the external sphincter.

Lower motor neuron damage at the sacral level produces fecal incontinence.

Damage to the descending pathways leading to the parasympathetic preganglionic neurons of the sacral cord produces fecal retention, but lesions in the sacral cord or the cauda equina paralyze the external sphincter muscle, which causes fecal incontinence. Isolated deficits in micturition and defecation are rare because their neural circuits are located so close to one another.

Denervation Hypersensitivity

Receptor up-regulation makes the denervated effectors hypersensitive.

Denervation of voluntary muscles causes paralysis and atrophy. Muscles and glands under autonomic control, however, remain functional following denervation but develop a hypersensitivity to their normal neurotransmitters and agonists. For example, patients with Horner's syndrome demonstrate miosis due to interruption of the autonomic pathway that innervates the ciliary muscles of the eye. When the patient is aroused, circulating levels of epinephrine increase and activate the denervated, but hypersensitive, ciliary muscles. In patients with Horner's syndrome, denervation hypersensitivity can be tested by dripping a 0.1% epinephrine solution into the conjuctival sac of the eye. Epinephrine at this dilution has no effect on healthy individuals, but it produces pupillary dilation in patients with sympathetic denervation. In this example, prior to the injury, the number of catecholaminergic receptors was maintained within normal limits by the nerve whose activity suppressed the expression of the receptor genes for the neurotransmitter. Following nerve damage there are fewer active muscles, so the number of receptors proliferate, making the muscles hypersensitive.

GENERAL ORGANIZATION OF THE NEUROENDOCRINE SYSTEM

The combined and coordinated actions of the hypothalamus and hypophysis regulate a host of vital behavioral and endocrine processes. The hypothalamus is capable of targeting specific viscera and glands through autonomic and somatic motor pathways. More sweeping effects are mediated by hormones secreted either by the hypothalamus or by other endocrine sites controlled directly or indirectly by the hypothalamus (e.g., pituitary, gonads, adrenal medulla). Neuroendocrine secretion of each hormone consists of a three-tier hierarchy involving the brain, the pituitary, and the peripheral glands.

> Autonomic regulation requires that the hypothalamus, the pituitary, and a target organ operate as a unit.

Hypothalamus

The hypothalamus constitutes only 4 g, or 0.5%, of the brain, but it is a critically important part of the brain. With the exception of the cerebral cortex, whose large size easily dwarfs the hypothalamus, no other area of the brain is involved in as many diverse functions. In keeping with its obligation to maintain homeostasis, the hypothalamus regulates food intake, water and electrolyte balance, body temperature, and blood pressure. The hypothalamus also helps regulate the body's circadian rhythm and sleep-waking cycles, orchestrates numerous reproductive and maternal behaviors, and mobilizes the body's response to stressors. The pervasive effects of the hypothalamus derive from its widespread connections with other parts of the CNS as well as its neurohormonal control of the hypophysis.

As part of the diencephalon, the hypothalamus is bounded rostrally by the lamina terminalis and caudally by its border with the midbrain, expressed as a straight line between the posterior edges of the mammillary nuclei and the posterior commissure. Laterally, the hypothalamus approaches the substantia innominata (rostrally) and the internal capsule (caudally). The hypothalamic sulcus separates the hypothalamus from the dorsal thalamus.

Within these small confines, the hypothalamus contains approximately a dozen nuclei; most are small and poorly differentiated and are named according to their positions relative to the floor of the diencephalon or the third ventricle. For both clarity and functional reasons, the hypothalamus typically is divided into coronal and sagittal zones.

> In the coronal plane, the hypothalamus consists of periventricular, middle, and lateral segments.

When viewed in the coronal plane, the hypothalamus contains periventricular, middle, and lateral segments. The periventricular segment is subjacent to the thin shell of neurons that line the third ventricle. Many of the neurosecretory cells that regulate hormone release from the adenohypophysis are located in nuclei within the periventricular segment. The middle zone, whose lateral boundary is marked by the fibers of the fornix, contains several nuclei as well as distinct populations of magnocellular and parvicellular neurons closely related to the pituitary. The lateral segment is a poorly differentiated region whose connections with the cerebral cortex, the amygdala, and other hypothalamic and brainstem nuclei enable it to integrate autonomic regulation with behavior.

> As a general rule, nuclei within the anterior hypothalamus contribute to parasympathetic activities, whereas posterior hypothalamic sites participate in sympathetic functions.

In the sagittal plane, the hypothalamus is divided into anterior (supraoptic), middle (tuberal), and posterior (mammillary) regions (Figure 13.10). The rostrocaudal boundaries of the anterior hypothalamus are the lamina terminalis and the caudal border of the optic chiasm, respectively. The middle hypothalamus surrounds the infundibular recess of the third ventricle between the optic chiasm and the mammillary bodies. The mammillary bodies, which form two prominent lumps on the basal surface of the diencephalon, mark the posterior hypothalamus. The supraoptic, tuberal, and mammillary regions of the

> In the sagittal plane, the hypothalamus consists of anterior, middle, and posterior zones.

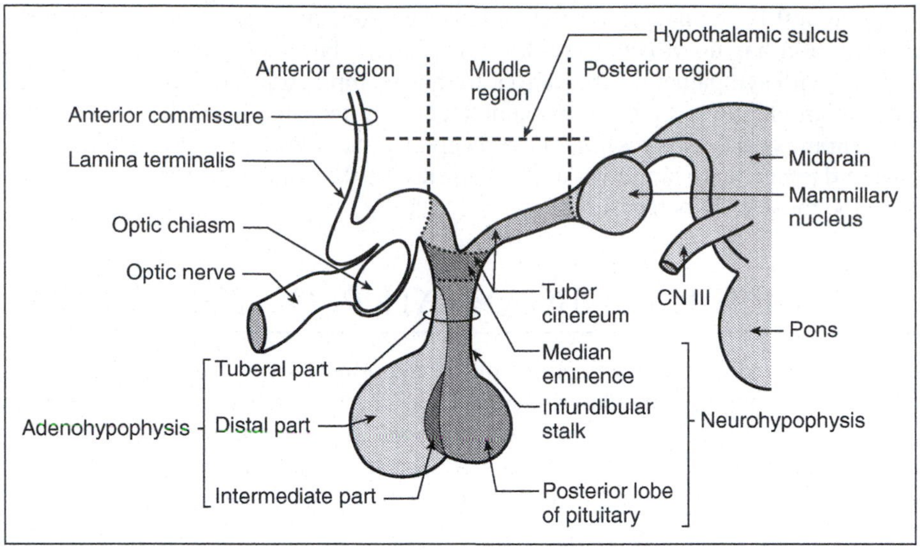

FIG. 13.10. Sagittal View of the Hypothalamus and Hypophysis. The hypothalamus consists of anterior, middle, and posterior regions. The hypophysis is divided into anterior (adenohypophysis) and posterior (neurohypophysis) parts.

hypothalamus lie caudal to the preoptic area, which for functional reasons is typically discussed with the hypothalamus, even though it is a telencephalic derivative.

Magnocellular neurons in the SON and PVN synthesize and release vasopressin and oxytocin. Parvicellular neurons secrete hypophyseal-releasing hormones.

Anterior (Supraoptic) Hypothalamus and Preoptic Area. The anterior hypothalamus contains four nuclei: the supraoptic nucleus (SON), the paraventricular nucleus (PVN), the suprachiasmatic nucleus, and the anterior nuclei (see Figures 13.10 through 13.12). Magnocellular neurons of the PVN and SON synthesize the hormones vasopressin and oxytocin. Vasopressin (antidiuretic hormone) decreases water secretion by the kidneys. Oxytocin promotes maternal behavior and induces uterine contractions and ejection of milk by the mammary glands. Parvicellular neurons in the PVN and SON modulate autonomic tone through direct descending projections to the dorsal motor nucleus of the vagus, the NST, the nucleus ambiguus, the respiratory neurons in the ventrolateral medulla, and

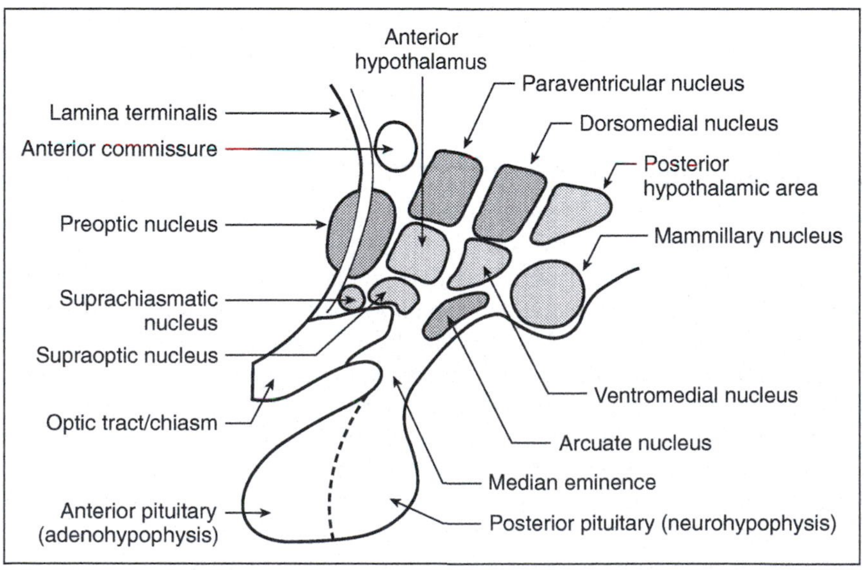

FIG. 13.11. The Hypothalamic Nuclei Viewed in the Sagittal Plane.

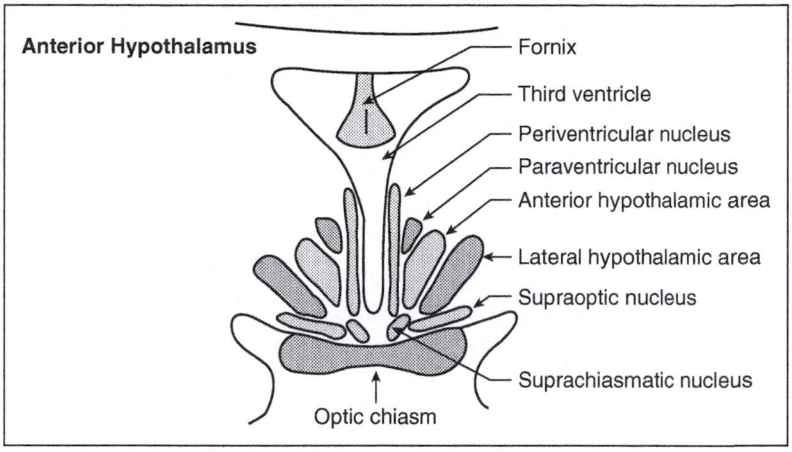

FIG. 13.12. Diagram of the Anterior Hypothalamus in the Coronal Plane.

the sympathetic neurons in the intermediolateral cell column. These descending hypothalamic axons form part of the medial forebrain bundle, a loose fiber ensemble that courses through the lateral hypothalamus between the septal area and the dorsolateral tegmentum of the medulla. Other parvicellular neurons in the PVN synthesize releasing hormones that are axoplasmically transported through the tuberoinfundibular tract and released into the portal veins and capillaries that supply the cells of the anterior pituitary. The hypothalamic-hypophyseal portal system is described below.

The small, densely staining suprachiasmatic nucleus, from its perch on the superior surface of the optic chiasm, works in concert with the pineal gland to synchronize the body's circadian clock with the ambient day-night light cycle. Information regarding the day-night cycle is conveyed from the retina to the suprachiasmatic nucleus by a small fraction of fibers in the optic tract. Circadian rhythms are discussed in more detail in Chapter 15.

> The **suprachiasmatic nucleus** helps synchronize the body's circadian rhythm.

The nondescript area lying between the third ventricle and the more anterior basal nucleus of Meynert is called the preoptic area. Medial and lateral divisions of the preoptic area have been identified, but the functions of the lateral area are not well understood. Neurons in the medial preoptic area, like some neurons in the arcuate nucleus, periventricular nucleus, and lateral hypothalamus, synthesize gonadotropin-releasing hormone (GnRH). The tuberoinfundibular tract transports GnRH to the hypophyseal portal system, where pituitary gonadotropes in the adenohypophysis release luteinizing hormone and follicle-stimulating hormone. The preoptic area also participates in temperature regulation and may contribute to fever production by detecting circulating cytokines. In general, stimulation of the preoptic area and the anterior hypothalamus produces parasympathetic effects such as vasodilation, sweating, pupillary constriction, decreases in blood pressure and heart rate, and increased intestinal peristalsis and gastrointestinal secretion.

> The **preoptic area** participates in temperature regulation.

Two important circumventricular organs are located near the lamina terminalis: the organum vasculosum of the lamina terminalis (OVLT) and the subfornical organ (SFO). The attenuated blood-brain barrier in the OVLT and SFO enable their constituent neurons to detect proteins, hormones, and other blood-borne chemicals. For example, neurons in the SFO and the OVLT respond directly to dehydration-induced osmotic changes and indirectly to hypotension caused by hypovolemia.

> **Hypovolemia:** an abnormally low blood volume

Middle or Tuberal Hypothalamus. The middle hypothalamic area contains the arcuate nucleus in the periventricular zone, the dorsomedial and ventromedial nuclei in the medial zone, and the lateral hypothalamic nucleus in the lateral zone (see Figures 13.10, 13.11, and 13.13).

The arcuate nucleus is located at the base of the third ventricle along the dorsal margin of the median eminence and infundibular stalk. Like other parvicellular secretory hypothalamic nuclei, the arcuate nucleus modulates hormone secretion by the anterior

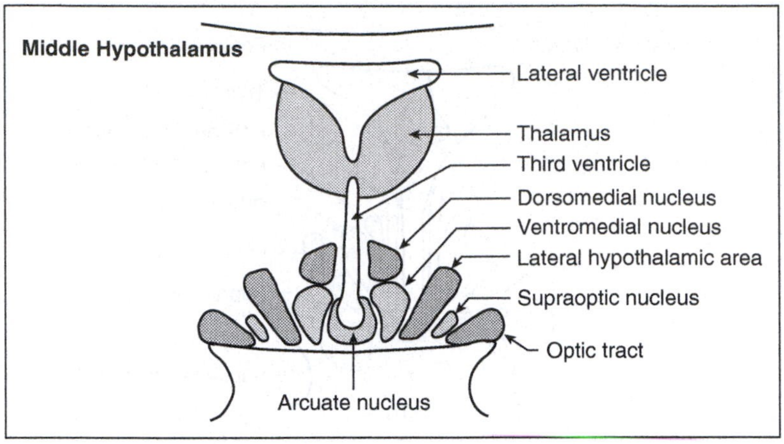

FIG. 13.13. Diagram of the Tuberal Hypothalamus in the Coronal Plane.

pituitary. Electrical stimulation of the dorsomedial nucleus produces unusually intense, but poorly focused, aggression called sham rage. The ventromedial and lateral hypothalamic nuclei contribute to the complex distributed system that regulates food intake (see below). In addition to feeding, the widespread and often reciprocal connections between the lateral hypothalamus and the cerebral cortex, the basal forebrain, and the brainstem contribute to a variety of autonomic functions and behavior.

The infundibulum is attached to the tuberal region of the hypothalamus.

The middle hypothalamus lies directly above the median eminence and the infundibulum, the tubular stalk linking the hypothalamus to the peduncular pituitary gland. The supraopticohypophyseal tract and the hypothalamic-hypophyseal portal system, which run through the infundibular core, enable the hypothalamus and hypophysis to work in concert.

Lateral Hypothalamus = LH = **L**ess **H**ungry (following damage)

Ventromedial Hypothalamus = VMH = **V**ery **M**uch **H**ungry (following damage)

Ingestive Behavior. Many studies have demonstrated that rats with lesions of the lateral hypothalamus do not eat (aphagia) or drink (adipsia) and without investigator intervention would eventually die. Lesions of the ventromedial hypothalamus have the opposite effect: uncontrolled eating (hyperphagia) and drinking (polydipsia) that lead to obesity. Division of the hypothalamus into a lateral feeding nucleus and a ventromedial satiety nucleus received further support from electrical stimulation experiments. More recent experiments, however, have shown that some of the initial results were due to inadvertent damage to fibers of passage. Although the field has abandoned the simplistic view of hunger and satiety centers, there is little doubt that the hypothalamus is intimately involved in regulation of feeding and drinking.

Sales of the serotonin agonist **fenfluramine,** which decreases food intake, were halted by the FDA after concerns about its safety were raised.

Patients with **Prader-Willi syndrome** are obese.

Animal studies examining the role of the hypothalamus in feeding have implicated the lateral nucleus, the ventromedial nucleus, and the PVN. Microinjections of norepinephrine and neuropeptide Y into the PVN increase feeding, particularly of carbohydrates. Consumption of fat increases following central injections of the peptide galanin; opioids increase protein consumption. Feeding decreases following micro-injections of dopamine and serotonin, and increases following injections of serotonin antagonists. The lateral and ventromedial hypothalamus and the PVN may play a role in long-term weight regulation by monitoring systemic levels of the neuropeptides cholecystokinin (CCK) and ghrelin, as well as the protein leptin. Secretion of CCK by the duodenum and upper intestine terminates feeding and for this reason is considered a potential satiety signal. Interestingly, central administration of CCK also interrupts feeding. Leptin, a protein secreted by adipocytes, may be the sensory signal used by the hypothalamus for long-term weight regulation. Ghrelin, a peptide hormone secreted by the epithelial cells of the stomach, increases hunger and triggers secretion of growth hormone (somatotropin) from the anterior pituitary. Blood concentrations of ghrelin are elevated in patients with anorexia nervosa and Prader-Willi syndrome.

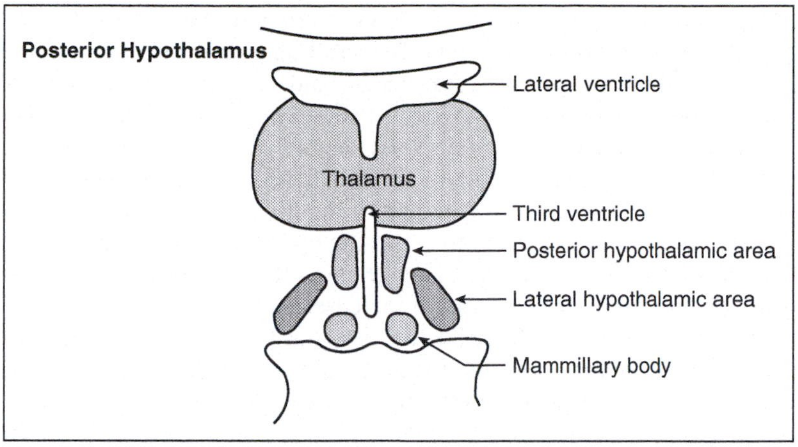

FIG. 13.14. Diagram of the Posterior Hypothalamus in the Coronal Plane.

The sensory, autonomic, and endocrine connections of the PVN enable it to participate in a host of feeding-related activities. Projections from the NST to the PVN convey visceral information from the gastrointestinal tract, liver, and pancreas. The PVN also receives projections from other hypothalamic nuclei, various nuclei of the limbic system (amygdala, bed nucleus of the stria terminalis), and noradrenergic and dopaminergic areas in the brainstem. Release of thyroid-stimulating hormone and corticotropin-releasing hormone by the parvicellular neurons of the PVN affects metabolism, whereas secretion of vasopressin by the magnocellular neurons of the PVN modulates water retention. Efferent projections from parvicellular neurons in the PVN to the brainstem and spinal cord affect hormone release by the pancreas (insulin, glucagon) and catecholamine release by the adrenal medulla.

Posterior or Mammillary Hypothalamus. The posterior hypothalamus includes the mammillary bodies, the posterior hypothalamic area, and the caudal part of the lateral hypothalamic area (Figure 13.14; see also Figures 13.10 and 13.11). The mammillary bodies are the hypothalamic component of the Papez circuit, an elaborate multinuclear pathway that plays a role in emotion. Surrounding the mammillary bodies is the posterior hypothalamic area, a poorly defined region that merges caudally with the mesencephalic reticular formation.

The posterior hypothalamic area complements the thermoregulatory actions of the anterior hypothalamic area. In general, stimulation of the posterior hypothalamus produces sympathetic effects such as vasoconstriction, piloerection, shivering, pupillary dilation, increases in blood pressure and heart rate, and decreased intestinal peristalsis and gastrointestinal secretion, all of which take place during emergencies.

Temperature Regulation. Autonomic, endocrine, and behavioral responses that regulate body temperature are mediated by the anterior and posterior regions of the hypothalamus. Neurons in the preoptic area respond to changes in blood and skin temperature. Increased core body temperature triggers parasympathetic responses such as decreased metabolism, increased sweating, and peripheral vasodilation. Sympathetic responses to decreased core temperature include vasoconstriction, piloerection, and heat generation through shivering; all are mediated by projections from the preoptic area to the posterior hypothalamus. These sympathetic actions may be supplemented by appropriate changes in thyroid-stimulating hormone production by the anterior pituitary and epinephrine secretion by the adrenal medulla that generate heat though increased cellular metabolism. These physiologic responses usually are supported by appropriate behavioral responses such as closing a window, adjusting the room thermostat, or putting on a sweater. Damage to the preoptic area prevents vasodilation and sweating and ultimately produces hyperthermia.

Fever, an increase in the body's normal core temperature of 98.6°F (37°C), is the normal hypothalamic response to illness. Bacterial and viral infections, immune reactions, trauma, inflammation, metabolic diseases, and dehydration are just a few of the many causes of fever. Endogenous pyrogens—that is, chemicals produced inside the body such as cytokines (interferon, tumor necrosis factor) that fight infection—also induce fever. Indeed, the list of pyrogenic stimuli is so broad, fever has little diagnostic value. Although most patients consider fever to be part of the illness, it is, in fact, a signal that the body is fighting back. The hypothalamus raises the body's core temperature by increasing metabolism (muscle shivering) and reducing heat loss through the skin with vasoconstriction and piloerection. As core temperature increases, the body begins to thermoregulate around a higher set point, ~100–101°F (37.8°–38.3°C), because fevers above 101°F (38.3°C) may cause seizures, and temperatures above 104°F (40°C) may damage the nervous system. Heat loss is achieved through vasodilation, sweating, and hyperventilation. As the illness resolves and the pyrogenic stimulus abates, the body's normal thermal set point is restored and the fever clears.

The **fornix** is the primary efferent pathway of the hippocampal formation.

Afferent and Efferent Projections of the Hypothalamus. The hypothalamus has extensive and usually reciprocal connections with many forebrain structures including the septal area, amygdala, hippocampus, thalamus, cerebral cortex, brainstem, and spinal cord. The main afferent projections of the hypothalamus are carried by the fornix, the ventral amygdalofugal pathway, the stria terminalis, and the medial forebrain bundle.

The massive C-shaped fornix is the largest and most easily recognized fiber tract within the diencephalon (see Chapter 3 and Figures 3.6 to 3.9; see Chapter 14 and Figure 14.1). The fornix originates within the subiculum and hippocampus and exits the posterior hippocampal formation as a thin sheet of axons called the alveus. As the alveus ascends toward the splenium of the corpus callosum, it becomes thicker and forms the fimbria. During the fimbria's passage rostrally beneath the body of the corpus callosum, it assumes a new name: the fornix. At this point a small contingent of fibers crosses to the opposite fornix, forming the hippocampal commissure. Further rostrally at the level of the interventricular foramen, the fornix sweeps ventrally toward the anterior commissure and divides into two parts. The small precommissural limb, containing axons that originated in the hippocampus, terminates in the septal area, the preoptic area, and the anterior hypothalamus. The larger postcommissural limb, which originates in the subiculum, projects primarily to the medial mammillary nucleus.

The hypothalamus and amygdala are reciprocally connected by the stria terminalis and the ventral pathways (VAFP, VAPP).

The anterior commissure is an excellent landmark for the substantia innominata and the VAFP/VAPP.

The hypothalamus and the amygdala are reciprocally connected by the stria terminalis, the ventral amygdalofugal pathway (VAFP), and the ventral amygdalopetal pathway (VAPP). The stria terminalis, which originates in the corticomedial amygdaloid nuclei, runs dorsally and rostrally in the groove between the thalamus and the caudate nucleus in the lateral ventricle. Most fibers of the stria terminalis terminate in the bed nucleus of the stria terminalis, but others continue caudally and synapse in the septum, the preoptic area, and the anterior and ventromedial hypothalamus. Projections from the basolateral amygdala to the lateral hypothalamus form the ventral amygdalofugal pathway (VAFP). Instead of taking the circuitous, embryologically derived route through the lateral ventricle, the VAFP enters the lateral hypothalamus by coursing directly through the substantia innominata (see Chapter 14; Figure 6.1A). Some of the more anterior fibers of the VAFP destined for the preoptic area form the diagonal band of Broca.

There are so many fibers joining and departing the medial forebrain bundle along its course that, at the microscopic level, it must look like a frayed rope.

Many hypothalamic connections with the forebrain and brainstem form part of the medial forebrain bundle, a loose ensemble of ascending and descending fibers that run through the lateral hypothalamus. Forebrain areas connected to the hypothalamus by the medial forebrain bundle include the septal area, the amygdala, the basal nucleus of Meynert, and the subiculum. As the medial forebrain bundle courses through the lateral hypothalamic area, some axons depart and other axons join until the composite tract exits the hypothalamus caudally and terminates in the brainstem tegmentum and central gray. Serotonergic, dopaminergic, and noradrenergic projections from the brainstem enter the hypothalamus through the medial forebrain bundle.

The efferent projections of the mammillary bodies form the mammillothalamic and mammillotegmental tracts. The mammillothalamic tract projects to the anterior nucleus of the thalamus, the first leg of the circuitous, multisynaptic pathway that began and eventually returns to the hippocampal formation (see Chapter 14). This circuit may contribute to memory retrieval and emotion. The mammillotegmental tract links the mammillary bodies with the locus ceruleus, the pontine parabrachial nucleus, the central gray, the dorsal motor nucleus of the vagus, the NST, and the spinal cord.

Other ascending and descending autonomic pathways between the hypothalamus and the brainstem are too diffuse for visual identification, but they are important nonetheless. Ascending projections from the NST to the hypothalamus relay afferent information from carotid baroreceptors and chemoreceptors as well as numerous thoracic and abdominal viscera. Brainstem and spinal autonomic reflexes are modulated by descending projections from a variety of central structures, but most notably the hypothalamus. Various brainstem nuclei (e.g., dorsal motor nucleus of the vagus, NST) and the brainstem tegmentum receive direct projections from the cerebral cortex, the lateral and paraventricular nuclei of the hypothalamus, and the mammillary nuclei, as well as indirect projections from the amygdala, the hippocampus, and the limbic lobe. Descending projections to the spinal cord also originate in the hypothalamus and brainstem reticular formation. Destruction of these descending autonomic pathways by tumors and strokes within the periaqueductal gray, lateral tegmentum, or spinal cord produces Horner's syndrome (see above and Chapter 5).

Damage to descending autonomic pathways produces Horner's syndrome.

Pituitary Gland

The pituitary gland or hypophysis resembles a small sack suspended from the ventral surface of the diencephalon into its bony case, the sella turcica (see Figure 13.10). The stalk-like infundibulum provides a structural and functional link between the hypothalamus and the underlying pituitary gland. The pituitary consists of anterior (adenohypophysis) and posterior (neurohypophysis) lobes, which differ dramatically in terms of their development, anatomy, and function. The adenohypophysis develops as an outpouch from the underlying ectoderm of Rathke's pouch, originally part of the roof of the palate. As the immature adenohypophysis migrates dorsally, it fuses with the cells of the neurohypophysis, which forms as an evagination of the hypothalamic floor.

The **adenohypophysis** is a derivative of non-neural ectoderm; the **neurohypophysis** develops from neuroepithelium.

The pituitary gland releases stimulating and, in some cases, inhibitory hormones that act on the body, the viscera, or other endocrine glands such as the gonads, the adrenals, and the thyroid (Table 13.2). In most cases, hormone secretion by the adenohypophysis is controlled by releasing and inhibitory hormones synthesized in the hypothalamus and then transported through the hypothalamic-hypophyseal portal system to the anterior hypophysis. In other cases, such as vasopressin and oxytocin, the hormones are synthesized in the hypothalamus and then transported axoplasmically by the supraopticohypophyseal tract to the posterior hypophysis, where they are released directly into the systemic circulation.

The hypothalamus is connected to the pituitary gland by the hypothalamic-hypophyseal portal system and the supraopticohypophyseal tract.

Hypothalamic-Hypophyseal Portal System and the Tuberoinfundibular Tract. Release of hormones synthesized and stored within the adenohypophysis is controlled by regulatory hormones synthesized and released by the hypothalamus. These regulatory hormones are axoplasmically transported by the tuberoinfundibular tract to their axon terminals that line an elaborate capillary bed in the median eminence. This capillary bed is the "headwater" of the hypothalamic-hypophyseal portal system that flows to the adenohypophysis (Figure 13.15). The so-called portal system consists of two capillary beds: one in the median eminence and a second one in the anterior lobe of the pituitary. The two capillary beds are connected by the long portal veins that run the length of the infundibulum. The portal system provides the vascular link between the synthesizing and regulatory areas in the hypothalamus and the secretory cells of the adenohypophysis that ultimately release the appropriate pituitary hormones into the systemic circulation.

The **adenohypophysis** operates at the behest of the hypothalamus.

The **portal system,** consisting of two capillary beds connected by long portal veins, connects the hypothalamus with the anterior pituitary.

The neurohypophysis also has a close relationship with the hypothalamus, but unlike the adenohypophysis, this relationship is not based on releasing hormones. Instead, the

The **supraopticohypophyseal tract** connects the hypothalamus with the posterior pituitary.

TABLE 13.2 Adenohypophyseal Hormones

Hypothalamus		Adenohypophysis			
Location of Secretory Neurons	**Releasing Hormone**	**Secretory Cells**	**Hormone Released**	**Target Organ**	**Effect**
Parvicellular PVN	Thyrotropin-releasing hormone (TRH)	Thyrotropes	Thyroid-stimulating hormone (TSH; thyrotropin)	Thyroid gland	Release of triiodothyronine (T3) and thyroxin (T4)
Parvicellular PVN	Corticotropin-releasing hormone (CRH)	Corticotropes	Adrenocorticotropic hormone (ACTH)	Adrenal cortex	Release of cortisol promotes growth, aids in recovery from stress and injury
Arcuate nucleus	Growth hormone–releasing hormone (somatocrinin; GHRH)	Somatotropes	Somatotropin Growth hormone	Widespread	Growth
Periventricular anterior hypothalamus	Growth hormone–inhibiting hormone (somatostatin; GHIH or SS)	N/A	N/A	GHRH neurons in the hypothalamus	Suppresses somatotropin release
Anterior hypothalamus Preoptic area Arcuate nucleus	Gonadotropin hormone–releasing hormone (GnRH; also called luteinizing hormone–releasing hormone [LHRH])	Gonadotropes	Luteinizing hormone (LH) Follicle-stimulating hormone (FSH)	Gonads	Ovulation Production of sex hormones Promotes follicle growth
Arcuate nucleus	Prolactin inhibitory factor (PIF; dopamine)	Lactotropes	Prolactin	Mammillary glands Immune system	Milk synthesis and release Maternal behavior

The link between the anterior pituitary and the hypothalamus is vascular; the connection between the hypothalamus and the posterior pituitary is neural.

hormones vasopressin and oxytocin are synthesized by the magnocellular neurons of the SON and PVN and then transported by the supraopticohypophyseal tract to the posterior hypophysis (see Figure 13.15). Because axons of the supraopticohypophyseal tract terminate on fenestrated capillaries within the posterior hypophysis, they secrete vasopressin and oxytocin directly into the systemic circulation.

Adenohypophyseal Hormones. Because hormones are typically associated with specific endocrine glands, the differences between hormones are often more salient than their similarities. From a regulatory standpoint, however, hormone secretion is remarkably similar across the endocrine system. Hormone secretion by each target organ (e.g., thyroid gland, gonads) is triggered by a unique stimulating hormone released by the adenohypophysis. For example, cortisol is released by the adrenal cortex after adrenocorticotropin is secreted by the adenohypophysis. Adrenocorticotropin secretion, in turn, is regulated by neurons in the hypothalamus that use a releasing hormone to signal the adenohypophysis that the body requires cortisol. This three-tier chemical cascade involving the hypothalamus, hypophysis, and a target organ is repeated, with some variation of course, for each hormone (see Table 13.2).

Thyroid-Stimulating Hormone (TSH). Hormones released by the thyroid gland affect fat and carbohydrate metabolism, which has implications for body temperature, brain function, body weight, and growth, as well as a host of autonomic functions including heart rate, blood pressure, and gastric motility. Release of the thyroid hormones thyroxin (T4) and triiodothyronine (T3) is under both endocrine and neural control. The endocrine limb relies on circulating levels of TSH, or thyrotropin, which is secreted by thyrotropes

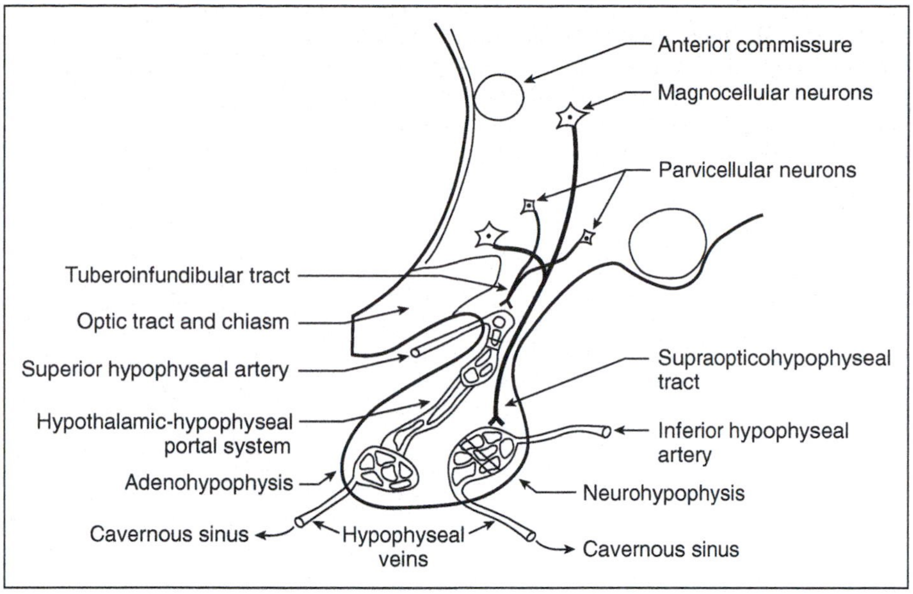

FIG. 13.15. Diagram of the Hypothalamic-Hypophyseal Portal System and Supraopticohypophyseal Tract. Oxytocin and vasopressin synthesized in the magnocellular neurons of the supraoptic and periventricular nuclei are transported axoplasmically along the supraopticohypophyseal tract to the neurohypophysis. Oxytocin and vasopressin enter the systemic circulation through fenestrated capillaries of the hypophyseal veins. The two sets of double lines in this figure represent the capillary beds separating the arterial and venous circulations. Regulatory hormones synthesized in the parvicellular neurons of the hypothalamus are released at axon terminals that line the capillary bed within the anterior part of the median eminence. After transport through the long portal veins to the adenohypophysis, these hypothalamic hormones regulate release of pituitary hormones into the systemic circulation.

located in the adenohypophysis. Secretion of TSH, in turn, is regulated by thyrotropin-releasing hormone (TRH), which is produced by parvicellular neurons of the PVN and transported to the adenohypophysis through the hypothalamic-hypophyseal portal system. Thyroid hormone synthesis (and possibly secretion) is also influenced by the autonomic nervous system, which regulates blood flow to the thyroid gland. Daily TRH and TSH secretion is pulsatile, occurring once every 60–160 minutes, and varies as a function of the circadian rhythm.

PVN → TRH → adenohypophysis → TSH → thyroid → T3 and T4

> **Hypothyroidism** = sluggishness and obesity; **hyperthyroidism** = nervousness and weight loss

A deficiency in TSH produces an underactive thyroid gland (hypothyroidism) and lower circulating levels of T3 and T4. Hypothyroidism, by lowering the body's metabolic rate, produces lethargy, obesity, and sluggish autonomic function in adults and cretinism in children. Cretinism is characterized by physical and mental retardation. Excess T3 and T4 production (hyperthyroidism) promotes weight loss, tachycardia, and nervousness. To avoid these problems, thyroid hormone production is maintained within narrow limits by an elaborate, multilevel, negative feedback system (Figure 13.16). Neurons in the PVN and thyrotropes in the adenohypophysis each respond to circulating levels of T3. As blood levels of T3 increase, TRH production by the PVN decreases, thereby lowering TSH output from the pituitary. Down regulation of TSH is reinforced by the pituitary thyrotropes, which also detect circulating levels of T3. Conversely, low levels of circulating T3 up-regulate TRH and TSH secretion by the hypothalamus and the pituitary, respectively. Figure 13.16 shows how circulating levels of T3 and T4 regulate TSH release and ultimately their own levels in the blood.

Adrenocorticotropic Hormone (ACTH, Adrenocorticotropin or Corticotropin). During periods of psychological and physical stress (e.g., trauma, infection, hemorrhage,

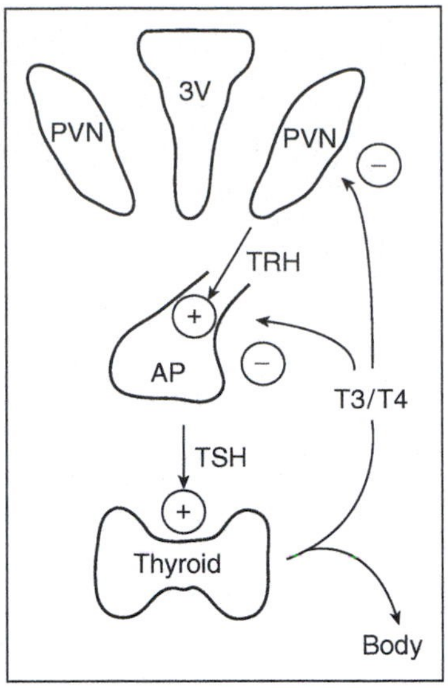

FIG. 13.16. Regulation of TRH and TSH Levels by Circulating Levels of T3 and T4. 3V = third ventricle; AP = anterior pituitary; PVN = paraventricular nucleus; TRH = thyrotropin-releasing hormone; TSH = thyroid-stimulating hormone; T4 = thyroxin; T3 = triiodothyronine.

Cortisol protects the body from stress.

hyperthermia), the adenohypophysis releases ACTH into the systemic circulation, which increases steroidal hormone production by the adrenal cortex. Cortisol, the primary glucocorticoid released by the adrenal cortex, protects the body from the adverse effects of stress by making carbohydrates, amino acids, and fats available for glucose or protein synthesis that may be required to mount a successful defense.

Release of ACTH by the adenohypophysis is regulated by secretion of corticotropin-releasing hormone (CRH) from the parvicellular neurons in the PVN. Like the other pituitary-releasing hormones, CRH is transported through the hypothalamic-hypophyseal portal system to the adenohypophysis, where it activates corticotropes that release ACTH into the systemic circulation.

PVN → CRH → adenohypophysis → ACTH → adrenal medulla → cortisol

Pituitary tumors that increase ACTH secretion or tumors of the adrenal cortex trigger excess cortisol production and produce Cushing's disease. Patients with Cushing's disease are in a constant state of metabolic high alert, trying to repair stress-induced damage that is not present. These patients are hypertensive and have rampant protein catabolism that causes muscle weakness. As part of this persistent stress response, they mobilize unneeded energy stores that, if left untreated, may exhaust islet cells in the pancreas and cause diabetes mellitus.

Circulating levels of cortisol provide negative feedback that regulates ACTH release.

Patients with atrophy of the adrenal cortices develop Addison's disease and demonstrate symptoms related to a diminished glucocorticoid (cortisol) and mineralocorticoid (aldosterone) production. Low cortisol levels cause muscle weakness, hypotension, and weight loss due to sluggish glucose, fat, and protein mobilization. The inability of the body to mobilize energy stores to repair stress-induced damage usually creates a life-threatening crisis for the Addison's patient. Loss of aldosterone production causes excessive urine production, which places the Addison's patients at risk of dehydration and death if left untreated for even a week. Cortisol levels are normally kept in check by up-regulation and down-regulation of ACTH production by cortisol-induced negative feedback within the hypothalamus and the pituitary.

Growth Hormone (Somatotropin). The hormone somatotropin is essential for development of the bones, connective tissue, the viscera, and the reproductive organs. Unlike TSH, which targets a single organ, somatotropin has widespread effects. Somatotropin release from the somatotropes in the adenohypophysis is regulated by a growth hormone–releasing hormone (GHRH or somatocrinin) and a growth hormone–inhibitory hormone (GHIH or somatostatin [SS]). The releasing and inhibiting hormones are synthesized in the hypothalamus—GHRH in the arcuate nucleus and SS in the periventricular region of the anterior hypothalamus. Axons from both GHRH-containing and SS-containing neurons terminate in the median eminence where both hormones are released into the portal circulation that flows to the anterior hypophysis. Secretion of GHRH increases following physical and emotional stress and feeding. Elevated GHRH levels trigger SS release, which ultimately terminates somatotropin discharge.

Arcuate nucleus → GHRH → adenohypophysis → somatotropin → body, organs, and so on

During childhood, somatotropin promotes bone and tissue growth; in adults, growth hormone enhances protein synthesis and maintains cellular integrity throughout the body. Overproduction and underproduction of growth hormone in children produces gigantism and dwarfism, respectively. Children with low levels of growth hormone may be given recombinant growth hormone to promote growth. In adults, overproduction of growth hormone causes acromegaly, a gross distortion and enlargement of the bones that is most noticeable in the face (protruding jaw), hands, and feet.

Gonadotropins (Luteinizing Hormone (LH); Follicle-Stimulating Hormone (FSH)). Reproduction depends on the coordinated actions of the hypothalamus, pituitary, and gonads. For both males and females, the impetus for this complicated neuroendocrine cascade arises from the hypothalamus, which prompts the pituitary to release the two gonadotropins that act on the gonads. The two gonadotropins, LH and FSH, have similar effects on the gonads of the female and the male. In the female, LH promotes ovulation and production of the sex hormones estrogen and progesterone, which, in turn, support the secondary sex organs (e.g., uterus, cervix) and development of other sex-related characteristics (e.g., breast development). In the male, LH stimulates testosterone synthesis, supports the secondary sex organs (penis, prostate), and triggers expression of the secondary male traits (e.g., facial hair, increased muscle mass). As its name implies, FSH stimulates follicular growth in the ovaries; in males, FSH initiates spermatogenesis in the testes.

Synthesis of gonadotropins within the gonadotropes of the anterior hypophysis is governed by gonadotropin-releasing hormone (GnRH; also called luteinizing hormone-releasing hormone [LHRH]). Following synthesis of GnRH by neurons in the anterior hypothalamus, the preoptic area, and the arcuate nucleus, the gonadotropins are released into the portal circulation. Circulating levels of testosterone, estrogen, and progesterone are kept in check through the negative feedback they provide to the GnRH neurons of the hypothalamus and the gonadotropes of the pituitary. Hypogonadotropic hypogonadism (Kallmann's syndrome) is caused by a failure to secrete gonadotropic hormones due to a gene deletion that prevents proper prenatal migration of GnRH neurons from the olfactory placode to the hypothalamus.

> Patients with **Kallmann's syndrome** are anosmic because they lack olfactory receptor neurons.

Anterior hypothalamic areas → GnRH → adenohypophysis → LH & FSH → gonads

Prolactin. The role of prolactin in development of the mammillary glands and milk synthesis and secretion is well known, but it has other effects throughout the body, most notably in the immune system. Unlike the pituitary hormones described above, prolactin secretion by lactotropes in the anterior pituitary is not under the control of a hypothalamic releasing factor. Instead, prolactin secretion by the anterior pituitary must be inhibited by dopamine (prolactin inhibitory factor [PIF]) released into the portal system by neurons in the arcuate nucleus. Because prolactin secretion is regulated by a hypothalamic braking factor instead of a releasing factor, section of the infundibulum increases circulating levels of prolactin. Prolactin release is also triggered by TRH, GRH, vasoactive intestinal polypeptide, and estrogen. Postpartum production of prolactin triggered by suckling contributes to maternal behavior and suppresses the reproductive cycle.

Arcuate nucleus → PIF → adenohypophysis → mammillary glands

Neurohypophysis Hormones. The neurohypophysis, unlike the adenohypophysis, does not synthesize hormones and thus does not rely on the hypothalamus for either releasing or inhibitory hormones. There are, however, two hormones that are synthesized in the hypothalamus and released by the neurohypophysis into the systemic circulation: vasopressin (also called antidiuretic hormone [ADH]) and oxytocin. Vasopressin and oxytocin are synthesized in separate populations of magnocellular neurons in the PVN and SON and transported by the supraopticohypophyseal tract to the neurohypophysis. In the neurohypophysis, oxytocin and vasopressin are released into the blood through fenestrated capillaries. Although vasopressin and oxytocin are structurally similar nonapeptides, they have vastly different functions.

Vasopressin, which is sometimes referred to as arginine vasopressin (AVP), increases water retention by the kidney.

Drinking and antidiuresis are triggered by increased serum osmolarity.

Drinking and antidiuresis are triggered by hypotension caused by hypovolemia.

Vasopressin (Antidiuretic Hormone) and Regulation of Water Balance. When the body is water depleted, vasopressin increases water retention by the kidney, which, in turn, helps preserve serum osmolarity and maintain blood pressure and blood volume until thirst-induced drinking restores homeostasis.

Water lost through perspiration, respiration, urination, and defecation increases serum osmolarity and triggers a cascade of physiological and behavioral events that gradually restore fluid homeostasis (Figure 13.17). When osmoreceptors located in the SFO, the OVLT, and the adjacent medial preoptic area detect increases in serum osmolarity, they activate magnocellular neurons in the SON and PVN, which release vasopressin from the neurohypophysis. Patients with hypothalamic tumors that destroy the magnocellular neurons of the PVN and SON are unable to secrete vasopressin, the only known antidiuretic hormone. As a consequence, these patients produce copious amount of urine (polyuria) with low osmolarity, and they consequently have low blood volume (hypovolemia). The excessive water loss caused by polyuria triggers thirst and water consumption (polydipsia). This condition, known as diabetes insipidus, is treated by vasopressin replacement. Other projections from the SFO and OVLT to the parvicellular neurons of the PVN increase blood pressure indirectly through their descending influence on the autonomic areas of the brainstem and spinal cord.

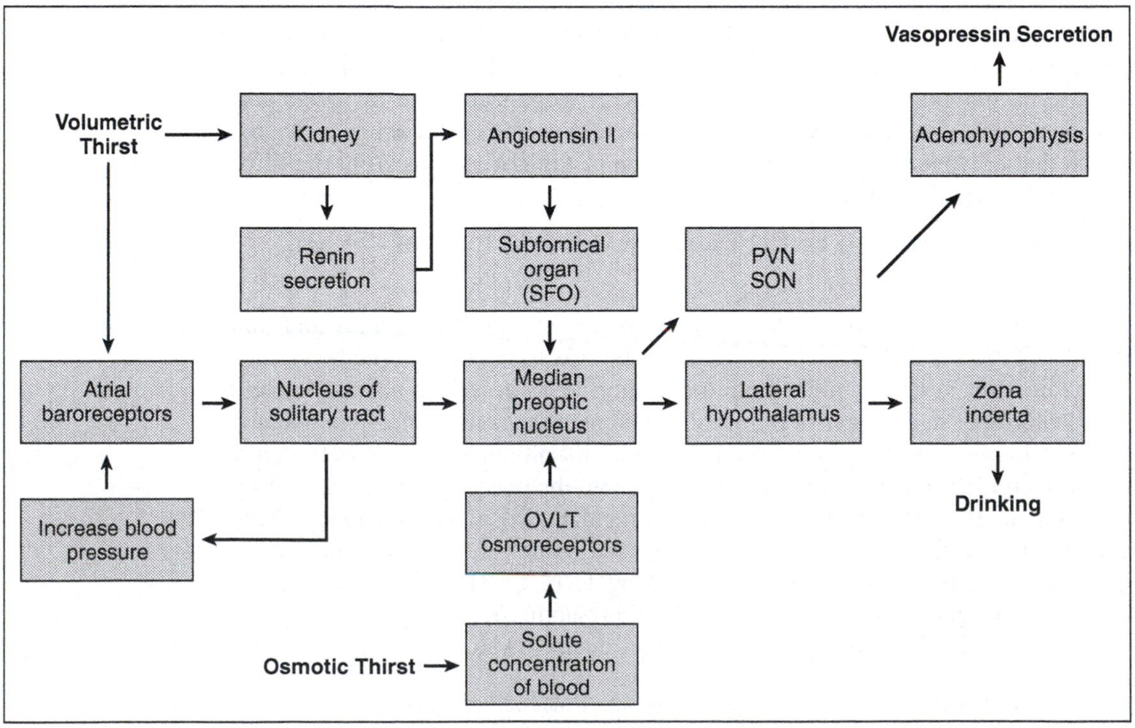

FIG. 13.17. Neural Circuitry Associated with Hypovolemic and Osmotic Regulation of Thirst. NST = nucleus of the solitary tract; OVLT = organum vasculosum of the lamina terminalis; PVN = paraventricular nucleus of the hypothalamus; SON = supraoptic nucleus.

Hypovolemia caused by hemorrhage, or excessive vomiting or diarrhea, is corrected in two ways. First, hypovolemic hypotension stimulates the baroreceptors, which, in turn, activate the NST. Projections from the NST to the SON and the PVN stimulate vasopressin release, whose antidiuretic actions limit further water loss through urination. The second and more important corrective action is initiated by the kidney, which secretes renin. Renin initiates an enzymatic cascade that increases serum levels of angiotensin II, a potent vasoactive peptide. Angiotensin II releases aldosterone from the adrenal cortex, which raises blood pressure by reducing sodium loss through kidney filtration. Angiotensin II also triggers vasopressin secretion by its direct action on the SFO.

> **Aldosterone** improves conservation of sodium by the kidneys.

Hypotension and serum hyperosmolarity have an additive effect on vasopressin release, but serum osmolarity is the more effective antidiuretic stimulus. Although conserving the body's fluid resources is important, restoration of fluid homeostasis ultimately requires that the patient drink water. Water depletion and serum hyperosmolarity produce thirst, an unpleasant sensation that triggers drinking. Lesion experiments have demonstrated that the integrity of the median preoptic area is critical for the initiation of drinking.

Oxytocin. Oxytocin causes uterine contractions during childbirth; pitocin, a synthetic analog of oxytocin, is used to induce labor in women who are several weeks past term. In postpartum women, suckling triggers oxytocin release, which, in turn, initiates milk ejection from the breast (let-down) and contractions of the uterus that restore both its size and shape. Oxytocin also may promote maternal behavior. The natriuretic properties of oxytocin promote sodium secretion by the kidney during periods of hyperosmolarity.

> Oxytocin contracts the smooth muscle of the uterus during childbirth, releases milk from the mammary glands following parturition, and promotes secretion of Na^+.

RESOLUTION OF CLINICAL CASE

All of this patient's symptoms are consistent with mass effects caused by a pituitary adenoma. Polyuria and polydipsia were caused by inadequate production of vasopressin. Diabetes mellitus, which also causes polyuria and polydipsia, was ruled out because the urine had a low specific gravity and only a nominal amount of glucose. The second set of blood tests suggested that the patient's fatigue was caused by an abnormally low level of thyroxin, presumably due to a lack of thyroid-stimulating hormone. The visual field defect and headache were caused by the tumor pressing against the crossing fibers of the optic chiasm. The MRI scan revealed a tumor around the infundibular stalk. The patient was given hormone replacement therapy and scheduled for surgery to remove as much of the tumor as possible. Following radiation therapy, he may have near normal vasopressin and thyroid-stimulating hormone production and improved eyesight.

REVIEW QUESTIONS

Directions: For each of the following questions, choose the **one** best answer.

1. What are the neurotransmitters used by the preganglionic and postganglionic neurons of the parasympathetic nervous system (PNS), respectively?
- **A.** Acetylcholine and norepinephrine
- **B.** Epinephrine and norepinephrine
- **C.** Norepinephrine and acetylcholine
- **D.** Acetylcholine and acetylcholine
- **E.** Acetylcholine and glutamate

2. Where are the receptors for the baroreceptor reflex are located?
- **A.** Organum vasculosum of the lamina terminalis (OVLT)
- **B.** Subfornical organ (SFO)
- **C.** Nucleus of the solitary tract (NST)
- **D.** Lungs
- **E.** Carotid sinus

3. A deficiency in which of the following causes diabetes insipidus?
- **A.** Thyroid-stimulating hormone (TSH)
- **B.** Corticotropin-releasing hormone (CRH)
- **C.** Insulin
- **D.** Vasopressin
- **E.** Thyroxin

4. What type of urinary problems ensue following a complete transection of the sacral spinal cord?
- **A.** Automatic bladder that fills to capacity before emptying automatically
- **B.** Atonic bladder that is difficult, if not impossible, to empty voluntarily

C. Uninhibited bladder that empties when full, but is under the patient's control
D. Empty bladder that drains urine as it fills
E. Inhibited bladder that empties only when it is filled to capacity

5. Where does the vagus nerve, which contains afferent projections from the thoracic and abdominal viscera, terminate?
A. Dorsal motor nucleus of the vagus
B. Nucleus ambiguus
C. Edinger-Westphal nucleus
D. Lateral hypothalamus
E. NST

6. The efferent projections of the PNS emerge from which parts of the spinal cord?
A. Cranium and lumbar
B. Cervical and lumbar
C. Cervical and sacral
D. Cervical and thoracic
E. Cranium and sacral

7. Hyperphagia may be caused by damage to which part of the hypothalamus?
A. Supraoptic nucleus of the hypothalamus
B. Ventromedial nucleus of the hypothalamus
C. Lateral nucleus of the hypothalamus
D. Anterior hypothalamus
E. Posterior hypothalamus

8. Which of the following neural events triggers a compensatory increase in heart rate?
A. Increased neural activity in the dorsal motor nucleus of the vagus
B. Increased baroreceptor activity
C. Increased neural activity in the NST
D. Decreased baroreceptor activity in the carotid sinus
E. Decreased sympathetic tone

9. Which of the following functions would be affected by changes in the firing rate of the magnocellular neurons in the supraoptic and paraventricular nuclei?
A. Food and water intake
B. Temperature regulation
C. Oxytocin and antidiuretic hormone release
D. Secretion of hormone releasing factors
E. Modulation of the adenohypophysis

10. Which of the following functions is modulated by the suprachiasmatic nucleus?
A. Circadian rhythm
B. Thirst
C. Blood pressure
D. Temperature regulation
E. Feeding

ADDITIONAL READING

Classic Literature

Cannon WB: *The Wisdom of the Body*. 2nd ed. New York, NY: Norton, 1932.

Dale HH: Pharmacology and nerve endings. *Proc Royal Soc London Ser B* 28:319–332, 1935.

Langley JN: *The Autonomic Nervous System*. Cambridge: Heffer & Sons, 1921.

Reviews and Landmark Research Articles

Appenzeller O, Oribe E: *The Autonomic Nervous System: An Introduction to Basic and Clinical Concepts*. 2nd ed. Amsterdam: Elsevier, 1997.

Benarroch EE: The central autonomic network: functional organization, dysfunction, and perspective. *Mayo Clin Proc* 68:988–1001, 1993.

Camina JP: Cell biology of the ghrelin receptor. *J Neuroendocrinol* 18:65–76, 2006.

Coggeshall, RE. Law of separation of function of the spinal roots. *Physiol Rev* 60:716–755, 1980.

Costa M, Brookes SJ: The enteric nervous system. *Am J Gastroenterol* 89:Suppl 8:S129–137, 1994.

de Groat WC, Steers WD: Neural control of the urinary bladder and sexual organs. In: Bannister R. *Autonomic Failure*. New York, NY: Oxford University Press, 1988:196–222.

de Groat WC, Yoshimura N: Mechanisms underlying the recovery of lower urinary tract function following spinal cord injury. *Prog Brain Res* 152:59–84, 2006.

Elfvin LG, Lindh B, Hokfelt, T: The chemical neuroanatomy of sympathetic ganglia. *Ann Rev Neurosci* 16:471–507, 1993.

Furness JB, Costa M: *The Enteric Nervous System*. Edinburgh: Churchill Livingstone, 1987.

Janig W: Neurobiology of visceral afferent neurons: neuroanatomy, functions, organ regulations and sensations. *Biol Psychol* 42:29–51, 1996.

Lowey AD, Spyer KM, eds: *Central Regulation of Autonomic Function*. New York, NY: Oxford University Press, 1990.

Parent A: *Carpenter's Human Neuroanatomy*. Baltimore, MD: Williams & Wilkins, 1996.

Pick J: *The Autonomic Nervous System*. Philadelphia, PA: J. B. Lippincott, 1970.

Swanson LW: The hypothalamus. In: Bjorklund A, Hokfelt T, Swanson LW. *Handbook of Chemical Neuroanatomy*. Amsterdam: Elsevier, 1987.

Swanson LW, Sawchenko PE: Magnocellular integration: organization of the paraventricular and supraoptic nuclei. *Ann Rev Neurosci* 6:269–324, 1983.

INTERNET RESOURCES

Colorado State University
Endocrine System
http://arbl.cvmbs.colostate.edu/hbooks/pathphys/endocrine/index.html
Hypothalamus and Pituitary Gland
http://arbl.cvmbs.colostate.edu/hbooks/pathphys/endocrine/hypopit/index.html

The Diabetes Insipidus Foundation
http://www.diabetesinsipidus.org/

Dysautonomia Foundation, Inc.
http://www.familialdysautonomia.org/whatisfd.htm

Timothy C. Hain, MD
Orthostatic Hypotension
http://www.dizziness-and-balance.com/disorders/medical/orthostatic.html

Loyola University
Circumventricular Organs
http://www.meddean.luc.edu/lumen/MedEd/Neuro/Circumventricular.html

National Dysautonomia Research Foundation
http://www.ndrf.org/ans.htm

National Institute of Neurological Disorders and Stroke
Dysautonomia Information Page
http://www.ninds.nih.gov/disorders/dysautonomia/dysautonomia.htm
Pituitary Tumors Information Page
http://www.ninds.nih.gov/disorders/pituitary_tumors/pituitary_tumors.htm

National Institutes of Health (MedlinePlus)
Pituitary Disorders
http://www.nlm.nih.gov/medlineplus/pituitarydisorders.html

New York Medical College
Orthostatic Hypotension
http://www.nymc.edu/fhp/centers/syncope/orthostatic_hypotension.htm

The Pituitary Foundation
http://www.pituitary.org.uk/

University of Wisconsin
Hypothalamus
http://www.neuroanatomy.wisc.edu/coursebook/neuro2(2).pdf

Washington University School of Medicine
Hypothalamus and Autonomic Nervous System
http://thalamus.wustl.edu/course/hypoANS.html

Wikipedia, the Free Encyclopedia
Autonomic Nervous System
http://en.wikipedia.org/wiki/Autonomic_nervous_system

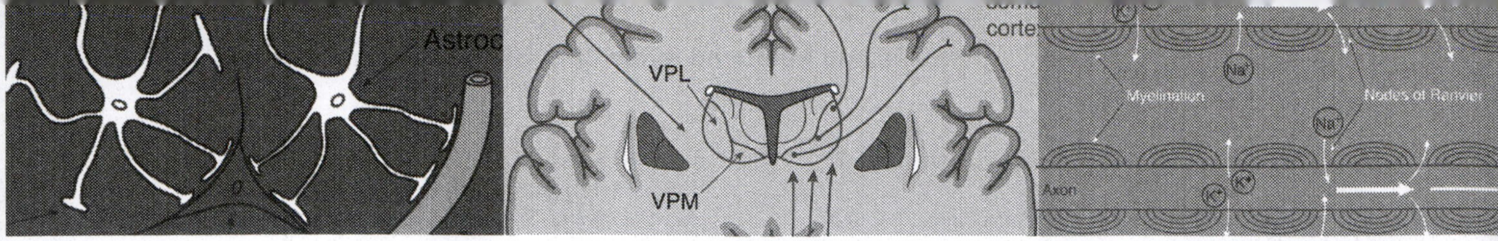

CHAPTER 14

Limbic System

INTRODUCTION OF CLINICAL CASE

An 18-year-old woman experienced recurring seizures that gradually increased in frequency. The patient reported that seizure onset was characterized by unpleasant visceral sensations and a feeling of fear or dread. Initially, the motor symptoms consisted of repetitive movements of the lips and tongue, but more recently the seizures included clonic, bilateral twitching of the face. Following these seizures, the patient appeared confused for 30 to 60 minutes. An electroencephalogram (EEG) revealed focal slowing and sharp waves or spikes in the temporal lobe.

INTRODUCTION TO THE LIMBIC SYSTEM

The function of many forebrain structures is unclear because they are part of an interconnected neural system that mediates complex behaviors such as cognition and emotion. Such is the case with the amygdaloid complex, a multinuclear structure in the temporal lobe that plays a critical role in regulating emotional behavior. Similarly, the hippocampal formation is necessary for memory formation, but its neural mechanisms are poorly understood.

No single neural structure can mediate complex processes such as motivation, memory, or emotion. The autonomic, cognitive, and behavioral responses associated with these processes are mediated by a distributed system of interacting neural structures that include the amygdaloid complex, the hypothalamus, the basal forebrain (i.e., septal nucleus, substantia innominata, basal nucleus of Meynert), the nucleus accumbens and ventral striatum, the prefrontal and cingulate cortices, and a collection of somatic and autonomic motor nuclei in the brainstem. Thus, the amygdaloid complex and other limbic structures act as an interface between the cerebral cortex and autonomic structures such as the hypothalamus and parts of the brainstem.

HISTORICAL VIEWS OF THE LIMBIC SYSTEM

In contrast to other cortical lobes, the limbic lobe is not demarcated by distinct fissures but is a synthesis of the cortical structures surrounding the limbus, or rim, of the corpus callosum (Figure 14.1). Defined by Paul Broca in 1878, the limbic lobe includes the subcallosal area, the cingulate gyrus, the parahippocampal gyrus, and the underlying hippocampal formation. James Papez, who observed emotional disturbances among patients who had sustained damage in this area, proposed a specific function for the limbic lobe in the 1930s. Based on his observations and knowledge of brain morphology, Papez proposed a closed neural circuit that linked the hippocampus and cingulate gyrus for the purpose of expressing emotional behaviors. According to Papez, the hippocampus organizes emotional "programs" and communicates them to the hypothalamus via the fibers of the fornix. In response, the hypothalamus executes these emotional programs via pathways to other parts of the limbic lobe. Thus, the mamillothalamic tract conveys emotional information to the anterior nucleus of the thalamus, which projects to the cingulate cortex via the thalamocortical radiations. Papez also believed that the cingulate cortex represents the anatomical site for conscious experience of emotions just as certain cortical areas represent the neural substrate for sensory perception. In view of evidence that the cingulate cortex projects to the parahippocampal gyrus and the underlying hippocampus via the fibers of the cingulum, the Papez circuit represented a neural loop in which information reverberated in successive, recurrent cycles.

In the 1950s, Paul MacLean recognized that the limbic lobe is connected to many subcortical structures that regulate visceral functions. To make sense of these anatomic relationships, he developed the concept of a "limbic system" to explain how emotional affect may influence autonomic responses. According to MacLean, the hypothalamus uses

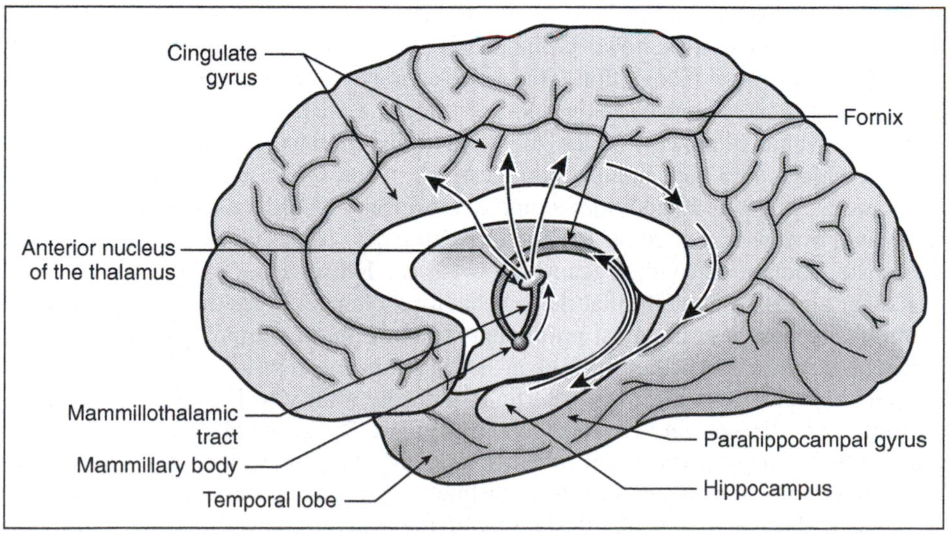

FIG. 14.1. Papez Circuit. The Papez circuit consists of a series of anatomical projections that permit reverberating interactions between the cingulate gyrus and hippocampal formation. Large arrows indicate the sequence of information flow that was proposed by James Papez.

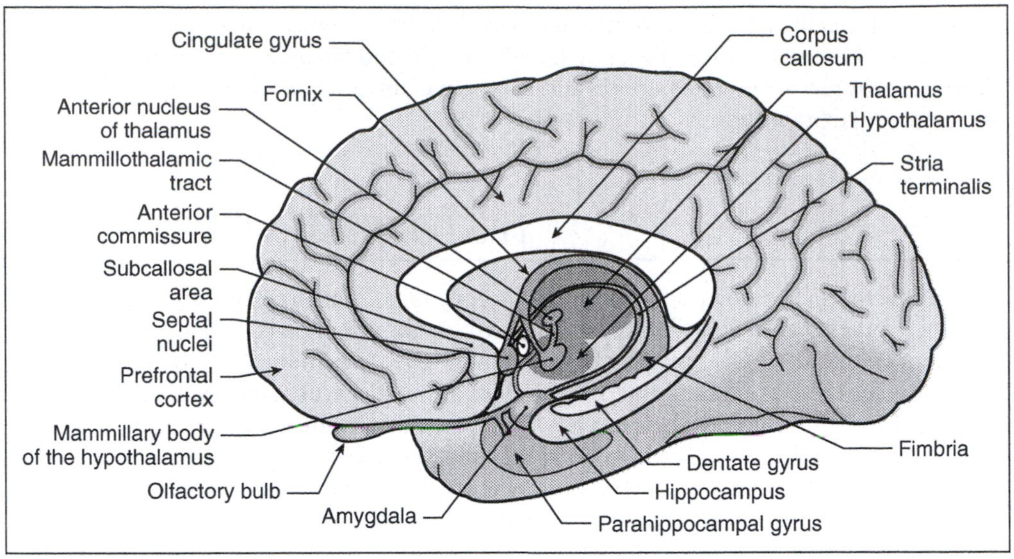

FIG. 14.2. Major Structures in the Limbic System. The limbic system is composed of several cortical and subcortical structures located along the medial aspect of the brain. The amygdaloid complex and its connections regulate emotional behavior. The hippocampus and its connections consolidate information into long-term memory.

information received from a variety of limbic areas to coordinate the autonomic responses associated with different emotional states. In MacLean's view, the major subcortical nuclei in the limbic system include the amygdala, the septal nucleus, the nucleus accumbens, the substantia innominata, the hypothalamus, and the anterior and mediodorsal nuclei of the thalamus (Figure 14.2).

Klüver-Bucy Syndrome

Klüver-Bucy syndrome:
- Placid behavior
- Visual agnosia
- Oral tendencies
- Hypersexuality

In the late 1930s, Heinrich Klüver and Paul Bucy showed that temporal lobe removal, which disrupts the Papez circuit, has profound effects on the social and emotional behaviors of rhesus monkeys. In those experiments, bilateral temporal lobotomy produced tame monkeys that were unafraid of humans and did not vocalize or show fearful reactions to snakes. Subsequent studies, however, indicated that this apparent tameness was due to a general deficit in visual recognition. Thus, monkeys with temporal lobe lesions fail to recognize a wide range of behaviorally relevant stimuli, a phenomenon known as visual agnosia or "psychic blindness." Such monkeys indiscriminately place a wide range of inanimate objects into their mouth and ingest fish, meat, feces, and other substances that normal monkeys avoid. In addition, temporal lobectomy disturbs normal sexual behavior, as indicated by repeated attempts to copulate with other species or with inanimate objects. This constellation of behaviors became known as the Klüver-Bucy syndrome.

Klüver and Bucy thought that these behavioral changes were due to loss of the hippocampus, because it is the most prominent structure in the temporal lobe. More recent studies, however, indicate that the Klüver-Bucy syndrome is produced by removal of the amygdala alone. Amygdalectomy interferes with the ability to link past experiences to stimuli that have important behavioral consequences. The amygdala receives sensory information from many cortical and subcortical areas, and it plays a crucial role in associating behaviorally significant stimuli with their social and emotional consequences. In this context, the behavioral manifestations of the Klüver-Bucy syndrome represent an inability to make appropriate sensory-affective associations.

Patients with amygdaloid lesions exhibit behavioral changes that are remarkably similar to those observed in nonhuman primates. In humans, for example, amygdala damage causes visual, auditory, and tactile agnosia and increases the tendency to sniff objects and place them in the mouth. As in non-human primates, damage to the human amygdala increases inappropriate sexual behavior, which may take the form of suggestive remarks and ill-conceived attempts to make sexual contact. Because amygdalectomy reduces anxiety and causes complacency, it was often used to treat some individuals who had a history of violent behavior. This form of psychosurgery, however, has been discontinued. Nonetheless, both clinical and experimental evidence indicates that amygdala damage interferes with the ability to link sensory stimuli to past social or emotional experiences. Larger lesions that damage the amygdala, hippocampus, and the entorhinal and perirhinal cortices cause amnesia. Furthermore, when most of the temporal lobe is damaged, patients exhibit nonfluent aphasia because Wernicke's area is affected (see Chapters 6 and 8).

NEURAL REGULATION OF EMOTIONAL BEHAVIOR

Afferent projections from the association cortex provide the amygdaloid complex with visual, somatosensory, auditory, and visceral information. In addition, the amygdaloid complex has dense, reciprocal connections with the hypothalamus and several brainstem nuclei that enable coordination of a wide range of autonomic responses (Figure 14.3). Hence, these widespread afferent and efferent connections are consistent with the view that the amygdala receives the critical information needed to execute the neural interactions that subserve emotion, mood, personality, and other psychological processes. Not surprisingly, neurochemical imbalances in the amygdaloid complex and related structures have been implicated in anxiety, depression, and other affective disorders.

Anatomy of the Amygdaloid Complex

Classically, the amygdaloid complex is considered part of the basal ganglia because of its embryological origin. The functional role and anatomic connections of the amygdala, however, have prompted most modern neuroscientists to classify it as part of the limbic system. Located underneath the uncus in the rostromedial part of the parahippocampal gyrus, the amygdaloid complex is composed of several distinct nuclei that vary in neuronal composition and anatomical connectivity. Moreover, because of the amygdala's close proximity to the hippocampal formation, temporal lobe damage usually affects both of these structures (Figure 14.4).

Nuclear Organization. Based on its connectivity and neurochemical composition, the amygdaloid complex can be subdivided into more than a dozen nuclei. Because the

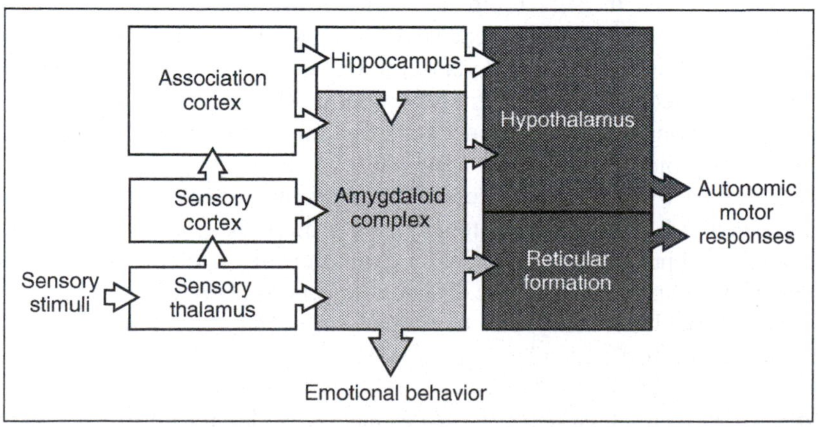

FIG. 14.3. Afferent and Efferent Connections with the Amygdala. The amygdala uses sensory information received from the cerebral cortex to coordinate autonomic responses with emotional behaviors.

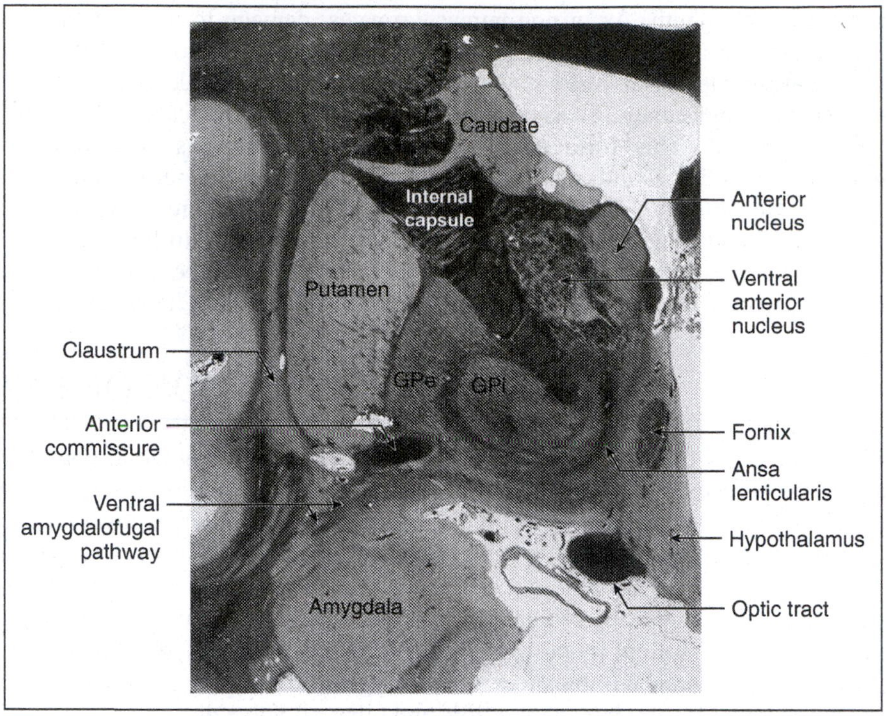

FIG. 14.4. The Amygdala. This photomicrograph shows a cross section of the amygdaloid complex with respect to the nucleus accumbens, the basal forebrain, and the basal ganglia. (Reprinted with permission from the late Dr. Malcolm B. Carpenter.)

nomenclature describing individual amygdaloid nuclei is inconsistent, however, many neuroanatomists prefer to organize them into basolateral and corticomedial groups.

Basolateral nuclei receive visual, auditory, and somatosensory inputs.

Basolateral Nuclei. In humans, the basolateral nuclei are located in the lateral and ventral two-thirds of the amygdaloid complex. The basolateral amygdaloid complex is considered a quasi-cortical structure because its anatomic features resemble the neocortex. Like the frontal cortex, the basolateral nuclei have reciprocal connections with the mediodorsal nucleus of the thalamus. The basolateral nuclei also have direct, sometimes reciprocal, connections with the prefrontal cortex, the cingulate gyrus, the insula, the parahippocampal gyrus, the subiculum, and adjacent gyri in the temporal lobe. Similar to the neocortex, the basolateral nuclei receive diffuse cholinergic projections from the basal nucleus of Meynert, which is located ventral to the anterior commissure. Finally, the basolateral nuclei project to motor areas in the frontal lobe and, like limbic cortical areas, send dense projections to the nucleus accumbens and ventral striatum.

Corticofugal projections from the temporal lobe, cingulate gyrus, and insula provide the basolateral nuclei with highly processed visual, auditory, somatosensory, and olfactory information (Figure 14.5). In addition to receiving projections from the mediodorsal thalamus, the basolateral nuclei receive projections from modality-specific thalamic nuclei such as the medial geniculate nucleus. These diverse connections provide a rich source of sensory information that enables the amygdala to evaluate the social and emotional significance of a wide range of stimuli.

Corticomedial nuclei receive olfactory and viscerosensory inputs.

Corticomedial Nuclei. Compared to the basolateral nuclei, the corticomedial nuclei are located dorsomedially and comprise only a third of the amygdaloid complex. Most afferent projections to the corticomedial nuclei originate from brain regions that are concerned with autonomic or viscerosensory functions. For example, the corticomedial nuclei receive olfactory inputs directly from the olfactory bulb and indirectly from the adjacent

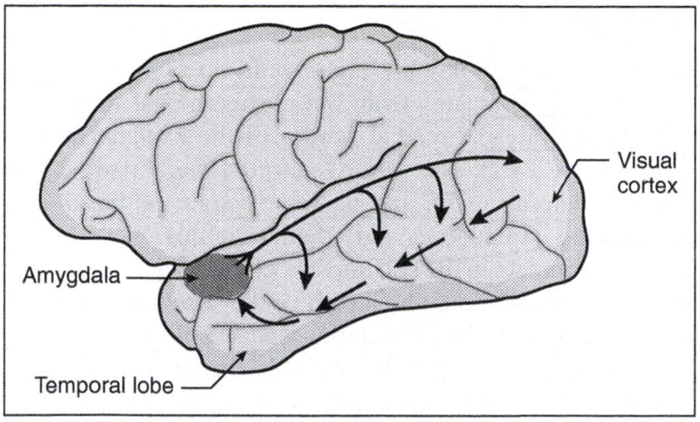

FIG. 14.5. Visual Projections to the Amygdala. Visual information is transmitted through successive regions of the occipital and temporal lobes before it reaches the amygdaloid complex. The amygdala sends feedback projections to the visual processing regions in the temporal and occipital lobes.

pyriform cortex. The parabrachial nucleus of the pons, which receives viscerosensory information from the caudal nucleus of the solitary tract, sends a dense projection to the central amygdaloid nucleus, which forms part of the corticomedial nuclei. The ventromedial and lateral hypothalamic nuclei also project to the corticomedial nuclei and, to a lesser extent, to the basolateral nuclei.

From an evolutionary perspective, the afferent connections of the corticomedial nuclei enable this part of the amygdaloid complex to evaluate the sensory properties of stimuli that are linked to survival and reproduction. Thus, olfactory information associated with food, predators, potential mates, and other stimuli are sent to the corticomedial nuclei. Ascending projections from the solitario-parabrachial pathway provide the amygdala with the essential visceral information needed to coordinate cardiovascular, respiratory, and other autonomic responses with specific emotional experiences.

Role of the Amygdala in Anxiety and Depression. The neurochemical composition of the amygdaloid complex has drawn the attention of neuropharmacologists who develop drugs for treating mood disorders such as anxiety and depression. In this regard, the amygdala contains a high concentration of the amino acid γ-aminobutyric acid (GABA), which acts as an inhibitory neurotransmitter in most parts of the central nervous system (CNS). Although GABAergic neurons are found in all amygdaloid nuclei, the basolateral nuclei are noteworthy because they contain a high density of GABA receptors that bind benzodiazepines (e.g., diazepam, or Valium™) and other anxiolytic drugs. Benzodiazepines are not direct GABA agonists, but they act synergistically to enhance GABA binding, thereby promoting the inhibitory effects of this neurotransmitter. In animals, direct infusion of benzodiazepines into the amygdala reduces conditioned fear and other behavioral signs of anxiety. Hence, the therapeutic benefit of the benzodiazepines is derived, in part, from their ability to enhance GABA-mediated inhibition in the amygdala. This mechanism suggests that the placid behavior observed in the Klüver-Bucy syndrome may, to some extent, represent a reduction in fear and anxiety.

Antidepressants modulate monoaminergic transmission in the amygdala.

The amygdaloid complex receives dense, serotonergic projections from the dorsal and median raphe nuclei in the brainstem. Ascending dopaminergic projections from the ventral tegmental area and noradrenergic projections from the locus ceruleus also terminate in the amygdala, especially in the central nucleus. These monaminergic pathways modulate neuronal excitability in several forebrain regions, including the amygdala. Given the amygdala's role in emotional behavior, it is not surprising that serotonin, dopamine, and norepinephrine have a strong influence on mood and other emotional behaviors. An imbalance in neurotransmitter release within the amygdaloid complex may lead to depression or other affective disorders. The clinical importance of the ascending serotonergic pathways is apparent from the large number of prescriptions for fluoxetine (Prozac™) and other antidepressant drugs that derive their therapeutic benefits by selectively blocking the synaptic reuptake of serotonin. Antidepressants are effective, in part, because of their pharmacologic actions in the amygdaloid complex and related parts of the limbic system.

Amygdalofugal Pathways

Basal forebrain includes the substantia innominata and the basal nucleus of Meynert.

The **corticomedial nuclei** give rise to the stria terminalis.

The **basolateral nuclei** give rise to the ventral amygdalofugal pathways.

Efferent projections from the amygdaloid complex are organized into two major pathways. One pathway, the stria terminalis, originates from the corticomedial nuclei and proceeds with the thalamostriate vein along the medial border of the caudate nucleus where it adjoins the thalamus (see Figure 14.2). The ventral amygdalofugal pathway, by comparison, originates from the basolateral nuclei and passes through the basal forebrain before it terminates in the lateral hypothalamus and other structures.

Most fibers in the stria terminalis terminate in the bed nucleus of the stria terminalis, an elongated collection of neurons that aggregate along the length of the stria terminalis as it arches rostromedially toward the septal nucleus. The remaining fibers project to the septal nucleus and to parts of the hypothalamus including the preoptic area, the anterior hypothalamus, the ventromedial hypothalamus, and the lateral hypothalamus. The central amygdaloid nucleus and the bed nucleus of the stria terminalis also send descending projections to assorted brainstem nuclei including the parabrachial nucleus, the nucleus of the solitary tract, the dorsal motor nucleus of the vagus, the periaqueductal gray region, the ventral tegmental area, the substantia nigra, and parts of the reticular formation. These brainstem regions and their descending projections mediate the cardiovascular, respiratory, and gastric responses associated with the expression of fear and other stress-related behaviors.

Fibers in the ventral amygdalofugal pathway proceed rostrally and medially as they pass through the substantia innominata. Many of these fibers make en passant synapses on acetylcholine-containing neurons in the basal nucleus of Meynert as they proceed toward the septal nucleus, hypothalamus, cingulate cortex, and olfactory areas. Cholinergic fibers from the basal forebrain terminate diffusely throughout the cerebral cortex and, by increasing the excitability of their postsynaptic targets, the basal forebrain increases cortical responsiveness to incoming sensory inputs. Hence, the ventral amygdalofugal pathway indirectly modulates cortical excitability. Other fibers of the ventral amygdalofugal pathway ascend to the medial prefrontal cortex either directly or indirectly via the mediodorsal nucleus of the thalamus. Thus, direct amygdalofugal projections to the prefrontal and cingulate cortical areas, as well as indirect projections through the basal forebrain and mediodorsal thalamus, provide parallel routes by which the amygdala may influence the cognitive aspects of emotional behavior (Figure 14.6). Finally, the amygdaloid complex sends axons to adjacent parts of the hippocampal formation, especially

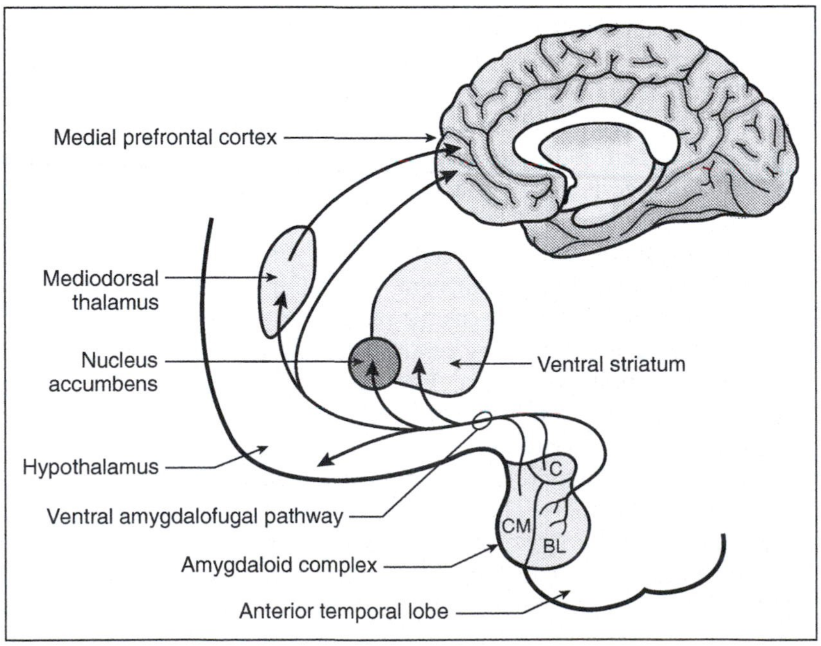

FIG. 14.6. Ventral Amygdalofugal Pathway. The basolateral (BL), corticomedial (CM), and central (C) amygdaloid nuclei project to the central striatum, nucleus accumbens, thalamus, and hypothalamus via the ventral amygdalofugal pathway. The amygdaloid nuclei also project to the prefrontal cortex both directly and indirectly via the mediodorsal thalamus.

the subiculum and entorhinal cortex. These latter projections allow emotional states to influence the neural mechanisms of learning and memory.

Nucleus Accumbens and Ventral Striatum

The nucleus accumbens lies lateral to the septal nucleus in the ventromedial part of the basal ganglia. Functional studies indicate that the nucleus accumbens and ventral striatum play an important role in motivation, and, consistent with this view, these regions receive dense projections from the basolateral amygdala via the ventral amygdalofugal pathway. The nucleus accumbens also receives projections from other limbic regions in the forebrain, especially the medial prefrontal cortex and the hippocampal formation.

The nucleus accumbens, the ventral striatum, and the medial prefrontal cortex are major targets of ascending dopaminergic fibers that originate from the ventral tegmental area. Dopaminergic neurons in the ventral tegmental area and their forebrain targets comprise a medial subset of limbic structures known as the mesolimbic system. Projections from the central amygdaloid nucleus to the ventral tegmental area enable the amygdaloid complex to activate the dopaminergic pathways and their forebrain targets.

Mesolimbic Dopamine and the Neural Basis of Reward. The mesolimbic dopamine system and its projections to the nucleus accumbens play a critical role in the subjective experience of pleasure and its rewarding effects. The search for a neural substrate for pleasure began in earnest after the discovery of intracranial self-stimulation by James Olds and Peter Milner in 1954. They found that rats implanted with stimulating electrodes would press a bar to deliver brief pulses of electrical current to specific brain regions. Electrical stimulation of the mesolimbic dopamine system was so rewarding that rats would give up eating and sleeping to self-stimulate this brain region. Following lesions of the mesolimbic dopamine system or infusions of dopamine antagonists into the nucleus accumbens, the rate of intracranial self-stimulation is greatly attenuated.

Mesolimbic dopamine system: dopaminergic projections from the ventral tegmental area to the nucleus accumbens, ventral striatum, and medial prefrontal cortex

There is considerable debate regarding the exact function of the mesolimbic dopamine system. Consistent with a proposed role in motivation and feelings of pleasure, synaptic release of dopamine increases significantly when animals are presented with food or the opportunity to engage in sexual behavior. Dopamine release is also triggered by stimuli that were previously associated with a reward or by novel cues that are encountered during exploration. Hence, dopamine mediates the pleasurable or reinforcing properties of many stimuli, but it also maintains alertness and increases psychological vigilance in novel situations that demand concentration.

Drugs of Abuse. Psychomotor stimulants such as amphetamine and cocaine produce an increase in dopaminergic transmission in the nucleus accumbens and other targets of dopamine-containing terminals. The motivation to use these drugs and the potential for addiction are related to the pleasurable sensations that accompany dopaminergic transmission in the nucleus accumbens. This view is based on behavioral studies demonstrating that animals will work for the opportunity to drink water laced with amphetamine or cocaine. Furthermore, if low doses of dopamine antagonists are systemically injected into a trained animal, the animal will work at a higher rate to obtain a dose of amphetamine or cocaine that overcomes the partial block of dopamine transmission. When higher doses of dopamine antagonists are administered, however, animals stop working for amphetamine or cocaine because the postsynaptic antagonist effectively blocked dopamine transmission. In addition to working for the opportunity to drink diluted solutions of cocaine or amphetamine, animals are easily trained to self-administer infusions of these drugs directly into the nucleus accumbens. This suggests that dopamine release in the nucleus accumbens alone is sufficient to maintain drug-taking behavior. Consistent with this suggestion, the rewarding properties of these drugs can be blocked by direct focal infusions of dopamine antagonists into the nucleus accumbens.

Drugs of abuse increase mesolimbic dopamine transmission.

Other classes of commonly abused drugs, such as alcohol, nicotine, and heroin, also increase dopaminergic transmission in the mesolimbic system. Although this effect may mediate some of their reinforcing properties, these drugs of abuse act on a multitude of neurochemical systems throughout the brain. Hence, these additional pharmacologic properties make it difficult to pinpoint the precise mechanisms or sites that mediate their rewarding properties.

Despite the physiologic and social costs of drug abuse, the mesolimbic system serves an important function in normal behavior. In essence, the mesolimbic system rewards an organism for engaging in behaviors that enhance success and survival. Sensory information funneled into the amygdaloid complex enables the recognition of stimuli that are behaviorally significant. Subsequent activation of the efferent projections from the amygdala coordinates a variety of autonomic responses; those that activate the mesolimbic dopaminergic system produce feelings of elation when a tangible reward is obtained. Hence, this neural mechanism increases the probability of behaviors that lead to natural rewards, such as food, water, and sex, which are needed for the survival of both the individual and the species. In humans, rewarding experiences also accompany the attainment of abstract goals that involve the expenditure of considerable energy over long periods of time. In the case of drug abuse, however, the intense sensations of instant pleasure that accompany drug administration merely reward the drug-taking behavior. Consequently, drug abuse disrupts and circumvents those behaviors needed to achieve long-term goals. Furthermore, chronic use of psychomotor stimulants and related drugs of abuse alter the synaptic terminals of dopamine neurons and have other deleterious morphologic effects that interfere with the reward mechanisms of the limbic system.

HIPPOCAMPUS

The hippocampus was originally thought to play a major role in the expression of emotional behavior because patients with severe damage to the hippocampus and surrounding temporal lobe showed clear signs of emotional disturbance. Subsequently, it became evident that most of the emotional changes produced by temporal lobe lesions were a consequence of damage to the amygdaloid complex. Although the hippocampal formation has a role in emotional expression, selective damage to this structure indicates that it has a specific role in learning and the formation of memory.

Anatomy of the Hippocampal Formation

"Hippocampus," from Greek, means "sea horse."

The hippocampal formation is a collection of laminated structures that lie below the parahippocampal gyrus on the ventral aspect of the temporal lobe (Figure 14.7). Located immediately caudal to the amygdaloid complex, the hippocampal formation extends along the inferior horn of the lateral ventricle until it reaches the splenium of the corpus callosum. The hippocampal formation includes the dentate gyrus, the hippocampus proper, the subiculum, and the entorhinal cortex. The sigmoid configuration of these structures resembles the shape of a seahorse, which is called a hippocampus in Greek.

Dentate Gyrus and Hippocampus Proper. When viewed in transverse section, the dentate gyrus and hippocampus proper consist of interlocking C-shaped structures (Figure 14.8). Both structures contain three cortical layers, which define them as phylogenetically older allocortex.

The dentate gyrus contains a densely packed layer of granule cells that is easily seen in most histologic preparations of the hippocampal formation. The external side of the granule cell layer is encircled by the molecular layer, which contains a dense plexus of incoming axons, their terminals, and the dendrites extending from the granule cells. The polymorphic layer of the dentate gyrus, which lies within the hilus of the granule cell layer, contains interneurons, glia, and axons arising from the granule cells.

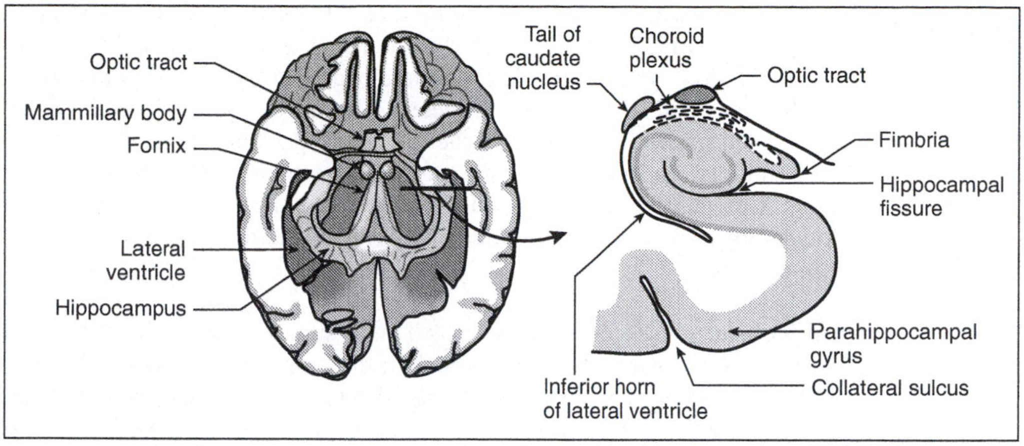

FIG. 14.7. Hippocampal Formation. Diagram of the hippocampus after removing the ventral half of the temporal lobe. A transverse section through the rostral part of the hippocampus is shown on the right.

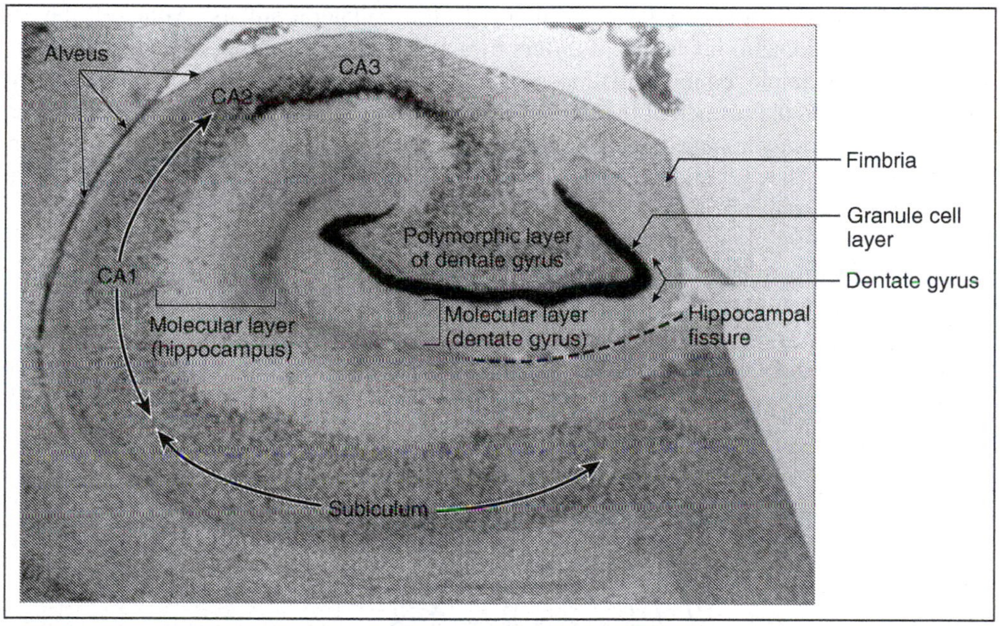

FIG. 14.8. Hippocampus Proper and Dentate Gyrus. This photomicrograph illustrates the laminar structure of the dentate gyrus and the cornu Ammonis (CA) subfields of the hippocampus. (Reprinted with permission from the late Dr. Malcolm B. Carpenter.)

The hippocampus proper, which lies between the dentate gyrus and the subiculum, consists of a thick layer of pyramidal cells sandwiched between the more superficial polymorphic layer and a deeper molecular layer. As shown by Figure 14.8, the molecular layers of the hippocampus and dentate gyrus are continuous with each other. Apical dendrites from the pyramidal cells extend into the molecular layer of the hippocampus where they receive synaptic inputs from the dentate gyrus. The polymorphic layer contains the axons and basal dendrites extending from the pyramidal neurons. The polymorphic layer is separated from the inferior horn of the lateral ventricle by a thin sheath of myelinated axons called the alveus, which contains the projection fibers originating from the hippocampus and subiculum.

Cornu Ammonis is Ammon's horn.

The hippocampus is divided into subfields that vary in their cytologic appearance: CA1, CA2, and CA3. According to this nomenclature, in which CA stands for cornu Ammonis (Ammon's horn), the CA3 subfield begins at the polymorphic layer of the dentate gyrus and extends for several millimeters. The largest pyramidal cells in the hippocampus are located in the CA3 subfield where they are packed into a relatively thick layer. The CA2 subfield is a short transitional region between the more extensive CA3 and CA1 subfields. Compared to the CA2 and CA3 subfields, the cell density of the CA1 subfield is noticeably lower and the pyramidal cell layer gradually becomes thicker as it approaches the subiculum.

Subiculum. The subiculum is located in the superior part of the parahippocampal gyrus, partially buried within the ventral bank of the hippocampal fissure. The subiculum forms the transition between the trilaminar hippocampus and the six layers of the entorhinal cortex. Like the dentate gyrus and the hippocampus proper, the three-layered subiculum has a distinct layer of pyramidal neurons located between a superficial molecular layer and a deeper polymorphic layer. Pyramidal neurons in the subiculum provide most of the projections from the hippocampal formation to the septal nucleus, the mammillary body, the nucleus accumbens, and the anterior nucleus of the thalamus.

Entorhinal Cortex. The entorhinal cortex occupies the inferior part of the parahippocampal gyrus and extends laterally almost to the collateral sulcus. Although the entorhinal cortex contains six layers, it differs from traditional neocortex in several respects. Layer II, for example, contains distinct aggregates of large pyramidal neurons that form visible bumps on the surface of the parahippocampal gyrus. The pyramidal cells of layers III and V are closely apposed to each other because layer IV is virtually absent in the entorhinal cortex. The pyramidal neurons in layers II and III of entorhinal cortex provide the major route for transmitting information to the hippocampus.

Intrinsic Circuits in the Hippocampal Formation. One of the defining characteristics of the hippocampal formation is the serial flow of information through each of its components (Figure 14.9). The entorhinal cortex begins this multisynaptic circuit by projecting to the granule cells of the dentate gyrus. These entorhinal projections, which are called the perforant pathway because they perforate the hippocampal fissure, terminate on granule

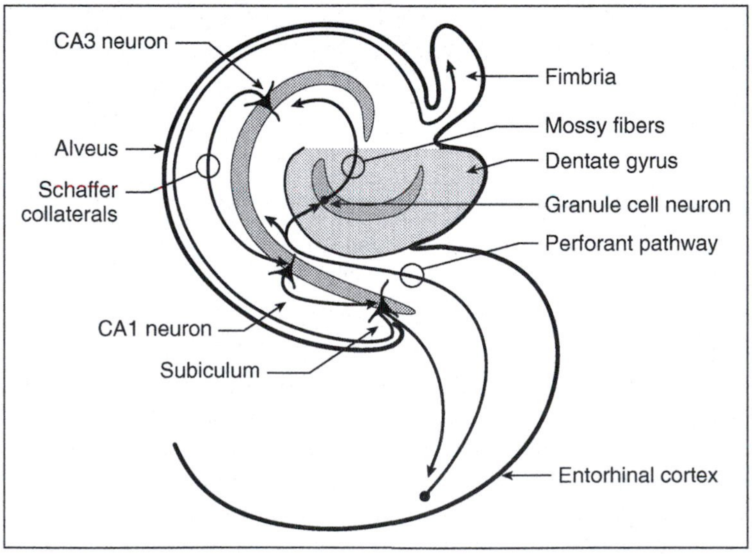

FIG. 14.9. Intrinsic Hippocampal Circuits. The hippocampal formation contains a unidirectional circuit that transmits information from the entorhinal cortex, to the dentate gyrus, to CA3, to CA1, and finally to the subiculum.

cell dendrites in the molecular layer. The granule cells send a dense projection of axons, or mossy fibers, to the molecular layer of the CA3 subfield where they synapse on the apical dendrites of the pyramidal neurons. Axons from the CA3 pyramidal neurons bifurcate into two branches, one of which departs the hippocampus and enters the alveus to form the fibers of the fornix. The other collateral branches, known as Schaffer collaterals, project to pyramidal neurons in the CA1 subfield. The CA1 pyramidal neurons project to the subiculum, which completes the multisynaptic loop through the hippocampal formation by projecting to the entorhinal cortex.

As the perforant pathway proceeds to the dentate gyrus, its axons form en passant synapses with the distal dendrites of pyramidal neurons in CA1 and CA3, but there is no other opportunity for feedback processing within the hippocampal formation. The serial, feed-forward progression of information throughout the hippocampal formation is emphasized by the total absence of feedback projections from CA3 to the dentate gyrus and by a similar lack of projections from CA1 to CA3. Furthermore, all output from the dentate gyrus is transmitted to the CA subfields; the dentate gyrus does not project to any other brain region.

This unidirectional flow of information through the hippocampal formation is conveyed entirely by excitatory connections. The perforant pathway, the mossy fibers, the Schaffer collaterals, and the efferent projections from CA1 and the subiculum use glutamate as an excitatory neurotransmitter. Although GABAergic inhibitory interneurons are present in the deeper parts of the granule cell layer of the dentate gyrus and in the polymorphic layers of the hippocampal CA fields, glutamate is the main neurotransmitter in each part of the hippocampal formation. The predominance of excitatory glutamatergic transmission renders the hippocampus vulnerable to seizure activity, which can quickly spread to neighboring parts of the temporal lobe and then to widespread cortical regions.

The **hippocampus** is susceptible to seizures because it contains few inhibitory neurons.

Neural Plasticity in the Hippocampus

To learn new information or to remember events of the past, the nervous system must have the capacity for plasticity. In other words, the morphologic structure of the nervous system must change to acquire new memories. The most likely mechanism for plasticity involves the selective strengthening and weakening of synaptic connections. In 1949, Donald Hebb hypothesized that the synapses between connected neurons would become stronger if both neurons discharged synchronously over an extended period. This view, known as Hebb's postulate, is widely regarded as the major mechanism that underlies learning. Synaptic changes represent a normal function of the brain that occurs continuously throughout each person's life. Consistent with its role in memory, numerous experiments have demonstrated synaptic plasticity in the hippocampus.

Neurons that fire together, wire together.

Most of our knowledge about hippocampal plasticity has been obtained from studies conducted on rodents. When the rodent hippocampal formation is sectioned transversely, the multisynaptic pathways that interconnect the dentate gyrus with the hippocampus proper remain intact. Thus, when thin slices of the hippocampal formation are placed in a warm and oxygenated solution of artificial cerebrospinal fluid, the pyramidal neurons in CA3 and CA1 have normal membrane potentials and will respond to electrical stimulation of the perforant pathway or the Schaffer collaterals. This experimental technique has been used extensively to reveal the cellular events that mediate neural plasticity.

Long-Term Potentiation. When Schaffer collaterals are electrically stimulated in a hippocampal slice, the orthodromic impulses excite the CA1 pyramidal neurons (Figure 14.10). If the electrical stimulus is delivered only once or twice per minute, the amplitude of the CA1 excitatory postsynaptic potential (EPSP) remains constant. If many electrical pulses are quickly administered as a tetanic stimulus, however, a subsequent test stimulus produces a much larger EPSP in CA1. This potentiation in the size of the postsynaptic response may persist for several hours; therefore, this phenomenon is called long-term potentiation (LTP). Synaptic potentiation is limited to those synapses that are activated repeatedly by tetanic stimulation. For example, if two stimulating electrodes were used to activate separate

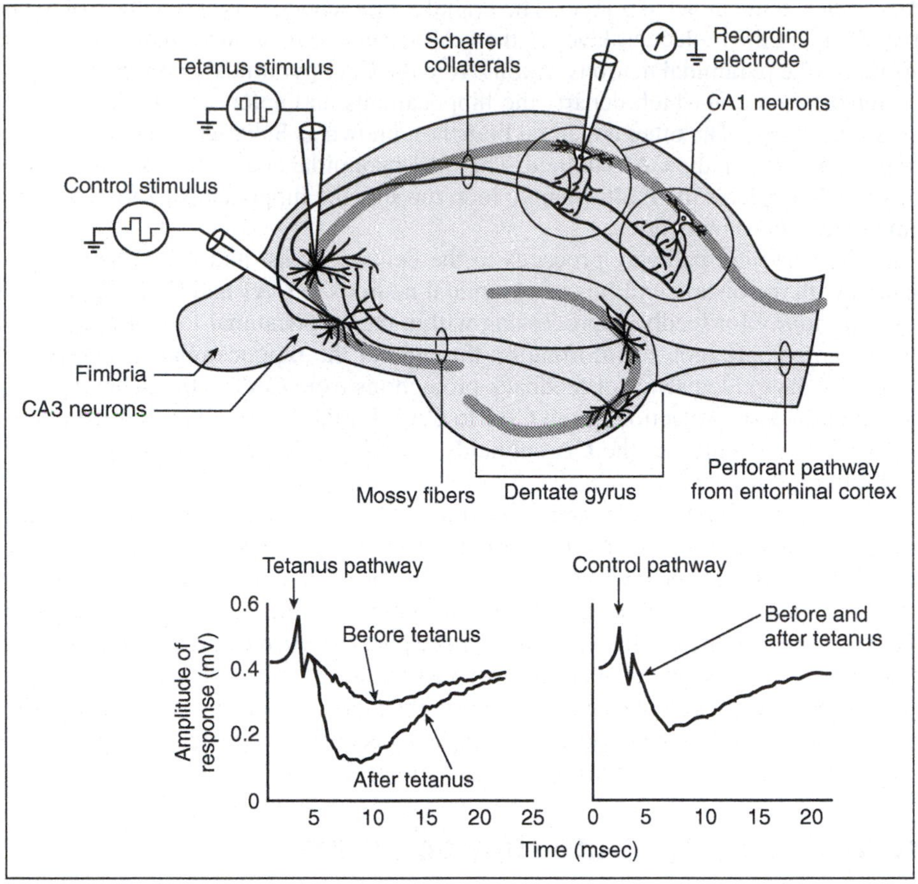

FIG. 14.10. Long-Term Potentiation. This diagram shows a slice of the rodent hippocampus in which a pair of stimulating electrodes is positioned at different sites in the CA3 subfield and an extracellular recording electrode is positioned in the CA1 subfield. When either part of the CA3 subfield is stimulated with a brief electrical pulse, CA1 neurons show a well-defined response. Following tetanic stimulation of one CA3 region, however, the CA1 response is potentiated when a brief pulse is applied to the same pathway. The CA1 response to pulse stimulation of the other CA3 subfield does not change.

populations of Schaffer collaterals with a test stimulus, but tetanic stimulation was administered by only one of these electrodes, LTP would appear only in the pathway that received high-frequency stimulation (Figure 14.10). It is thought that selective potentiation of certain synapses, but not others, may mediate normal learning.

Synaptic responses in the hippocampus can be potentiated without using tetanic stimulation, but only if the presynaptic and postsynaptic neurons are excited simultaneously. To demonstrate this effect, an intracellular electrode is used to briefly depolarize a CA1 neuron while a single electrical pulse is applied to the Schaffer collaterals. After several trials of pairing postsynaptic depolarization with activation of the Schaffer collaterals, the synaptic connections become potentiated. In this paradigm, however, synaptic potentiation appears only when the presynaptic and postsynaptic neurons are co-activated within an interval of 100 milliseconds (ms) or less.

Synaptic plasticity is induced by tetanic stimulation.

Although many neuroscientists believe that LTP is necessary for behavioral conditioning and other types of associative learning, few studies have demonstrated a specific linkage between behavioral learning and LTP. The best evidence for such a linkage is shown by studies in which pharmacologic blockade of LTP impairs acquisition of new memories without interfering with established memories. Furthermore, the temporal properties of LTP and its demonstration within the hippocampus, which is necessary for memory consolidation, suggest that LTP represents the most likely synaptic process for mediating the formation of new memories.

Long-Term Depression. Learning and memory are probably not mediated exclusively by increases in synaptic efficacy. If neural plasticity manifested itself only as an increase in synaptic strength, eventually all synapses would attain a maximum level of efficacy, and it would be difficult to encode new information. Some patterns of electrical stimulation, however, produce a decrease in synaptic efficacy. For example, if Schaffer collaterals are stimulated at low frequencies (~1 hertz) for an extended period, a subsequent test stimulus elicits a weaker or depressed postsynaptic response in the CA1 subfield. This change may persist for several hours and can reverse the effects of LTP. Although the relationship between synaptic depression and learning is not understood, it is clear that synaptic strength can be attenuated in the hippocampus under certain circumstances.

Cellular Basis for Hippocampal Plasticity. The discovery of synaptic plasticity in the hippocampus has prompted considerable research to determine its cellular basis. These studies have demonstrated that blockade of glutamatergic transmission prevents LTP because this synaptic process depends on the activation of a specific glutamate receptor, the *N*-methyl-D-aspartate (NMDA) receptor (see Chapter 2).

LTP depends on activation of glutamate NMDA receptors.

The postsynaptic effects of glutamate depend on the types of glutamate receptors that are activated. If the neuron is at its resting membrane potential, glutamate binding to non-NMDA receptors allows an influx of sodium ions (Na^+). Glutamate is unable to activate NMDA receptors because NMDA-gated channels are blocked by magnesium ions (Mg^{2+}) when the membrane potential is negative (Figure 14.11). When the membrane potential is depolarized, however, Mg^{2+} is expelled and glutamate is able to activate the NMDA receptors and trigger an influx of both Na^+ and calcium ions (Ca^{2+}).

An influx of Ca^{2+} is critical for the induction and maintenance of LTP. An increase in intracellular Ca^{2+} promotes LTP, whereas Ca^{2+} chelators (compounds that sequester Ca^{2+} from the cytoplasm) effectively block the induction of LTP. The influx of Ca^{2+} activates two types of protein kinases (enzymes that phosphorylate certain protein molecules):

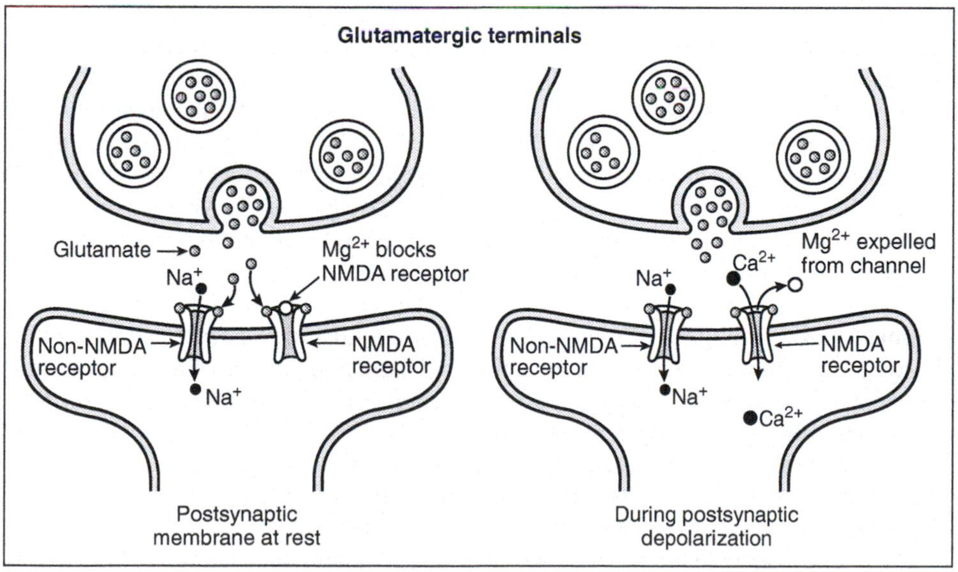

FIG. 14.11. ***N*-Methyl-D-Aspartate (NMDA) Receptors.** Magnesium ions (Mg^{2+}) block NMDA receptors when the postsynaptic membrane is in its resting potential. Depolarization of the postsynaptic membrane removes the Mg^{2+} block and allows glutamate to activate NMDA receptors, which allow an influx of sodium (Na^+) and calcium (Ca^{2+}) ions.

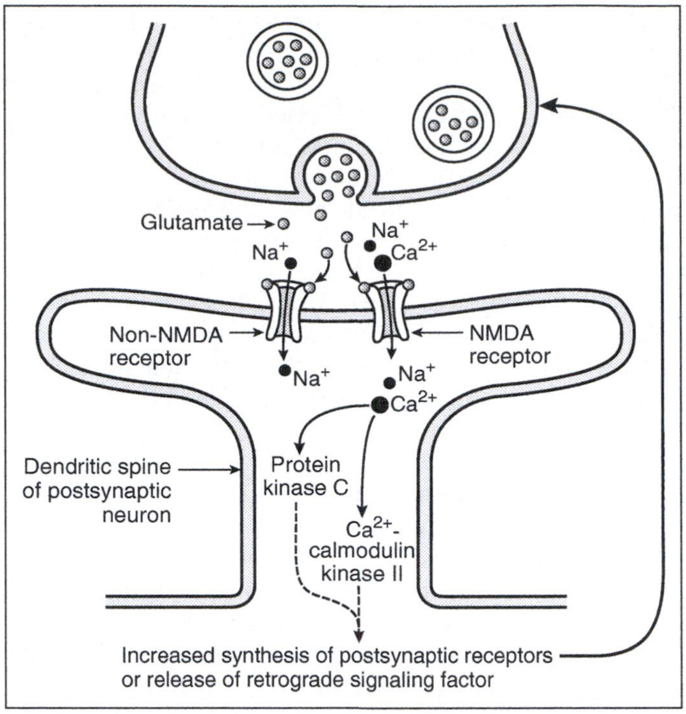

FIG. 14.12. Molecular Basis of Long-Term Potentiation (LTP). LTP depends on glutamatergic activation of *N*-methyl-D-aspartate (NMDA) receptors and the subsequent increase in calcium ion (Ca^{2+}) influx. Increased levels of Ca^{2+} activate protein kinase C and Ca^{2+}-calmodulin kinase II. These Ca^{2+}-dependent enzymes may cause the metabolic machinery of the neuron to synthesize more glutamate receptors or release a retrograde signal, which acts on the presynaptic terminal. Na^+ = sodium ion.

Ca^{2+}-calmodulin-dependent protein kinase and protein kinase C (Figure 14.12). These Ca^{2+}-activated proteins trigger changes in gene expression that lead to increased protein synthesis and production of more postsynaptic glutamate receptors. Other evidence suggests that the postsynaptic neuron produces nitric oxide, which directs the presynaptic terminal to release more glutamate in response to incoming action potentials.

Regardless of the exact mechanisms by which Ca^{2+} induces LTP, the properties of LTP are reflected in the dynamics of the NMDA receptor. Thus, LTP is induced by high-frequency stimulation because the tremendous increase in the synaptic release of glutamate depolarizes the postsynaptic neuron enough to remove the Mg^{2+} block. Alternatively, LTP can be induced by pairing weak presynaptic stimulation with direct depolarization of the postsynaptic cell, because this also removes the Mg^{2+} block.

Temporal Lobe Epilepsy. Epilepsy is a neurologic disorder that is mediated by dysfunctional, synchronous, and rhythmic activity of large populations of neurons. Although epileptic seizures may occur throughout the cerebral cortex, most seizures are initiated in the hippocampus or in the adjacent temporal lobe. The propensity of the hippocampus for initiating seizures is directly related to the ease with which synaptic excitation can be potentiated in this brain region. Thus, the same mechanisms that mediate LTP may, under certain conditions, lead to excessive and uncontrollable neuronal activity.

Kindling is the repetitive electrical stimulation of the amygdala, which leads to seizures.

The relationship between synaptic potentiation and seizure initiation is illustrated by kindling studies in which a weak electrical stimulus is delivered to the amygdaloid complex once a day. Initially, this stimulation does not elicit seizure activity or behavioral convulsions. After several daily kindling sessions, however, the same electrical stimulus evokes a full-blown seizure that is accompanied by convulsions. The pattern of hippocampal seizures elicited by kindling in animals is remarkably similar to the seizure activity seen in human epilepsy.

Epileptic seizures in humans can be caused by trauma, tumors, infections, ischemia, and vascular malformations. Although no consensus has developed regarding how these factors alter the cellular and metabolic functions of hippocampal neurons, substantial evidence indicates that an increase in the extracellular concentration of potassium (K^+) (10-12 mM compared to a normal concentration of 3-5 mM) makes hippocampal neurons more excitable. The role of increased extracellular K^+ has received attention because certain forms of epilepsy are associated with low levels of adenosine triphosphate (ATP) and Na^+-K^+-adenosine triphosphatase (ATPase), both of which are needed to maintain the differential concentrations of Na^+ and K^+ across neuronal membranes. An increase in extracellular K^+ effectively shifts the K^+ reversal potential (E_K) more positive and, by causing a decrease in K^+ efflux, leads to partial depolarization of the resting membrane potential (see Chapter 2). Any diminishment in K^+ efflux also reduces the amplitude of $GABA_B$-mediated inhibitory potentials that normally promote additional K^+ efflux. Furthermore, a brief burst of action potentials in hippocampal neurons is immediately followed by a large hyperpolarization, or afterhyperpolarization, to prevent sustained repetitive firing. Because the afterhyperpolarization is mediated by a Ca^{2+}-dependent K^+ efflux, any reduction in K^+ outflow also interferes with the inhibition provided by the afterhyperpolarization. The net effect of all of these changes is to increase the excitability of hippocampal neurons.

Epilepsy occurs in the hippocampus because it potentiates reverberating excitatory activity.

Given its capacity for potentiating excitatory responses and its unidirectional circuit of excitatory connections, excessive activity in any part of the hippocampus can spread to the entorhinal cortex and then escape to other parts of the cerebral cortex. The behavioral manifestations of seizure activity in the cerebral cortex depend on the specific location and size of the affected area. Focal seizures that affect a small region of the motor cortex, for example, may produce mild twitching in a limb; more generalized seizures across a larger expanse of the cortex may lead to sensory hallucinations, uncontrollable convulsions, and loss of consciousness.

ROLE OF THE HIPPOCAMPUS IN MEMORY

Memory is a specific cognitive function that underlies our ability to learn new information. Neural plasticity is necessary for learning and memory, and different forms of neural plasticity appear in various structures including the hippocampus and cerebral cortex. Much of our knowledge about the role of the hippocampus in learning and memory comes from clinical studies that correlate psychological performance with neuropathological findings.

Memory Classifications

Neuroscientists have classified memory into two broad categories: declarative memory and procedural memory. Declarative memory is concerned with the conscious storage and retrieval of semantic information such as the meaning of words, famous dates in history, names of acquaintances, and the specific events that transpire during personal experience. Declarative memory is often assessed by presenting a list of items to an individual and then determining, after a delay interval, the number of items that can be recalled.

Procedural memory is concerned with the acquisition of motor, cognitive, and perceptual skills that improve in speed and accuracy through repetition. For example, typing and playing tennis are motor skills that are perfected with practice. Once learned, these skills can be performed after long time intervals because the brain has "memorized" the motor programs that specify the timed sequence of muscle activity needed to perform these tasks. By comparison, the ability to read mirror-reversed words is an example of a cognitive skill that improves because of procedural memory. Thus, procedural memory is demonstrated by the retention of improved performance on a specific set of procedures that involve either physical or cognitive manipulations.

Declarative memories are encoded by language or visual images.
Procedural memories are encoded by repetitive motor or cognitive performance.

The division of memory into procedural and declarative categories is appropriate from an anatomical perspective because different neural systems store these types of

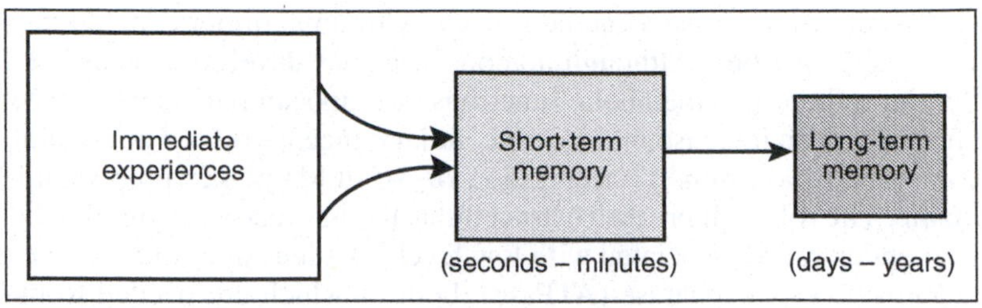

FIG. 14.13. Time Course of Memory. How memory is stored depends on how long the information is needed. Only a fraction of our perceptual experiences are stored in short-term memory for a period of several seconds or minutes. Only a fraction of the information in short-term memory is consolidated into long-term memory for days, weeks, or years.

memory. The cerebellum, basal ganglia, and both motor and premotor cortices are critical for the long-term storage of procedural memories. By comparison, declarative memories depend on interactions between the hippocampus and the surrounding cortical areas in the temporal lobe. Selective damage to one of these systems can affect one category of memory processing without affecting the other.

Temporal Classifications

Consolidation is the transfer of short-term memory into long-term memory.
Retrieval is the process that brings memory into consciousness.

Memories are also classified by the time period over which they persist (Figure 14.13). Immediate memory, which is the ability to hold a thought for a brief instant, provides us with our sense of the present. Short-term memory, which involves retention of information for a few minutes, is frequently used to perform a specific task, but is rapidly forgotten after the task is completed. Memorizing a phone number and then forgetting it after completing the call is an example of short-term memory that is sometimes called working memory. Finally, information that can be retrieved after an interval of several days, weeks, months, or years is stored in long-term memory.

The ability to form and retrieve a memory involves several distinct processes. The process by which information is transferred from short-term memory into long-term memory is called consolidation. Some evidence indicates that consolidation depends on physical changes in synaptic connections, such as the construction of new synapses or a change in the strength of existing synapses. The act of remembering refers to the process by which information is retrieved from long-term storage and brought into consciousness (declarative memory) or expressed as a motor skill (procedural memory). Thus, consolidation, long-term storage, and subsequent retrieval refer to distinct aspects of memory that involve separate mechanisms and brain regions.

Amnesia

Anterograde amnesia is the inability to establish new memory because of a defect in consolidation.
Retrograde amnesia is the inability to retrieve information from long-term memory.

Forgetting is a normal process that occurs over time in all individuals. For most of us, unimportant facts are soon forgotten, but we remember significant details and can easily recall information that is actively memorized for testing purposes. In some individuals, however, memory loss is due to a pathologic process that disrupts specific neural mechanisms. In these cases, the loss of memory is classified as anterograde or retrograde amnesia. Anterograde amnesia is an inability to establish new memories (i.e., consolidation has been impaired) after some precipitating event or illness; retrograde amnesia is characterized by difficulty in retrieving information that had been consolidated (i.e., stored) in long-term memory.

Anterograde Amnesia. The classic example of anterograde amnesia is represented by the case of H.M., a 27-year-old man who received a bilateral medial temporal lobectomy to alleviate intractable epileptic seizures. Since the age of 16, H.M. had suffered major seizures characterized by generalized convulsions, tongue-biting, urinary incontinence, and a loss of consciousness. Despite receiving heavy doses of different anticonvulsants, these attacks gradually increased in frequency and severity to the point where H.M. was unable to maintain a normal life.

When anticonvulsants are unsuccessful in managing temporal lobe seizures, the hippocampus and surrounding structures can be removed to reduce seizure activity. For this reason, H.M. underwent surgery in which the amygdala, uncus, parahippocampal gyrus, and the anterior two-thirds of the hippocampus were removed bilaterally. This surgery was performed in 1953, before it was known that the hippocampus was necessary for establishing memories. After he recovered from his operation, however, it was clear that H.M. suffered from severe anterograde amnesia.

Approximately 19 months after his surgery, H.M. was tested on several psychological tasks to determine the precise nature of his amnesia. The severity of his memory defect was immediately apparent because H.M. was unable to recall any details of his life since the operation and was not even aware that he had received an operation. Despite his memory impairment, H.M. achieved an intelligence quotient (IQ) score of 112 on the Wechsler-Bellevue Intelligence Scale, which was similar to his preoperative score of 104. Furthermore, H.M. showed no deficits in perception, abstract thinking, reasoning ability, or motor learning.

On tests that measured declarative memory, H.M. failed to remember any new stories or memorize word pairs that were presented to him a few minutes earlier. Whenever his attention turned to a new task, H.M. was unable to recall the preceding task in which he had been engaged. Even though these deficits indicate a profound loss of short-term and long-term memory, H.M. was able to recall events that occurred prior to his operation. Indeed, when presented with pictures of celebrities, H.M. was able to identify those people who were famous prior to his surgery. His ability to retrieve memories established before bilateral removal of the temporal lobes indicates that the hippocampus and surrounding cortical regions do not store information or participate in the retrieval process. Instead, the inability to establish new declarative memories suggests that a major function of the hippocampus and surrounding temporal cortex is to consolidate semantic information into long-term memory.

> **Causes of anterograde amnesia:**
> - Temporal lobe damage
> - Head trauma

Retrograde Amnesia. By definition, retrograde amnesia means that a patient is unable to recall events that occurred prior to some precipitating event. In contrast to anterograde amnesia, which is produced by focal damage in the temporal lobe, retrograde amnesia is typically produced by global pathologic processes in the cerebral cortex. Because long-term memories are stored in a distributed fashion throughout the cortex, any event that causes cortical dysfunction may interfere with the retrieval of long-term memory. Consistent with this view, retrograde amnesia can be precipitated by head trauma, electroconvulsive therapy, or generalized lesions produced by Alzheimer's disease.

> **Causes of retrograde amnesia:**
> - Alzheimer's disease
> - Head trauma
> - Electroconvulsive shocks

Head Trauma. Patients may exhibit varying degrees of amnesia while recovering from a loss of consciousness caused by a severe head injury. Victims of head trauma are unable to remember events that immediately preceded the injury (retrograde amnesia) and may have difficulty recalling events that transpired soon after consciousness was regained (anterograde amnesia). In either case, the severity and duration of amnesia are directly related to the amount of brain trauma or damage. With a minor concussion, amnesia is rare, but following a severe contusion (i.e., bruise) of the brain, anterograde and retrograde amnesia may persist for several days or weeks. These patients gradually recover their memories of the events surrounding the injury until, eventually, no further recovery is apparent. The last memories that are restored are those closest in time to the trauma; unfortunately, events immediately preceding severe head trauma are never recalled because this information was never consolidated into long-term memory.

Electroconvulsive Therapy. Many patients suffering from epilepsy become depressed and, ironically, their depression is often temporarily alleviated by an epileptic seizure. This discovery prompted psychiatrists to treat depressed individuals by administering electrical shocks to the head to produce a full-blown seizure. Electroconvulsive therapy (ECT) is an

> **ECT** interferes with memory consolidation.

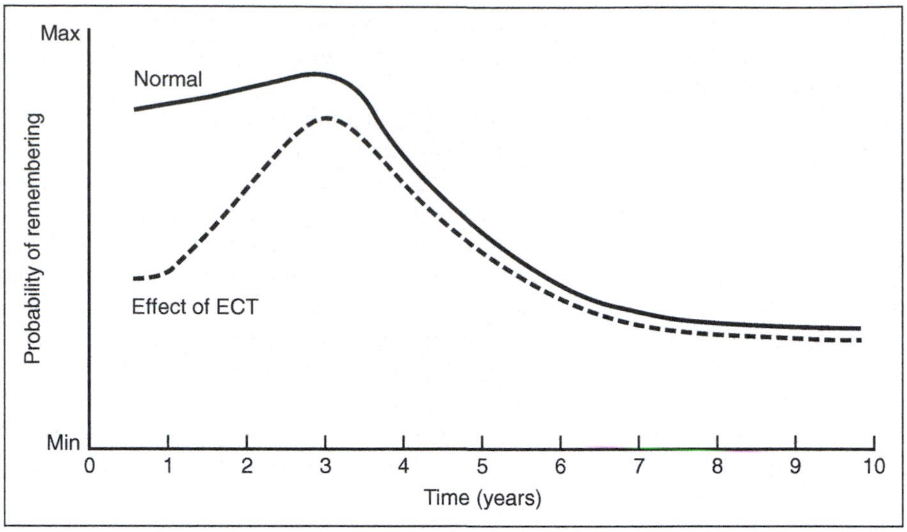

FIG. 14.14. Amnesia Produced by Electroconvulsive Therapy (ECT). In normal individuals, television programs that were broadcast 1–3 years earlier had a high probability of being remembered. The probability for recalling earlier programs gradually declined over a period of several years. Depressed patients who were subjected to electroconvulsive shock therapy showed a significant decrease in the probability of remembering programs that were televised 1–3 years earlier. (Graphs based on data appearing in Squire LR, et al: Retrograde amnesia: temporal gradient in very long-term memory following electroconvulsive therapy. *Science* 187:77–79, 1975.)

effective treatment for severe depression, but it produces anterograde and retrograde amnesia.

Controlled studies of the effects of ECT on memory indicate that recent memories are more easily disrupted than older memories (Figure 14.14). In one study, depressed patients were asked to identify the names of television programs that were shown for only 1 year between 1957 and 1972. Different sets of TV programs were presented to each patient before and after receiving ECT, and the proportion of identified shows was plotted as a function of the time since each program was on the air. Results from this study indicated that memory for the programs declined over time and followed a pattern of forgetting that is observed in all individuals. Administration of ECT disrupted the ability to name the most recent programs but had little effect on the memory for programs seen several years earlier. These results suggest that memory formation is a prolonged process and ECT interferes with the ability to retrieve memories that are still labile but does not affect the retrieval of memories that are established for more than 2 years. With further passage of time, however, even stable memories gradually degrade and become more difficult to retrieve.

Neural Substrate of Memory

The case of H.M. indicates that the hippocampus and surrounding temporal cortex are necessary for memory consolidation, but this case study does not reveal the site of long-term memory storage. Accumulating evidence suggests that memories related to a specific sensory modality are stored in different cortical areas that are connected with the primary sensory cortex for that modality. Visual memory, for example, appears to be distributed throughout the inferior temporal gyrus, which receives visual information needed for object recognition and the perception of visual patterns (see Chapter 11).

The precise neural mechanisms and pathways by which the hippocampus consolidates information in the cerebral cortex have not been fully established. The prevailing view holds that perceptual information is conveyed by sensory association cortex to the hippocampus where it is transformed before it is returned to those association areas via

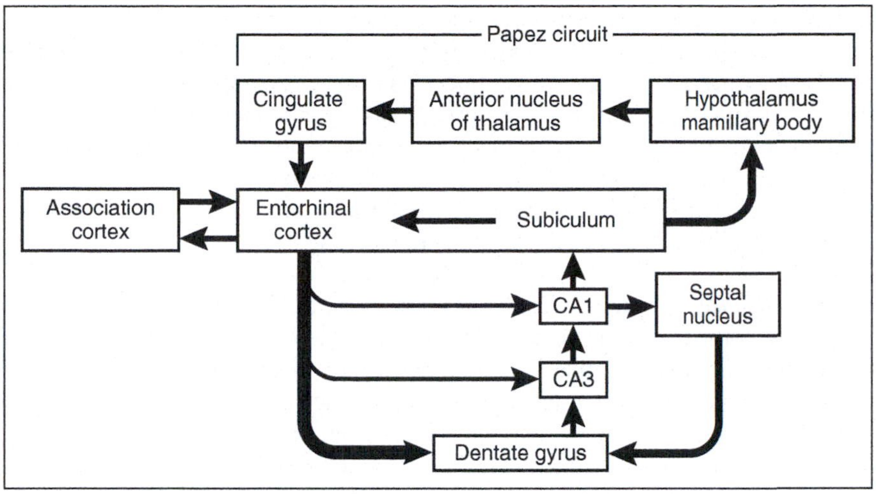

FIG. 14.15. Connections of the Hippocampal Formation. This diagram shows the main cortical and subcortical connections with the hippocampal formation.

the cortical projections of the subiculum and entorhinal cortex. The hippocampal formation is also interconnected with a variety of subcortical structures within the diencephalon and basal forebrain (Figure 14.15). The importance of these structures in memory has been demonstrated by several clinical cases, but their precise role in learning and memory has not been elucidated.

Cortical Hippocampal Connections. Extensive regions of the cerebral cortex project directly to the subiculum and entorhinal cortex or to adjacent parts of the parahippocampal gyrus (Figure 14.16). The cingulate gyrus sends a major projection to the entorhinal cortex via the cingulum, a thick bundle of fibers buried below the cingulate gyrus. Additional projections to the entorhinal cortex and subiculum originate from the dorsolateral prefrontal cortex (Brodmann areas 9, 10, and 46), the medial frontal cortex (Brodmann areas 25 and 32), and the orbitofrontal cortex. In the temporal lobe, the superior temporal gyrus, the perirhinal cortex, and the temporal pole all project to the entorhinal cortex. Finally, olfactory information reaches the hippocampal formation via projections from the piriform cortex and the periamygdaloid cortical area.

With the exception of the perforant pathway, efferent connections of the subiculum and entorhinal cortex have not been studied in detail. It is known that the entorhinal cortex

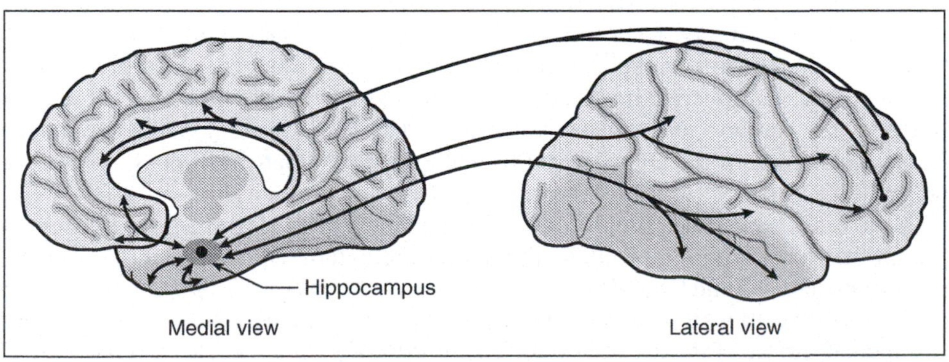

FIG. 14.16. Long-Term Memory Storage in the Cerebral Cortex. Widespread regions of the cerebral cortex have reciprocal connections with the hippocampus, which may mediate the consolidation of short-term memory into long-term memory.

and subiculum project to the perirhinal cortex, the cingulate gyrus, and the orbitofrontal cortex, but other long-range cortical projections are likely to exist as well. In addition, the entorhinal cortex has dense reciprocal connections with the parahippocampal gyrus, which projects to widespread regions in the temporal, parietal, and frontal lobes. Hence, connections with the parahippocampal gyrus provide a major route by which the hippocampus influences diverse parts of the cerebral cortex. Consistent with this, damage to the parahippocampal gyrus and surrounding temporal lobe produces effects similar to those produced by selective damage to the hippocampus alone.

Alzheimer's disease is characterized by an age-related pathologic decline in attention, reasoning, and memory.

Alzheimer's Disease. Patients with Alzheimer's disease illustrate the importance of the cerebral cortex for memory. Typically seen in older adults, Alzheimer's disease is a progressive neurologic disorder that is characterized by severe memory impairment and a progressive decline in attention, orientation, abstract reasoning, and language skills. Although all individuals show some mental deterioration with advancing age, the cognitive deficits produced by Alzheimer's disease are much more severe and debilitating. Furthermore, in contrast to medial temporal lobe damage, Alzheimer's disease interferes with the retrieval of distant memories.

The memory deficits associated with Alzheimer's disease are correlated with a significant loss of neurons in the hippocampus, subiculum, entorhinal cortex, and association cortex. Additional neuropathology is characterized by a reduction in cholinergic neurons in the basal forebrain (i.e., substantia innominata and basal forebrain of Meynert), which has widespread projections to the cerebral cortex. The loss of cholinergic neurons is also characterized by a concomitant decline in cholinergic markers (i.e., choline O-acetyltransferase) throughout the cerebral cortex. Although there is no cure for Alzheimer's disease, the pharmacologic treatments that have the most benefit for delaying memory loss during the earliest stages of Alzheimer's disease involve drugs that enhance cholinergic transmission in brain. For an in-depth description of Alzheimer's disease and related disorders, see Chapter 16.

Subcortical Hippocampal Projections. The septal nucleus is one of the few subcortical regions that projects to the hippocampal formation (see Figure 14.15). Most of the neurons in the medial septal nucleus that project directly to the hippocampus via the fornix are cholinergic and, thus, comprise a portion of the basal forebrain cholinergic system. These septohippocampal projections terminate most densely in the dentate gyrus, subfield CA3, the subiculum, and the entorhinal cortex.

Information that has strong emotional significance is usually consolidated into long-term memory. Consistent with this fact, the basolateral nuclei of the amygdaloid complex send a modest set of projections to the entorhinal cortex and the subiculum. Connections between the amygdala and hippocampus are reciprocal, but the amygdala exerts considerably more influence on the hippocampus than vice versa.

Consistent with the fact that a state of wakefulness is necessary to memorize information, several ascending projections from the brainstem terminate in the hippocampal formation. Thus, the hippocampus receives dopaminergic innervation from the ventral tegmental area, serotonergic innervation from the mesencephalic raphe nuclei, and noradrenergic innervation from the locus ceruleus. These modulatory pathways innervate widespread regions of the hippocampal formation but terminate most densely in the dentate gyrus.

Nearly all subcortical projections from the hippocampal formation are conveyed through the fornix. These projections originate from pyramidal neurons in the subiculum and in subfields CA3 and CA1. The axons from these neurons form a thin sheath, the alveus, that covers the ventricular surface of the hippocampus before emerging as the fimbria on the dorsomedial surface of the dentate gyrus. The fimbria proceeds caudally and medially with the hippocampus and lateral ventricle until it thickens to form the fornix, which arches under the splenium of the corpus callosum. At this point, some fibers in the fornix cross the midline as the hippocampal commissure, which interconnects the CA3 subfields of both hemispheres. The remaining fibers in the fornix proceed rostrally under the corpus callosum until they form the columns of the fornix, which enter the diencephalon between the interventricular foramen and the anterior commissure. The columns of the fornix divide into precommissural and postcommissural pathways. The smaller, precommissural fornix contains fibers arising from subfields CA3 and CA1, and these terminate in the septal nucleus, the nucleus accumbens, and the medial frontal cortex. The more numerous fibers of the postcommissural fornix originate from the subiculum and terminate in either the mammillary body of the hypothalamus or the anterior nucleus of the thalamus.

Korsakoff's Syndrome. Korsakoff's syndrome is a form of amnesia that is correlated with bilateral lesions in the mammillary bodies and mediodorsal nucleus of the thalamus. The cause of Korsakoff's syndrome is attributed to prolonged thiamine deficiency, which develops during chronic alcoholism (thiamine absorption is impaired in alcoholics). Patients with Korsakoff's syndrome are unable to remember recent events and tend to fabricate information to fill in the missing memory. Korsakoff's syndrome often appears with Wernicke's syndrome, another form of dementia induced by chronic alcoholism, which is associated with an ataxic gait and dysfunctional eye movements. Many neurologic problems occur in chronic alcoholics, and for this reason, Korsakoff's syndrome does not provide a clear picture of the relationship between amnesia and neuropathology. Nonetheless, autopsy findings from patients who had only the amnestic syndrome of Korsakoff's suggest that specific nuclei within the diencephalon play an important role in memory.

Wernicke's syndrome is not the same as **Wernicke's aphasia.**

RESOLUTION OF CLINICAL CASE

This clinical case describes symptoms that are typical of temporal lobe epilepsy. This form of epilepsy, which is the most common type in adults, involves paroxysmal events in the amygdala, hippocampus, and parahippocampal gyrus. Temporal lobe epilepsy often begins in late childhood or adolescence, and although its cause is usually unknown, a history of febrile (fever-induced) seizures is common. Several criteria are used to classify seizures according to their severity. Partial seizures denote epileptiform activity within a focal region of cortex, whereas general seizures involve widespread cortical regions in both hemispheres. Consciousness is always preserved during a simple seizure but is impaired during a complex seizure. An aura usually precedes a complex-partial seizure, and the patient's description of the aura can be helpful in determining the focus of the epileptiform activity. Hence, an aura may have well-defined sensory characteristics such as visual, auditory, or olfactory hallucinations or may consist of general feelings of fear, detachment, or a sense of déjà vu. Complex-partial seizures are often marked by repetitive motor activity or automatisms that affect the oral musculature (e.g., lip-smacking, tongue-biting, jaw movements). A loss of consciousness during a complex seizure is typically followed by a variable and prolonged period of confusion.

Epileptic seizures usually recur and will increase in frequency and severity if left untreated. Successive seizures may cause brain damage and atrophy of the affected cortical sites, presumably due to the excitotoxic effects associated with excessive discharge of glutamatergic neurons (see Chapter 2). For this reason, patients diagnosed with epilepsy must be treated to prevent further seizures. Scalp electrodes can display dysfunctional electrical activity that develops spontaneously among populations of cortical neurons, and a routine EEG may detect a specific epileptic syndrome even in the absence of behavioral symptoms.

No cure exists for epilepsy, but a variety of drugs are available to eliminate seizures or reduce their frequency. Because the propagation of seizure activity depends on excitatory neurotransmission, most drugs used in the treatment of epilepsy are anticonvulsants that act by attenuating neuronal excitability. Many anticonvulsant drugs inhibit neurons directly because they are GABAergic agonists (e.g., phenobarbital, valproic acid), whereas others reduce excitability by stabilizing the membrane conductance of Na^+ (e.g., carbamazepine, phenytoin). Patients who continue to have debilitating seizures after trying different classes of anticonvulsant drugs usually undergo surgical resection of the epileptic focus to control their seizures.

REVIEW QUESTIONS

Directions: For each question, choose the **one best** answer.

1. What symptoms are most likely to be produced by a focal lesion in the amygdaloid complex?
A. Agnosia
B. Amnesia
C. Anxiety
D. Aphasia
E. Automatism

2. Which neurotransmitter and nucleus are associated with subjective feelings of pleasure?
A. Acetylcholine—basal nucleus of Meynert
B. Dopamine—nucleus accumbens
C. γ-Aminobutyric acid (GABA)—amygdala
D. Glutamate—hippocampus
E. Serotonin—hypothalamus

3. What psychoactive drug produces its therapeutic benefit by increasing serotonergic transmission in the amygdala?
A. Amphetamine (Adderall)
B. Phenytoin (Dilantin)
C. Phenobarbital (Donnatal)
D. Fluoxetine (Prozac)
E. Diazepam (Valium)

4. What brain region is most likely to be damaged in a chronic alcoholic?
A. Entorhinal cortex
B. Mediodorsal thalamus
C. Nucleus accumbens
D. Prefrontal cortex
E. Septal nucleus

5. Which anatomical sequence best represents the flow of activity through the limbic system?
A. Amygdala → mediodorsal thalamus → cingulate gyrus → entorhinal cortex → amygdala
B. Amygdala → mediodorsal thalamus → prefrontal cortex → hypothalamus → amygdala
C. Entorhinal cortex → dentate gyrus → CA3 → CA1 → subiculum → entorhinal cortex
D. Subiculum → CA1 → CA3 → dentate gyrus → entorhinal cortex → subiculum
E. Subiculum → cingulate gyrus → anterior thalamus → mammillary bodies → subiculum

6. What cognitive process is impaired by hippocampal damage?
A. Attention
B. Consolidation
C. Memory retrieval
D. Motor learning
E. Visual recognition

7. What brain region is the most critical for long-term storage and retrieval of declarative memory?
A. Nucleus accumbens
B. Hippocampal formation
C. Amygdaloid complex
D. Cerebral cortex
E. Hypothalamus

8. Which neural structure and fiber system are associated with each other?
A. Amygdala and stria terminalis
B. Nucleus accumbens and perforant pathway
C. Hypothalamus and cingulum
D. Dentate gyrus and fornix
E. Cingulate gyrus and subiculum

9. Which of the following behavioral phenomena are associated with NMDA receptor activation?
A. Memory retrieval
B. Temporal lobe epilepsy
C. Memory consolidation
D. Depression
E. Retrograde amnesia

ADDITIONAL READING

Classic Literature

Klüver H, Bucy PC: Preliminary analysis of functions of the temporal lobes in monkeys. *Arch Neurol Psychiat* 42:979–1000, 1939.

Lashley KS: In search of the engram. *Symp Soc Exp Biol* 4:454–482, 1950.

MacLean PD: Some psychiatric implications of physiological studies on the frontal temporal portion of the limbic system. *Electroencephal Clin Neurophysiol* 4:407–418, 1952.

Papez JW: A proposed mechanism of emotion. *Arch Neurol Psychiat* 38:725–743, 1937.

Scoville WB, Milner B: Loss of recent memory after bilateral hippocampal lesions. *J Neurol Neurosurg Psychiat* 20:11–21, 1957.

Reviews and Landmark Research Articles

Adolphs R, Tranel D, Damasio H, Damasio AR: Fear and the human amygdala. *J Neurosci* 15:5879–5891, 1995.

Aggleton JP: The contribution of the amygdala to normal and abnormal emotional states. *Trends Neurosci* 16:328–333, 1993.

Alvarez P, Zola-Morgan S, Squire LR: Damage limited to the hippocampal region produces long-lasting memory impairment in monkeys. *J Neurosci* 15:3796–3807, 1995.

Bliss TVP, Collinridge GL: A synaptic model of memory: long-term potentiation in the hippocampus. *Nature* 361:31–39, 1993.

Bliss TVP, Lomo T: Long-lasting potentiation of synaptic transmission in the dentate area of the anaesthetized rabbit following stimulation of the perforant path. *J Physiol* 232:331–356, 1973.

Cahill L, McGaugh JL: Mechanisms of emotional arousal and lasting declarative memory. *Trends Neurosci* 21:294–299, 1998.

Davis M: The role of the amygdala in fear and anxiety. *Ann Rev Neurosci* 15:353–375, 1992.

Eichenbaum H: A cortical-hippocampal system for declarative memory. *Nat Rev Neurosci* 1:41–50, 2000.

Engert F, Bonhoffer T: Dendritic spine changes associated with hippocampal long-term synaptic plasticity. *Nature* 399:66–70, 1999.

Kauer JA, Malenka RC, Nicoll RA: A persistent postsynaptic modification mediates long-term potentiation in the hippocampus. *Neuron* 1:911–917, 1988.

Kempermann G, Kuhn HG, Gage FH: More hippocampal neurons in adult mice living in an enriched environment. *Nature* 386:493–495, 1997.

LeDoux JE: Emotion circuits in the brain. *Ann Rev Neurosci* 23:155–184, 2000.

Malenka RC, Kauer JA, Zucker RS, Nicoll RA: Postsynaptic calcium is sufficient for potentiation of hippocampal synaptic transmission. *Science* 242:81–84, 1988.

McNamara JO: Cellular and molecular basis of epilepsy. *J Neurosci* 14:3413–3425, 1994.

Mulkey RM, Malenka RC: Mechanisms underlying induction of homosynaptic long-term depression in area CA1 of the hippocampus. *Neuron* 9:967–975, 1992.

Pedley TA, Scheuer ML, Walczak TS: Epilepsy. In: Rowland LP. *Merritt's Textbook of Neurology.* Baltimore, MD: Williams & Wilkins, 1995:845–868.

Schafe GE, Nader K, Blair HT, LeDoux JE: Memory consolidation of Pavlovian fear conditioning: a cellular and molecular perspective. *Trends Neurosci* 24:540–546, 2001.

Squire L: Memory and the hippocampus: a synthesis from findings with rats, monkeys, and humans. *Psych Rev* 99:195–231, 1992.

Squire LR, Ojemann JG, Miezen FM, Petersen SE, Videen TO, Raichle ME: Activation of the hippocampus in normal humans: a functional anatomical study of memory. *Proc Natl Acad Sci USA* 89:1837–1841, 1995.

Squire LR, Slater P, Chace P: Retrograde amnesia: temporal gradient in very long-term memory following electroconvulsive therapy. *Science* 187:77–79, 1975.

Zola-Morgan S, Squire LR: The primate hippocampal formation: evidence for a time-limited role in memory storage. *Science* 250:288–290, 1990.

Zola-Morgan SM, Squire LR: Neuroanatomy of memory. *Ann Rev Neurosci* 16:547–563, 1993.

INTERNET RESOURCES

Alzheimer's Research Foundation
http://www.alzheimers-research.org/

American Epilepsy Society
http://www.aesnet.org/

American Psychological Association
http://www.apa.org/topics/homepage.html

BrainSource.com
Brain Injury, Rehabilitation, Neuropsychology, and Learning
http://www.brainsource.com/

National Institutes of Health (MedlinePlus)
Memory
http://www.nlm.nih.gov/medlineplus/memory.html#nlmnihresources

National Society for Epilepsy
http://www.epilepsynse.org.uk/

PatientPlus
Memory Problems and Their Assessment
http://www.patient.co.uk/showdoc/40024840/

PsychEducation.org
Brain Tours
http://www.psycheducation.org/emotion/introduction.htm#Tours

University of California, San Francisco
Memory and Aging Center
http://memory.ucsf.edu/Education/Topics/memory.html

Washington University
Limbic System
http://thalamus.wustl.edu/course/limbic.html

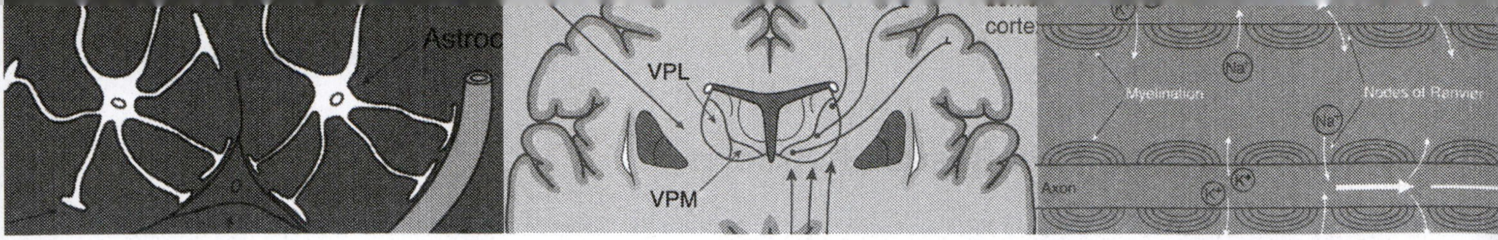

CHAPTER 15

Sleep, Coma, and Brain Death

INTRODUCTION OF CLINICAL CASE

A 58-year-old man was seen by his family physician because of constant sleepiness that interfered with his work and other activities. The patient stated that he rarely slept well and that his sleep was often punctuated by a series of awakenings. His wife confirmed this remark. She hastened to add that her husband snored loudly when he fell asleep and that a silent period lasting 30 or 40 seconds followed each series of snores. Examination revealed enlargement of the patient's adenoids and tonsils, but all other findings were normal. The patient was generally healthy, but he had gained 30 lbs since his last office visit; his weight was now in the top quartile for someone of his age and height. His physician referred him to a sleep clinic where he was scheduled for polysomnography.

OVERVIEW OF SLEEP

The human nervous system cannot remain in a waking state for prolonged periods of time without suffering adverse effects. We require regular periods of sleep that consume approximately one-third of our life span. While we are sleeping, our normal sense of consciousness is suspended as we experience dreams and other sensations that revitalize the central nervous system (CNS). Despite the restful feeling acquired from a good night's sleep, the sleep state is not mediated by a simple decrease in neuronal activity throughout the brain. Rather, sleep is an active process that involves dynamic changes in the pattern of neural activity in the neocortex, diencephalon, and certain brainstem nuclei.

Disruption of sleep is a common complaint heard by many physicians. Approximately 15% of the population has a chronic sleeping problem, and another 20% suffers from occasional bouts of insomnia. Insufficient sleep is an enormous public health problem underscored by the fact that 5%–10% of all adults habitually use hypnotic medications to fall asleep. Furthermore, industrialization has increased the number of night workers whose sleep patterns are severely disrupted. One consequence of this lifestyle is an increase in major accidents during the night, such as the nuclear incidents at Chernobyl and Three Mile Island, when the urge to sleep is strongest.

Neural Activity and Electroencephalography

In 1928, Hans Berger demonstrated the feasibility of monitoring human cortical activity with electrodes placed on the scalp. This procedure, called electroencephalography, is widely used to characterize the global features of cortical activity during wakefulness and different stages of sleep.

As discussed in Chapter 1, membrane potentials are small (less than 100 mV), and they are observed only when a microelectrode is placed near the neuron. However, when a large population of cortical neurons is excited simultaneously, the massive flow of ionic current can be detected by electrodes located on the overlying scalp. A record of these electrical signals, called an electroencephalogram (EEG), represents the time course of changes in the summed electrical activity of large populations of cortical neurons. The neural activity recorded on the scalp is produced primarily by changes in subthreshold postsynaptic membrane potentials, not action potentials. Action potentials are too brief to make a significant contribution to the EEG unless a large number of cortical neurons discharge at precisely the same time.

Scalp electrodes detect only local changes in neural activity and must be placed at several sites over the frontal, parietal, temporal, and occipital lobes to obtain a complete EEG record (Figure 15.1). Electroencephalography is routinely performed to determine whether epileptic seizure activity originates from the hippocampus, the surrounding limbic structures, or other cortical regions. For this reason, EEG electrodes are sometimes placed on the sphenoid bone or in the nasopharynx to detect paroxysmal events in the medial temporal lobe.

The EEG is used in the diagnosis of sleep disorders and epilepsy.

Changes in EEG activity related to sensory stimuli are called evoked potentials or event-related potentials (ERPs). Depending on the modality of the stimulus, ERPs appear in one of the primary cortical regions that receive direct sensory projections from the thalamus. Cutaneous stimulation, for example, produces somatosensory-evoked potentials (SEPs) in the contralateral parietal cortex. Similarly, tones or flashes of light produce ERPs in the auditory or visual cortices, respectively. In patients who have sustained damage to a cranial nerve or to one of the ascending sensory pathways, the cortical ERPs for that particular modality are substantially smaller.

Sensory stimuli produce evoked potentials in the EEG.

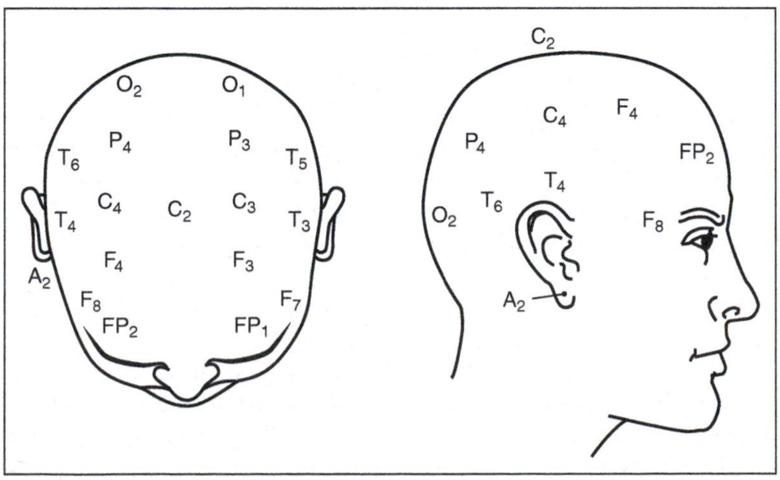

FIG. 15.1. Standard Electroencephalogram (EEG) Recording Sites. Top and side views of the human scalp showing the location of electrodes for electroencephalography. A = auricle; C = central; F = frontal; FP = frontal pole; O = occipital; P = parietal; T = temporal.

TABLE 15.1 Classification of EEG Activity

Classification	Frequency	Level of Arousal
Beta waves	14-40 Hz	Alert, eyes open
Alpha waves	8-14 Hz	Quiet waking, eyes closed
Theta waves	4-8 Hz	Drowsy, sleep stages 1 and 2
Delta waves	0.5-4 Hz	Deep sleep, stages 3 and 4

States of Consciousness Correlated with EEG Activity. Changes in EEG amplitude and frequency indicate the dynamic activity of the cerebral cortex. As such, the EEG record provides a reliable indicator of the changes in cortical physiology that transpire during wakefulness or different stages of sleep (Table 15.1). During the alert waking state, for example, neuronal activity throughout the cerebral cortex is desynchronized. Although neuronal discharges within specific cortical circuits are tightly coordinated as they perform sensory and other cognitive functions, most cortical neurons discharge at different times as they process different types of information. Thus, an EEG recorded from an alert individual with both eyes open is characterized by desynchronized activity comprised of low-amplitude, high-frequency waves. The waking EEG typically contains frequencies between 14 and 40 hertz (Hz), a bandwidth known as the beta range. During quiet resting with the eyes closed, the EEG shows prominent oscillations at 8-14 Hz, which are classified as alpha waves. During sleep, EEG activity slows, and larger amplitudes become more prominent as an increasing number of cortical neurons oscillate synchronously in the theta (4-8 Hz) or delta (0.5-4 Hz) frequency ranges.

Clinical Evaluation of Sleep

To evaluate a patient's sleeping behavior, it is necessary to monitor several physiologic parameters in a specially equipped laboratory. In addition to recording EEG activity, a typical sleep laboratory records an electro-oculogram (EOG) to detect rapid eye movements (REMs) and an electromyogram (EMG) to record changes in muscle tone. This ensemble of records, known as a polysomnogram, provides the critical elements for characterizing sleep patterns in most individuals. Most sleep studies also measure changes in nasal airflow, respiratory movements, body temperature, and postural changes in body position.

Wakefulness: fast frequency, small-amplitude EEG waves
NREM sleep: slow frequency, large-amplitude EEG waves

Sleep Stages. A typical night's sleep is composed of a sequence of stages that are characterized by distinct shifts in the frequency and amplitude of the EEG (Figure 15.2). In a healthy adult, normal sleeping behavior follows a cyclic pattern in which the individual descends into deeper stages of non-rapid eye movement (NREM) sleep followed by progressively longer periods of REM sleep.

Large-amplitude spikes in stage 2 sleep are called **K complexes.**

Slow-wave sleep consists of delta waves (0.5-4 Hz).

NREM Sleep. When an individual rests quietly with eyes closed, the EEG contains low-voltage, alpha (8-14 Hz) rhythms. After the individual becomes drowsy, sleep onset is marked by a gradual shift to stage 1 sleep, which is characterized by the presence of theta (4-8 Hz) waves and slow, rolling eye movements. Stage 1 represents a brief transition from wakefulness to sleep, and it usually does not reappear during the course of a night's sleep. As a person descends more deeply into stage 2 sleep, the EEG gradually becomes slower and is periodically interrupted by episodes of higher-frequency sleep spindles and large-amplitude spikes that resemble the letter K (see Figure 15.2). Sleep spindles, which represent interactions between the thalamus and cerebral cortex, contain 12-14 Hz waveforms that persist for 1–2 seconds. Later, in stage 3, sleep spindles occur less frequently and slow EEG waves increase in amplitude. Delta (0.5-4 Hz) waves appear irregularly in stage 3 sleep but are the main component of the EEG pattern during stage 4 of NREM sleep. In fact, stage 4 sleep is called "slow-wave sleep" because this deep level of sleep is composed almost entirely of slow, high-amplitude delta rhythms.

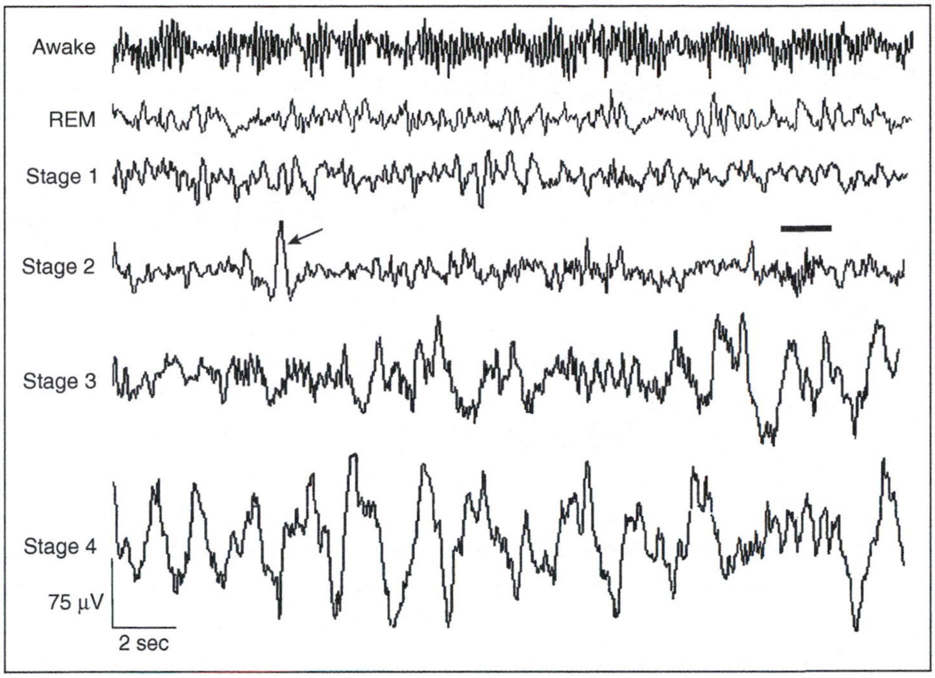

FIG. 15.2. Cortical Activity during Different Stages of Sleep. The electroencephalogram (EEG) recordings illustrate the different patterns of cortical activity associated with wakefulness and the different stages of sleep. The arrow in stage 2 indicates the presence of a K complex; the horizontal bar indicates a sleep spindle. (EEG recordings provided courtesy of Dr. Edward Bixler, Pennsylvania State University.)

Total sleep deprivation disrupts homeostatic functions and leads to death. The chronic loss of NREM sleep is thought to be a major factor in this process because selective deprivation of REM sleep alone does not produce serious problems. Despite the obvious physiologic importance of NREM sleep, its functions remain unknown. Consistent with its restorative and revitalizing effects, slow-wave sleep reduces cerebral blood flow by 40% and produces a similar decline in oxygen consumption. This metabolic decrease is matched by a small but significant decrease in core body temperature. Indeed, a strong correlation exists between the circadian changes in body temperature and the propensity for sleep.

REM (paradoxical) sleep: fast-frequency, small-amplitude EEG waves that resemble the waking state

REM Sleep. At the end of each slow-wave sleep period, the EEG and other parameters show abrupt changes that signal the transition to REM sleep (Figure 15.3). During REM sleep, the EEG shows high-frequency, low-amplitude activity that resembles

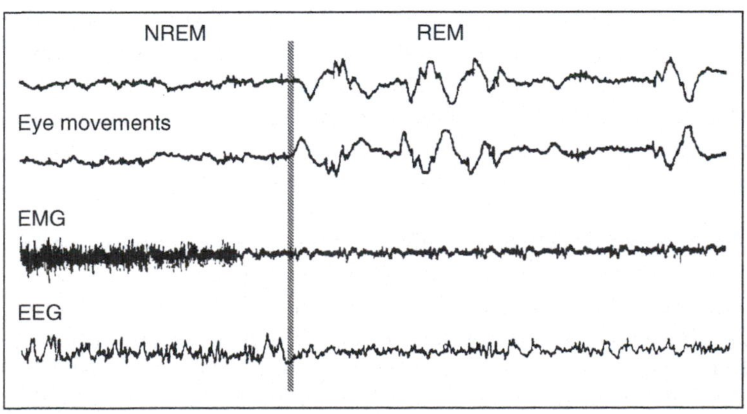

FIG. 15.3. Transition to REM Sleep. The onset of a REM sleep period is marked by a sharp decrease in electromyogram (EMG) activity and the appearance of rapid eye movements as indicated by the electro-oculogram (EOG). The electroencephalogram (EEG) waves shift to a lower amplitude and faster frequency. (Adapted from Kales A, Kales JD: *Evaluation and Treatment of Insomnia*. New York, NY: Oxford University Press, 1984.)

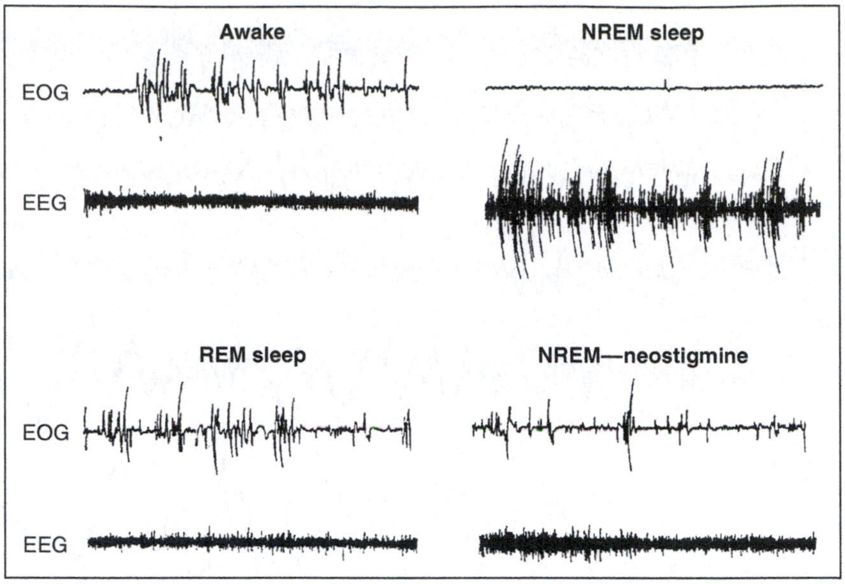

FIG. 15.4. Wakefulness, NREM, and REM Sleep States. One-minute polygraphic recordings from a feline illustrate differences in the states of wakefulness, NREM sleep, and REM sleep. An injection of neostigmine, an acetylcholinesterase inhibitor, into the medial pontine reticular formation induces a REM-like sleep state. EOG = electro-oculogram; EEG = electroencephalogram. (Courtesy of Dr. Ralph Lydic, University of Michigan.)

the desynchronized pattern of the waking state. Cerebral metabolism, which is measured by cerebral blood flow and glucose consumption, increases 30%–40% over the resting wakeful state. For these reasons, REM sleep is often called paradoxical or active sleep.

REMs are mediated by a burst of activity in the pons, lateral geniculate nucleus, and occipital cortex, which are called PGO spikes.

As indicated by its name, REM sleep is characterized by rapid eye movements that are superimposed on a background of slower, rolling eye movements. The eye movements of REM sleep are driven by phasic bursts of neuronal activity that originate in the pontine tegmentum. Neuronal recordings from experimental animals during REM sleep indicate that rapid eye movements are correlated with bursts of neuronal discharges in the pons and numerous sites in the visual system including the oculomotor and lateral geniculate nuclei, as well as the occipital cortex. Although recordings from the pons and lateral geniculate nucleus have been conducted only in experimental animals (Figure 15.4), pontogeniculate-occipital (PGO) spikes are considered an essential component of REM sleep in humans. Many parameters of REM sleep, including changes in respiration, heart rate, and cerebral blood flow, are mediated by projections from the pontine tegmentum to sites located more caudally in the pons and medulla.

Dreams occur during **REM sleep.**

Unlike the waking state or the NREM sleep stages, REM sleep is associated with a profound loss of skeletal muscle tone. Only the extraocular muscles, the respiratory muscles, and the muscles controlling the middle ear remain active during REM sleep. The ability to regulate body temperature is lost, in part, because of the general paralysis of striated muscles. Furthermore, REM sleep is accompanied by a global suppression of sympathetic activity, one sign of which is pupillary constriction. All of these signs are consistent with a general reduction in homeostatic functions during the REM sleep stage.

Sleep studies on human volunteers indicate that almost all dreams occur during REM sleep. More than 75% of human subjects awakened from REM sleep state that they were in the midst of a vivid dream. When awakened from NREM sleep, however, subjects often report having thoughts or other mental experiences, but only a small percentage state that they were dreaming. Given the role of the lateral geniculate nucleus and striate cortex in mediating vision, PGO spikes are likely to represent physiological correlates of the visual images that are perceived during a dream.

Rhythmic Pattern of NREM and REM Sleep. The sequence of EEG activity during a night's sleep follows a predictable pattern (Figure 15.5). After sleep onset, the EEG shows a regular stepwise descent from stage 1 to stage 4 that usually takes about 60 minutes. The first abrupt shift from the slow-wave sleep of stage 4 to the desynchronized pattern of REM sleep occurs about 70–90 minutes after sleep onset. After the first REM sleep episode, which lasts only about 10 minutes, EEG activity returns to stage 2 and then

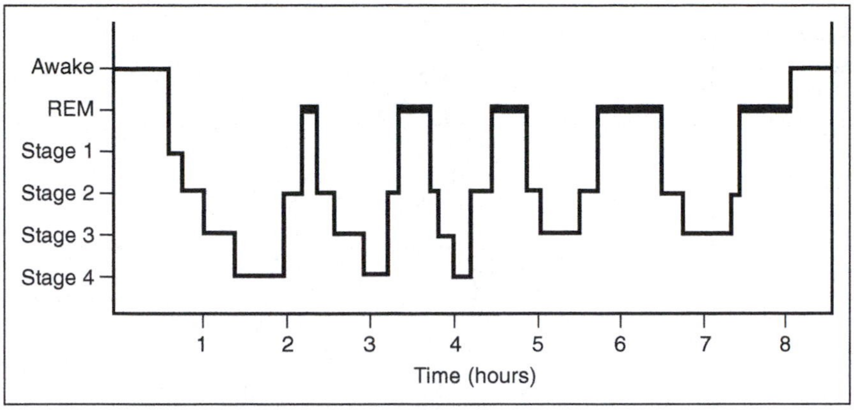

FIG. 15.5. Periodic Pattern of Sleep. During a night of sleep, EEG activity shifts between the different stages of slow-wave sleep and REM sleep at regular intervals.

descends through stages 3 and 4 of NREM sleep. A second REM episode appears about 90 minutes after the start of the first REM period. This alternating cycle between REM and NREM sleep is usually repeated four or five times during the course of a night's sleep. With the exception of the first REM period, most REM episodes last 20–30 minutes and a complete cycle of REM and NREM sleep takes about 90 minutes. With each successive cycle, however, the proportion of NREM sleep devoted to stage 4 declines and, by the end of the night, REM sleep may commence without passing through stage 4.

Neuroanatomy of Sleep

Slow EEG waves reflect synchronized oscillations of thalamic and cortical neurons.

The changes in cortical activity that accompany the different stages of sleep are initiated by ascending projections from the thalamus and specific parts of the brainstem. The high-voltage, slow waves of activity in the EEG during stages 2, 3, and 4 of NREM sleep are mediated by reverberating oscillations of synchronized activity between the thalamus and cerebral cortex. Subsequent desynchronization of EEG activity during REM sleep occurs because thalamocortical synchronization is disrupted by depolarizing influences ascending from specific nuclei in the brainstem.

Thalamocortical Interactions and Cortical Synchronization. The slow cortical oscillations of NREM sleep are a product of thalamic and cortical circuits working in concert with the intrinsic membrane properties of their constituent neurons. As indicated by Figure 15.6, the thalamocortical circuit that mediates EEG oscillations during slow-wave sleep is composed of three types of neurons. Thalamocortical neurons, which are located in almost all thalamic nuclei, project to widespread parts of the cerebral cortex, including sensory, motor, and association areas. Thalamocortical neurons also have collateral axons that terminate in the thalamic reticular nucleus, a slender nucleus on the lateral surface of the thalamus that is composed exclusively of GABAergic neurons that project to other parts of the thalamus (see Chapter 6). In essence, the reticular nucleus provides a recurrent inhibitory circuit that suppresses activity in thalamocortical neurons. Finally, excitatory corticothalamic neurons, which are located in the deep layers of the cerebral cortex, project to both the reticular nucleus and the thalamocortical relay neurons.

The biophysical properties of the thalamocortical projection neurons play a critical role in maintaining the slow oscillations that characterize NREM sleep in stages 3 and 4. As shown in Figure 15.7, the membrane potentials of thalamocortical neurons oscillate between hyperpolarized and depolarized states during deep NREM sleep. When a thalamocortical neuron is strongly hyperpolarized by GABAergic inputs from the thalamic reticular nucleus, specific ion channels are activated that allow an inward, depolarizing flow of cations. Called hyperpolarization current (I_h) because it begins during the hyperpolarized state, the small depolarization produced by I_h leads to activation of voltage-regulated calcium (Ca^{2+}) channels and a massive influx of Ca^{2+} ions into the hyperpolarized neuron. Known as a low-threshold spike (LTS) because it is evoked by a small depolarizing current

FIG. 15.6. Thalamocortical Circuits. Slow-wave sleep activity in the EEG is mediated by interactions between neurons of the thalamus and cerebral cortex. The cerebral cortex and the thalamocortical relay nuclei have reciprocal excitatory connections and collateral projections to the reticular nucleus of the thalamus. The reticular nucleus contains GABAergic neurons that inhibit the thalamocortical relay neurons.

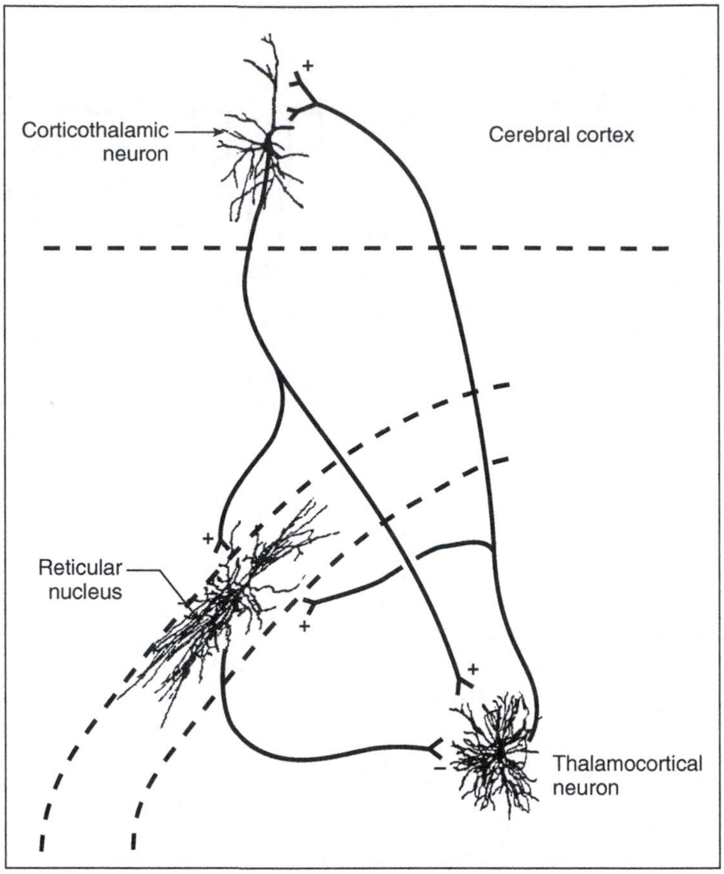

FIG. 15.7. Delta Frequency Thalamocortical Rhythms. This trace shows rhythmic changes in the membrane potentials of a thalamocortical relay neuron. Following activation of the hyperpolarization current (I_h), the low-threshold spike (LTS) is mediated by a massive influx of calcium (Ca^{2+}). The Ca^{2+}-mediated LTS is of much longer duration than the sodium (Na^+)-mediated burst of action potentials. The LTS oscillates at a frequency of 1-4 Hz because of the voltage-regulated membrane currents (I_h and Ca^{2+}) and the interactions between the thalamocortical relay neurons and the inhibitory neurons of the reticular nucleus.

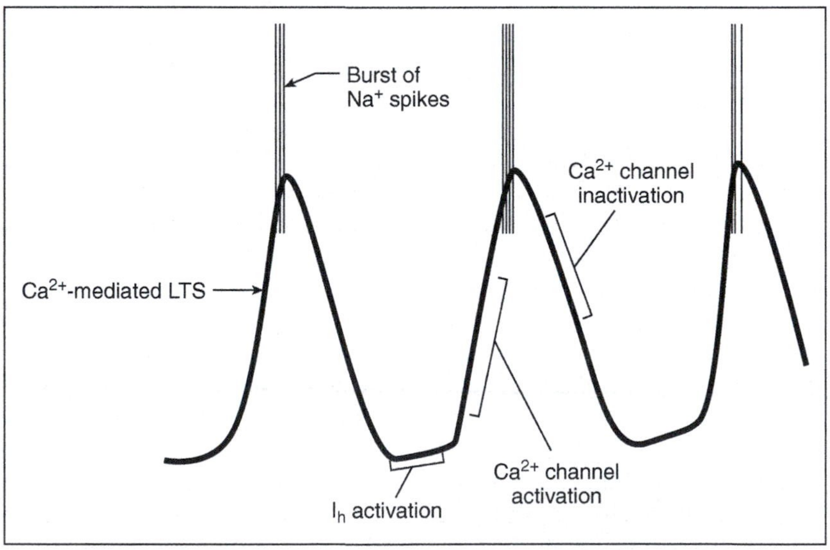

(i.e., I_h), the Ca^{2+}-mediated LTS depolarizes the membrane potential sufficiently to produce a burst of sodium (Na^+)-driven action potentials that inactivate the Ca^{2+} channels and prevent further Ca^{2+} influx.

Pacemaker neurons in the reticular nucleus control thalamocortical oscillations.

Low-threshold Ca^{2+} spikes occur at regular intervals because of the sequential interplay between thalamocortical neurons and the inhibitory neurons of the thalamic reticular nucleus. A shown by Figure 15.6, thalamocortical neurons excite the inhibitory neurons of the reticular nucleus. The GABAergic reticular nucleus neurons inhibit the thalamocortical relay neurons at the same time that their Ca^{2+} channels are inactivated. Consequently, the thalamocortical neurons become silent, and this loss of excitatory input causes the reticular neurons to become inactive. Removing the reticular-driven inhibition leads to activation of the hyperpolarization current, I_h, and this evokes another cycle of calcium influx and a low-threshold spike (see Figure 15.7). Hence, the intrinsic membrane properties of thalamocortical neurons, along with their reciprocal interactions with the reticular nucleus, produce the slow (0.5-4 Hz) delta rhythms that are observed during stage 4 of NREM sleep.

Slow-frequency delta oscillations can also occur during wakefulness, but only if parts of the cerebral cortex are damaged. Following trauma to the head, EEG recordings are sometimes used to determine whether neural activity is normal in all parts of the cerebral cortex. Head trauma may produce delta wave rhythms at a few recording sites in an awake patient even though the EEG patterns at other sites have desynchronized activity. The delta rhythms represent slow oscillations between the thalamus and those cortical areas that are partially surrounded by regional damage. These delta rhythms may emerge during wakefulness if the cortical damage prevents some of the lateral interactions that would normally contribute to desynchronized activity. Hence, the selective loss of lateral cortical interactions allows ascending thalamocortical inputs to dominate the cortical activity that borders the damaged region.

Delta waves are also produced by pharmacologic agents that promote GABAergic transmission. Benzodiazepines, for example, are often prescribed to treat insomnia because they induce sleep by enhancing GABAergic inhibition in the thalamus and other brain regions. By augmenting the inhibitory interactions between the reticular nucleus and the thalamocortical neurons, benzodiazepines induce thalamic oscillations that are transmitted to the cerebral cortex via the thalamocortical pathways.

Benzodiazepines induce sleep by enhancing GABAergic transmission in the thalamus.

Ascending Brainstem Pathways and Cortical Desynchronization. Cortical desynchronization during REM sleep is mediated by increased activity in a set of ascending pathways that originate in the brainstem near the pons-midbrain junction. The first suggestion that such pathways might desynchronize cortical activity was provided by the work of Moruzzi and Magoun in 1949. Using anesthetized cats, they showed that electrical stimulation of the reticular formation shifts the EEG from slow-wave activity to high-frequency desynchronized activity. Furthermore, destruction of the ascending pathways from the rostral reticular formation produced behavioral stupor that was accompanied by low-frequency EEG waves in the delta range. These results led Moruzzi and Magoun to propose that ascending excitatory projections from the brainstem reticular formation system must mediate the desynchronized activity observed in the forebrain during wakefulness.

A large body of evidence indicates that cortical desynchronization and other aspects of REM sleep are controlled by projections from the brainstem (Figure 15.8). For example, cortical desynchronization is initiated by ascending projections from the pedunculopontine tegmental (PPT) and laterodorsal tegmental (LDT) nuclei, both of which are cholinergic and project to the thalamus and the nucleus basalis. The PPT and LDT also send cholinergic projections to the medial part of the pontine reticular formation (mPRF), which projects to the thalamus and uses excitatory amino acid neurotransmitters to depolarize thalamocortical neurons. In addition to these ascending projections, descending projections from the pontomedullary reticular formation inhibit the motor neurons in the spinal cord and prevent the skeletal muscles from contracting during REM sleep.

Involvement of the cholinergic LDT and PPT nuclei in REM sleep is supported by many experimental findings. The onset of REM sleep is immediately preceded by increased activity in the LDT and the PPT, and lesions of these nuclei reduce REM sleep. Furthermore, direct application of cholinergic agonists into the mPRF produces cortical desynchronization and other signs of REM-like sleep (see Figure 15.4). These facts corroborate evidence showing that mPRF neurons are excited by acetylcholine and discharge more frequently during REM sleep. Hence, the shift from EEG synchronization to desynchronization during REM sleep is mediated by prolonged thalamic depolarization triggered by activation of ascending projections from the mPRF. Direct cholinergic projections from the LDT and PPT nuclei to the thalamus may also contribute to EEG desynchronization, but their primary role is to initiate REM sleep by ascending projections

The LDT and PPT nuclei contain "REM-on" neurons; the mPRF contains "effector" neurons.

FIG. 15.8. Brainstem Regulation of REM Sleep. Sagittal diagram of the brain showing the cholinergic laterodorsal tegmental (LDT) and pedunculopontine tegmental (PPT) nuclei, both of which project to the medial pontine reticular formation (mPRF). Together the LDT/PPT and mPRF activate the thalamus and the nucleus basalis in the forebrain. In turn, the thalamus and nucleus basalis send widespread excitatory projections to the cerebral cortex. Additional nuclei in the pons and medulla send descending projections to the brainstem that inhibit the motor neurons in the anterior horn, thereby producing muscle atonia during REM sleep.

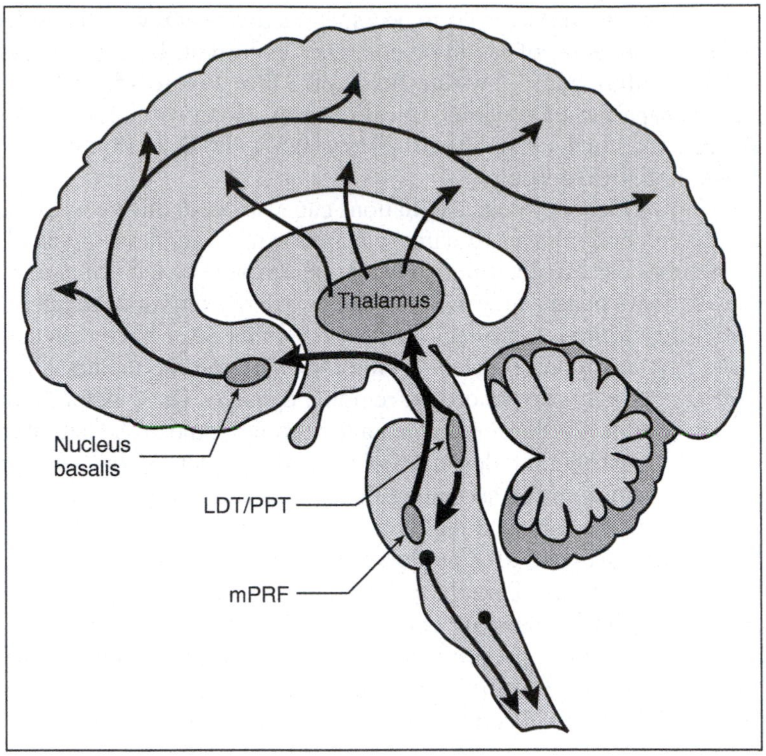

from the mPRF. Consistent with this mechanism, neurons in the LDT/PPT nuclei serve as "REM-on" neurons, whereas those in the mPRF are considered "effector" neurons for REM sleep.

The locus ceruleus and the dorsal raphe nucleus contain "REM-off" neurons.

The periodic nature of REM sleep is controlled by brainstem nuclei that inhibit the REM-on neurons of the PPT and LDT nuclei. Physiology studies have shown that noradrenergic neurons in the locus ceruleus and serotonergic neurons in the raphe nuclei are virtually silent during REM sleep but become increasingly active just before the end of each REM sleep episode. Furthermore, direct infusion of serotonin inhibits neuronal activity in the LDT/PPT nuclei. These findings suggest that serotonergic and noradrenergic neurons in the brainstem act as "REM-off" neurons. According to many neurophysiologists, the pattern of periodic changes in the activity of REM-on and REM-off neurons suggests that reciprocal connections between these groups of neurons may control the duration of NREM and REM sleep periods (Figure 15.9).

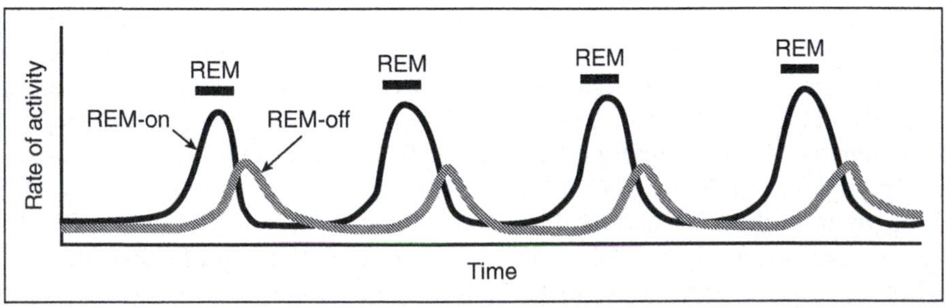

FIG. 15.9. Relative Activity of REM-on and REM-off Neurons. The REM-on cholinergic neurons of the laterodorsal tegmental (LDT) and pedunculopontine tegmental (PPT) nuclei show periodic changes that control the onset and duration of REM sleep. The end of the REM sleep period coincides with increasing activity of REM-off noradrenergic neurons in the locus ceruleus and REM-off serotonergic neurons in the dorsal raphe nucleus.

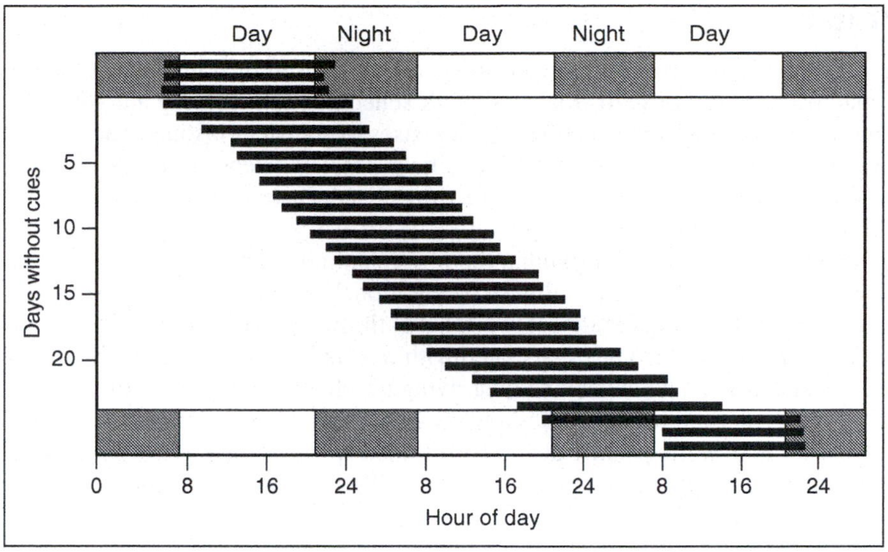

FIG. 15.10. Circadian Rhythms. When cues about the time of day are removed, human subjects maintain a regular cycle of waking and sleeping, but each cycle lengthens to 25 or 26 hours. The circadian pattern returns to a normal 24-hour cycle when time cues are reinstated. Horizontal bars represent waking hours.

Circadian Rhythms

In humans and most other vertebrates, sleep and other behavioral activities follow a circadian pattern. Although these behaviors are strongly influenced by alternating cycles of day and night, the brain has intrinsic mechanisms for maintaining circadian rhythms. When human subjects are placed in environments without clocks, windows, or other cues that indicate the time of day, they continue to sleep at regular intervals that follow a relatively normal circadian rhythm (Figure 15.10). In the absence of external temporal cues, however, the sleep-wake cycle usually lengthens to 25 or 26 hours. Based on this evidence, humans appear to have an internal clock that is reset each day and can be adjusted by seasonal changes in the onset and duration of daylight.

Circadian rhythms are controlled by the suprachiasmatic nucleus of the hypothalamus. Located above the optic chiasm, the suprachiasmatic nucleus receives direct collateral projections from fibers in the optic nerve that convey information about the onset, intensity, and duration of daylight. In turn, the suprachiasmatic nucleus projects to the pontine tegmentum and other brainstem areas that control the different stages of sleep.

The **suprachiasmatic nucleus** is a biologic clock that paces **circadian rhythms.**

The role of the suprachiasmatic nucleus as a biologic clock is indicated by animal studies showing that circadian rhythms are severely disrupted when this structure is damaged. Although the total amount of REM and NREM sleep is unaffected following removal of the suprachiasmatic nucleus, these sleep periods occur randomly and are not linked to nocturnal intervals. Suprachiasmatic nucleus control of the circadian rhythm appears to involve cyclic changes in hormonal activity. After removing the suprachiasmatic nucleus, circadian rhythms are lost but can be reestablished by transplanting a suprachiasmatic nucleus from another animal. Given that synaptic connections between the donor and host tissues are not present, hormone diffusion from the transplanted tissue must account for the immediate recovery of the circadian rhythm.

SLEEP DISORDERS

More than 50 specific types of sleep disorders have been identified, and each one can be classified into one of the following categories: (1) insomnias, (2) hypersomnias, (3) parasomnias, and (4) rhythm disruptions. The insomnias involve problems with initiating and maintaining sleep, whereas hypersomnias are characterized by excessive sleep or drowsiness. The parasomnias encompass a broad set of undesirable sleep-related behaviors such as sleepwalking and nocturnal enuresis (bed-wetting). Rhythm disruptions involve changes in circadian rhythm such as those caused by changing time zones (i.e., jet lag). Some of the more common sleep disorders are described in the following sections.

Insomnia

Insomnia, or an inability to obtain adequate sleep, can be caused by a number of factors. Insomnia may occur in response to an altered work schedule (i.e., working a night shift), stress, or merely drinking too much coffee. Other cases of transient insomnia are caused by the emotional upheaval associated with a specific event. Persistent insomnia may have many underlying causes including chronic pain, drug abuse, gastroesophageal reflux, respiratory difficulty, or psychiatric illness.

When a patient complains of insomnia, the physician must determine whether sleep disruption is symptomatic of another illness or emotional problem. It is estimated that emotional disturbances account for almost two-third of the insomnias. Chronic anxiety and depression, for example, are strongly associated with insomnia and can exacerbate the inability to sleep, and this can potentiate the underlying psychopathology. Polysomnograms from depressed patients indicate that they obtain less slow-wave sleep and enter REM sleep much earlier than normal individuals. Unfortunately, many depressed patients are not properly diagnosed and are prescribed sleeping pills instead of antidepressants (see Chapter 17).

> The EEG of an insomniac patient rarely shows any striking abnormality.

Many insomniacs are awakened by events that they cannot identify. The most common cause is periodic limb movement disorder (PLMD), which is characterized by jerking leg movements that occur during NREM sleep. These leg movements, which consist of a triple flexion involving the ankle, knee, and hip, last only 2–3 seconds and occur periodically for several minutes. In contrast to movement disorders that are inhibited by sleep (e.g., extrapyramidal tremors, chorea), the leg jerks associated with PLMD are present during sleep. Patients with PLMD are unaware of these leg movements because they are sleeping, but eventually the leg movements cause them to be awakened. Hence, proper diagnosis of PLMD requires that their sleep behavior be evaluated by polysomnography. Insomnia produced by periodic leg movements is usually treated with clonazepam, a benzodiazepine with sedative effects.

Unfortunately, many patients complaining of chronic insomnia show no irregularities in their polysomnograms. Compared to the amount of delta activity recorded in their EEGs, most insomniacs underestimate the amount of sleep that they obtain. In fact, when insomniacs are awakened from a deep sleep (as indicated by the presence of delta waves in the EEG), many of these patients claim that they were not sleeping but were lying awake when the experimenter aroused them. Hence, insomniacs may sleep as much as a normal person, but do not experience the same quality of sleep. Some studies, however, indicate that insomniacs experience more intermittent awakenings than normal. This view is consistent with evidence suggesting that benzodiazepines are effective hypnotics because they reduce the number of awakenings in the course of a night's sleep.

Restless Legs Syndrome

> In RLS, the loss of sleep is secondary to unpleasant somatic sensations that generate voluntary leg movements.

Restless legs syndrome (RLS) is characterized by unpleasant paresthetic sensations (e.g., burning, tingling, or the feeling of crawling insects) in one or both legs. The intensity of the sensations may vary from uncomfortable to painful, and patients report an uncontrollable urge to move their legs to obtain relief. These sensations increase when the patient lies down or tries to relax. Consequently, patients with RLS have constant leg movements during the day and have difficulty falling asleep and staying asleep during the evening. About 80% of patients with RLS also develop PLMD (see "Insomnia"); in contrast to RLS, which is characterized by voluntary movements, the sudden jerky leg movements associated with PLMD are involuntary.

The cause of RLS is not known. A family history for RLS is present in about 50% of cases, which suggests a genetic basis for some forms of the disorder. Persons with low iron levels or anemia have a higher incidence of RLS and show noticeable improvement when the low iron levels or anemia are corrected. In many cases, RLS is associated with certain lifestyle factors, and altering these conditions can reduce symptoms. For example, mild cases of RLS can often be managed by avoiding caffeine, alcohol, and tobacco. In addition, RLS symptoms can be reduced by massage, regular exercise, and hot baths or heating pads. In more severe cases of RLS, physicians prescribe medications to alleviate the symptoms. Dopaminergic agents are usually tried first, but benzodiazepines, opioids, and anticonvulsants have also been used.

Sleep Apnea

Apnea is a temporary cessation in breathing.

Sleep apnea is characterized by a sleeping individual who ceases to breathe for periods of 15–30 seconds. Due to the lack of air intake, blood oxygen levels fall and carbon dioxide levels rise significantly. The extreme change in the concentration of these blood gases stimulates the respiratory centers in the brainstem, which causes the individual to make several loud, gasping snores immediately before they awaken. This increase in air intake returns the blood gases to normal levels and allows the person to resume sleeping until the cycle is repeated. Because of the constant shifting between periods of sleep and arousal, the individual is unrefreshed upon awakening and feels a pervasive sleepiness throughout the day.

Sleep apnea is usually associated with loud, periodic snoring. A series of three to six loud snores or gasps followed by a silent period of 20–50 seconds is repeated throughout the night. This pattern characterizes the obstructive sleep apnea (OSA) syndrome in which the airway collapses and airflow ceases despite persistent respiratory effort. Abnormalities such as narrow nasal passages, a deviated nasal septum, enlarged adenoids or tonsils, an enlarged tongue, or temporomandibular joint problems may cause OSA. This syndrome occurs more frequently among men than women, and it is most common among overweight adults between 40 and 60 years of age. Approximately two-thirds of the patients diagnosed with OSA are obese, and their symptoms are exacerbated by alcohol consumption or sleep deprivation.

Sleep apnea is associated with an increased risk of sudden death during sleep. Sleep apnea may occur in infants and has been proposed as a factor in sudden infant death syndrome (SIDS). The incidence of sleep apnea among the elderly is high, perhaps 30% among persons greater than 65 years of age. Sleep apnea is more common in adults who have chronic obstructive pulmonary disease and systemic hypertension, and it is associated with a variety of cardiac arrhythmias that occur during sleep.

A polysomnogram is necessary to diagnose sleep apnea and to determine whether it is obstructive or central in origin. Obstructive apnea is characterized by respiratory effort in the absence of airflow caused by a blocked airway. Central apnea is due to a lack of respiratory effort, presumably because the brainstem respiratory centers are inhibited; the airway remains open, but there is no airflow because the diaphragm does not contract. The distinction between central and obstructive apnea can be determined by monitoring respiratory movements. Some individuals have a mixed apnea involving both central and obstructive components.

Narcolepsy

Narcolepsy represents the intrusion of REM sleep into the waking state.

Cataplexy involves the complete loss of muscle tone without affecting consciousness.

Narcolepsy is a neurologic disorder characterized by drowsiness and sudden sleep attacks that occur at inappropriate moments during the day. These attacks last 5–30 minutes and may strike without warning while the patient is eating, speaking, or even driving. Thus, narcolepsy poses a serious health risk because these patients are prone to accidental injury while operating a car or other types of machinery.

The first sign of narcolepsy is excessive sleepiness, which typically emerges between 15 and 30 years of age. Patients with narcolepsy need to sleep more frequently than normal individuals; the narcoleptic sleep attack is essentially a minisleep that intrudes into the waking state. In addition to sleep attacks, narcoleptic patients also exhibit cataplexy, but this symptom may have a delayed onset of several months or years. Cataplexy is precipitated by strong emotional behaviors (e.g., laughing or crying) and consists of an abrupt loss of muscle tone without a change in consciousness. During a cataplexic episode, the patient's head falls forward, the arms drop, and the knees buckle because all of the muscles except those needed for respiration are completely paralyzed.

Many of the behavioral symptoms of narcolepsy are similar to those of REM sleep. Thus, narcoleptic patients exhibit sleep paralysis, a global paralysis of voluntary muscles during the entry into sleep or on awakening from sleep. During these periods, narcoleptic patients experience both auditory and visual hallucinations. Collectively, the presence of cataplexy, sleep paralysis, and sensory hallucinations resemble the muscle atonia and dream state that normal individuals experience during REM sleep. The possibility that narcolepsy might represent the intrusion of REM sleep into the waking state is strongly suggested by polysomnographic recordings showing that narcoleptic patients enter the REM sleep state almost directly from the waking state. For diagnostic purposes, the presence of a sleep-onset REM period is considered the hallmark of narcolepsy.

The neural mechanisms underlying narcolepsy are unknown. Damage to the upper brainstem or ventral hypothalamus has sometimes produced narcoleptic symptoms, but the neuropathologic findings in narcoleptic patients have been inconsistent. Narcolepsy has a genetic basis that is associated with inheritance of a class II antigen of the major histocompatibility complex on chromosome 6. The major histocompatibility complex is a cluster of genes that encode the molecules in the immune system responsible for recognizing antigens. Several pairs of monozygotic twins have been identified that are discordant for this disease, however, which suggests that environmental factors may also play a role.

Despite a lack of knowledge concerning the neural basis of narcolepsy, cataplexy can be controlled by medications that enhance synaptic transmission of the putative REM-off neurons. Tricyclic antidepressants, which block the reuptake of norepinephrine and serotonin, prevent cataplexy but have little effect on sleep attacks. Instead, excessive sleepiness is treated by psychomotor stimulants (e.g., methylphenidate, amphetamine) that elevate alertness by increasing the synaptic release of catecholamines. Prolonged use of stimulants has serious side effects, however, so their use should be minimized by scheduling daytime naps at appropriate times.

INTRAOPERATIVE AWARENESS

Intraoperative awareness refers to instances in which patients awaken from general anesthesia during surgery but are unable to inform the surgeon of their conscious state. In the United States, the incidence of intraoperative awareness is at least 1 in every 1000 surgeries that are performed under general anesthesia. In these cases, surgical patients are usually helpless because they are paralyzed and are being ventilated. Consequently, they cannot speak or make any movement that would alert the surgeon to their conscious state. More importantly, inadequate anesthesia means that these patients can perceive pain. As one might expect, intraoperative awareness is a terrifying experience that has serious emotional and psychological repercussions. In fact, most patients who experience intraoperative awareness develop post-traumatic stress disorder and require psychological counseling.

Intraoperative awareness occurs when the anesthetic is inadvertently discontinued or the anesthetic dosage is not sufficient to maintain the patient in an unconscious state. The incidence of intraoperative awareness varies with surgical procedures and is highest for trauma, cardiac, and emergency obstetrical surgeries. Furthermore, patients with certain pulmonary or cardiovascular diseases have an increased risk for intraoperative awareness. Finally, patients with a history of chronic exposure to alcohol, benzodiazepines, opioids, or related drugs are less sensitive to anesthesia and require greater amounts of anesthesia to be maintained in an unconscious state.

Anesthesiologists and medical organizations are adopting measures to reduce the incidence of intraoperative awareness. Stricter regulations on the use and maintenance of anesthesia monitors, vaporizers, and infusion pumps have reduced the incidence of intraoperative awareness to its present level (1 in 1000). Many institutions, but not all, have begun using EEG recordings to monitor the patient's cortical activity before, during, and upon recovery from general anesthesia. Because raw EEG waveforms are difficult to interpret on a moment-to-moment basis, most institutions that use EEG recording during surgery rely on pattern recognition software to measure multiple features of the EEG record and to generate a single number, the bispectral index, that indicates the likelihood that the patient is conscious.

COMA AND BRAIN DEATH

The loss of consciousness that accompanies sleep is a normal and self-regulating process. In instances such as fainting, loss of consciousness may represent a temporary reduction in cerebral blood flow that can be easily treated (see Chapter 13). In almost all other cases, however, loss of consciousness is a serious condition produced by brain damage, drug overdose, hypothermia, or certain types of toxic-metabolic disorders. The comatose patient represents the ultimate challenge to the capabilities of the attending neurologist.

Neural Basis of Consciousness

Patients who are awake and aware of their surroundings are said to be conscious. This implies that the person has the capacity to perceive, learn, and engage in purposeful behavior. Because the conscious state is inherently introspective and, therefore, not easily accessible to scientific study, the biologic basis of consciousness is uncertain. Nonetheless, extensive study of patients with brain damage indicates that human consciousness depends on interactions between three distinct systems in the brain (Figure 15.11). Cognitive functions, such as perception, memory, language, and the capacity to plan and execute motor behaviors, are mediated by the cerebral cortex, basal ganglia, and the sensory-specific nuclei of the thalamus. The mechanisms for regulating attention, motivation, and emotional behavior reside in the hypothalamus, basal forebrain, hippocampus, amygdala, cingulum, and septal nuclei. Activation and arousal of both the cognitive and limbic systems are mediated by a third neural system comprised of the ascending projections from the reticular formation, the intralaminar nuclei of the thalamus, and the posterior hypothalamus.

The division of consciousness into distinct functional systems suggests that consciousness has both qualitative and quantitative dimensions. Although certain structures within these systems may have specific neurologic functions, they are widely distributed throughout the neuraxis, and the functional boundaries between them are imprecise. Thus, even focal damage may affect more than one of these systems. Regardless of whether consciousness is affected by global or focal abnormalities, its character can change either partially or completely.

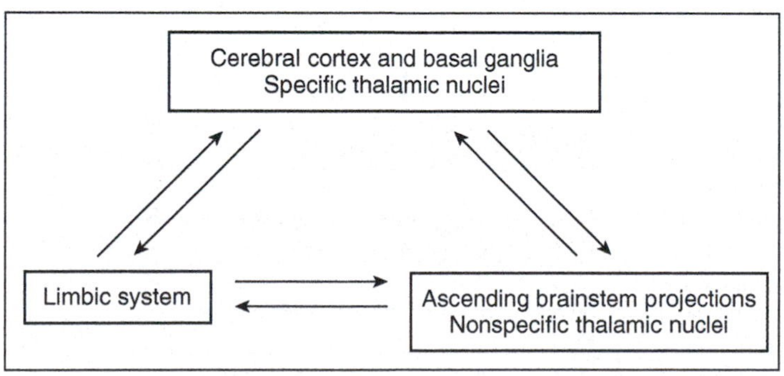

FIG. 15.11. Neural Substrate Underlying Consciousness. Consciousness is an emergent property that depends on complex interactions between distinct systems within the brain. High-level cognitive functions (e.g., perception, awareness) are derived from processes in the telencephalon and the sensory-specific pathways of the thalamus. Affect, mood, attention, and motivation depend on structures in the limbic system. Rostral projections from the brainstem and the nonspecific nuclei of the thalamus arouse the telencephalic and limbic structures.

Comatose States and Other Global Impairments in Consciousness

An isoelectric or flat EEG trace usually indicates brain death.

The terms "coma" and "comatose" are used to describe a state in which a patient cannot be aroused by internal or external stimuli. In contrast to concussion or syncope, a coma persists for a minimum of one hour. Comatose patients have no awareness of themselves or their environment. The EEG shows abnormal patterns and, if the coma deepens, the electrical activity of the EEG gradually decreases and may disappear. With the exception of patients who are deeply anesthetized or suffering from severe hypothermia, the loss of EEG activity indicates brain death.

Most comatose patients that survive gradually become arousable within one month of the precipitating event, but this recovery might progress no further than a vegetative or minimally conscious state. In fact, more than 15,000 patients in the United States are in a vegetative state and another 100,000 patients are classified as being minimally conscious. Alternatively, recovery from the comatose state may progress more completely to a normal conscious state, but this is unpredictable and may require several prolonged stages of physiological improvement.

Vegetative State. Patients in a vegetative state have not regained conscious awareness, but their EEG contains rhythmic activity resembling sleep-wake cycles. In addition, they may open their eyes spontaneously and might not require ventilation because the brainstem circuits that mediate these functions are still intact. Hence, patients in a vegetative state are described as being awake, but they are not conscious of themselves or their surroundings. Structural brain damage is often present in these individuals as revealed by computerized tomography (CT) or magnetic resonance imaging (MRI). The vegetative state is considered permanent and irreversible if it persists more than 3 months after nontraumatic brain damage (e.g., in response to hypoxia) or more than 12 months after a traumatic brain injury. In the permanent vegetative state, the patient has suffered "cognitive death" because only the neural mechanisms that subserve autonomic functions remain intact.

Minimally Conscious State. Within the last decade, the term "minimally conscious" has been used to describe patients who have greatly diminished consciousness but are not in a vegetative state (Figure 15.12). To fit this description, patients must show some limited awareness of themselves or their environment. This usually consists of following simple commands that extend beyond reflexive behaviors. For example, most minimally conscious patients exhibit purposeful eye movements that pursue or fixate on stimuli consistently. These patients may also respond to threatening gestures or have some

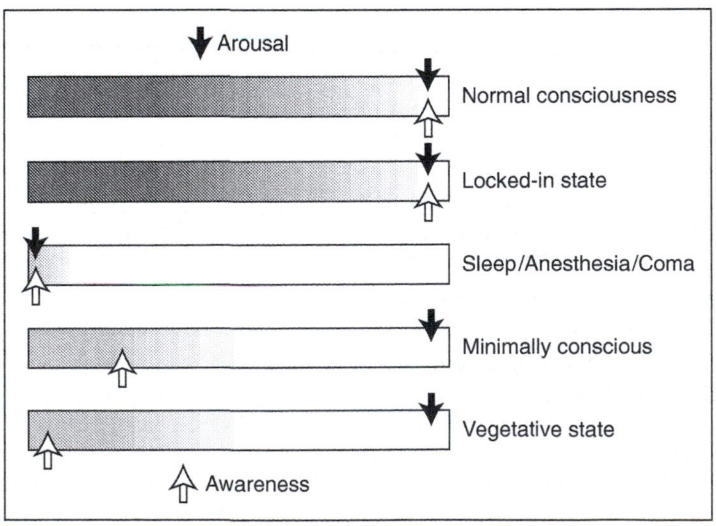

FIG. 15.12. Arousal and Awareness Levels in Different States of Consciousness. Awareness of self and environment is present during normal consciousness or in the locked-in state, but it is significantly reduced in other states of consciousness. Loss of both awareness and arousal is a defining property of the comatose state. Gray gradients represent the presence of individual variations in the degree of consciousness in different states. (Adapted from Laureys S, Owen AM, Schiff ND: Brain function in coma, vegetative state, and related disorders, *Lancet Neurol* 3:537–546, 2004.)

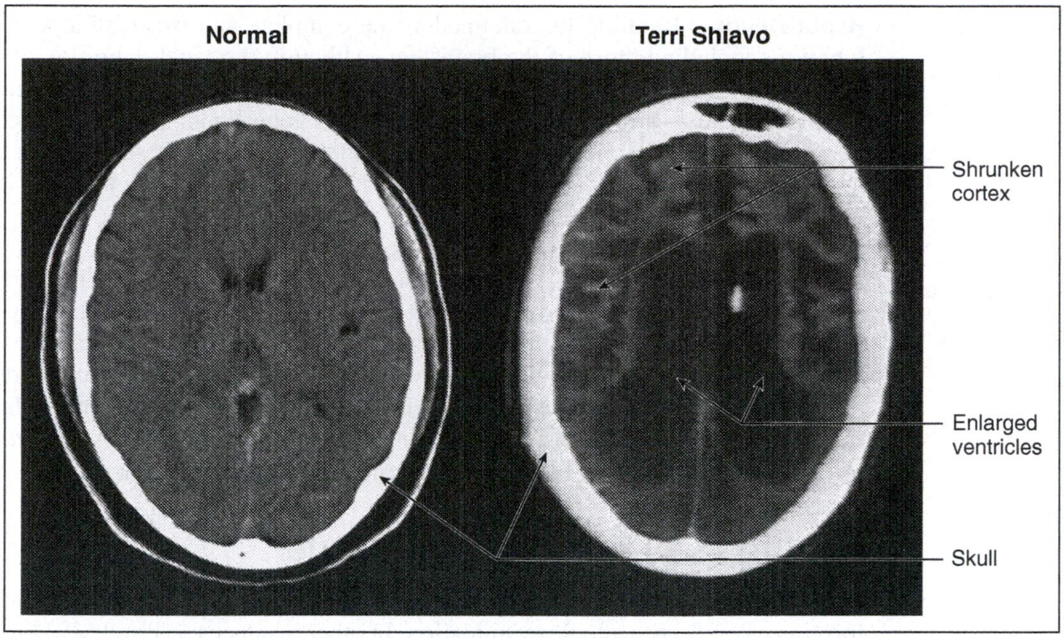

FIG. 15.13. Brain Damage in a Patient in a Permanent Vegetative State. CT scans of a normal 25-year-old (left) and the brain of Terri Schiavo (right) in 2002. The CT scan of Ms. Schiavo reveals severe atrophy and shrinkage of the cerebral cortex with greatly enlarged ventricles. (CT scans provided courtesy of the late Dr. Ronald Cranford, University of Minnesota.)

intelligible speech. While patients in a minimally conscious state are more likely to show improvement than those in a vegetative state, many patients remain in a state of minimal consciousness permanently.

The differential diagnosis of a vegetative or minimally conscious state is based on clear neurologic and behavioral criteria. However, patients in a vegetative state exhibit reflexive responses and other signs of arousal (e.g., spontaneous eye movements and EEG cycles) that are sometimes mistaken for behaviors associated with minimal consciousness. This has caused some confusion about the classification of some patients and has prompted debates about the legal and ethical treatment of patients in a permanent vegetative state. In the highly publicized case of Terri Schiavo, for example, a sustained period of anoxia led to global brain damage that was revealed by CT scans and a flat EEG (Figure 15.13). Several neurologists examined Ms. Schiavo and concluded that she never demonstrated any sign of conscious awareness and was in a permanent vegetative state, but video recordings of her spontaneous eye movements and other reflexive behaviors raised public doubt about her diagnosis and cognitive status. Because of uncertainty about which patients will recover from a state of unconsciousness, the Schiavo case raised public awareness about the issues surrounding the care of patients with severe brain damage and brought attention to our incomplete understanding of the neural mechanisms of consciousness. Current research is aimed at addressing this shortcoming by using functional MRI, positron emission tomography, and related imaging techniques to determine the location of residual brain function in patients who have severe brain damage and are in a vegetative or minimally conscious state.

Stupor. The term "stupor" is sometimes used to describe a state in which a patient must receive constant noxious stimulation, such as shouting or shaking, to remain awake. Stupor caused by structural damage to the brain is associated with many abnormal clinical signs, whereas stupor caused by a chemical poisoning resembles a state of deep sleep. The EEG pattern is abnormal in patients with stupor and can easily be distinguished from the EEG patterns that represent normal sleep.

Brain Death. Brain death is defined as the complete and irreversible loss of all brain functions including those of the brainstem. Although the legal definition of brain death varies among different countries, brain death is indicated clinically by the loss of all brainstem reflexes and the presence of continuous apnea in an individual who is in a state of persistent coma. Hypothermia, neuromuscular blockade, and severe drug intoxication must always be ruled out. When required by law, a brain dead individual exhibits a flat or isoelectric EEG record at all tested sites.

Patients who are conscious, but completely paralyzed, are in a **"locked-in state."**

Locked-In State. Patients with bilateral disruption of the corticospinal and corticobulbar tracts are paralyzed but can have full conscious awareness. Such patients are said to be "locked-in" because they cannot move and cannot easily communicate with others. The locked-in state can be caused by trauma as well as by severe postinfectious polyneuritis of the descending motor pathways. Lesions that spare consciousness almost always spare the oculomotor pathways originating from the midbrain. Thus, locked-in patients can communicate only by blinking or making selected eye movements.

Diagnosis of the Comatose State

Some cases of coma are quickly diagnosed after obtaining an accurate history and performing a careful neurologic examination. In other instances, CT and MRI brain scans are necessary to determine the location of brain damage, and an EEG is indispensable for discerning coma from epilepsy or other conditions caused by infectious or metabolic disorders. Coma is sometimes difficult to distinguish from severe hysteria, depression, or drug overdose, and this requires that the physician exclude drug use or other possible causes. On rare occasions, coma is considered erroneously in cases in which the patient is in the locked-in state.

Coma can be distinguished from deep sleep on the basis of several criteria (Table 15.2). Whereas a person in a deep sleep can be aroused by vigorous and sustained external stimulation, this is not the case with a comatose individual. A comatose person does not exhibit REM activity, circadian rhythms, or any periodic changes that characterize normal sleep. Finally, normal sleep is an active process associated with fluctuations in the metabolic activity of the brain. In the comatose state, however, cerebral metabolism falls significantly below the levels observed during deep slow-wave sleep (Figure 15.14).

SEPs and BAEPs are used to evaluate comatose patients.

The measurement of somatosensory and auditory ERPs is useful for evaluating comatose patients. Somatosensory-evoked potentials (SEPs) are induced by electrically stimulating the median or peroneal nerves. Electrodes placed over the spinal column, the brainstem, and the scalp reveal the presence of distinct waves or potentials that correspond to the sequential activation of the spinal cord, thalamus, and cerebral cortex. Auditory stimuli produce a similar series of waves known as brainstem auditory-evoked potentials (BAEPs), which represent sequential waves of activity from the auditory nerve (wave I) to the cochlear nuclei (wave II), the superior olives (wave III), the lateral lemnisci (wave IV), and finally the inferior colliculi (wave V) (see Chapter 8). The latency

TABLE 15.2 Differences between Coma and Sleep

	Coma	Sleep
Behavior	Not arousable	Arousable to wakefulness
Movements	Reflex responses	Spontaneous turning, eye movements
EEG activity	REM activity absent	Periodic REM and NREM
Evoked potentials	Abnormal BAEPs	Normal BAEPs and SEPs
Cortical metabolism	Declines 50%–60%	Fluctuates with REM and NREM

Note. EEG = electroencephalogram; REM = rapid eye movement; BAEPs = brainstem auditory-evoked potentials; SEPs = somatosensory-evoked potentials.

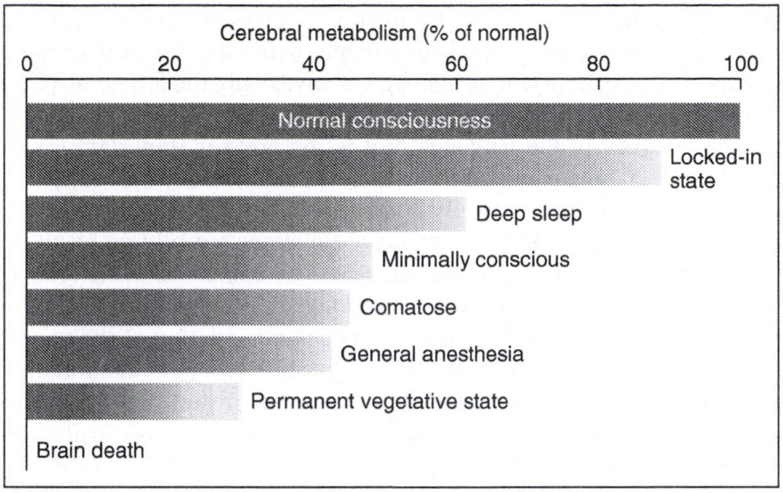

FIG. 15.14. Cerebral Metabolism in Different States of Consciousness. The rate of cerebral metabolism is depressed in unconscious patients. Gray gradients indicate the presence of individual variation in metabolism for different states. (Adapted from Laureys S, Owen AM, Schiff ND: Brain function in coma, vegetative state, and related disorders, *Lancet Neurol* 3:537–546, 2004.)

and size of the SEPs and BAEPs help determine the brain regions that are functionally intact and those that are damaged. Because SEPs and BAEPs are resistant to anesthetics, they retain relatively normal waveforms even at drug doses that cause an isoelectric or flat EEG. Changes in the latency of SEPs, in particular, have value in predicting the outcome of coma. Comatose patients that lose cortical SEPs have never survived; bilateral disappearance of the SEPs usually precedes brain death by as much as 24 hours. By comparison, individuals who have normal bilateral SEPs shortly after injury or asphyxia have a 90% chance of regaining consciousness.

Principal Causes of Coma

The causes of coma can be divided into two major categories: structural lesions and toxic-metabolic disorders (Table 15.3).

Structural Lesions Associated with Coma. Coma may result from destruction or compression of critical areas in the brainstem-diencephalic arousal system caused by trauma, hemorrhage, or neoplasms. In addition, the brainstem-diencephalic system can also be affected indirectly by the gradual enlargement of an intracranial mass or tumor that is located some distance away (see Chapter 3). Both types of structural lesions are classified with respect to the tentorium, the dural sheet located between the occipital lobe and the cerebellum.

TABLE 15.3 Coma Classifications and Their Causes

Type of Coma	Neural Structures Affected	Causes
Structural-supratentorial	Bilateral cortex and thalamus	Large infarcts, tumors, hemorrhages, neoplasms, brain herniation through tentorial notch
Structural-infratentorial	Midbrain-pontine junction	Infarcts, hemorrhages, neoplasms, trauma, uncal herniation
Toxic or metabolic	Global and diffuse	Drugs, poisons, anoxia, hypoglycemia, hepatic or renal failure, encephalitis

Supratentorial lesions produce coma by compressing the brainstem.

Supratentorial Lesions. Coma is not frequently produced by cortical lesions unless the damage is both extensive and bilateral. In patients with large cortical wounds, the incidence of coma is nearly 30% when the damage involves only the left hemisphere, but only 10% when the damage is restricted to the right hemisphere. These differential findings suggest that the integrity of the language processing areas is important for maintaining global consciousness. Coma is more likely with cortical hemorrhage because it is accompanied by massive cerebral swelling. By comparison, cortical lesions caused by embolic strokes may affect sensory, motor, and language functions but seldom result in coma.

Supratentorial lesions often affect consciousness by compressing the brain through the tentorial notch. Progressive enlargement of a tumor or other intracranial mass increases the downward pressure on the brainstem, which causes herniation of the medial temporal lobe (uncal herniation) and protrusion of the medulla through the foramen magnum (see Figure 5.32). Uncal herniation invariably affects the rostral brainstem, including the oculomotor nerve, and this loss of parasympathetic influence produces ipsilateral mydriasis (pupillary dilation). Eventually, compression of the rostral brainstem damages the ascending pathways that regulate consciousness. If the supratentorial lesion is unilateral, differential compression of the descending corticospinal tracts may cause asymmetrical limb movements and deep tendon reflexes. Continued downward pressure on the caudal brainstem and its intrinsic nuclei leads to abnormal respiratory patterns including Cheyne-Stokes breathing (rhythmic waxing and waning in the depth of respiration), hyperventilation, and apnea.

Most infratentorial lesions produce coma by damaging the pontine and mesencephalic tegmentum.

Infratentorial Lesions. Substantial data support the concept of a distributed nonspecific arousal system that originates from the central paramedian region of the lower thalamus, mesencephalon, and rostral pons. In most cases where coma is produced by an infratentorial lesion, noninvasive imaging techniques indicate widespread damage to the central tegmental area of the midbrain that usually extends into the thalamus, pons, or both regions. Damage restricted to only one segment of the neuraxis (i.e., the pons or the midbrain) rarely produces coma. Moreover, infratentorial lesions that produce coma frequently spare the ascending sensory pathways and their relay nuclei in the brainstem. Thus, coma does not result merely from the loss of ascending sensory influences on the diencephalon.

Vascular lesions resulting in coma are more likely to involve both the thalamus and mesencephalon. Such lesions are especially likely following occlusion of the perforating vessels arising from the basilar artery, the posterior cerebral arteries, and the posterior communicating arteries. Damage to the posterior thalamus alone may cause severe coma if the lesion is bilateral and involves the paramedian thalamus and related areas such as the posterior intralaminar nuclei, the central median nuclei, and the medial dorsal nuclei.

Patients who survive extensive damage to the rostral brainstem may persist in a coma for a prolonged period. These patients eventually regain cyclic patterns of arousal and nonarousal in their EEG activity that is characteristic of a vegetative state; this pattern does not follow the cyclic activity between NREM and REM that is observed in normal sleep. Patients who sustain severe damage to the pontine-mesencephalic junction may exhibit desynchronized EEG activity in the alpha range that is called "alpha coma." In these patients, however, attempts to link particular EEG patterns to the integrity of specific neural structures have been disappointing. Although some patients may show EEG synchronization, which suggests the activation of neural structures involved in sleep, most neurologists regard coma as a pathologic process that disrupts the neural mechanisms controlling the sleep-wake cycle.

Virtually no individual has survived extensive damage to the caudal brainstem. Because the medulla and lower pons regulate respiration and cardiovascular functions, damage to this region usually causes immediate death. In rare cases in which the patients are ventilated and do not die immediately, they are usually paralyzed due to loss of the descending pyramidal tracts. These patients do not descend into a comatose state; they remain conscious because of damage to areas in the caudal brainstem that must become active to induce sleep. Until death ensues, these patients are in a "locked-in state" and can communicate only by making a series of coded eye movements.

Toxic-Metabolic Disorders. Coma can be produced by many conditions that cause global neural depression. Metabolic coma usually has a gradual onset and can be caused by brain anoxia, ischemia, hypoglycemia, or exposure to a variety of drugs and poisons. The most common symptoms that precede metabolic coma include tremor, loss of postural control, and myoclonic limb movements (non-rhythmic jerks). Ocular movements are rarely affected unless the coma is severe.

RESOLUTION OF CLINICAL CASE

A polysomnogram revealed that the patient's excessive sleepiness was caused by OSA. Despite making respiratory movements, the patient periodically ceased breathing during sleep because his airway became obstructed, possibly due to his enlarged adenoids and tonsils. Although surgical removal of the adenoids and tonsils might cure his problem, a more conservative approach would be to prescribe a weight-loss program in combination with continuous positive pressure of the nasal passages. Among obese patients who have moderate cases of OSA, weight loss alone is often successful. In more severe cases, an increase in nasal air pressure is the most effective treatment for managing OSA. Such patients wear a tight-fitting mask that delivers pressurized air to keep the airways expanded between breaths.

REVIEW QUESTIONS

Directions: For each of the following questions, choose the **one best** answer.

1. What signs characterize deep NREM sleep?
A. PGO spikes
B. K spike complexes
C. Muscle atonia
D. Increased cerebral metabolism
E. EEG waves in the delta frequency range

2. What brain region initiates REM sleep?
A. Pedunculopontine and laterodorsal tegmental nuclei
B. Medial pontine reticular formation
C. Suprachiasmatic nucleus
D. Dorsal raphe nuclei
E. Locus ceruleus

3. Severe coma results from damage to which of the following brain regions?
A. Medulla
B. Basal ganglia
C. Anterior thalamus
D. Right cerebral hemisphere
E. Pontine-mesencephalic junction

4. Which of the following conditions is most likely to cause coma?
A. Cerebral infarction
B. Uncal herniation after a subdural hematoma
C. Occlusion of the medial striate artery
D. Contusion of the cerebellum
E. Transient ischemic attack

5. Which of the following is a general characteristic of normal sleep?
A. Apnea
B. Cataplexy
C. Long latencies (>50 ms) of somatosensory-evoked potentials (SEPs)
D. Fluctuations in cerebral metabolism
E. Diffuse slowing of EEG activity below 8 Hz for several hours

6. A patient who periodically falls asleep during the day, often in response to emotional stimuli, is likely to have which of the following conditions?
A. Insomnia
B. Narcolepsy
C. Cognitive death
D. Obstructive sleep apnea (OSA)
E. Circadian rhythm disorder

7. A patient undergoes surgery during general anesthesia. In addition to recording heart rate, blood pressure, and other standard parameters, the patient is monitored for possible signs of consciousness. Which of the following findings is most likely to suggest intraoperative awareness?
A. Bilateral somatic evoked potentials
B. Theta frequency EEG waves with large amplitude K spike complexes
C. Eye movements
D. Low-amplitude beta frequency EEG waves
E. Delta wave EEG synchronization

8. What is the neural mechanism by which benzodiazepines induce sleep?
A. Activation of the LDT/PPT nuclei
B. Enhancement of GABAergic transmission in the thalamus
C. Inhibition of the mPRF
D. Enhancement of cholinergic transmission in the cerebral cortex
E. Activation of the nucleus basalis

ADDITIONAL READING

Classic Literature

Aserinsky E, Kleitman N: Regularly occurring periods of eye motility, and concomitant phenomena during sleep. *Science* 118:273–274, 1953.

Jouvet M: Neurophysiology of the states of sleep. *Physiol Rev* 47:117–177, 1967.

Moruzzi G, Magoun HW: Brain stem reticular formation and activation of the EEG. *Electroenceph Clin Neurophysiol* 1:455–473, 1949.

Reviews and Landmark Research Articles

Buzsaki G, Bickford RG, Ponomareff G, Thal LJ, Mandel R, Gage FH: Nucleus basalis and thalamic control of neocortical activity in the freely moving rat. *J Neurosci* 8:4007–4026, 1988.

Colwell CS, Michel S: Sleep and circadian rhythms: do sleep centers talk back to the clock? *Nature Neurosci* 10:1005–1006, 2003.

Erman MK: Therapeutic options in the treatment of insomnia. *J Clin Psychiat* 66:18–23, 2005.

Giacino J, Whyte J: The vegetative and minimally conscious states: current knowledge and remaining questions. *J Head Trauma Rehabil* 20:30–50, 2005.

Hobson JA, Pace–Schott EF: The cognitive neuroscience of sleep: neuronal systems, consciousness and learning. *Nat Rev Neurosci* 3:679–693, 2002.

Kales A, Kales JD: *Evaluation and Treatment of Insomnia*. New York, NY: Oxford University Press, 1984.

Laureys S, Owen AM, Schiff ND: Brain function in coma, vegetative state, and related disorders. *Lancet Neurol* 3:537–546, 2004.

Lydic R, Biebuyck JF, eds: *Clinical Physiology of Sleep*. Bethesda, MD: American Physiological Society, 1988.

McCarley RW: Sleep, dreams and states of consciousness. In: Conn PM, ed. *Neuroscience in Medicine*. Philadelphia, PA: JB Lippincott, 1995:537–553.

McCarley RW, Nelson JP, Hobson JA: Ponto-genicululo-occipital (PGO) burst neurons: correlative evidence for neuronal generators of PGO waves. *Science* 201:269–272, 1978.

McCormick DA, Pape H-C: Noradrenergic and serotonergic modulation of a hyperpolarization-activated cation current in thalamic relay neurons. *J Physiol* 431:319–342, 1990.

——: Properties of a hyperpolarization-activated cation current and its role in rhythmic oscillation in thalamic relay neurons. *J Physiol* 431:291–318, 1990.

Mistlberger RE: Circadian regulation of sleep in mammals: role of the suprachiasmatic nucleus. *Brain Res Brain Res Rev* 49:429–454, 2005.

Plum F: Coma and related global disturbances of the human conscious state. In: Jones EG, Peters A, eds. *Cerebral Cortex: Normal and Altered States of Function*, vol 9. New York, NY: Plenum Press, 1991:359–425.

Schiff ND, Plum F: The role of arousal and "gating" systems in the neurology of impaired consciousness. *J Clin Neurophysiol* 17:438–452, 2000.

Schiff ND, Rodrguez-Moreno D, Kamal A, Kim KH, Giacino JT, Plum F, Hirsch J: MRI reveals large-scale network activation in minimally conscious patients. *Neurology* 64:514–523, 2005.

Steriade M, Dossi R, Nunez A: Network modulation of a slow intrinsic oscillation of cat thalamocortical neurons implicated in sleep delta waves: cortically induced synchronization and brainstem cholinergic suppression. *J Neurosci* 11:3200–3217, 1991.

Steriade M, Jones, EG, Llinas RR: *Thalamic Oscillations and Signaling*. New York, NY: J Wiley and Sons, 1990.

Steriade M, McCarley RW: *Brainstem Control of Wakefulness and Sleep*. New York, NY: Plenum Press, 1990.

Steriade M, McCormick DA, Sejnowski TJ: Thalamocortical oscillations in the sleeping and aroused brain. *Science* 262:679–685, 1993.

INTERNET RESOURCES

American Academy of Sleep Medicine
http://www.aasmnet.org/

American Association of Nurse Anesthetists
Considerations for Intraoperative Awareness
http://www.aana.com/

American Clinical Neurophysiology Society
http://www.acns.org/

American Insomnia Association
http://www.americaninsomniaassociation.org/home.htm

American Sleep Apnea Association
http://www.sleepapnea.org/

Anesthesia Awareness Campaign
http://www.anesthesiaawareness.com/index2.ivnu

Coma Recovery Association, Inc.
http://comarecovery.org/

National Institutes of Health (MedlinePlus)
Sleep Disorders
http://www.nlm.nih.gov/medlineplus/sleepdisorders.html

Narcolepsy Network
http://www.narcolepsynetwork.org

National Center on Sleep Disorders Research
http://www.nhlbi.nih.gov/about/ncsdr/index.htm

National Sleep Foundation
http://www.sleepfoundation.org/

NINDS Restless Legs Syndrome Fact Sheet
http://www.ninds.nih.gov/disorders/restless_legs/detail_restless_legs.htm

NINDS Coma and Persistent Vegetative State Information Page
http://www.ninds.nih.gov/disorders/coma/coma.htm

Restless Legs Organization
http://www.restlesslegs.com/

Sleep and Health Journal
http://www.sleepandhealth.com/

Stanford School of Medicine
Center for Narcolepsy
http://med.stanford.edu/school/Psychiatry/narcolepsy/

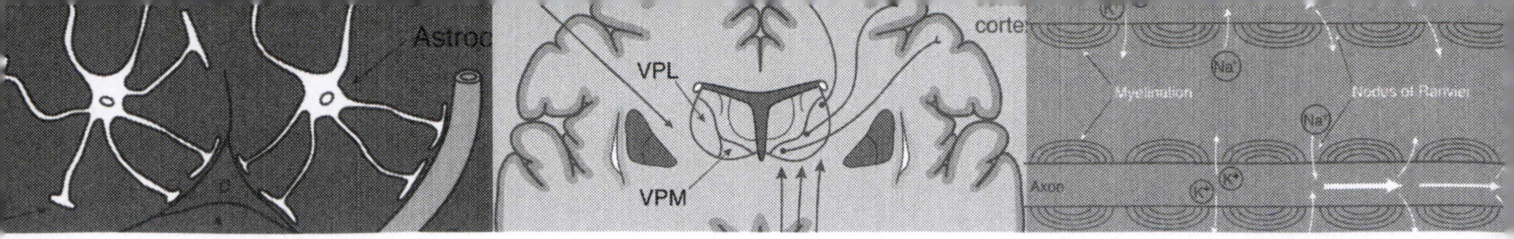

CHAPTER 16

Life Span Development of the Brain

INTRODUCTION OF CLINICAL CASE

A boy weighing 6 lb, 10 oz was born to a 31-year-old obese, diabetic woman whose first child has spina bifida. Even though the mother was not planning to have another baby, her gynecologist prescribed 4000 mcg of folic acid daily to reduce the chances of an unplanned pregnancy producing another child with a neural tube defect. The physical examination of the newborn was normal except for a small dimple and tuft of hair on his back near the waist. Ultrasound and imaging studies were ordered.

OVERVIEW

Development is a lifelong process.

Development of the nervous system is a lifelong process that begins within several weeks of conception, continues through childhood, and persists to a lesser degree through adulthood and old age. The earliest stages of neural development are initiated by a genetic blueprint and elaborated upon by intrinsic cellular and molecular interactions. Neural proliferation and migration takes place prior to synapse formation and is therefore not shaped by the individual's physical or social interactions with the outside world. Growth of the nervous system following birth, by comparison, is guided primarily by experience. Neurons and neural circuits required for successful interaction with the environment are retained while others are discarded. Even though neural growth and elaboration are virtually complete by age 25, new synapses and, to a lesser degree, new neurons, form throughout life.

PRENATAL DEVELOPMENT

Neurulation and Development of the Neural Tube

Through a process called gastrulation, the first embryonic cells differentiate into three germinal layers: ectoderm, mesoderm, and endoderm. On day 16, gastrulation transforms the mesoderm immediately below the ectodermal layer into the notochord. Over the next 2 days, the notochord changes from an indentation called the primitive pit into an elongated invagination known as the primitive streak. The notochord and the primitive streak define the longitudinal axis of the embryo, and on day 18, they produce the inductive signal that prompts the ectoderm to differentiate into the neural plate. Most of the neural precursor cells that form the central nervous system originate in the neural plate.

The nervous system develops from ectoderm.

As the neural plate grows longitudinally, its lateral edges thicken and arch medially as they fold around the neural groove, the hallmark of the keyhole stage of development (Figure 16.1). With further elaboration, these folds approach one another at the midline and fuse. Fusion of the neural folds begins on day 20 at the cervical cord and spreads both rostrally and caudally until the entire neural plate has been converted into a tube, a

Primary neurulation: formation of the neural tube

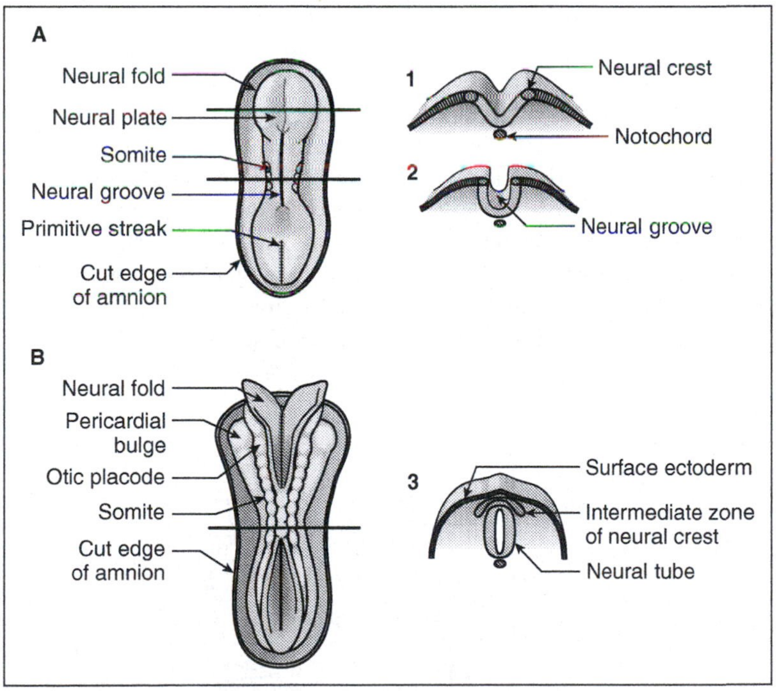

FIG. 16.1. Development of the Neural Tube. (A) The keyhole stage is marked by the development of the neural groove, the precursor of the neural tube. Formation of the neural groove is induced by the underlying notochord along the midline of the embryo. As cross sections 1 and 2 show, the neural groove first develops in the center of the embryo. (B) Closing of the neural groove forms the neural tube (cross section 3). Closure of the neural tube begins in the center of the embryo and spreads to both ends. Cross section 3 shows the closed neural tube with neural crest located dorsally.

FIG. 16.2. Cross Section of the Neural Tube. The alar (dorsal) and basal (ventral) plates are separated from one another by the sulcus limitans.

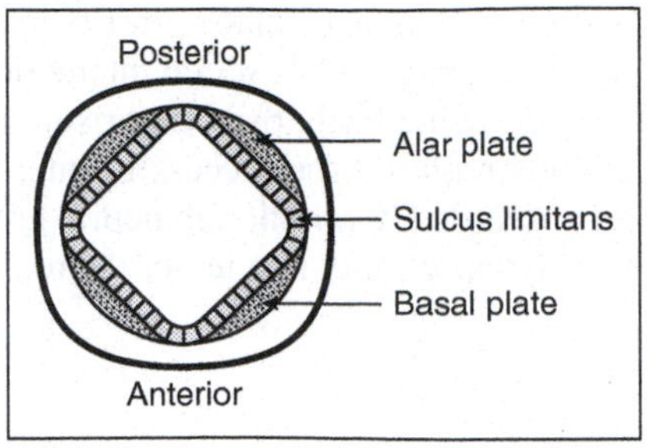

process called primary neurulation. Formation of the neural tube pinches off a small cluster of cells called the neural crest. As the neural crest cells migrate from the neural tube, they develop into the ganglia of the cranial nerves (V, VII, IX, and X), dorsal roots, and the autonomic nervous system. Some of the neural crest cells also form the enteric nervous system, the neurosecretory cells of the adrenal gland, the Schwann cells of the peripheral nervous system, and the meninges (see Figure 16.1)

Motor and sensory nuclei are separated by the **sulcus limitans.**

By the fourth postnatal week, a longitudinal groove called the sulcus limitans has developed in the neural tube wall (Figure 16.2). The sulcus limitans divides the neural tube into a dorsal alar plate and a ventral basal plate. With further differentiation, sensory and motor neurons develop from the alar and basal plates, respectively. This functional partition is best illustrated postnatally in the spinal cord where sensory and motor functions are mediated by the dorsal and ventral horns, respectively. The sulcus limitans is an important landmark in the brainstem as well because it marks the sensory/motor partition between the cranial sensory and motor nuclei (see Chapter 5).

Primary neurulation forms the entire CNS rostral to the sacral spinal cord; the sacral and coccygeal segments are formed by secondary neurulation. Secondary neurulation begins on day 20 when a cell mass, the caudal eminence, forms caudal to the immature neural tube. By day 42 the caudal eminence has developed a central canal and fused with the proximal lumbar cord.

At birth, the spinal cord ends at L3.

During early prenatal development, the spinal cord extends to the caudal tip of the vertebral column (Figure 16.3). Later, as growth of the vertebral columns outpaces that of the central nervous system, the caudal tip of the spinal cord gradually recedes from the end of the spinal canal. At birth, the spinal cord ends at the L3 vertebra, but by adulthood, the caudal tip of the spinal cord extends only as far as the L1-L2 vertebrae. This mismatch forces the nerve roots from the lumbar, sacral, and coccygeal segments to descend within the lumbar cistern before exiting the spinal canal below the vertebra for which each is named. Use of the lumbar cistern for spinal taps was discussed in Chapter 4.

FIG. 16.3. Relationship between the Spinal Cord and the Vertebral Column. (A) During early embryologic development. (B) At birth. (C) In the adult.

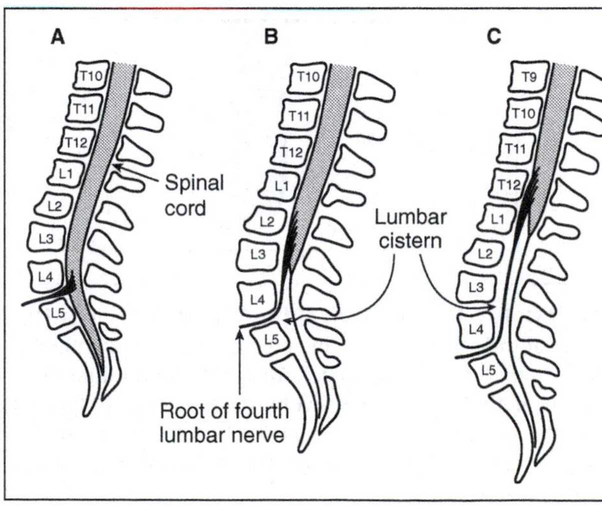

Neural Induction

Differential growth along the dorsal-ventral axis of the neural tube is induced by two proteins secreted by nearby non-neural cells: sonic hedgehog and bone morphogenetic protein. Sonic hedgehog triggers early embryologic development of the notochord from mesodermal cells and later promotes differentiation of motor neurons, interneurons, and floor plate cells within the ventral half of the neural tube. Bone morphogenetic protein, which is secreted by nearby ectodermal cells, triggers differentiation of dorsal horn cells into interneurons, roof plate cells, and neural crest cells.

Differential neural growth along the rostral-caudal axis is induced by proteins unique to the forebrain (e.g., follistatin, noggin, chordin) and hindbrain (fibroblast growth factor, retinoic acid). These proteins play an important role in the gene expression that controls embryologic development. For example, expression of the Hox gene, which controls segmental development of the caudal brainstem, is driven by mesodermal release of retinoic acid. Prenatal imbalance in retinoic acid disrupts Hox gene expression and causes serious craniofacial abnormalities.

Retinoic acid is a derivative of vitamin A.

Teratogenesis: birth defects caused by exogenous factors

Brain Vesicles and the Ventricular System

A thin membrane called the lamina terminalis closes the rostral end of the neural tube at the anterior neuropore by day 24; closure of the posterior neuropore takes place on day 26. The lumen of the neural tube is the embryonic predecessor of the ventricular system of the brain and the more caudal central canal of the spinal cord.

Following closure of the anterior neuropore, the rostral half of the neural tube dilates into three chambers or primary brain vesicles: the prosencephalon (forebrain), the mesencephalon (midbrain), and the rhombencephalon (hindbrain; Figure 16.4A). Two distinct flexures that form by the end of week 4 have a lasting impact on the shape of the CNS. The more pronounced of the two is the cephalic flexure, a sharp bend in the mesencephalon that turns the long axis of the telencephalon perpendicular to the brainstem. The less severe bend at the junction of the rhombencephalon and spinal cord is called the cervical flexure.

The **cephalic flexure** bends the brain 90°.

By week 5, the telencephalic flexure divides the prosencephalon into the telencephalon and the diencephalon. Similarly, the pontine flexure splits the rhombencephalon into the metencephalon and the myelencephalon (Figures 16.4B and 16.5). The metencephalon develops into the pons and cerebellum; the myelencephalon becomes the medulla. The only primary vesicle that does not subdivide during development is the mesencephalon, which forms the midbrain (Figure 16.6).

Growth and elaboration of the primary brain vesicles determine the size and shape of the brain's ventricles (Figure 16.7). For example, as the cerebellum develops from the alar

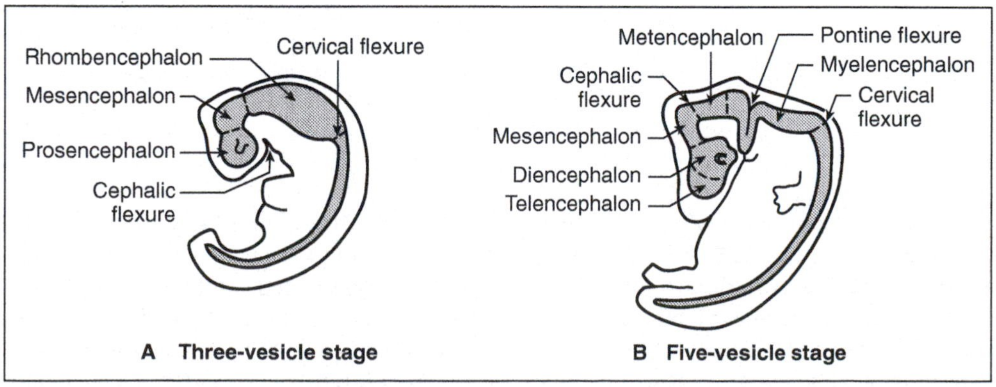

FIG. 16.4. Three-Vesicle (A) and Five-Vesicle Stages (B) of Embryonic Development.

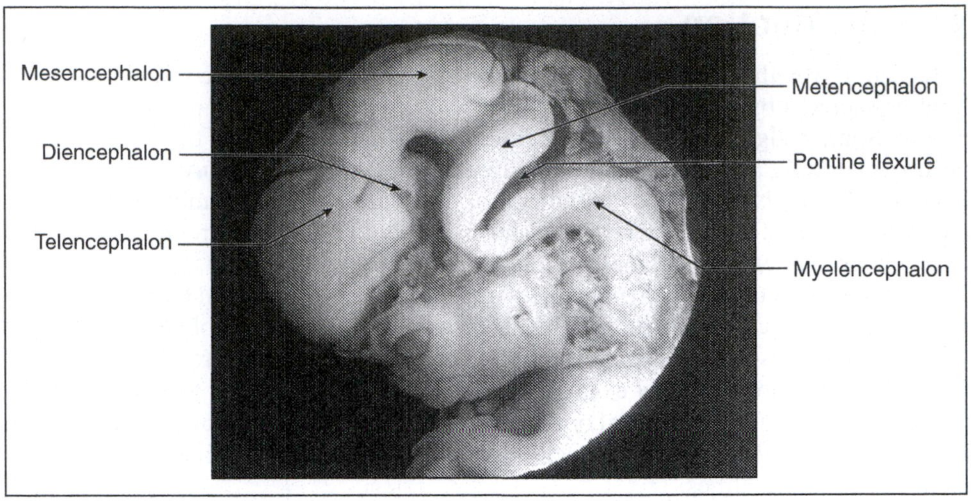

FIG. 16.5. The In Situ Brain of an 8-Week-Old Embryo. (Courtesy of the late Dr. Malcolm B. Carpenter)

FIG. 16.6. Divisions of the Embryonic and Adult Nervous System.

Embryonic divisions		Adult divisions
Prosencephalon	→	Telencephalon; Diencephalon
Mesencephalon	→	Mesencephalon
Rhombencephalon	→	Metencephalon; Myelencephalon

FIG. 16.7. Ventricular System as Seen from Above during Late Embryonic Development.

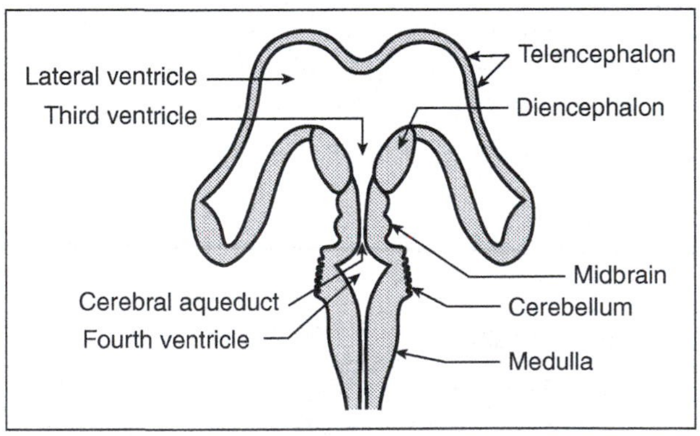

plate, the central canal widens into the fourth ventricle. The small, nearly round cerebral aqueduct, by comparison, reflects the modest growth of the mesencephalon. In the diencephalon, the third ventricle is compressed into a vertically oriented slit during proliferation of the thalamus and hypothalamus. The most profound changes to the ventricular system are caused by the explosive growth of the cerebral hemispheres, which form the bulk of the telencephalon. The lateral ventricle assumes the shape of a ram's horn as the telencephalon gradually envelopes the underlying diencephalon. Despite these changes in the shape and size of the ventricular system, it remains a continuous system—cerebrospinal fluid

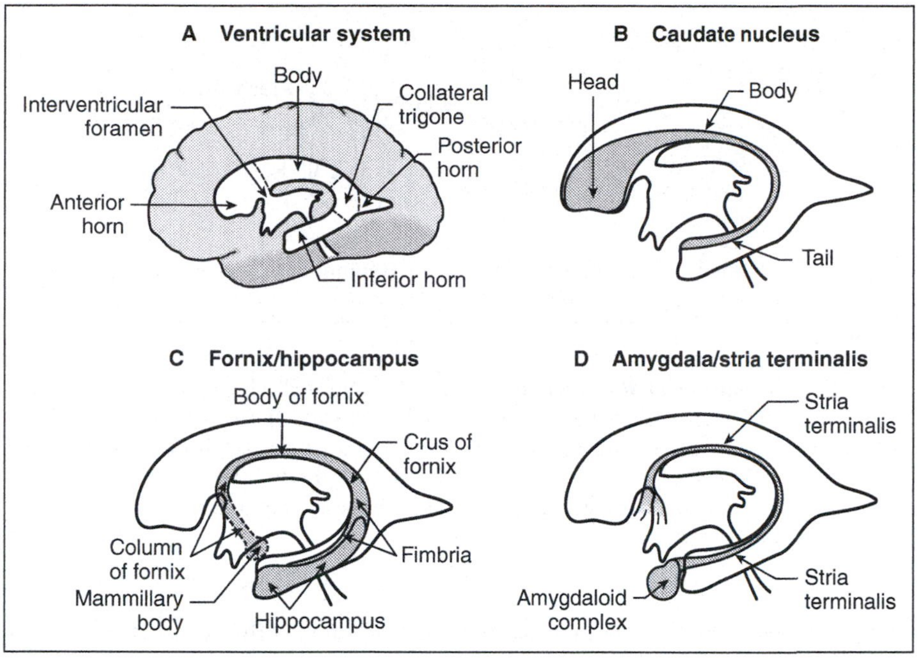

FIG. 16.8. Sagittal View of the Internal Structure of the Cerebrum. (A) The ventricular system. (B) Caudate nucleus. (C) Fornix, hippocampus, and fimbria. (D) Amygdala and stria terminalis. (Adapted with permission from Haines DE: *Fundamental Neuroscience.* New York, NY: Churchill Livingstone, 1997:214.)

produced in the lateral ventricles flows into the third and fourth ventricles and finally into the subarachnoid space, where it is resorbed by the venous system (see Chapter 3).

Development of the Forebrain

The telencephalic vesicles grow into the cerebral hemispheres and the underlying basal ganglia (see Figure 16.7). Development of the telencephalon spreads from the lamina terminalis first rostrally and then caudally, the latter growth being more pronounced. Eventually the telencephalon covers the dorsal aspects of the diencephalon, the mesencephalon, and the cerebellum. As caudal expansion of the telencephalon pulls the lateral ventricle into a pronounced C shape, closely associated structures such as the caudate nucleus, fornix, stria terminalis, and choroid plexus assume the same arched shape (Figure 16.8).

Growth of the cerebral cortex also follows a rostral-to-caudal sequence, beginning in the frontal lobe before spreading caudally through the parietal and occipital lobes. Rapid development of the frontal lobe traps and gradually buries the more slowly growing insular cortex within the depths of the lateral sulcus. Final interment of the insula commences near the time of birth as the temporal lobe increases in size.

The surface of the cerebral cortex is initially flat and featureless, but it gradually develops dozens of folds and grooves called gyri and sulci, respectively. The central (Rolando) and lateral (Sylvius) sulci are already visible at birth; many more will appear over the next 2 years. Folding the cerebral cortex into gyri and sulci maximizes the amount of neocortex within the limited confines of the calvarium.

Gyrencephalic brains have gyri and sulci. **Lissencephalic** brains are flat.

Clinical Aspects of Neurulation: Neural Tube Defects

Complete closure of the neural tube is essential for normal development of the nervous system. Incomplete closure of the neural tube or either neuropore causes a neural tube defect that may produce severe neurologic deficits. Women who are planning to get pregnant

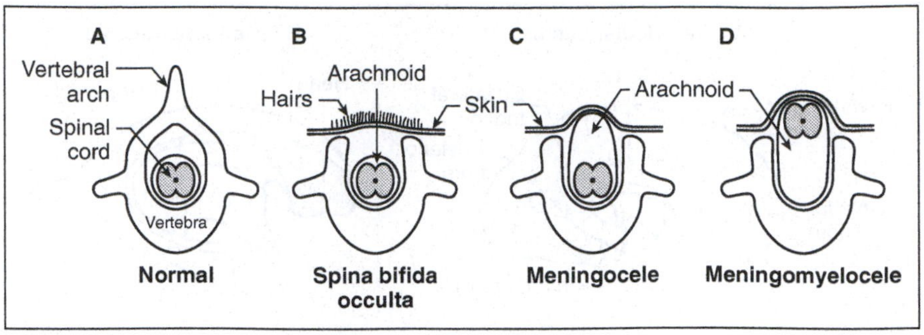

FIG. 16.9. Formation of the Vertebral Arch. (A) Normal. (B) Spina bifida occulta. Although the vertebral arch is missing, neither the arachnoid nor the spinal cord have herniated through the defect. One marker for spina bifida occulta is a patch of hair on the overlying skin. (C) Meningocele. Herniation of the arachnoid through the vertebral defect. (D) Meningomyelocele. Herniation of the spinal cord and arachnoid through the vertebral defect makes this the most serious form of spina bifida.

are often advised to supplement their multivitamin regimen with folic acid, which reduces the incidence of neural tube defects.

Anencephaly: no forebrain

Encephalocele: cyst-like cavity

Failure of the anterior neuropore to close prevents formation of the telencephalon and leaves the hindbrain poorly developed, a condition known as anencephaly. Most anencephalic infants are stillborn or die shortly after birth. Faulty closure of the anterior neuropore or congenital abnormalities of the brain and meninges are also associated with cranial defects that cause the brain to herniate into a cyst-like cavity called an encephalocele or a cranium bifidum. The neurologic consequences of an encephalocele are determined by the type of herniation present. In a cranial meningocele, the herniation is limited to the meninges, which can be excised. Meningoencephaloceles are more serious and difficult to treat because both brain tissue and meninges have been extruded through the cranial defect. The most serious type of herniation is the menigohydroencephalocele, in which the meninges, brain, and part of the ventricular system are extruded.

Arnold-Chiari malformations are the most common congenital cerebellar defect.

Arnold-Chiari malformations represent a different type of congenital brain herniation in which the medulla and cerebellar vermis protrude through the foramen magnum. All patients with encephaloceles are at risk of hydrocephalus, paresis and paralysis, and urologic problems, even if they have had a successful reconstructive surgery.

Worldwide, 60 million women are at risk for delivering babies with spina bifida.

Spina bifida: incomplete closure of the neural tube or posterior neuropore

Incomplete closure of the posterior neuropore or the neural folds in the caudal half of the neural tube causes spina bifida, a malformation of the vertebral column in which one or more vertebral arches remain open (Figure 16.9). Spina bifida is the most common permanent disabling birth defect, but the neurologic consequences of spina bifida vary widely. Spina bifida occulta occurs in 15%–40% of the population, but it has no clinical significance because the defect is not accompanied by meningeal or neural herniation (Figure 16.9B). The vertebral defect may be marked by a dimple and a patch of coarse hair on the overlying skin. Herniation of the meninges through the vertebral defect is called spinal bifida with meningocele (Figure 16.9C). The most serious form, spina bifida with meningomyelocele, includes meningeal and spinal cord herniation (Figure 16.9D). Unfortunately, meningomyeloceles account for 96% of spina bifida cases that present with herniation, most often of the cauda equina. Although most symptoms of spina bifida are caused by mechanical stress placed on the spinal cord or spinal nerves, mental retardation, hydrocephalus, and meningitis are frequent comorbid conditions.

Development of Neurons and Glia

Neurogenesis: neuron birth

The adult brain contains approximately 100 billion neurons, and, aside for some in the hippocampus and the olfactory bulb, all of these neurons develop before birth in a process call neurogenesis. It is not known why the ability to create new neurons is virtually lost at birth,

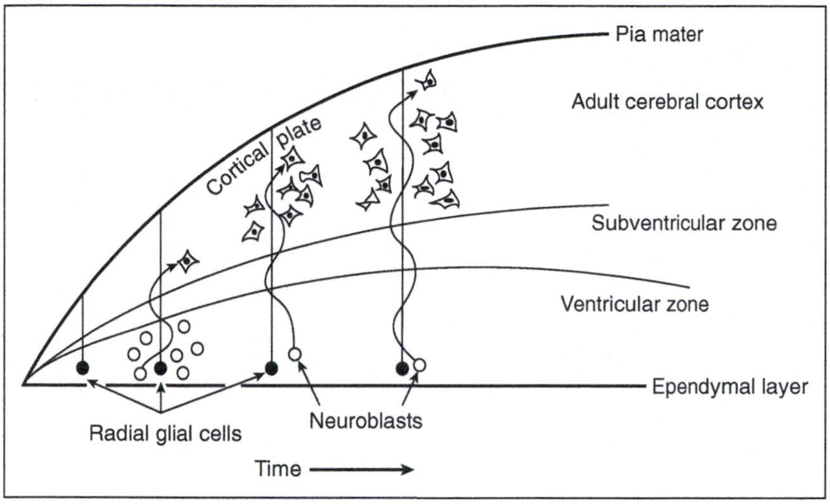

FIG. 16.10. Development of Cerebral Cortex. The cortical plate thickens as immature neuroblasts migrate from the ventricular zone toward the pial surface. The first neurons to reach the cortical plate form the deep layers of the cerebral cortex. The superficial layers of the cerebral cortex form later as newly formed neurons migrate through the previously established deep cortical layers.

but the implications are clear. The vast majority of neurons that succumb to postnatal disease, trauma, and aging are not replaced.

Neurons in the central and peripheral nervous systems receive structural and metabolic support from glial calls. Glia are 10–50 times more numerous than neurons and develop from the same embryonic precursor cells. Development of neurons and glia are best understood in two systems: the neural crest and the cerebral cortex.

Neural crest cells exposed to bone morphogenetic protein during migration to the periphery develop into neurons of the cranial, dorsal root, and autonomic ganglia. Glial growth factor, a cell surface protein on these neurons, suppresses neurogenesis of the precursor cells remaining in the neural crest. These neural crest cells develop into Schwann cells that provide the myelin coat for the first batch of neurons that developed from the neural crest.

Neurons migrate to the cortical surface by climbing a radial glial scaffolding.

The cerebral cortex develops from the inside out.

During the first trimester, neurons and glia of the cerebral cortex develop from precursor cells located in the ventricular zone adjacent to the epithelial wall of the neural tube (Figure 16.10). The first cells to emerge from the ventricular zone are the radial glia, whose apical process climbs to the outer surface of the immature telencephalic vesicle. As radial glial cells divide, they form new radial glia and neuroblasts. The neuroblasts, after moving away from the ventricular zone into the subventricular zone, differentiate into neurons that climb the radial glial scaffolding that stretches to the pial surface. The neurons that develop first form the deep layers of the cerebral cortex; neurons born later must migrate through the established cells to reach the superficial cortical layers. Thus, the cerebral cortex develops from the inside out. Cortical neurogenesis is almost complete by the end of the second trimester and, with few exceptions, no new neurons are added to the cortical mantle afterwards. Indeed, the brain as a whole will never have more neurons than it has by the end of the sixth month of gestation.

As neurogenesis begins to wane during the latter part of the second trimester of pregnancy, gliogenesis begins. Initially, precursor cells in the ventricular zone develop into astrocytes. As gliogenesis shifts to oligodendrocytes during the third trimester, myelination begins in the large sensory and motor tracts. When oligodendrocyte development ends, the remaining radial glial cells develop into astrocytes.

Cerebellar cortical development begins when the Purkinje cells generated from the ventricular zone of the fourth ventricle migrate radially and form an irregular layer called

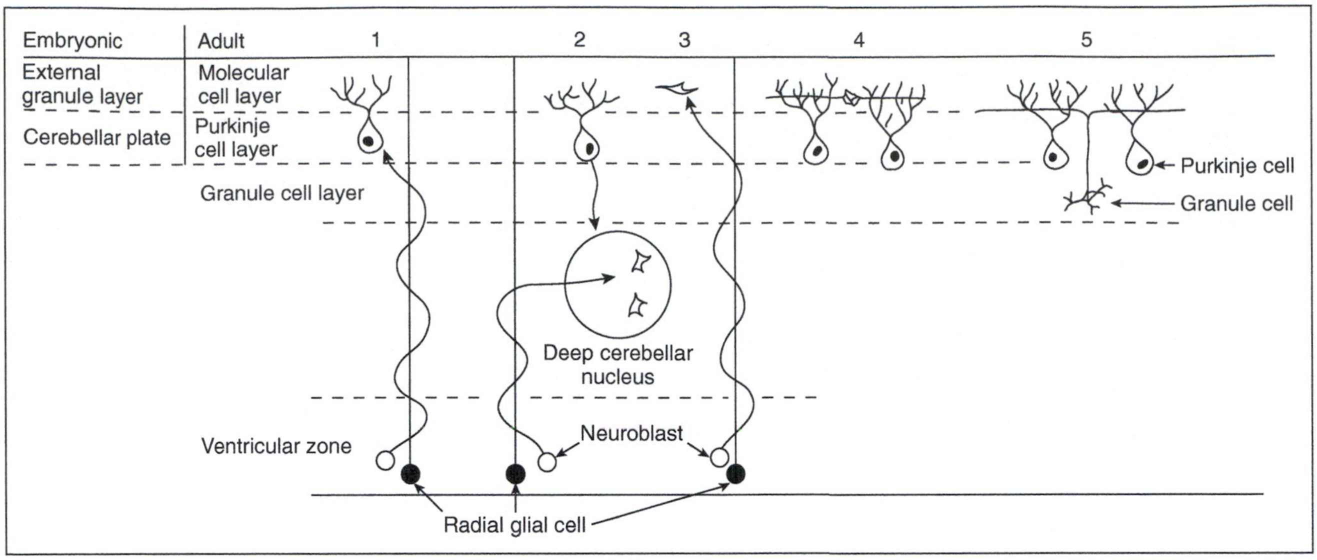

FIG. 16.11. Development of Cerebellar Cortex. (1) Following development of radial glia cells in the ventricular zone, neuroblasts climb the glial scaffolding, develop into Purkinje cells, and form the cerebellar plate layer of the cerebellar cortex. The cerebellar plate will become the Purkinje cell layer in the adult. (2) Other neuroblasts ascend and form the deep cerebellar nuclei. (3) After the Purkinje cells are in place, neuroblasts destined to become granule cells ascend the radial glia fibers and accumulate next to the pial surface in the external granule layer, the adult predecessor of the molecular layer. (4) Each granule cell sprouts an apical axon that bifurcates and grows parallel to the pial surface. As both axons grow, they establish synapses with the apical dendrites of the Purkinje cells. (5) As the granule cells mature, the proximal part of the axon elongates, which enables the soma to descend through the Purkinje cell layer and establish the granule cell layer.

The cerebellum develops from the outside in.

the cerebellar plate (Figure 16.11). As the cerebellum grows, the Purkinje cells level off into the single-cell layer characteristic of the adult brain. After the Purkinje cells have formed and established their axonal connections, the granule cells develop from progenitor cells located along the rhombic lip of the metencephalon. The granule cells migrate past the Purkinje cells and form a superficial stratum called the external granule layer. After the granule cell axons establish synaptic contact with the apical dendrites of the Purkinje cells, their somas descend through the cerebellar plate and form the granule cell layer observed in adults. Granule cells continue migrating from the embryonic external granule layer to the mature granule cell layer for at least 2 years following birth. When this process is complete, the molecular layer will occupy the position initially held by the granule cells and will contain the Purkinje cell dendrites and the T-shaped axons of the granule cells.

Axonal and Dendritic Growth and Guidance

When neurons first arrive in the cerebral cortex, they have no axons or dendrites. Despite their obvious functional differences, axons and dendrites develop similarly. Axons and dendrites, which are both considered neurites, begin growing after the soma has become polarized. Although neurite growth is genetically predisposed, it must be triggered by a series of signaling molecules. Neurite growth toward distant targets is guided by a spade-like tip called the growth cone. Growth cones contain numerous motile, finger-like projections called filopodia that forge through the neuropil. The filopodia are not only mechanical wedges, but also chemosensors that guide neurite growth.

Growth cones guide axons and dendrites through the neuropil.

Trophic factors attract axonal and dendritic growth.

The growth cone chemosensors enable axons and dendrites to detect attractive and repulsive factors that promote growth toward their targets. These molecules are either cell surface markers or molecules dissolved in the extracellular matrix. Growth cones follow the concentration gradients of these soluble attractant or repulsive molecules to guide themselves through the neuropil to their destinations.

Cell Surface Markers. Molecules that promote neurite growth are classified as calcium-dependent or calcium-independent. The calcium-*dependent* promoters are the cadherins, a diverse group of membrane-spanning glycoproteins. Cadherins are located on the surface of growth cones as well as on the neurons and glia that the fledging neurites grow through. The calcium-*independent* promoters include the cell adhesion molecules (CAMs), of which there are two major types. Neuron-glial cell adhesion molecules (Ng-CAM) promote axon growth along existing pathways marked by the presence of astrocytes and Schwann cells. Axons growing toward a common destination are assembled into bundles or fasciculi by neural cell adhesion molecules (N-CAMs).

Cell surface markers promote and guide neurite growth.

Molecules in the Extracellular Matrix. Neurite growth is also promoted by extracellular molecular markers such as laminin and fibronectin. Binding of laminin or fibronectin to receptors on the filopodia called integrins triggers a cascade of intracellular calcium and inositol triphosphate-based events within the growth cones that support neurite growth and extension. Neural migration is also guided by members of the semaphorin family that act as chemorepellants.

Synaptogenesis

Contact of the axonal filopodia with the target neuron triggers a series of structural changes on both the presynaptic and postsynaptic membranes. The axonal filopodia retract and are transformed into presynaptic membrane where preassembled synaptic vesicles and receptors immediately migrate. The filopodia on the postsynaptic membrane disappear and are replaced by dendritic spines, which are eventually stocked with the receptors and second-messenger systems required for neural transmission.

Neurotrophic Support and Apoptosis

The genetic code that guides neurogenesis does not specify how many neurons should constitute the central nervous system or exactly how those neurons should be interconnected. Instead, the embryonic nervous system generates more neurons, axons, dendrites, and synapses than the mature nervous system will ever need and then, based upon the person's experience, prunes the unnecessary elements. Neurons and their connections survive (1) if they are used routinely during the individual's physical, social, and emotional interactions with the outside world, and (2) if they receive trophic support from their postsynaptic targets (i.e., neurons, muscles, or glands). The neurons that retain their afferent innervation and postsynaptic neurotrophic support survive into adulthood because they contribute to the well-being of the individual.

Trophic factors sustain neurons and synapses.

The first rule of neuron survival: Use it or lose it.

The pioneering studies on neurotrophins conducted by Levi-Montalcini and Hamburger in the 1950s demonstrated that removal of a limb bud in a chick embryo led to a loss of spinal motor neurons. Replacing the limb before the motor neurons died saved them; grafting an extra limb onto the embryo increased the number of spinal motor neurons. Based upon these and other studies, they concluded that the limb buds contain a neurotrophic agent that sustains the presynaptic motor neurons. Subsequent studies by other investigators have shown that neural growth factor (NGF) is only one member of a larger family of neurotrophins that support presynaptic neurons in the central nervous system.

Even though neurotrophins are critical for neuronal survival, postsynaptic cells contain only a limited supply of NGF. Because neurotrophins are a limited resource in the target cells, the supply of NGF determines how many presynaptic neurons can converge onto the target cell. In this way, neurotrophins ensure that each target cell is innervated by the correct number of afferent neurons and that each afferent neuron innervates the proper number of target cells. After the presynaptic and postsynaptic relationships have been firmly established in the adult, neurotrophins modulate axonal sprouting and retraction to match the changing needs of the individual. Neurons deprived of trophic support die through an active process called programmed cell death or apoptosis. Neurotrophins also suppress so-called death genes that destroy neurons as well as activate survival genes that prevent apoptosis.

Apoptosis: programmed cell death

During gestation and early childhood, neurons can be rewired with relative ease and thus rescue functions that would otherwise be lost following brain damage. For this reason, the oversupply of neurons in the immature nervous system provides a hedge against irreversible traumatic brain injury. Indeed, serious neurological insults that occur during the perinatal period often produce only a transient deficit. As this neural surplus disappears during early childhood, the window of recovery closes as well.

CHILDHOOD DEVELOPMENT (BIRTH–AGE 12)

> The newborn is not notable for its abilities, but rather for its potential.

At birth, the basic outline of the nervous system is complete. The major structures are in place, as are most of the critical circuitry and synapses, yet the newborn remains a "work in progress." Even though programmed cell death begins during the third trimester, the newborn brain contains at least twice as many neurons as the adult brain. These excess neurons will be pruned over the next two decades as the brain gradually assumes its adult form.

The Role of Experience in Childhood Brain Development

> Each brain is customized by the user, for the user.

Prenatal neurogenesis and neural migration take place prior to synapse formation and thus are not shaped by the individual's interactions with the outside world. During the latter part of gestation, when the baby begins moving in utero, as well as during childhood and adolescence, the cellular composition, the axonal and dendritic organization, and the synaptic organization of the brain are modified by the individual's experience.

Some complex behaviors emerge only if the individual has specific experiences not only early in life but also during relatively circumscribed stages of development called critical periods. Imprinting, the tendency for newly hatched chicks to follow the first large moving object they encounter, is a prime example. In order for imprinting to take place, the encounter must occur within several days of hatching; other behaviors and developmental milestones have their own critical periods. Development of binocular vision, learned affective behavior, and acquisition of language are three examples of how human development relies on critical periods.

> The two eyes compete for space in primary visual cortex.

Development of Binocular Vision. The ocular dominance columns in visual cortex that mediate binocular (stereoscopic) perception develop during the first 6 weeks of life. In a series of seminal experiments, David Hubel and Torsten Wiesel demonstrated that ocular dominance columns fail to develop in newborn animals that do not experience normal binocular visual stimulation during this critical period. In one experiment, an animal deprived of visual stimulation in one eye during the critical period lost sight in that eye. Neurons in primary visual cortex of these animals responded to stimulation of the open eye, but not to stimulation of the eye that had been closed. Surprisingly, other animals that were deprived of visual stimulation in both eyes had near normal vision. Examination of the neurons in visual cortex activated by the sighted eye indicated that their synaptic territories had expanded at the expense of the dormant neurons innervated by the closed eye. Based on these data, Hubel and Wiesel concluded that monocular deprivation places cortical development of the areas innervated by the deprived eye at a competitive disadvantage with respect to the open eye.

In another experiment, one of the extraocular eye muscles was surgically altered to misalign the eyes (strabismus) and cause double vision. In strabismus, stereoscopic vision is lost because the cortical projections from corresponding areas of the two eyes are not in register. Following this manipulation, neurons in visual cortex responded to stimulation of one eye or the other, but none responded to stimulation of both eyes. It is unlikely that these animals viewed the world stereoscopically.

The implications of this research are clear for babies born with a congenital cataract or strabismus. A cataract is an opacity (cloudiness) of the lens that blocks most light from entering the eye. To assure normal visual development in the affected eye, it is imperative that the cataract be surgically removed before the critical period for cortical development has expired.

Children with congenital strabismus are unable to effectively utilize the affected eye and will eventually favor the opposite eye. Unless the child is forced to use the affected or so-called "lazy eye," binocular vision may be lost. If surgical correction of the misalignment is possible, that should be done. If the underlying problem cannot be corrected, a patch should be worn over the good eye periodically to force the child the use the affected eye. Intermittent use of the affected eye will promote even development of visual cortex for each eye. Because overuse of the patch might jeopardize vision in the good eye, treatment of strabismus should be supervised by a trained professional. Cataracts or strabismus that develop after the critical period has closed will interfere with sight but will not cause permanent injury to the visual system.

Learned Affective Behavior. Pioneering studies by Harlow in nonhuman primates demonstrated that early bonding between an infant and its mother is indispensable for later development of normal affective behavior. In one of these seminal studies, infant monkeys were reared in a cage with two surrogate mothers. One surrogate was a simple wire mesh frame with a wooden head; the other was identical but had a terry cloth cover. The infant monkeys spent more time with the cloth-covered surrogate mother, even if milk was available from the plain surrogate. Initial behavioral observations suggested that the monkeys raised with the cloth-covered surrogate had normal social skills, but later it was determined that courtship behavior of both the males and the females was dysfunctional and usually ineffective. Females that were able to get pregnant delivered healthy babies, but the mothers either neglected or abused them. Even more extreme behaviors were observed in other monkeys reared without a surrogate mother. These monkeys engaged in endless stereotypic rocking behavior, ignored external stimulation, stared aimlessly into space, and were terrorized when exposed to other infants. Some of these behaviors have also been observed in children raised in social and maternal isolation.

> Early maternal deprivation has permanent deleterious effects.

Language Development. Children begin speaking between the ages of 9 and 12 months, and for the next 5 years their language skills grow by leaps and bounds. In some unfortunate cases, infants have been raised in social isolation for as long as 14 years, during which time they had virtually no exposure to spoken language. After these children were rescued and even with professional tutoring, they never developed normal language skills. School districts that once delayed foreign language instruction until high school now introduce these classes in elementary school. Unfortunately, the window for language development begins to close before children have completed grade school; by puberty, the critical period for language acquisition is virtually over. After the critical period has ended, social isolation has no effect on language.

> The critical window for language is virtually closed by age 10.

THE ADOLESCENT BRAIN

Birth provides a convenient and indisputable "time zero" for early child development, but there is no such marker for adolescence. Because social, sexual, physical, and neural maturity each have their own timetables, there is little agreement about the age bracket that constitutes adolescence. If adolescence is defined as the final period of rapid growth before the adult plateau is reached, the onset should be around age 13. The endpoint of adolescence is even more difficult to define. Although the physical growth that defines adolescence tapers after age 20, development of the central nervous system clearly continues into the mid-20s, and by some estimates until age 30.

Children enter adolescence dependent upon their parents; they leave adolescence as independent adults. Adolescents acquire adult stature and sexual maturity years before they are able to consistently act like responsible adults. Some experts believe the teenagers' penchant for engaging in novel and risky behavior prepares them for the physical, social, romantic, and financial challenges of the adult world; other experts, more

> Adolescence is a period of intense social, intellectual, and emotional development.

commonly known as parents, worry about the high morbidity and mortality rates of teens. Whether risk-taking behavior is adaptive or just another way for adolescents to develop a life independent of their parents, it is clear that adolescent behavior can not be blamed entirely on "raging hormones." The brain is equally culpable. The adolescent brain is not physically mature and does not perform like an adult brain. One area of the brain that matures during adolescence is the prefrontal cortex. The prefrontal cortex manages many behaviors that are the hallmarks of adult behavior such as planning, impulse suppression, setting priorities, decision making, and understanding the consequences of one's actions.

During childhood, neurons grow larger and develop more elaborate axonal and dendritic trees. This growth is partly responsible for brain size peaking near the onset of adolescence (females at 11.0 years, males at 12.5 years). Brain size shrinks over the next decade, led by the prefrontal cortex, which undergoes the pruning that took place in the rest of the brain during pre-adolescence. As in the perinatal period and childhood, adolescent experience provides the use-it-or-lose-it incentives responsible for neuronal survival. Structural imaging studies have shown that the cerebral cortex loses 15% of it mass during adolescence; most of that loss occurs in the prefrontal cortex. This loss of cortical grey matter is accompanied by increases in intrahemispheric and interhemispheric white matter. Even though it is not known whether this decrease in volume represents neurons, neuropil, or synapses, it is clear that the prefrontal cortex undergoes significant reorganization. If the prolonged maturation of the prefrontal cortex plays a role in the latent expression of adult-like behavior, as most scientists believe, it may also contribute to the risk-taking behavior of adolescents.

Many social, cultural, and religious institutions and practices have been blamed for adolescent experimentation with drugs, sex, and alcohol; add the brain to the list of responsible parties. During adolescence, dopamine levels are high, but dopamine receptors are low in the nucleus accumbens, an area of the ventral forebrain intimately involved with motivation and reward gratification. Thrill-seeking behavior may represent the adolescent solution to the body's need for reward gratification. Although the relationship is correlational, as the nucleus accumbens matures near the end of adolescence, the incidence of risky behavior decreases.

ADULT NEUROGENESIS

For decades it was widely accepted that mammalian neurogenesis ended at birth. In 1962 Joseph Altman demonstrated that neurogenesis is a lifelong process in the hippocampus of the rat. Adult neurogenesis was firmly established in animals before Peter Eriksson demonstrated in 1998 that neurogenesis also takes place in the adult hippocampus of humans. In this study, patients with throat carcinomas received a single injection of a synthetic form of thymidine, BrdU, which is incorporated into developing cells. The doctors used BrdU cell labeling to stage the throat carcinomas of these patients and optimize their medical care. These patient provided informed consent for a brain autopsy to be performed following their death. The patients were 57–72 years old at the time of death, yet each showed newborn BrdU-labeled neurons in the hippocampus. This study generated a great deal of excitement in the lay press; unfortunately, stem cells are not widely distributed in the adult brain.

> Lifelong neurogenesis continues in the olfactory bulb.

Neural stem cells are located in the subventricular zone and the subgranular zone of the hippocampus in the adult. The neuroblasts in the subventricular zone migrate to the olfactory bulb where they develop into interneurons in the granular and glomerular layers. Neuroblast migration to the olfactory bulb follows the rostral migratory stream propelled by chain migration. In chain migration, the neuroblasts are assembled into long chains that repeatedly slide past each other. The chains of neuroblasts travel through a tube constructed by astrocytes that also originate in the subventricular zone. It is unclear why neurogenesis has been preserved in the olfactory system while so many other areas of the brain have lost their ability to replace spent neurons. Nevertheless, olfactory neurogenesis is an important model for neuronal replacement that may lead to new therapeutic treatments for brain damaged individuals.

Prenatally, hippocampal stem cells are located in a narrow band called the subgranular zone, which is sandwiched between the granule cell layer of the dentate gyrus and hilus (CA4) of the hippocampus. Just as during embryologic development, only a fraction of the precursor cells that develop into neurons survive and establish synaptic connections within the dentate gyrus and the CA3 hippocampal field. The neurons that do survive are believed to be those nurtured by the individual's experience. The surviving neurons do not replace dying older cells but rather produce a net increase in the size of the dentate gyrus. With advancing age, the dentate gyrus shrinks as the rate of cell death increases and the pace of neurogenesis slows. The precise contribution of these latecomers is unknown but is presumed to involve some aspect of memory formation.

Neural Plasticity in the Adult Brain

Neurogenesis is not a viable option for recovery of function for most of the adult brain. Adults show limited recovery following central nervous system damage; most is mediated by axonal sprouting and reactive synaptogenesis of neurons adjacent to the affected area.

Studies on peripheral denervation have illustrated the plastic ability of the brain. In a series of landmark experiments, Merzenich showed that the response properties of neurons in primary somatosensory cortex change dramatically following finger amputation. The neurons that once responded to tactile stimulation of an amputated finger begin responding to stimulation of the adjacent digits after about 10 days. Similar results have been obtained in visual cortex following focal retinal damage. In both systems, the loss of normal peripheral innervation creates a temporary void that is eventually filled by horizontal projections from neurons in the adjacent cortex. Neural expansion into the denervated cortical area enables the brain to more fully utilize its resources, but it does not restore sensation to the missing finger or retinal area. To the contrary, activation of the neurons once innervated by an amputated finger, arm, or foot may be responsible for phantom limb pain.

THE ELDERLY BRAIN

Brain size and weight decrease 2%–3% per decade during adulthood, but the behavioral effects of these losses are seldom apparent until the individual reaches old age. It was once thought that the decrease in brain size and weight was due to a loss of neurons, but more recent studies indicate that neuron shrinkage and myelin thinning are the more likely causes. Brain shrinkage can be detected on CT and MRI films as widened sulci and a wider brain/skull space, which may be accompanied by enlarged ventricles. In normal adults, brain shrinkage occurs most often in the frontal lobes, which may account for some of the normal cognitive slowing and memory impairment observed in the elderly. These deficits may force certain compromises in lifestyle, but they seldom interfere with work or social activities.

> The number of neurons in the brain remains relatively stable throughout adulthood.

Senile Dementia

Senile dementia is characterized by severe, progressive memory and cognitive impairment that interferes with work and activities of daily living. Cognitive slowing and memory impairment are normal in the aged; senile dementia, on the other hand, is a pathological condition and not an inevitable part of aging. The deficits associated with senile dementia are diverse, but most involve memory, language, problem solving, attention, and perception as well as executive functions such as planning and organization. Alzheimer's disease accounts for 60%–70% of all dementias; other causes include cardiovascular disease, Parkinson's disease, Huntington's disease, drug toxicity and alcoholism, prion disease (Creutzfeldt-Jacob disease, or "mad cow disease"), AIDS, syphilis, and brain tumors.

> **Dementia:** severe, progressive decline in memory and cognitive function

> **Alzheimer's disease** is responsible for 60%–70% of all cases of dementia.

Alzheimer's Disease

Alzheimer's disease is a pathological process that affects about 7% of the population over age 65 and as many as 40% of those older than 80. Like the other dementias, Alzheimer's disease is characterized by progressive intellectual deterioration and, in its early stages, may be difficult to distinguish from other dementias. This distinction must be made, however,

> Histopathological testing is the only definitive test for Alzheimer's disease.

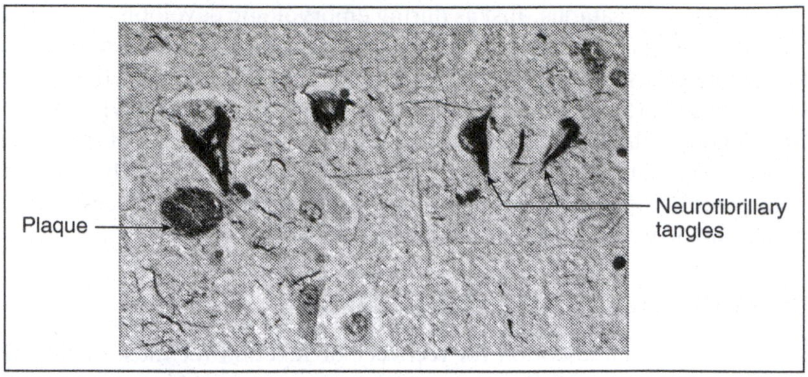

FIG. 16.12. Neurofibrillary Tangles and Plaque in the Cerebral Cortex of an Alzheimer's Disease Patient. (Courtesy of Dr. Javad Towfighi, Professor, Pennsylvania State University College of Medicine, Hershey, Pennsylvania.)

because unlike Alzheimer's disease, some of the others dementias respond well to treatment. Unfortunately, the only definitive diagnostic test for Alzheimer's disease requires a histopathological examination of the brain. Typically, the diagnosis of Alzheimer's disease is based on the patient's history, testimony from family, neuropsychological testing, laboratory testing, and neuroimaging.

Senile plaques and **neurofibrillary tangles** are the histological hallmarks of Alzheimer's disease.

Brain Abnormalities. In Alzheimer's disease, the brain of the patient shows a unique pattern of damage highlighted by inclusions called neurofibrillary tangles and senile plaques (Figure 16.12). As neurons besieged by tangles and plaques die, wasting of the gyri causes the sulci to widen (Figure 16.13). Neurofibrillary tangles are dense, twisted filamentous masses of the protein tau that form in the soma and proximal dendrites of the affected neurons. Senile plaques are extracellular accretions of the peptide A beta amyloid, which is derived from the amyloid precursor protein (APP) encoded by a gene on chromosome 21. Individuals with mutations of the APP gene have a genetic predisposition for Alzheimer's disease. Other genetic risk factors for Alzheimer's disease include mutations on chromosome 14 (presenilin 1 gene), chromosome 1 (presenilin 2 gene), and chromosome 19 (ApoE). Unfortunately, these genes indicate a predisposition, rather than a diagnostic marker, for Alzheimer's disease.

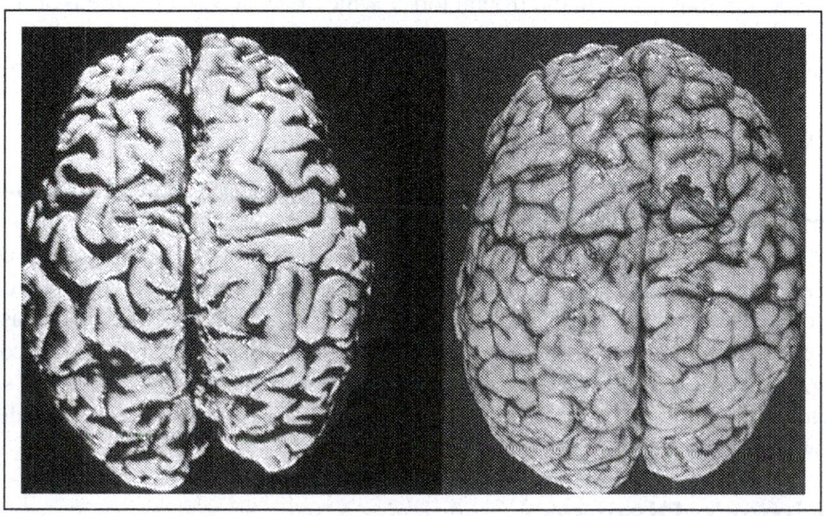

FIG. 16.13. Impact of Alzheimer's Disease on Brain Mass. Left: The brain of a patient who died with Alzheimer's disease. Right: The brain of a patient who was not suffering from Alzheimer's disease at the time of death. Anterior is to the top. (Courtesy of Dr. Javad Towfighi, Professor, Pennsylvania State University College of Medicine, Hershey, Pennsylvania.)

Neuronal damage in Alzheimer's disease follows a characteristic pattern. Neocortex and entorhinal cortex are the first and most severely affected areas, but substantial damage is also present in the hippocampus (CA1, CA2 fields). Neuronal damage in the entorhinal cortex and hippocampus is most likely responsible for the memory deficits that are hallmark of Alzheimer's disease. Other damage is present in the cholinergic nuclei of the ventral forebrain that project to the cerebral cortex: the nucleus basalis, the medial septal nucleus, and the diagonal band of Broca. Neural degeneration is also found in the amygdala, the locus ceruleus, and the raphe nuclei.

The memory deficits in Alzheimer's disease are caused by damage to the entorhinal cortex and the hippocampus.

Treatment and Prognosis. There is no cure for Alzheimer's disease. Medical care emphasizes alleviation of symptoms such as depression, delusions, hallucinations, agitation, and sleep disorders. Because some symptoms of Alzheimer's disease are probably caused by the loss of cholinergic innervation of the cerebral cortex and the hippocampus, several cholinesterase inhibitors have been approved as treatments. Cholinesterase inhibitors may offer short-term improvement of cognition, memory, and speech; unfortunately, these drugs do not stop disease progression. Survival time varies from a decade to as little as a few years if the patient is older than 80. Although death is usually caused by other unrelated age-related illnesses (e.g., heart attack, stroke), aspiration pneumonia is fairly common among these patients.

There is no cure for Alzheimer's disease.

RESOLUTION OF CLINICAL CASE

The dimple and tuft of hair are telltale signs of spina bifida. Because the mother was obese and diabetic and had previously delivered a child with a neural tube defect, this was a high-risk pregnancy. The folic acid supplement was a prudent precaution because neural tube defects form within 4 weeks of conception, before most women realize they are pregnant. For women whose fetuses are at high risk of neural tube defects, prenatal screening is usually performed. Prenatal blood tests can detect maternal levels of alpha-fetoprotein, a reliable marker for neural tube defects. If alpha-fetoprotein levels are high, the test is usually repeated on the amniotic fluid. Faulty closure of the vertebral arches can be detected prenatally with ultrasound. The postnatal imaging studies would confirm the diagnosis that the doctors in this case probably made prior to delivery. Many otherwise normal adults born with spina bifida occulta have no permanent neurological problems. In the more serious forms of spina bifida, the dura (meningocele) or dura plus either spinal nerves or spinal cord (meningomyelocele) herniate through the defective vertebral arch.

REVIEW QUESTIONS

Directions: For each of the following questions, choose the **one best** answer.

1. What neurologic defect is caused by failure of the anterior neuropore to close?
- **A.** Spina bifida
- **B.** Anencephaly
- **C.** Syringomyelia
- **D.** Meningomyelocele
- **E.** Hydrocephalus

2. All neurons in the CNS develop from precursor cells located where?
- **A.** Subventricular zone
- **B.** Neural crest
- **C.** Primitive streak
- **D.** Lamina terminalis
- **E.** Primary brain vesicles

3. Choose the temporal sequence that correctly describes the order in which the following structures emerge.
- **A.** Astrocytes, oligodendrocytes, neuroblasts, radial glial cells, neurons
- **B.** Oligodendrocytes, astrocytes, neuroblasts, radial glial cells, neurons
- **C.** Neuroblasts, neurons, radial glial cells, oligodendrocytes, astrocytes
- **D.** Radial glial cells, neuroblasts, neurons, astrocytes, oligodendrocytes
- **E.** Neurons, radial glia cells, astrocytes, oligodendrocytes, neuroblasts

4. Many areas of the brain mature during adolescence. Which one undergoes the largest transformation?
A. Somatosensory cortex
B. Cerebellum
C. Motor cortex
D. Prefrontal cortex
E. Visual cortex

5. How does early experience promote development of the central nervous system?
A. By triggering different critical periods
B. By signaling the end of primary neurulation
C. By releasing cell adhesion molecules
D. By facilitating neurogenesis
E. By pruning synapses

6. Neurogenesis occurs from cradle to grave in which of the following areas of the brain?
A. Cerebellum
B. Hippocampus
C. Hypothalamus
D. Neural crest
E. Neuroectoderm

7. Which of the following is an example of apoptosis?
A. Neural pruning
B. Synaptogenesis
C. Neural migration
D. Development of the radial glial lattice
E. Neurogenesis

8. What causes memory impairment in Alzheimer's disease?
A. Damage to the hippocampus and entorhinal cortex
B. Loss of myelin in the large fiber tracts of the forebrain
C. Neuron shrinkage and widened cortical sulci
D. Disruption of neurogenesis within the subventricular zone
E. Damage to the amygdala

ADDITIONAL READING

Classic Literature

Altman J, Das GD: Autoradiographic and histologic evidence of postnatal neurogenesis in rats. *J Comp Neurol* 124:319–335, 1965.

Erickson PS, Perfilieva E, Bjork-Eriksson T, Alborn AM, Nordborg C, Peterson DA, Gage FH: Neurogenesis in the adult human hippocampus. *Nat Med* 4:1313–1317, 1998.

Hamburger V, Levi-Montalcini R: Proliferation, differentiation, and degeneration in the spinal ganglia of the chick embryo under normal and experimental conditions. *J Exp Zool* 111:457–502, 1949.

Harlow HF: The nature of love. *Am Psychol* 13:673–685, 1958.

Hebb DO: *The Organization of Behavior: A Neurophysiological Theory*. New York, NY: John Wiley and Sons, 1949.

Hubel DH: Exploration of primary visual cortex: 1955–1978. *Nature* 299:515–524, 1982.

Hubel DH, Wiesel T: Binocular interaction in striate cortex of kittens reared with artificial squint. *J Neurophysiol* 28:1041–1059, 1965.

Kaplan MS, Hinds JW: Neurogenesis in the adult rat: electron microscopic analysis of light radioautographs. *Science* 197:1092–1094, 1977.

Penfield W: Neuroglia: normal and pathological. In: Penfield W, ed. *Cytology and Cellular Pathology of the Nervous System*. New York, NY: Hoeber, 1932:423–479.

Sperry RW: Effect of 180 degree rotation of the retinal field on visuomotor coordination. *J Exp Zool* 92:263–279, 1943.

Wiesel T: Postnatal development of the visual cortex and the influence of environment. *Nature* 299:582–591, 1982.

Reviews and Landmark Research Articles

Alvarez-Buylla A, Lois C: Neuronal stem cells in the brain of adult vertebrates. *Stem Cells* 13:263–272, 1995.

Dahl RE: Adolescent brain development: a period of vulnerabilities and opportunities. *Ann NY Acad Sci* 1021:1–122, 2004.

Giedd J, Blumenthalm J, Jeffries N, Castellanos F, Liu H, Zijdenbos A, Paus T, Evan A, Rapoport J: Brain development during childhood and adolescence: a longitudinal MRI study. *Nat Neurosci* 2:861–863, 1999.

Kempermann G: *Adult Neurogenesis*. New York, NY: Oxford University Press, 2006.

Kozorovitskiy Y, Gould E: Adult neurogenesis: a mechanism for brain repair. *J Clin Exp Neuropsych* 25:721–732, 2003.

Levi-Montalcini R: The nerve growth factor 35 years later. *Science* 237:1154–1162, 1987.

McConnell SK: The determination of neuronal fate in the cerebral cortex. *Trends Neurosci* 12:342–349, 1989.

Merzenich MM, Nelson RJ, Stryker MP, Cynader MS, Schoppmann A, Zook JM: Somatosensory cortical map changes following digit amputation in adult monkeys. *J Comp Neurol* 224:591–605, 1985.

Noctor SC, Flint AC, Weissman TA, Dammerman RS, Kriegstein AR: Neurons derived from radial glial cells establish radial units in neocortex. *Nature* 409:714–720, 2001.

Purves D, Lichtman W: Elimination of synapses in the developing nervous system. *Science* 210:153–157, 1980.

Rakic P: Neurogenesis in adult primate neocortex: an evaluation of the evidence. *Nat Rev Neurosci* 3:65–71, 2002.

Ralik P: Principles of neural cell migration. *Experientia* 46:882–891, 1990.
Reynolds BA, Weiss S: Generation of neurons and astrocytes from isolated cells of the adult mammalian central nervous system. *Science* 255:1707–1710, 1992.
Sanes DH, Reh TA, Harris WA: *Development of the Nervous System*. New York, NY: Academic Press, 2006.

INTERNET RESOURCES

Allyn and Bacon
Neurogenesis
http://www.abacon.com/pinel/hot_sept.html

Alzheimer's Association
www.alz.org

Alzheimer's Foundation of America
http://www.alzfdn.org

HD Lighthouse
Neurotrophins
http://www.hdlighthouse.org/research/drugs-supps/updates/1206neurotrophins.php

National Institute on Aging (NIA)
Alzheimer's Disease
http://www.nia.nih.gov/alzheimers

Society for Neuroscience
Axon Guidance, Brain Reorganization, Child Abuse and the Brain, Neural Migration
http://apu.sfn.org/index.cfm?pagename=brainBriefings_chrolongical

Spina Bifida Association
http://www.sbaa.org/site/PageServer?pagename=index

Stem Cell World
http://stemcellworld.tripod.com/index.html

Temple University
Neuroembryology
http://isc.temple.edu/neuroanatomy/lab/embryo_new/

Videohelp (David Boshell)
Neuroembryology
http://www.videohelp.com/~vitualis/med/Neuroembryology.html#top

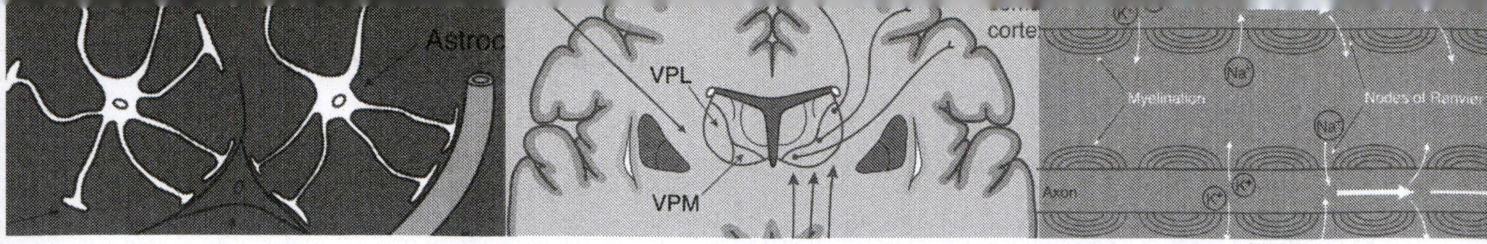

CHAPTER 17

Neural Basis of Anxiety and Depression

INTRODUCTION OF CLINICAL CASE

The husband of a 33-year-old woman was deeply concerned about his wife's health and mental attitude. A few months previously she had re-entered the job market when their youngest child entered grade school. Initially she was enthusiastic about her new job, but recent changes in her behavior indicated that something was wrong. She missed several days of work and had difficulty concentrating and performing routine tasks. Although she had a reputation as an outstanding cook, she no longer enjoyed cooking meals. In fact, she frequently expressed a lack of appetite at meal times and had lost a noticeable amount of weight. Even though she complained about being tired all the time, she did not sleep well at night. Her husband finally persuaded her to see her doctor. Except for her loss of weight, the doctor's physical examination found no remarkable health problems, and her hemoglobin, hematocrit, and blood cell counts were normal. The woman filled out a questionnaire used for psychiatric screening and, based on her answers, she was referred to a psychiatrist.

OVERVIEW

Anxiety, depression, and other mood disorders affect 20%–25% of the general population each year. Besides having a profound impact on the lifestyle of patients and their families, these disorders are associated with severe morbidity and mortality. Depression, for example, is the leading cause of suicide, yet nearly two-thirds of all depressed individuals do not receive treatment. This is unfortunate because more than 80% of depressed patients who receive proper treatment, including medication and/or psychotherapy, show clear signs of improvement within 6 weeks.

Most depressed patients show mood improvement after several weeks of pharmacotherapy and/or psychotherapy.

Consistent with the large number of people who are diagnosed with mood disorders each year, more than 10% of the prescriptions in the United States are for psychoactive medications that affect mood and related cognitive processes. Although mood disorders are often triggered by stressful events that surround daily life, pharmacotherapy has gained widespread clinical acceptance because of evidence indicating that these disorders are associated with disturbances in neurochemical regulation. Despite our knowledge of brain physiology and its relationship to psychiatric illness, several challenges remain in developing optimal therapeutic treatments. Foremost among these, the precise etiology of most mood disorders is poorly understood. Emotional states represent the product of interactions between psychosocial events and neurobiological mechanisms, but the precise role that these factors play in the development of psychiatric illness has not been elucidated. Furthermore, even though mental disorders are classified according to well-defined behavioral and psychological criteria, groups of patients with the same diagnosis are characterized by neurobiological heterogeneity. Consequently, optimal therapeutic approaches require the development of treatments that are tailored to each individual.

Patients with the same mood disorder may have different neurobiological profiles.

NEUROBIOLOGICAL CORRELATES OF MOOD DISORDERS

A neurobiological basis for mood disorders has been established by converging pieces of information from multiple disciplines within the basic and clinical neurosciences. Neuropathology, neuroradiology, psychopharmacology, and molecular genetics have all contributed to the view that anxiety, depression, and other mood disorders are linked to functional processes within the brain. Although the precise cause of most mood disorders is not known, our increased understanding of neuropathic physiology over the past two decades has significantly improved the diagnosis and treatment of depression, anxiety, and other emotional states.

The neurobiological factors that contribute to anxiety and depression are strongly tied to the limbic system and other neural structures that subserve emotion, cognition, and behavior. Thus, studies of patients with severe anxiety or depression have revealed functional-structural changes in the prefrontal cortex, the ventral striatum, the hippocampus, the amygdala, and multiple parts of the cingulate gyrus. These studies have also implicated the monoaminergic systems that modulate neuronal responses in the prefrontal cortex, basal ganglia, and related brain regions. In addition, the hypothalamic-pituitary-adrenal (HPA) axis plays a critical role in mediating responses to stressful life events, and the regulation of this system is often distorted in patients with a mood disorder.

Monoaminergic Involvement

The earliest hypothesis on the biological basis of depression emphasized the importance of monoaminergic transmission in the brain. This relationship was first reported in the 1950s by Edward Freis, who treated hypertensive patients with reserpine because this drug depletes noradrenergic nerve terminals of their neurotransmitter stores. Reserpine lowered the blood pressure of hypertensive individuals, but its prolonged use caused them to become psychologically depressed. This finding suggested that monoamines are necessary to maintain a normal mood state and, in the late 1950s, prompted the hypothesis that depression is caused by a deficiency in monoaminergic transmission.

Monoamine hypothesis of depression: Depression is produced by a deficiency in monoaminergic transmission.

Monoamines:
- Dopamine (DA)
- Norepinephrine (NE)
- Serotonin (5-HT)

Monoaminergic systems:
- Diffuse forebrain projections
- G-protein-coupled receptors
- Neuromodulatory functions

The monoamines, which include norepinephrine (NE), dopamine (DA), and serotonin (5-HT), are neurotransmitters for neurons whose cell bodies reside in a small number of compact brainstem nuclei such as the locus ceruleus (NE), the substantia nigra (DA), and the raphe nuclei (5-HT). Monoaminergic neurons comprise a limited number of neurons in the brain (less than 0.001%) but have highly divergent collateral projections that innervate widely separated brain regions (Figure 17.1). Unlike most projection systems that terminate densely within circumscribed neural targets, the monoaminergic systems have diffuse projections that innervate extensive parts of the cerebral cortex, neostriatum, nucleus accumbens, and limbic structures such as the amygdala and hippocampus. Consistent with these diffuse projection patterns, the monoaminergic systems do not transmit discrete bits of information, but act as neuromodulators that alter the responsiveness of their postsynaptic targets to other neural inputs. In contrast to neurotransmitters such as glutamate or GABA, which produce fast postsynaptic responses by interacting with ionotropic receptors, the monoamines interact with G-protein-linked (metabotropic) receptors that activate the neuron's metabolic machinery to produce slow, long-term changes in synaptic function (see Chapter 2).

Drugs that affect monoaminergic transmission produce well-known alterations in mood and emotional behavior. In general, pharmacologic agents that deplete NE or block its postsynaptic receptors induce depression and behavioral sedation, whereas those that promote noradrenergic transmission are behavioral stimulants. Acute use of drugs such as amphetamine and cocaine, which increase dopaminergic transmission, enhances psychomotor activity and produces an elevation in mood. Hence, the behavioral and emotional effects of these drugs are consistent with the monoamine hypothesis of depression.

Depressed patients do no exhibit consistent decreases in monoamine levels.

Monoaminergic depletion produces depression and sedation.

Monoaminergic stimulation produces behavioral stimulation.

After several years of clinical testing, however, the monoamine hypothesis was eventually discredited because depressed patients did not exhibit reliable and consistent decreases in their monoamine levels. The monoamine hypothesis was also discarded because antidepressants require several weeks of continuous use to produce their therapeutic benefits; hence, their clinical efficacy could not be due to the fact that they produced an immediate increase in monoaminergic transmission. Nonetheless, the clear relationship between monoamine depletion and the induction of clinical depression was pivotal in the development of the first generation of antidepressant drugs in the late 1950s. These drugs act primarily by increasing noradrenergic transmission, either by blocking the synaptic reuptake of NE or by inhibiting its degradative enzyme, monoamine oxidase (MAO). Drugs that act mainly by increasing dopaminergic transmission were also tested for their antidepressant qualities, but they have limited benefit because they induce insomnia, irritability, and other symptoms associated with depression.

Changes in serotonergic transmission have also been linked to the pathophysiology of mood disorders. Statistical comparisons indicate that, on average, the cerebrospinal fluid (CSF) levels of 5-HT and its metabolites tend to be lower in depressed patients than in normal control subjects. Furthermore, among individuals who have previously suffered a depressive episode, a subsequent depletion of tryptophan always causes another depressive cycle. Collectively, these findings led to the development of selective serotonin reuptake inhibitors (SSRIs), which are among the most efficacious of all antidepressant medications.

Neuroanatomical Correlates of Mood Disorders

Stroke-induced depression is associated with damage to the prefrontal cortex and the basal ganglia on the left side.

Structural imaging studies of stroke victims have consistently demonstrated a strong relationship between ischemic strokes in certain brain regions and the prevalence of depression. After many studies in the 1970s showed that approximately 40% of all stroke patients become depressed, computed tomography (CT) was first used in the early 1980s to determine whether stroke-induced depression is associated with damage to specific brain regions. Even though CT imaging has relatively crude resolution, this noninvasive imaging technique indicated that most stroke victims who became depressed were characterized by damage to the prefrontal cortex and basal ganglia on the left side. Subsequent studies that used the increased spatial resolution of magnetic resonance imaging (MRI) confirmed this finding.

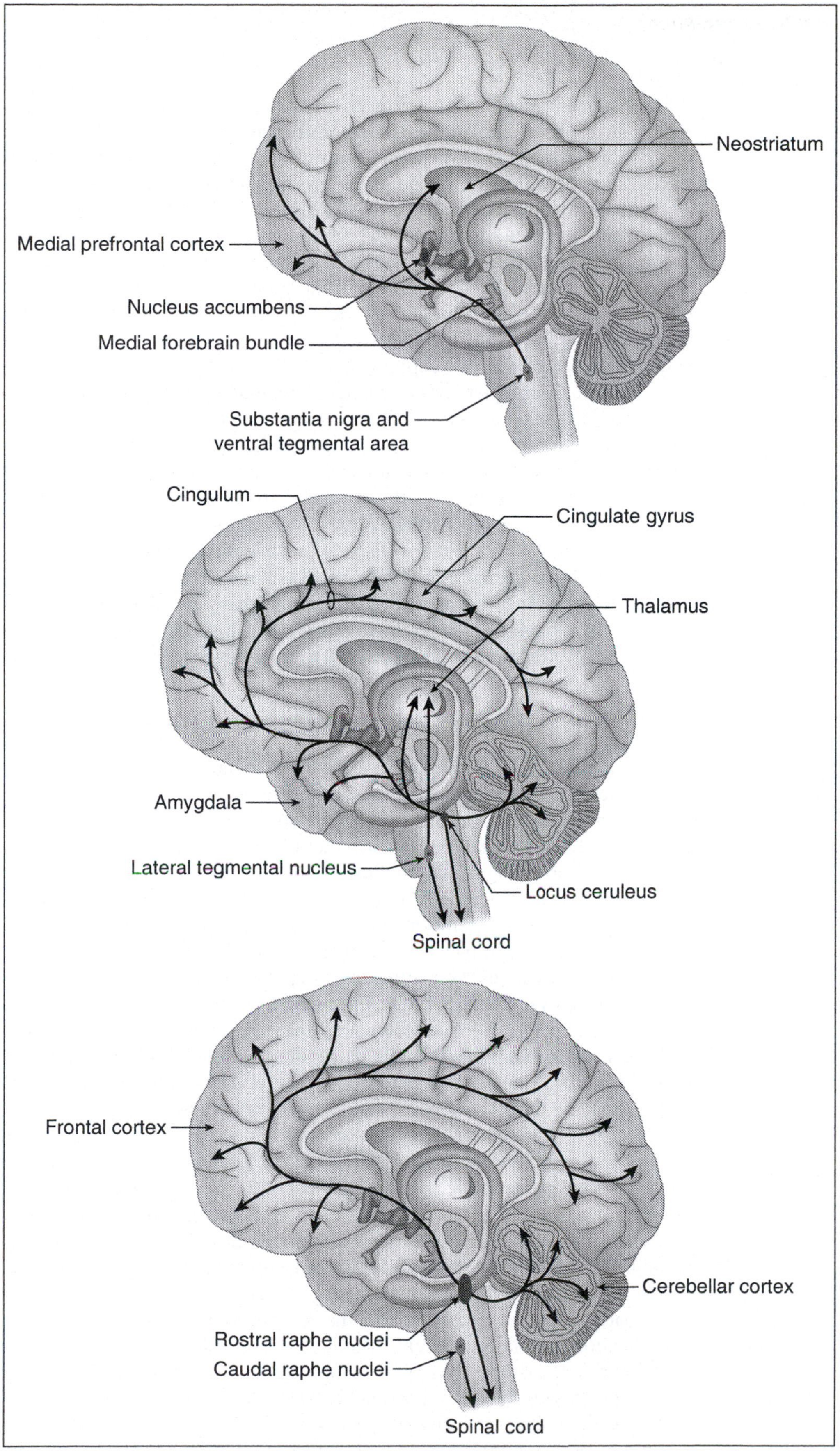

FIG. 17.1. Monoaminergic Regulation of Mood. Parasagittal diagrams of the dopaminergic (top), noradrenergic (middle), and serotonergic (bottom) pathways that regulate mood and arousal. Monoaminergic cell bodies are located in a small number of compact brainstem nuclei that project rostrally and innervate extensive parts of the forebrain. The dopaminergic pathways, which are critical for mediating reward, innervate fewer forebrain regions than the noradrenergic and serotonergic pathways. Additional noradrenergic and serotonergic pathways, which are not shown in this diagram, regulate the transmission of nociceptive information in the spinal cord.

Subsequent imaging studies of elderly patients who were depressed but had not suffered a stroke have also implicated the prefrontal cortex and basal ganglia. Late-onset depression is associated with larger ventricles, which suggests neuronal atrophy of the surrounding neural tissue including the basal ganglia. Lacunae or small pockets of fluid also appear in the basal ganglia of these patients. In addition, large numbers of small lesions are scattered throughout the white matter under the prefrontal cortex. Whereas lesions in the prefrontal cortex and basal ganglia are common in older people who do not suffer from depression, they are much more prevalent among those elderly individuals who are depressed. Furthermore, the topographic distribution of lesions in older, nonstroke patients who are depressed overlaps significantly with the neuropathology associated with post-stroke depression.

Stress-induced depression is associated with a smaller hippocampus and amygdala.

Structural imaging studies of younger individuals who are depressed have revealed abnormalities in the limbic system. For example, many patients with major depressive disorder have a noticeably smaller hippocampus and amygdala. In addition, depressed women who were victims of childhood abuse and had suffered from post-traumatic stress also have a smaller hippocampal volume. Both of these structural findings are probably related to the impact of stressful events on the HPA axis. Thus, stress increases secretion of corticotropin-releasing hormone (CRH) and cortisol, and many animal studies indicate that these glucocorticoids cause a decrease in hippocampal volume. Alternatively, the small hippocampal volume observed in some depressed individuals may represent a potential marker for vulnerability to depression. According to this view, a small hippocampus may represent a lack of the cognitive resources that are needed to manage stressful life events more effectively.

Functional Brain Changes Associated with Depression

Functional imaging enables visualization of regional changes in cerebral blood flow or glucose utilization.

Even though CT and structural MRI studies indicate that depression is often associated with structural abnormalities in the brain, the majority of depressive episodes are not linked to noticeable brain damage. In most instances, depression is associated with subtle changes in the functional mechanisms that mediate mood, emotion, and related cognitive processes. Such changes may include relative shifts in regional brain activity as well as more generalized changes in neural metabolism or neurotransmission. To assess these possibilities, positron emission tomography (PET) and other functional imaging techniques have been used to compare brain activation patterns in healthy subjects with those obtained from individuals who suffer from depression or anxiety. Most functional imaging techniques analyze changes either in regional cerebral blood flow (rCBF) or in glucose utilization, two physiologic parameters that are correlated with changes in neuronal activity. In addition, radioactive ligands that selectively bind to specific neurotransmitter receptors can be visualized to determine whether a mood disorder or subsequent pharmacotherapy has altered the density and distribution of these receptors.

Nearly all functional imaging studies of mood disorders have reported abnormal activity in the frontal cortex, basal ganglia, and limbic system, but many inconsistent results have also been reported. Although most of the discrepancies involve variations in the brain regions associated with a specific mood disorder, some involve opposite effects in the same brain region. For example, studies indicating that depression is associated with increased blood flow to one brain region have often been contradicted by reports showing decreased blood flow to the same region.

Apart from the technical factors that may account for such divergent results, patient classification is a major problem. Although depressed patients are classified according to strict behavioral criteria, the apparent homogeneous nature of their disorder may mask important underlying biological differences between individuals with the same diagnosis. Even a distinct category such as major depressive disorder can be further subdivided along a range of psychological and biological factors. For these reasons, most imaging studies on mood disorders have screened the subjects according to their family history, the inheritability of their disorder, their prior exposure to drugs and prescribed medications, as well as other factors. Conclusions derived from imaging studies conducted on well-defined, homogenous patient populations are considered to be the most reliable.

Longitudinal Imaging Studies. The earliest imaging studies of depression compared resting brain activity (i.e., rCBF) in normal subjects with the patterns observed in depressed patients. Unfortunately, this experimental design is not very sensitive for detecting possible changes in brain activity because rCBF may vary widely across both normal and depressed subjects. A within-subjects comparison, in which brain activity is measured in the same person in response to different manipulations, is more sensitive for detecting the effects of an experimental variable (e.g., a disease state) on rCBF.

Unfortunately, comparing functional brain images from the same individual before and after the onset of depression is usually not possible. Even if predepression images are obtained from individuals who have a high risk for depression, the interval between acquisition of the images (i.e., months or years) would raise doubts about whether the differences in brain activity were due to a change in mood state or other factors. In cases in which longitudinal imaging studies of depression have been conducted, brain activity was first visualized during the depressive episode and then subsequently when the patient's mood improved after using antidepressants or receiving other therapy. Both psychotherapy and the effects of antidepressants usually take several weeks to be effective, and the neural changes in that period represent both the improvement in mood state as well as other changes that might not be associated with resolution of the depression.

Mood disorders are often associated with functional abnormalities in the prefrontal cortex, the basal ganglia, and the limbic system.

Nonetheless, several studies indicate that a positive therapeutic outcome is highly correlated with changes in brain activity. The brain regions associated with improved mood vary across different studies, but such variation is consistent with a wide range of therapies (e.g., serotonin reuptake inhibitors, psychotherapy, electroconvulsive shock) that rely on different biological mechanisms for their effects. Despite this variation, studies that have directly compared the effects of antidepressants and psychotherapy have reported overlapping, but not identical, changes in brain activity. These studies suggest that depression is associated with abnormal activity in the prefrontal cortex and basal ganglia. Subsequent treatments with antidepressants or psychotherapy produced significant changes in these brain regions that were correlated with an improvement in mood. Some studies have also reported that mood improvement is associated with neural changes in the cingulate gyrus, the insula, and the inferior parts of the temporal lobe.

Effective treatment of depression is associated with functional changes in the prefrontal cortex and basal ganglia.

Emotional Provocation Studies. Many functional imaging studies have used "controlled provocation" to induce brain activity that simulates the neural responses to an emotional experience. In contrast to imaging studies that measure rCBF or metabolism when the subject is quietly resting and not engaged in a task, emotional provocation involves an explicit stimulus that evokes a specific mood state such as sadness or anxiety. In studies of depression, for example, subjects might be asked to recall a personal event that made them sad or, alternatively, might view a film clip that depicts a compelling tragedy. Using a within-subjects experimental design, rCBF or glucose metabolism is measured during alternate presentations of both emotional and neutral control stimuli. Hence, differences in neural activity during the two stimulus conditions indicate which brain regions are activated (or suppressed) during sadness and other experimentally induced moods.

Stimulus-induced sadness is linked to reciprocal changes in dorsal cortical (decreased CBF) and ventral limbic (increased CBF) brain regions.

In studies that have tested provocative stimuli on both normal and depressed individuals, the induction of transient sadness has produced comparable effects in both groups of subjects. Despite some discrepancies across studies, stimulus-induced sadness is usually associated with decreased blood flow to the dorsal lateral prefrontal and inferior parietal cortex. Simultaneously, blood flow also increases in multiple limbic regions including the amygdala, the hippocampus, the insula, and the ventral parts of the cingulate gyrus (Figure 17.2). Hence, in both normal and depressed individuals, sadness is correlated with reciprocal changes in blood flow to the dorsal cortical and ventral limbic regions of the brain. Successful treatments with antidepressant medications reverse this relationship during resting activity. Thus, in patients who recovered from depression, resting brain activity was significantly increased in the dorsal lateral prefrontal cortex but decreased in the ventral parts of the limbic system.

FIG. 17.2. **Neural Circuits That Regulate Mood.** Schematic diagram of the neural structures that regulate mood. Thin arrows represent connections that use the classical neurotransmitters, glutamate and GABA; thick arrows represent the neuromodulatory projections of the monoaminergic systems (DA, NE, and 5-HT). Brain regions that generally show increases or decreases in CBF during depression are indicated by plus and minus signs, respectively. GABA = γ-aminobutyric acid; DA = dopamine; NE = norepinephrine; 5-HT = serotonin; CBF = cerebral blood flow.

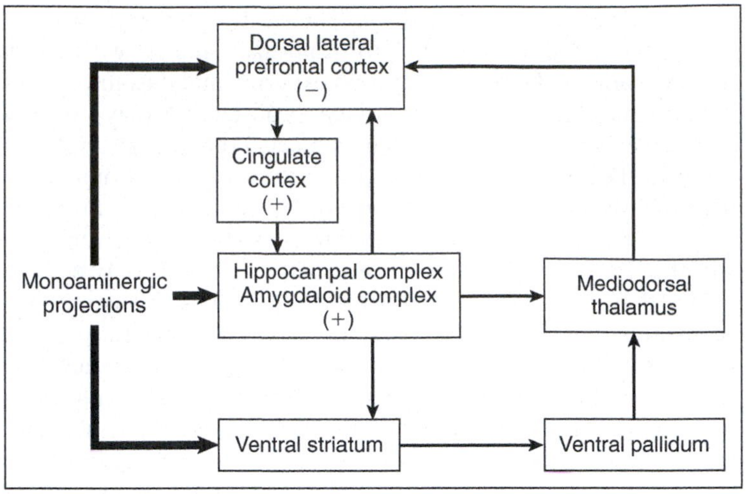

Stress and Depression

Stress precipitates depression in persons that are genetically predisposed to mood disorders.

Psychiatrists have long recognized that stressful life events may lead to depression, especially in persons with a family history of depression. Genetic susceptibility to environmental stressors has brought increased attention to the HPA axis and its role in mediating the acute and long-term biological responses to psychological stress (Figure 17.3). In addition, recent evidence suggests that stressful childhood experiences may cause persistent changes in the neuroendocrine system and related limbic circuits that sensitize people to subsequent stresses and increases their vulnerability to depression later in life. According to this view, persons with a genetic predisposition for depression are especially vulnerable to this sensitization.

FIG. 17.3. **Neuroendocrine System.** Schematic diagram that illustrates the neuroendocrine pathways responsible for secretion of several hormones from the brain and the periphery. The neuroendocrine system receives neural inputs from a variety of cortical and limbic pathways. This complex system is activated by physical and psychological stress, as well as by environmental factors such as circadian and seasonal rhythms. Adapted from RJ Hedaya: *Understanding Biological Psychiatry*. New York, NY: WW Norton & Co., 1996.

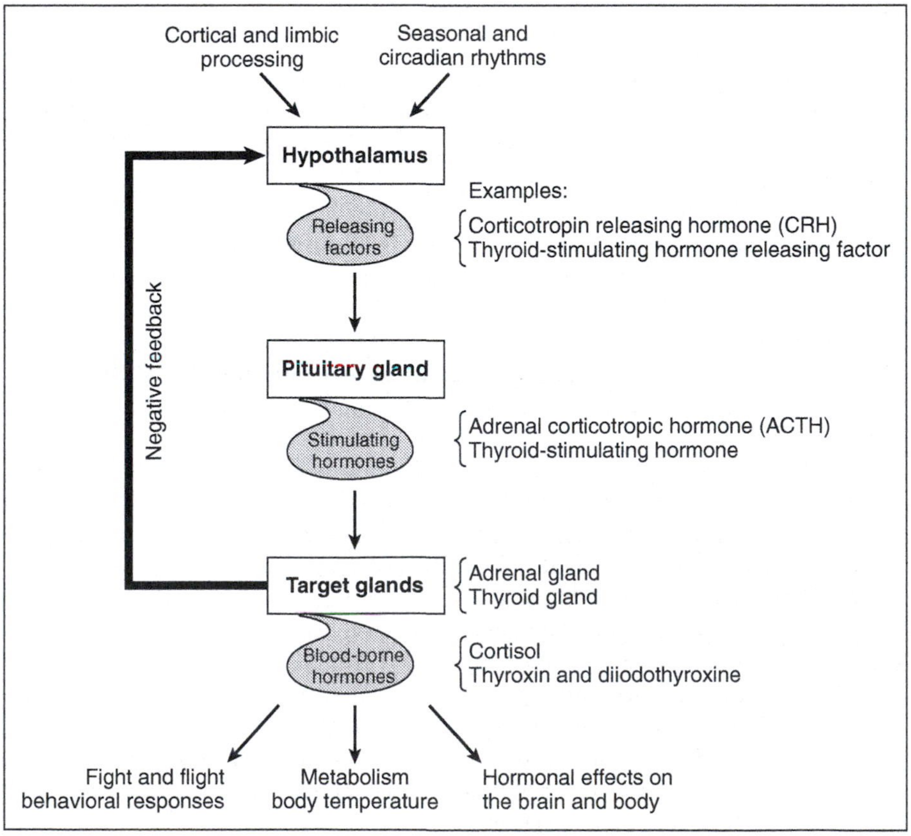

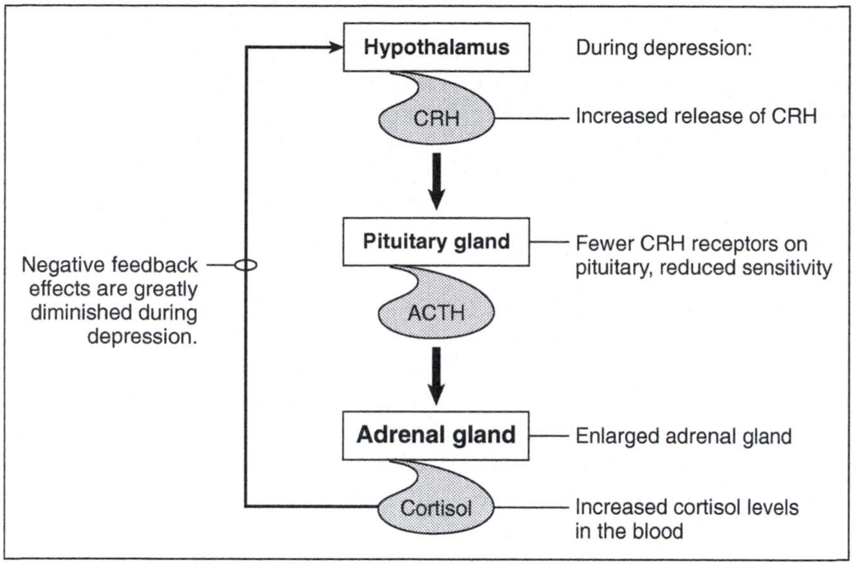

FIG. 17.4. Endocrine Responses Associated with Stress-Induced Depression. Neuroendocrine production of cortisol and other hormones is increased by chronic stress, which causes a decrease in the number of CRH (corticotropin-releasing hormone) receptors in the pituitary gland. ACTH = adrenocorticotropic hormone. Adapted from RJ Hedaya: *Understanding Biological Psychiatry*. New York, NY: WW Norton & Co., 1996.

In response to physical or psychological threats, the hypothalamus releases the neuropeptide CRH into the hypophysial portal system, which flows to the anterior pituitary gland (see Chapter 13 for a detailed review). Activation of CRH receptors in the pituitary stimulates the release of adrenocorticotropic hormone (ACTH) into the circulatory system, and this causes the adrenal glands to release cortisol, which has multiple actions on the brain and peripheral tissues. In addition, CRH-containing neurons and at least two classes of CRH receptors (i.e., CRH-R_1 and CRH-R_2) are found in multiple brain regions including the hypothalamus, amygdala, cerebral cortex, septal nuclei, and the bed nucleus of the stria terminalis. Neuropeptides such as CRH stimulate G-protein-coupled receptors that in turn initiate a cascade of chemical events that activate the synthesis of enzymes and other proteins needed to make membranes, receptors, and other structural components of the nervous system.

Stress and depression are associated with hyperactivity of the neuroendocrine system.

Several findings indicate that depression and other mood disorders are associated with chronic hyperactivity of the HPA axis (Figure 17.4). On average, depressed patients have higher concentrations of CRH in their CSF, but the number of CRH-R_1 receptors decreases. This result suggests that the increased levels of CRH cause the pituitary to synthesize fewer CRH-R_1 receptors. Such homeostatic mechanisms are common throughout the brain; synaptic changes in the concentration of a neurotransmitter or neuropeptide frequently cause an inverse effect on the number of receptors produced by the target cell. Nonetheless, even though the pituitary gland of a depressed person has fewer CRH-R_1 receptors, CRH is sufficiently elevated to cause an increase in the release of ACTH, and this activates the adrenal gland, which becomes enlarged and increases its production of cortisol. Increases in the amount of cortisol in the circulation should lead to negative feedback in the hypothalamus, but unfortunately it does not in depressed patients (see Figure 17.4). Instead, the effect of cortisol on the hypothalamus is reduced because the number of cortisol receptors in the hypothalamus declines in response to the chronically high levels of cortisol in the circulation.

In rats, maternal separation sensitizes the HPA axis to subsequent stimuli during adulthood.

Animal Model of Stress and Depression. Many animal studies suggest that early stressful experiences can sensitize the HPA axis and increase the vulnerability for depression in adulthood. For example, removing neonatal rat pups from their mothers leads to physiological and behavioral changes that parallel many of the clinical observations of depression. When compared with control animals, adult rats that endured maternal separation during the neonatal period show significant increases in plasma ACTH when they are startled by unexpected stimuli such as loud noises or sudden puffs of air. These animals also exhibit increased CRH concentrations in the locus ceruleus, hypothalamus, and amygdala, as well as decreased CRH receptor binding in the pituitary gland. These effects are observed only in those adult rats in which maternal separation occurred within a critical period, usually the first 2 weeks after birth. Maternal separation after that period does not cause a subsequent increase in the stress response of adult rats.

Maternal deprivation also alters other neural systems in ways that have a measurable impact on affective behavior. Maternal separation reduces the expression of both 5-HT_{1b} and $GABA_A$ receptors, as well as the expression of the DA transporter molecule. Consistent with an impaired DA reward system, maternal separation reduces consumption of sucrose, which normal rats readily ingest. This is significant because reduced food consumption and a decrease in behaviors associated with pleasurable experiences are hallmarks of human depression. Moreover, adults rats separated from their mothers early in life avoid spending time in open fields. Open field avoidance, which is a sign of anxiety in animals, is consistent with the reduction in 5-HT and GABA receptors that is produced by maternal deprivation. Antidepressants effectively reverse these anxiety-like behaviors and other changes that are evoked by maternal deprivation. Thus, antidepressant treatments restore sucrose consumption and reduce the CSF concentrations of CRH as well as the plasma levels of ACTH. Collectively, these results indicate that excessive activation of the HPA axis during early development has long-term consequences on behavior and its neurobiological correlates.

Clinical Studies of Stress and Depression. Depressed patients exhibit responses that are highly similar to the physiological changes observed in adult animals that have experienced maternal separation during early development. Thus, clinical depression is often associated with increased CSF concentrations of CRH and cortisol, as well as increased plasma levels of cortisol. Depressed patients show increases in the expression of CRH mRNA and a down-regulation (i.e., lower number and/or lower affinity) of CRH receptors in the pituitary. These parallel findings suggest that the physiological changes associated with human depression might be mediated by the same neuroendocrine mechanisms that were activated in rats by neonatal maternal separation.

> Childhood abuse produces changes in the neuroendocrine system that persist throughout life.

Several studies by Charles Nemeroff support this view. In one study, plasma levels of cortisol and ACTH were measured before, during, and after a stress test in which each subject delivered a public speech and then performed a difficult arithmetic problem. The subjects consisted of 4 groups of adult women: (1) healthy, normal adult women, (2) depressed women with no history of abuse, (3) non-depressed women who were abused as children, and (4) women who were depressed and had been abused as children. As shown in Figure 17.5, depressed women who were victims of child abuse showed increases in ACTH and cortisol that were larger than in the other groups. Furthermore, the mild responses in depressed women who were not abused as children were similar to those seen in the control subjects. This suggests that the large cortisol increases in the two groups of abused women were due to persistent neuroendocrine changes that were initiated by childhood stress and not by the depression itself.

In a subsequent study of the same women, CRH was administered intravenously to evoke an increase in plasma levels of ACTH. Although this CRH challenge produced a normal increase in ACTH in the normal, non-depressed subjects, the ACTH responses were significantly reduced in women who were depressed, regardless of their childhood history. More importantly, the cortisol response to ACTH stimulation was also diminished in women who were abused as children but were not depressed. Consistent with the view that childhood stress has a long-lasting impact on the reactivity of the neuroendocrine system, other studies have reported that adverse experiences during childhood are the most important variable for predicting high levels of CRH in the CSF.

> Stressful events during childhood change the neuroendocrine responses to stress in adulthood.

These neuroendocrine studies have significant clinical implications for understanding mood disorders. For some individuals, the physiological changes accompanying depression are influenced by stressful events that were first experienced during childhood or adolescence. According to this view, early life stressors cause the neuroendocrine system to produce excessive CRH, ACTH, and cortisol that leads to permanent structural changes in the nervous system, including a decrease in the number of CRH receptors in

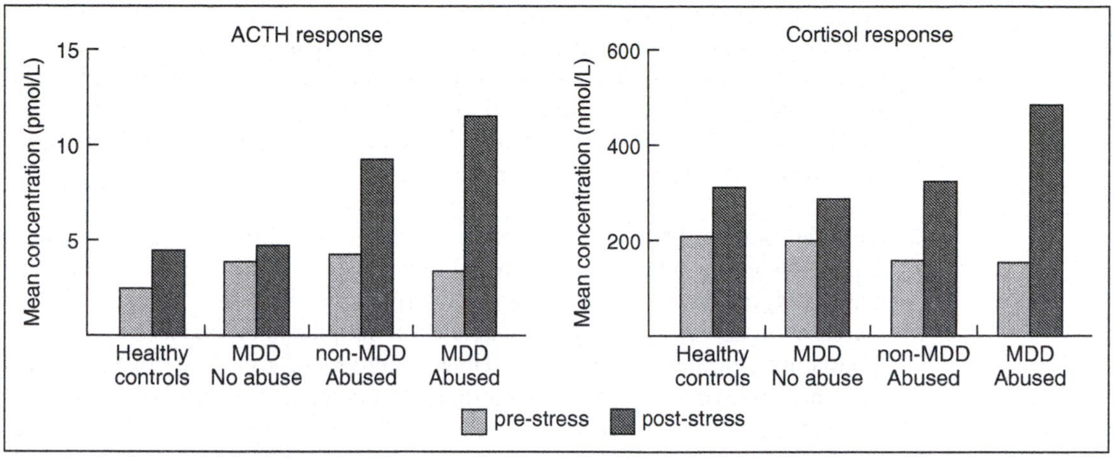

FIG. 17.5. Effects of Early Abuse on Endocrine Responses to Stress. Plasma levels of ACTH and cortisol were measured at 15-minute intervals from women who suffered experimental stress induced by public speaking and an arithmetic problem. Only the responses recorded immediately before the stress (pre-stress) and at the end of the 30-minute stressful period (post-stress) are shown. The subjects were divided into four groups: (1) no depression and no childhood abuse (healthy controls), (2) major depressive disorder and no abuse (MDD—no abuse), (3) no depression and childhood abuse (non-MDD—abused), and (4) major depressive disorder and childhood abuse (MDD—abused). Bar graphs based on data appearing in Heim, et al: Pituitary-adrenal axis responses to stress in women after sexual and physical abuse in childhood. *JAMA* 284:592–597, 2000.

the pituitary. Later, when the adult system is challenged by stressful events that cause a release of CRH, the ensuing production of ACTH and cortisol is greatly diminished because fewer CRH receptors are available to initiate the normal biochemical cascade of events.

These results have prompted additional research into the best treatments for depression and anxiety. In one study, for example, depressed patients were randomly assigned to three treatment groups: (1) antidepressants alone, (2) psychotherapy alone, and (3) a combination of antidepressants and psychotherapy. Whereas half the patients in the first two groups showed mood improvement, the combination of medication and psychotherapy helped three-fourths of the patients in the last group. These results were more easily interpreted, however, when the patient outcomes were analyzed with respect to their childhood experiences. For those individuals who had suffered stress during childhood (i.e., parental loss, neglect, or physical or sexual abuse), psychotherapy alone was more effective than antidepressant treatment alone and was nearly as effective as the combination of both therapies. This finding highlights the importance of using patient history to determine the most appropriate therapy for treating a mood disorder.

Inheritability of Depression

Although depression is not linked to a specific genetic defect like Huntington's disease, several lines of research indicate that depression has some degree of inheritability. A genetic basis for mood disorders was long suspected because depression and suicide are more prevalent in certain families. A meta-analysis of multiple twin studies indicates that the inheritability of major depressive disorder is 0.33, which means that if one twin becomes depressed the other twin has a 33% chance of developing depression. Additional studies have suggested that the inheritability of depression is greater among women than among men, which corresponds with the greater prevalence of depression among females in the general population.

A family history of mood disorders is a strong predictor for depression.

In contrast to Huntington's disease, which is expressed independently of environmental conditions, the phenotypic expression of depression is strongly influenced by psychosocial stress and other environmental events (e.g., financial circumstances, job loss).

The family environment is especially important, as indicated by many studies showing a correlation between familial dysfunction and the incidence of depression. Moreover, the likelihood of depression is strongly related to an interaction between adverse life events and a genetic susceptibility to mood disorders. Hence, individuals with a genetic vulnerability for developing a mood disorder may not show any signs of depression until they are confronted with stressful circumstances.

Genetic Mechanisms of Depression. The genetic influence on the vulnerability to depression could be exerted by several mechanisms. For example, slight changes in the genetic expression of the regulatory pathways that control neurotransmission could easily increase or decrease the synthesis, release, reuptake, or metabolism of one or more monoaminergic neurotransmitters. Hence, subtle shifts in the polygenetic regulation of these processes could produce deleterious effects on the regulation of mood, cognition, or other aspects of consciousness.

In the case of depression, the main neurotransmitter candidates likely to be affected by aberrant genes are NE and 5-HT. In fact, recent evidence suggests that polymorphism in the serotonin transporter (SERT) allele contributes to the genetic vulnerability for developing depression. Beginning in the 1980s, several studies reported that 5-HT reuptake is lower in the blood platelets of depressed patients and that this trait has a high degree of concomitance across monozygotic twins. Subsequent work indicated that the SERT allele exists in several forms, most commonly as a short "S" allele or as a long "L" allele, which differ by the number of repeated elements in the promoter region. The S and L forms yield different amounts of mRNA and, ultimately, the S form is associated with less of the serotonin transporter than the L form.

When an S allele is present in the SERT gene, vulnerability to depression increases.

Strong evidence for the involvement of the SERT gene in the expression of depression comes from a longitudinal study in which 847 individuals were examined at regular intervals between the ages of 3 and 26. The subjects were assessed according to their history of stressful events (related to finances, employment, health, interpersonal relationships, sexual and physical abuse, etc.) and by whether they suffered from one or more depressive episodes including attempted suicide. The results showed that stressful events during childhood were valid predictors of depression and suicide attempts in adulthood, but only for those individuals who had one or two S alleles for the SERT gene. Hence, the presence of the short allele of the SERT gene increases the vulnerability to depression for those adults who suffered stressful experiences during childhood.

These data do not mean that the SS form of the SERT gene causes depression, but that persons with the SS alleles are less equipped to deal with stress. Hence, for some people, depression represents the psychological outcome of an interaction between genetic vulnerability (SS alleles) and the environment (psychosocial stress). This view is consistent with data showing that mice with the SS alleles show greater stress-induced production of ACTH than mice with the LL alleles. Furthermore, rhesus monkeys that have the SS alleles show large reductions in CSF levels of the 5-HT metabolite, 5-hydroxy indole acetic acid (5-HIAA), but only when they are subjected to experimental stress. This latter result suggests that the stress-induced effects of the S allele are manifested, in part, by a decrease in serotonergic transmission.

Potential Markers of Mood Disorders: Endophenotypes

There is no physiological marker for depression.

Endophenotype: an endogenous or internal trait associated with a specific psychiatric illness

The neurochemical specificity of clinically effective antidepressants, as well as the inheritability of depression, has prompted a search for biological markers that could be used to diagnose this disorder. Unfortunately, even though mood disorders are correlated with certain biological profiles, there are no genetic, biochemical, or neuroanatomical markers that definitively identify those patients suffering from a specific mood disorder. Nonetheless, because some inheritable traits are associated with certain mental disorders, research on the biological basis of psychiatric illness has focused on identifying those endogenous traits or endophenotypes that might represent clues about the neurobiological mechanisms that underlie a specific psychiatric disorder.

Endophenotypes can be neurophysiological, biochemical, neuroanatomical, or cognitive in nature. An endophenotype does not represent a direct symptom of the disorder, but indicates a characteristic trait that is prevalent among patients who have been diagnosed with the disorder. Thus, the small hippocampal volume and other structural brain abnormalities observed in many depressed individuals represent examples of endophenotypes for major depression disorder. Because each endophenotype represents a single biological phenomena, the number of genes that regulate a particular endophenotype is fewer than those that influence a complete psychiatric entity. Hence, endophenotypic analysis represents a reductionistic approach for elucidating the biological processes that might contribute to the etiology of a specific psychiatric disorder.

Several potential endophenotypes have been identified for depression. Among the neurobiological parameters that have been proposed as potential endophenotypes for depression, those that have gained the most attention include changes in rapid eye movement (REM) sleep, structural and functional changes in the brain (see above), serotonergic dysfunction, and changes in the neuroendocrine system.

Sleep Cycles. Mood disorders are marked by obvious disruptions in sleep patterns that are characterized by diminished sleep, excessive sleep, or periods in which sleep is altogether absent (e.g., during the manic phase of bipolar disorder). One potential sign of clinical depression is indicated by the observation that depressed patients enter REM sleep more quickly than normal individuals (see Chapter 15 for a description of sleep stages). In addition, depressed patients have significantly less slow-wave sleep, as indicted by a deficit in non-REM sleep in stages 3 and 4. When depressed patients are successfully treated with a combination of antidepressants and psychotherapy, their electroencephalogram (EEG) sleep patterns return to normal. However, even though abnormal shifts in the distribution of REM and non-REM activity are often associated with depression, polysomnography (i.e., EEG sleep recording) is rarely used as a diagnostic tool because of the large variation in sleep responses that exist across both normal and depressed individuals. Hence, even though there are group differences in sleep behaviors between depressed and normal subjects, a quantitative measure of REM latency or other sleep parameters cannot identify an individual suffering from depression.

Serotonergic Markers. The intention to commit suicide represents an extreme psychological state and requires immediate psychiatric intervention. Hence, a definitive marker for this state would be very beneficial, and this has prompted studies of individuals who have attempted suicide. Compared to normal control subjects, suicidal patients have lower concentrations of 5-HIAA in their CSF and a higher concentration of 5-HT receptors on their blood platelets. Because neurons and other cells dynamically regulate the number of their neurotransmitter receptors in response to fluctuations in transmitter concentration, an increase in 5-HT receptors may represent a decline in serotonergic transmission. Although these findings initially suggested that a "suicide marker" may exist, other studies have found that individuals who committed homicide also have decreased levels of 5-HIAA in their CSF. This has prompted the view that increased aggressiveness, directed inward or outward, is associated with a decline in serotonergic transmission. In any event, 5-HIAA levels in both healthy and depressed subjects are highly variable; although group differences exist, there is no subthreshold value of 5-HIAA that reliably identifies a depressed individual.

Neuroendocrine Responses. As stated earlier, stressful psychosocial events have an impact on the neuroendocrine system, which consists of the hypothalamus, pituitary, and target glands in the periphery (see Figure 17.3). Because stress is often a contributing factor in the etiology of depression, changes in hormonal regulation may provide a potential marker for identifying a depressed person. This view has been supported by studies showing that CRH levels in the CSF are, on average, higher in depressed individuals. Furthermore, suicide victims and others suffering from severe depression have larger and heavier adrenal glands that can be detected by CT scans, presumably because the adrenal glands

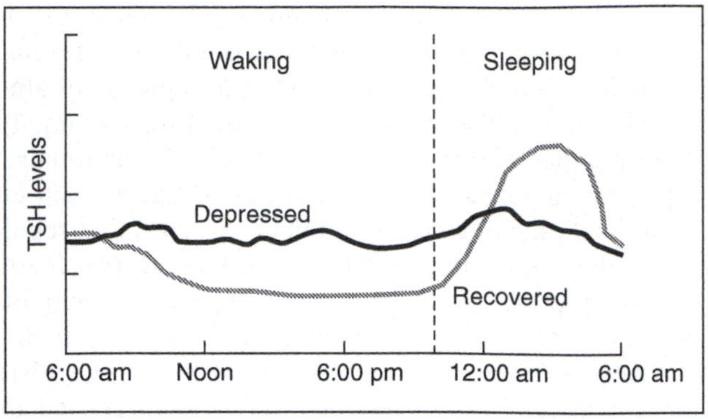

FIG. 17.6. Effect of Depression on Circadian TSH Secretions. The secretion of TSH from the pituitary gland normally fluctuates with the sleep-waking cycle. In depressed individuals, however, fluctuations in TSH are noticeably flattened. Following recovery from depression, the TSH cycle is restored to normal. Adapted from Souetre, et al: Twenty-four-hour profiles of body temperature and plasma TSH in bipolar patients during depression and during remission and in normal control subjects. *Amer J Psychiat* 145:1133–1137,1988.

become overactive and produce more cortisol in response to the increased release of CRH and ACTH (see Figure 17.4).

Cortisol production is not suppressed by dexamethasone in chronically depressed persons.

Dysfunctional neuroendocrine regulation can be determined by the dexamethasone suppression test (DST). In normal individuals, administration of a small dose of the steroid dexamethasone causes a decrease in the level of cortisol that can be detected in the blood 12 hours later. In approximately half of the patients suffering from severe depression, however, cortisol levels are not suppressed by dexamethasone administration. In these depressed individuals, vasopressin becomes the primary controller of the HPA axis, but the effect of vasopressin on cortisol production is not influenced by dexamethasone. Although the DST was studied as a possible diagnostic test for depression, subsequent studies indicate that cortisol suppression occurs in nondepressed individuals who are suffering from Cushing's disease, eating disorders, dementia, or other problems. Although there is no clear cutoff value for using the DST in the diagnosis of depression, additional findings suggest that the DST might be a sensitive indicator for persistent depression.

Depressed individuals also exhibit signs of hormonal dysfunction that are linked to sleep-wake cycles and other physiological rhythms. Consistent with the regulation of the hypothalamus and pituitary by seasonal and circadian rhythms (see Figure 17.3), most people exhibit daily patterns in body temperature and in the production of thyroid stimulating hormone (TSH). In depressed individuals, however, these daily cycles are significantly flattened (Figure 17.6). Successful treatment of depression with medications and/or psychotherapy restores the circadian changes in body temperature and TSH to their normal amplitudes.

THERAPEUTIC APPROACHES TO MOOD DISORDERS

Effective treatment of many mood disorders, especially depression, relies predominantly on psychoactive medications, psychotherapy, or a combination of medications and psychotherapy. Mood disorders are often treated successfully by pharmacologic intervention alone, but psychoactive drugs do not remove stress or other environmental factors that may contribute to the psychiatric illness. For this reason, psychotherapy is often used to help patients develop the cognitive and behavioral skills necessary to identify and resolve the issues that contributed to their illness. Psychotherapy is also beneficial in helping family members cope with the patient's illness.

Psychotherapy

Psychotherapy has a powerful effect on the nervous system even though it does not involve any direct physiological manipulation of the brain. Although psychotherapy has been used at least since the time of Freud, its potential for treating clinically depressed patients was not fully appreciated until the 1960s when Martin Seligman conducted a series of behavioral experiments on animal learning. His model of learned helplessness, which is widely recognized as the first animal model of depression, provides a compelling rationale for using behavioral and cognitive techniques to improve the functional status of depressed patients.

In his landmark study, Seligman placed three dogs in separate cages. The first dog that received electric shocks had been trained to perform a response that would turn the electric shock off. Electric shocks were also administered to a second dog, but this dog could not turn them off. Because the second dog did not have control over the shocks, it became depressed as indicated by immobility, whimpering, and other changes in its temperament. The third dog did not receive any shocks. In the second phase of the experiment, each dog was placed in a two-compartment enclosure in which the dog could move from one compartment to the other by jumping over a small hurdle. When each dog was shocked in one of the two compartments, it could escape the shock by jumping into the adjacent compartment. The second dog in the group, which had received inescapable shocks in the first phase of the study, never learned to escape the shock by jumping between compartments. Instead it remained immobile, showed no appetite, and developed abnormal sleep patterns and other behaviors. The other two dogs, however, quickly learned to jump over the hurdle to escape the shocks.

Depression may represent conditioned responses to uncontrolled, unpleasant events.

Based on these results, Seligman inferred that the second dog learned that it was unable to escape from shock in the first phase of the experiment and had generalized this helplessness to shocks occurring in the second phase of the experiment. Seligman tried to reverse this learned behavior in the third phase of the experiment by shocking the helpless dog and then carrying it to the safe compartment. After a few hundred trials in which the dog was shocked and then carried over the hurdle to the other compartment, the dog began jumping between the two compartments after receiving a shock. Although the dog eventually learned to escape the shock, it still exhibited helpless behaviors at certain times. This suggests that the dog's earlier experience with inescapable shock had altered its neural circuits and had partially interfered with its ability to learn new avoidance behaviors. In later studies, Seligman showed that he could prevent learned helplessness from developing by giving dogs experience in controlling their environment before the experiment began.

These animal studies are clinically significant for several reasons. First, they illustrate the concept of helplessness as a learned behavior. Unpleasant and uncontrollable events may elicit the belief that any action is futile and, faced with this inevitable outcome, the only appropriate course is to give up. Second, these studies demonstrate that behavioral conditioning can help reverse or prevent learned helplessness. Hence, a major aim of psychotherapy is to help depressed patients resolve their sense of helplessness by identifying the source of this belief and then determining the appropriate set of behaviors that will enable them to gain control and solve their problems.

Psychotherapy alters learned behaviors such as helplessness.

Psychotherapy and Functional Imaging. Direct comparison of the effects of psychotherapy and antidepressants on depression and other mood disorders has revealed that both types of therapy can be effective as judged by psychiatrists using the Hamilton Depression Rating Scale to assess the psychological and behavioral status of their patients. In fact, when both therapies are used in combination to treat depression, clinical efficacy usually increases. Such results have prompted an analysis of the effects of psychotherapy on brain activity to determine whether therapeutic effectiveness is associated with consistent changes in brain state.

When healthy, nondepressed subjects are asked to remember negative events and evaluate them in a more positive light, this experience is associated with an improved attitude about the event. In most imaging studies, this experience is associated with increased blood flow to the dorsal prefrontal cortex and decreased blood flow to the amygdala and orbitofrontal cortex. This is consistent with imaging studies showing a reciprocal relationship between these brain regions in which stimulus-induced sadness increases blood flow to the limbic brain regions and other ventral cortical areas, but decreases blood flow to the dorsal prefrontal cortex (see Figure 17.2). Together, these findings suggest that psychotherapy might exert its effect by increasing neural activity in brain regions associated

Psychotherapy alters brain activity.

with positive affect (dorsal prefrontal cortex) while decreasing it in regions associated with negative affect (limbic and ventral cortical areas).

Brain activity is altered in different ways by psychotherapy and pharmacotherapy.

Subsequent functional imaging studies have examined the effects of different psychotherapeutic approaches and compared them directly with the effects of pharmacotherapy. In one study, for example, one half of the depressed patients received psychotherapy and the other half received antidepressant medications. Both patient groups in this study were similar in their psychological and behavioral profiles, and both psychotherapy and pharmacotherapy were equally effective in treating depression. Contrary to most predictions, however, psychotherapy decreased the amount of activity in the dorsal prefrontal cortex and increased the activity in the ventral limbic and paralimbic regions (i.e., amygdala, hippocampus, and ventral cortical areas). This result was consistently produced by different psychotherapeutic methods (i.e., cognitive-behavioral therapy and interpersonal therapy). Antidepressants and psychotherapy were equally efficacious in terms of behavioral and psychological outcomes, but they did not produce identical changes in brain activity. Compared to psychotherapy, the effects of antidepressant medications on brain activity were more variable. In general, antidepressants activated the prefrontal cortex and basal ganglia, but suppressed the hippocampus, parahippocampal regions, and cingulate cortex. These results suggest that psychotherapy and antidepressants achieve their psychotherapeutic effects through different brain mechanisms.

Anxiety is associated with activation of the amygdala.

Behavioral treatments for anxiety disorders use behavioral desensitization to reduce patient fears to anxiogenic stimuli. Data from both animal and human studies indicate that fear is dependent on neural processing in the amygdala and ventral prefrontal cortex. In animals, for example, lesions of these regions prevent fear conditioning. Similarly, in humans, imaging studies have shown that conditioned fear responses are associated with activation of the amygdala. Hence, to the extent that psychotherapeutic intervention has a measurable impact on specific parts of the brain, desensitization and other anxiety treatments should suppress activation of the limbic system.

Both psychotherapy and pharmacotherapy reduce anxiety-induced activation of the limbic system.

Psychotherapy and pharmacotherapy are both used to reduce anxiety. Imaging studies that examined the neural correlates of anxiety have reported that fear of public speaking as well as phobic responses to spiders are both associated with activation of the amygdala, hippocampus, and surrounding parahippocampal regions. Direct comparisons of anxiolytics and psychotherapy indicate that successful treatment of fear and anxiety by either approach is associated with suppression of the ventral limbic and paralimbic regions.

Electroconvulsive Therapy

ECT is safe and effective for treating severe depression.

First used in 1934 to treat psychosis, electroconvulsive therapy (ECT) is an effective and safe method for treating depression and other mood disorders such as mania. The application of bilateral electric shocks to the temples produces grand mal seizure activity, which alleviates both depressive mood and suicidal ideation. Generally, ECT is administered in multiple sessions over a few weeks to be optimally effective. Although most theories concerning its mode of action have focused on increases in the synaptic release and turnover of catecholamines, GABA, or neuropeptides, the exact mechanism by which ECT elevates mood remains unclear. Because ECT has a stigma for both patients and physicians, it is generally considered to be the therapy of last resort and is used most frequently for patients who need a rapid medical response because they are suicidal or in extremely poor health. Approximately 100,000 patients in the United States with mood disorders are treated annually with ECT; the primary side effects are short-term confusion and loss of memory for events occurring around the time of ECT.

Pharmacotherapy: Antidepressants

Antidepressants increase monoaminergic transmission, but depressed patients do not show consistent decreases in monoamine levels or their receptors.

The initial discovery of antidepressants and their effectiveness in treating depression supported the view that this disorder might be caused by a deficiency in monoaminergic transmission. Subsequent clinical studies, however, failed to confirm this hypothesis. Thus, monoamine levels and their receptors are not consistently lower in depressed

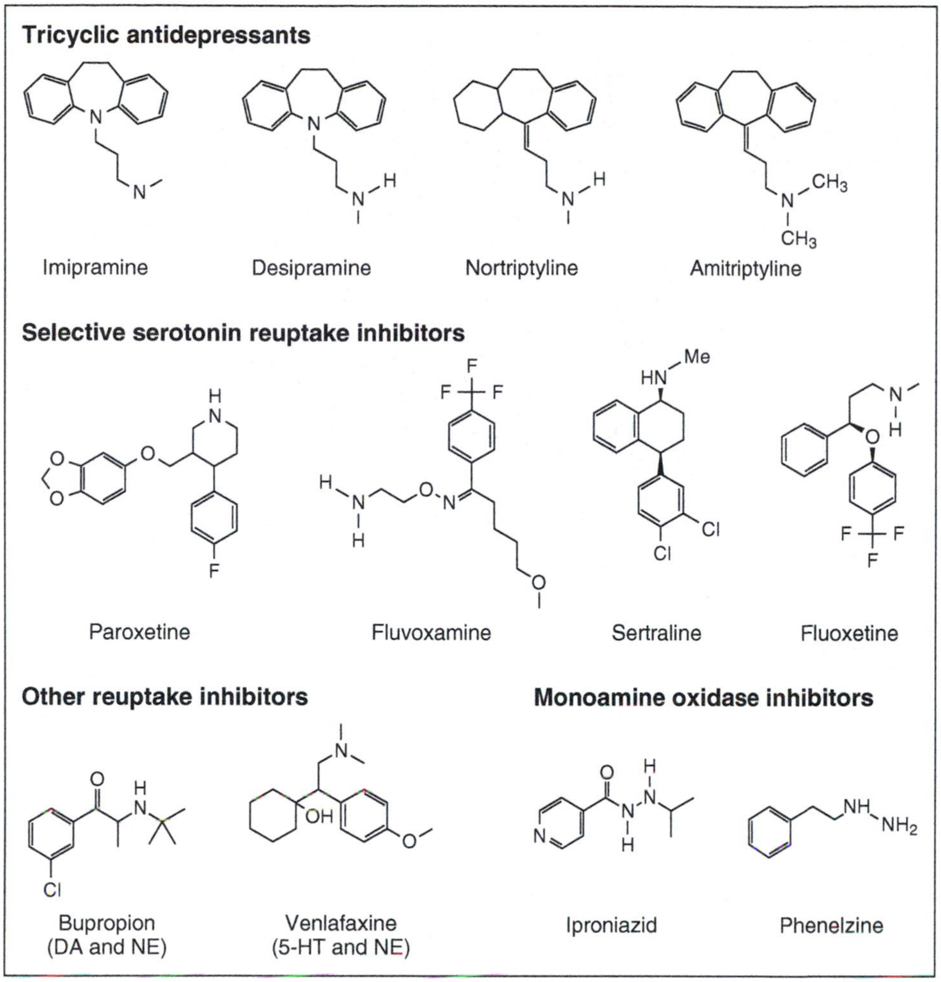

FIG. 17.7. Molecular Structure of Different Classes of Antidepressants. Tricyclic antidepressants have three contiguous carbon rings. By comparison, the molecular configurations of antidepressants that block 5-HT (serotonin) reuptake or inhibit MAO (monoamine oxidase) are more variable. DA = dopamine; NE = norepinephrine.

individuals than in control subjects. Despite this lack of a compelling biological explanation for the cause of depression, extensive clinical experience indicates that between 55% and 65% of all depressed individuals show improvement in mood following treatment with antidepressants alone. By comparison, the efficacy rate for placebo controls is usually no better than 15% to 20%.

Antidepressants were discovered serendipitously in 1951 when iproniazid, an MAO inhibitor, was used to treat patients with tuberculosis and was found to have mood-elevating properties. Since then, many antidepressants have been identified that increase neurotransmission at monoaminergic synapses. Different classes of antidepressants are named according to their mode of action (MAO inhibitors or SSRIs) or by their chemical structure (tricyclic antidepressants). As shown in Figure 17.7, the tricyclic antidepressants contain three contiguous carbon rings. The remaining antidepressants contain one or more carbon rings, but their molecular structures vary significantly even though they may have similar physiological mechanisms.

The majority of antidepressants increase monoaminergic transmission by acting at one of two presynaptic sites. Following the release of a monoamine neurotransmitter from a presynaptic terminal, the molecule is normally removed from the synaptic cleft by protein transporters that are embedded in the presynaptic membrane (Figure 17.8). Most

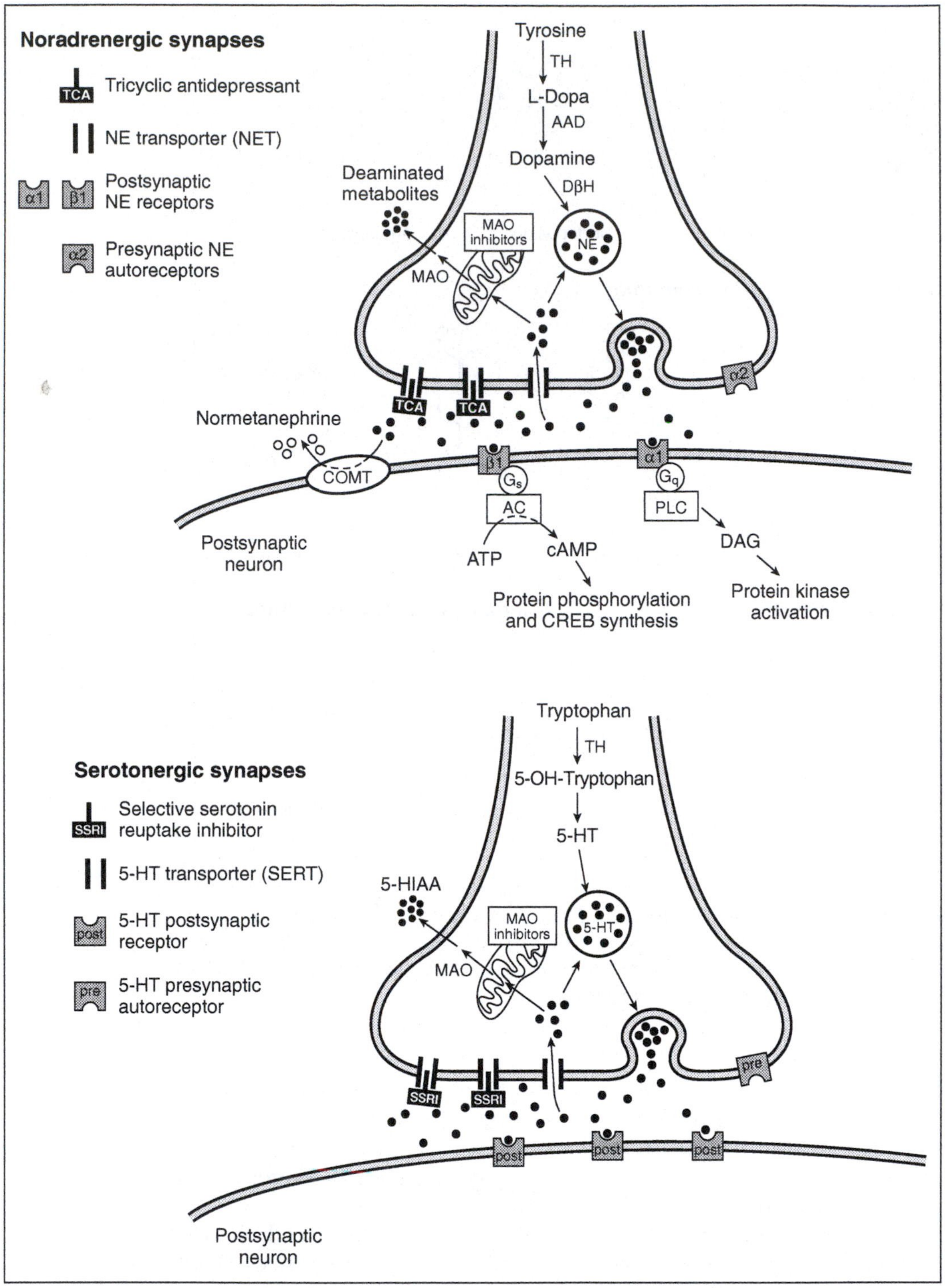

FIG. 17.8. Noradrenergic and Serotonergic Synaptic Mechanisms. Top and bottom diagrams illustrate the synaptic mechanisms for the synthesis and degradation of NE (norepinephrine) and 5-HT (serotonin). Antidepressants work either by blocking synaptic reuptake of the neurotransmitter or by inhibiting the degradative enzyme, monoamine oxidase (MAO). Both mechanisms increase the number of neurotransmitter molecules in the synaptic cleft. In addition, stimulation of postsynaptic G-protein-coupled receptors activates a series of enzymes and transcription factors that mediate the formation of membranes, receptors, and other structures necessary for remodeling synaptic connections. TH = tyrosine hydroxylase; AAD = aromatic amino acid decarboxylase; DBH = dopamine beta hydroxylase; COMT = catecholamine methyltransferase; AC = adenylate cyclase; PLC = phospholipase C; ATP = adenosine triphosphate; cAMP = cyclic adenosine monophosphate; DAB = diacylglycerol; 5-HIAA = 5-hydroxyindoleacetic acid.

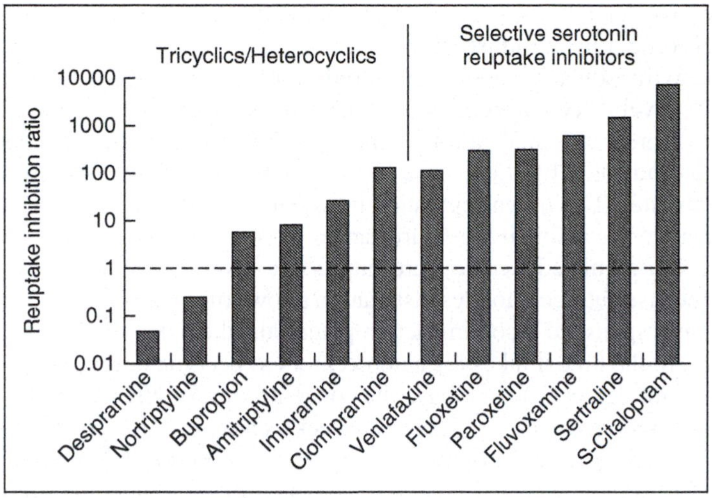

FIG. 17.9. Relative Potency of Antidepressants in Blocking NE and 5-HT Synaptic Reuptake. Each bar represents the relative inhibition of synaptic reuptake of NE and 5-HT; ratios are based on inhibition constants measured from radioactive ligand transport competition assays conducted on cell lines transfected with human genes for specific transporter proteins (NET and SERT). Antidepressants that act primarily by inhibiting NE reuptake have ratios <1, and those that act primarily by inhibiting 5-HT reuptake have ratios , >1. (Bar heights based on data appearing in Baldessarini: Drug therapy of depression and anxiety disorders. In: Brunton LL, ed. *Goodman and Gilman's The Pharmacological Basis of Therapeutics*, 11th ed. McGraw-Hill, 2006.)

antidepressants interfere with this removal step by blocking the presynaptic reuptake of either NE or 5-HT; this action effectively increases the concentration of these neurotransmitters in the synaptic cleft. As shown by Figure 17.9, most reuptake blockers are more potent in blocking synaptic reuptake of one monoamine, either NE or 5-HT. Despite this neurotransmitter specificity, some antidepressant medications inhibit synaptic reuptake of both NE and 5-HT to varying degrees.

Other antidepressants increase monoaminergic transmission by inhibiting MAO. After NE and 5-HT are transported back to the synaptic cytosol, they are either metabolized by MAO in the mitochondria or repackaged into synaptic vesicles (see Figure 17.8). Hence, inhibition of MAO allows more neurotransmitter molecules to be recycled for re-release into the synaptic cleft.

Development of Antidepressants. The behavioral effects of newly developed antidepressant drugs are often tested on an animal model of learned helplessness known as the forced swim test. In this test, a laboratory rat is placed in a pool of water. Typically the rat will swim vigorously for about 10 minutes and then give up. The rat does not drown, however, but is able to float. When the rat is tested in the pool of water on the next day, it gives up much faster, usually after a minute or two. On subsequent days, administration of an antidepressant drug causes the rat to swim for more than one or two minutes. Most effective antidepressant treatments, including ECT, MAO inhibitors, and tricyclic antidepressants, produce similar effects in the forced swim test. Unlike laboratory rats, however, depressed humans do not experience an immediate benefit after receiving antidepressants.

Delayed Clinical Effects of Antidepressants. Any explanation of the clinical mechanisms of antidepressants must contend with the discrepancy between their rapid pharmacological actions and their delayed clinical efficacy. Even though antidepressants produce significant increases in monoaminergic transmission within an hour of ingestion, they must be administered daily for 2–6 weeks before a significant improvement in mood is observed. Although the exact reason for this temporal discrepancy remains unclear, most

> Antidepressants must be used for 2–6 weeks to improve mood.

explanations have focused on synaptic plasticity and other dynamic events that occur in response to chronic drug administration.

When the extracellular synaptic concentrations of NE and 5-HT are elevated for a prolonged period, several secondary effects occur that may explain the delayed clinical efficacy of antidepressant medications. Initially, neurotransmitter receptors become desensitized as indicated by a decrease in the number of NE or 5-HT receptors on the synaptic membranes. This down-regulation in receptor number represents a normal homeostatic mechanism for maintaining neurotransmission within a specific functional range. Some of the down-regulated receptors are autoreceptors on the presynaptic membrane (see Chapter 2). Because autoreceptor desensitization allows more presynaptic release of a neurotransmitter in response to incoming action potentials, the delay in clinical efficacy could be due, in part, to the time it takes for autoreceptors to become desensitized.

Continued use of antidepressants causes prolonged stimulation of monoaminergic metabotropic receptors; this activates the genetic machinery that induces synaptic remodeling.

Given that antidepressants increase the concentration of NE and 5-HT in the synaptic cleft, their continuous use over several weeks causes prolonged stimulation of the postsynaptic receptors. Even though the number of receptors has declined, prolonged stimulation of G-protein-coupled receptors activates many genes that are critical in the remodeling of synaptic connections. As shown by Figure 17.8, ligand stimulation of the G-protein-coupled NE receptor activates cyclic AMP, protein kinase, and the cAMP response element binding protein (CREB). An important transcription factor, CREB induces gene expression of brain-derived neuronal growth factor (BDNF), a neuropeptide that promotes the synaptic growth of hippocampal and cortical neurons. Administration of BDNF to animals also produces behavioral effects that are similar to antidepressants. Hence, even though postsynaptic NE and 5-HT receptors are initially down-regulated by antidepressant therapy, their persistent stimulation gradually activates a cascade of intracellular genetic machinery that promotes synaptic remodeling, including the synthesis of new NE and 5-HT receptors.

The effectiveness of antidepressants may even depend on stimulating neurogenesis in the hippocampus, especially in the dentate gyrus. The hippocampus is one of the few brain regions in which new neurons are continuously generated throughout adulthood. Consistent with imaging studies showing that major depressive disorder is correlated with smaller hippocampal volumes, decreased neurogenesis in the hippocampus, which occurs in response to stress, may precipitate a depressive episode. This view is supported by animal studies showing that antidepressants increase the rate of neurogenesis in the hippocampus. In fact, if neurogenesis is completely blocked, antidepressants fail to alter behavior in animal models of depression. Hence, in an effort to develop new antidepressants, researchers have begun focusing on drugs that initiate neurogenesis.

The delayed clinical effects of antidepressants may partly explain why some depressed patients do not respond to pharmacologic intervention. If the clinical efficacy of an antidepressant depends on activating several genes that promote synaptic growth and neurogenesis, some patients may not respond because the medication did not sufficiently activate the postsynaptic genetic machinery, either because of receptor desensitization or other factors. In cases in which patients are resistant to one antidepressant, switching them to another antidepressant with different mechanisms of action can sometimes produce the desired therapeutic outcome, but this strategy is generally characterized by a low probability of success. By contrast, the effectiveness of an antidepressant is often improved by augmenting it with lithium.

Pharmacotherapy: Lithium

Lithium salts have been used as a sedative and, to a lesser extent, as an anticonvulsant throughout the 19th century. Although lithium use declined in the first half of the 20th century because of its toxic effects, lithium was rediscovered in 1949 when John Cade noticed that it had sedative effects on animals and was effective in treating psychiatric patients diagnosed with mania. Concerns about lithium's toxic effects on the heart delayed its widespread clinical use, but in 1970 lithium was finally approved by the United States Food and Drug Administration as an effective treatment for mania.

Based on substantial data reported over the last four decades, lithium is considered safe and effective in preventing the recurring episodes of bipolar disorder. Classified as a mood-stabilizing agent in patients who suffer from both mania and depression, lithium does not have any psychotropic effects in normal individuals. Although lithium and anticonvulsants such as carbamazepine and valproic acid are routinely used as mood stabilizers in bipolar disorder, these agents are rarely used alone in the treatment of unipolar depression. In cases in which a depressed individual responds suboptimally to antidepressant therapy, lithium has been used successfully as an adjunct to enhance the efficacy of the antidepressant.

Although many reports indicate that lithium suppresses protein kinase activity and has other regulatory actions in the brain, its mechanism of action in treating mania was a mystery for several years. Lithium may partly inhibit the synaptic release of NE and DA, but it has few effects on 5-HT and it does not alter catecholamine binding to postsynaptic receptors. Recent studies, however, indicate that lithium has multiple actions on glutamate transmission. Thus, lithium increases the presynaptic reuptake of glutamate and, consistent with removing excessive levels of glutamate from the synaptic cleft, lithium protects neurons from glutamate excitotoxicity (see Chapter 2). As part of this mechanism, lithium inactivates postsynaptic *N*-methyl-D-aspartate (NMDA) receptors and suppresses the glutamate-induced loss of cyclic AMP response binding protein and other regulatory agents in the postsynaptic neuron. These findings suggest that lithium keeps glutamate at a stable level in the synaptic cleft and has prompted the view that mania is due, at least in part, to excessive amounts of glutamate in the synaptic cleft.

Pharmacotherapy: Anxiolytics

The benzodiazepines are the most widely prescribed drugs for treating excessive anxiety. Anxiolytic drugs such as chlordiazepoxide (Librium), diazepam (Valium), and others act by binding to the $GABA_A$ receptor. Benzodiazepines alter the conformational structure of the GABA receptor, and this action increases the affinity of GABA for the GABA receptor. By promoting the binding of GABA to its postsynaptic receptor, benzodiazepine drugs enhance the inhibitory effects that are produced by GABAergic transmission. Benzodiazepines also enhance the binding of barbiturates to the GABA receptor; because of this synergistic effect, benzodiazepines should never be mixed with barbiturates or alcohol.

Benzodiazepines have a rapid onset of action that is associated with a mild elevation of mood. In general, the calming effects of the benzodiazepines are directly associated with their ability to enhance GABAergic inhibition of neuronal activity. Pharmacologic agents that block GABA receptors or benzodiazepine receptors produce anxiety and a propensity for convulsions.

Development of Anxiolytic Drugs. The development of anxiolytic drugs has been facilitated by the use of several animal models of anxiety. Most of these models exploit the propensity of rodents to stay in dark, secluded spaces. Thus, the open field test involves placing a laboratory mouse or rat in a well-lit enclosure and then measuring the amount of time that the animal spends along the perimeter of the enclosure or in the center of the field. Rodents generally prefer the perimeter of the enclosure much more than the open field. In the light/dark test, the animal is placed in a two-chamber box in which the dark chamber is connected to the lighted chamber by a tunnel. The test consists of measuring the proportion of time spent in the two chambers; most rodents prefer the dark chamber.

Administration of anxiolytic agents causes rodents to spend more time in either the open field or in the lighted chamber. Conversely, anxiety-provoking drugs that block GABAergic receptors or block the pharmacologic actions of an anxiolytic drug cause the animal to stay in more secluded areas. These behavioral tests have also been used to examine the effects of gene knockouts, such as those that prevent the formation of GABA receptors. As might be predicted, loss of GABA receptors reduces the time spent in a well-lit, open area, but manipulations that promote GABAergic transmission have the opposite behavioral effect.

DEPRESSIVE DISORDERS

Four major depressive disorders are recognized. The most common is major depressive disorder, which is sometimes called unipolar major depression. The other mood disorders include the bipolar disorders, cyclothymia, and dysthymia. Diagnosis of a specific mood disorder is based on strict criteria described in the *Diagnostic and Statistical Manual of Mental Disorders,* Fourth Edition-Text Revision (DSM-IV-TR), which is periodically revised and published by the American Psychiatric Association. An alternative handbook, *The International Statistical Classification of Disease and Related Health Problems*, is published by the World Health Organization and is used internationally.

Major Depressive Disorder

The most prevalent depressive disorder is major depressive disorder (MDD), which has a lifetime risk of 10%–15% for females and 6%–9% for males. The main symptoms that characterize MDD are depressed mood, diminished interest or pursuit of normal activities (anhedonia), significant weight loss, insomnia, fatigue and decreased energy, and an inability to concentrate or make decisions. Individuals suffering from MDD frequently have suicidal thoughts, and it is estimated that 15% of individuals with MDD actually commit suicide. Most patients with MDD respond to medication, psychotherapy, or a combination of these treatments. In severe cases in which the risk of suicide is high, ECT is administered because antidepressant medications have to be administered for several weeks before they become effective. Patients with MDD may show spontaneous improvement in mood, but they generally relapse into another depressive episode unless proper treatment is administered.

Bipolar Disorder

Bipolar disorder, which is sometimes called manic-depressive illness, is characterized by cyclic shifts in mood that alternate between depression and mania. Bipolar disorders are classified in two forms that differ in severity. The classic form of the illness, known as bipolar I disorder, is marked by recurrent episodes of dramatic mood swings epitomized by debilitating cycles of depression and extreme mania (Figure 17.10). Individuals with

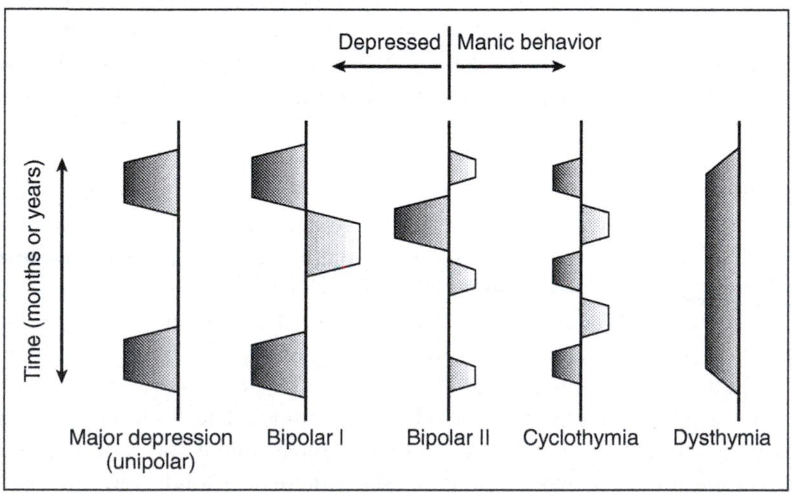

FIG. 17.10. Depressive Disorders. Mood changes in the direction of depression or mania are shown for several categories of depression. Individual patient profiles within each disorder may vary significantly with respect to duration, intensity, and the rate of cycling. Adapted from Kelsey and Nemeroff: Affective disorders. In: Enna SJ, Coyle JT, eds. *Pharmacological Management of Neurological and Psychiatric Disorders*. New York, NY: McGraw-Hill, 95–136,1998.

bipolar I disorder may lose contact with reality during the manic phase, can suffer from hallucinations, and sometimes require hospitalization. Because of the severity of this illness and the possibility of hallucinations, patients with bipolar I disorder are often misdiagnosed as having schizophrenia. Manic symptoms include restlessness, extreme irritability, racing thoughts, an excessive euphoric mood, decreased need for sleep, increased sexual drive, increased assertive behavior, poor judgment, and an unrealistic view of what is possible. The signs and symptoms appearing in the depressive phase of the bipolar disorders are similar to those described for MDD.

In bipolar II disorder, the manic-like phase is much milder than what is observed in bipolar I disorder and is referred to as hypomania. In fact, hypomania is usually manifested by an increase in energy and a decreased need for sleep.

Bipolar disorder: mood swings between mania and depression, the two poles of the mood continuum

Bipolar disorders represent a severe recurrent illness that usually requires long-term treatment. A combination of psychotherapy and medication are optimal for treating bipolar disorder, and this illness is best managed when treatment is continuous rather than episodic. Mood stabilizers, such as lithium, when used for extended periods of time are effective for treating both manic and depressive episodes. Anticonvusants such as valproate and carbamazepine also have mood-stabilizing effects and have been prescribed to manage severe bipolar episodes.

Cyclothymia

Patients with cyclothymia display alternating mood swings that are characterized by repeated cycles of depressive and hypomanic episodes, but each phase is milder than the episodes observed in bipolar disorder. Onset of cyclothymia, which normally appears in early adulthood, is so gradual that a definitive onset time is often difficult to determine. The symptoms are not as debilitating as those appearing in bipolar disorder, and most patients with cyclothymia can function in work and social situations, but at a reduced capacity. Most treatments for cyclothymia rely on psychotherapy and mood stabilizers such as lithium and anticonvulsants. Antidepressants are generally not used because they often increase the frequency of the hypomanic episodes, a phenomenon known as "cycling."

Dysthymia

As shown by Figure 17.10, dysthymia is a chronic mood disorder that persists continuously for at least 2 years. Characterized by a depressed mood most of the time, dysthymic individuals show at least two of the following symptoms: lack of appetite or overeating, insomnia, low energy, poor concentration, and feelings of helplessness. In contrast to MDD, dysthymic individuals do not show remission or other signs of episodic cycling. Dysthymic individuals usually require psychotherapy that is augmented with antidepressant medication.

ANXIETY DISORDERS

Irrational fears, tension, and pervasive worrying that persist for more than 6 months represent the common symptoms of all anxiety disorders. Although this general categorization is largely accurate, clinical research has led to the classification of several distinct anxiety disorders that are defined in the DSM-IV-TR. The psychological and behavioral symptoms that define specific anxiety disorders vary tremendously, and patients with an anxiety disorder may also suffer from depression, drug dependence, or another mental illness. Despite these complications, effective treatments have been developed for virtually every anxiety disorder that has been identified.

Generalized Anxiety Disorder

Persistent anxiety and worrying represent the essential feature of generalized anxiety disorder (GAD). Persons diagnosed with GAD exhibit excessive anxiety that is often focused on minor, everyday problems. The focus of their worry may shift from one issue to another and often includes worries about their finances, minor health issues, family interactions, minor problems in the workplace, and other issues that are normally handled with ease by most people. Patients diagnosed with GAD have difficulty concentrating on assigned tasks, show an exaggerated startle response, and suffer from insomnia. Minor physical complaints and symptoms often accompany this disorder including fatigue, headache, irritability, muscle twitches, and trembling. Most people with GAD can function in the workplace, although this becomes problematic in severe cases. About 2%–3% of the population suffers from GAD, with women being affected twice as often as men. Patients with GAD may also suffer from depression. Cognitive-behavioral therapy and medications, especially benzodiazepines, are used to treat GAD.

Panic Attacks

Patients who have panic disorder suffer from severe, sudden attacks of terror that are often associated with many physiologic symptoms including a pounding heart, profuse perspiration, weakness, and dizziness. They may also report nausea, chest pains, tingling sensations, and numbness. Psychologically, the patient is extremely fearful and has an overwhelming sense of doom and foreboding. In many cases, the panic attack causes the patient to believe they are suffering a heart attack and that they are about to die. Panic attacks afflict 1%–2% of the population annually, and they affect women more than men. Full-blown panic attacks can be disabling and will invariably evoke fear about when the next attack will occur. Patients also fear the stimuli associated with previous panic attacks, and this fear prompts avoidance behaviors that interfere with normal activities. Panic disorder is effectively treated by cognitive-behavioral therapy and antipanic medications, which form a subset of all antidepressants.

In left untreated, some patients gradually become fearful of an increasingly larger set of situations. As they avoid more and more environments associated with panic attacks, their interactions become more restrictive and they may ultimately limit themselves to only their home environment. This resulting fear of public spaces is known as agoraphobia. When agoraphobia develops, patients are usually treated by graduated exposure therapy combined with antidepressant medications, usually SSRIs.

Social Anxiety Disorder

Social anxiety disorder is characterized by excessive anxiety and fear of embarrassment in normal social settings. In some patients, the phobia is limited to specific situations, such as public speaking, and in others the phobia extends to a broad range of situations that involve other people. Stage fright represents a classic example that has afflicted well-known actors and actresses. The anxiety and apprehension associated with this disorder can produce intense discomfort and a variety of physical symptoms including blushing, profuse sweating, nausea, and difficulty speaking. In addition to interfering with work and other activities, social anxiety may interfere with the development of friendships. Social anxiety disorder affects approximately 3%–4% of the adult population and is equally likely in males and females. Although social anxiety disorder is associated with abnormal activity in the amygdala, the exact cause of this disorder has not been established. Effective treatment of social anxiety disorder relies primarily on medications such as SSRIs or benzodiazepines and, to a lesser extent, on cognitive-behavioral therapy.

Obsessive-Compulsive Disorder

Obsessive-compulsive disorder (OCD) represents a form of anxiety characterized by intrusive thoughts, ideas, images, or impulses (obsessions) that cause the patient to perform specific behaviors (compulsions) aimed at reducing or counteracting the anxiety associated with the obsession. Generally, the obsessions and compulsions occur repetitively to such an extreme degree that normal activities are disrupted. Most patients with OCD have both obsessions and compulsions. Common examples of OCD include excessive hand-washing to remove germs or repeatedly rearranging items in a precise, symmetrical configuration. The lifetime risk for OCD is 3%, but only a fraction of afflicted individuals are diagnosed and receive appropriate treatment. Usually OCD is treated by combining psychotherapy with an antidepressant medication that increases serotonergic transmission (SSRIs). Psychotherapies developed for treating OCD are aimed at reducing stress and anxiety, and they have focused on conditioning the patient to resist compulsions and stop unwanted thoughts in the presence of stimuli that trigger the compulsion.

Post-Traumatic Stress Disorder

Post-traumatic stress disorder (PTSD) is characterized by intense anxiety, fear, and related autonomic symptoms. As implied by its name, this disorder can almost always be traced to one event or a related series of events in which the patient either experienced severe physical trauma or witnessed its infliction on others. Events that may precipitate PTSD include natural disasters, violent crimes, assaults, automobile accidents, and wartime combat. Among children, inappropriate sexual contact can cause PTSD, even though no physical injury occurred. Although the lifetime prevalence of PTSD is less than 3% across all adults, nearly 30% of military personnel that are exposed to heavy combat suffer from PTSD. Patients with PTSD repeatedly relive the event as memory flashbacks, dreams, or stress reactions to stimuli associated with the original experience. Consequently, patients take steps to avoid all stimuli associated with the traumatic experience. Patients with PTSD often suffer from hyperarousal that is manifested by insomnia, inability to concentrate, and an exaggerated startle response.

> PTSD can always be traced to one or more traumatic events.

Severe traumatic events that precipitate PTSD have a significant impact on neural functions, especially on the amygdala and related parts of the limbic system such as the HPA axis. Fear conditioning and repeated exposure to stimuli associated with trauma activate the amygdala, hypothalamus, and locus ceruleus. Effective treatment for PTSD varies according to the circumstances that prompted the disorder and other factors. In general, pharmacological intervention with SSRIs is combined with different forms of psychotherapy including group therapy, cognitive-behavioral therapy, and techniques aimed at promoting desensitization and relaxation.

RESOLUTION OF CLINICAL CASE

Determining whether a patient is suffering from a mood disorder requires a complete patient history, a physical examination, and a psychological evaluation. The physician must determine whether the patient is taking any medications or has a medical condition that might produce symptoms resembling depression or other affective disorders. For this reason, the physician must know if the patient is taking opiates, steroids, beta-blockers, stimulants, sedatives, or cardiac drugs that contain reserpine. In addition, the physician should rule out neurological conditions such as Huntington's disease, Parkinson's disease, multiple sclerosis, dementia, and diseases of the endocrine system such as Cushing's disease. In this process, several lab tests are often requested: a complete blood count with hemoglobin and hematocrit levels, as well as studies of thyroid function, urinalysis, and an electrocardiogram. After ruling out potential non-psychiatric medical conditions, a psychological evaluation should be performed to determine what symptoms are present, when they began, and whether they have been treated previously. Many physicians use the Hamilton Depression Rating Scale for this purpose. The patient should also be asked if other family members have an affective disorder and what treatments were administered.

RESOLUTION OF CLINICAL CASE

In the clinical case for this chapter, a diagnosis of major depressive disorder was made. The psychiatrist informed both the patient and her husband that depression is a medical illness and not a character flaw. In addition to prescribing antidepressant medication, fluoxetine, the patient was scheduled for psychotherapy to identify any issues that distressed her. In this particular case, the patient identified several stressful issues surrounding her new job, including problematic interactions that had occurred with some of her colleagues. Eventually, after taking antidepressants for several weeks and learning different coping strategies for handling interpersonal conflicts, the woman's mood improved.

REVIEW QUESTIONS

Directions: For each of the following questions, choose the **one best** answer.

1. A patient with post-stroke depression is most likely to have damage in which brain region?
- **A.** Prefrontal cortex
- **B.** Amygdaloid complex
- **C.** Locus ceruleus
- **D.** Hippocampus
- **E.** Mediodorsal thalamus

2. A screening questionnaire suggests that a patient might be suffering from depression. What physiological test or biochemical marker would confirm a diagnosis of depression?
- **A.** Elevated levels of CRH in the CSF
- **B.** Reduced levels of the serotonin metabolite, 5-HIAA
- **C.** A deficit in slow-wave non-REM sleep activity
- **D.** Cortisol suppression in response to dexamethasone administration
- **E.** There is no definitive marker for establishing depression.

3. What result is most likely in a functional imaging study of unipolar depression?
- **A.** Decreased glucose metabolism in the amygdaloid complex
- **B.** Enlargement of the lateral ventricles
- **C.** Decreased blood flow to the dorsal lateral prefrontal cortex
- **D.** Increased activity in the locus ceruleus
- **E.** Decreased blood flow to the hippocampus

4. What set of neuroendocrine responses are associated with stress-induced depression?
- **A.** Increased CSF levels of both CRH and cortisol
- **B.** Decreased CSF levels of CRH and an increased adrenal gland
- **C.** Increased plasma levels of ACTH and a decreased adrenal gland
- **D.** Increased CRH receptors on the pituitary and an increased adrenal gland
- **E.** Increased CSF levels of CRH and an increased ACTH response to a CRH challenge

5. What evidence most strongly indicates that inheritability is a factor in clinical depression?
- **A.** A family history of suicide is the best predictor for developing depression.
- **B.** A family history of mood disorders indicates vulnerability to depression.
- **C.** The likelihood of depression among monozygotic twins is 33%.
- **D.** The short allele of the serotonin transporter gene is highly correlated with depression.
- **E.** Family members with depression respond best to the same antidepressants.

6. What pharmacologic properties of antidepressants best explain their delayed clinical efficacy?
- **A.** Inhibition of monoamine oxidase
- **B.** Increased synaptic concentrations of monoamines
- **C.** Autoreceptor desensitization
- **D.** Monoamine activation of metabotropic receptors
- **E.** Reuptake blockade of monoamines

ADDITIONAL READING

Classic Literature

Freis ED: Mental depression in hypertensive patients treated for long periods with large doses of reserpine. *New Engl J Med* 251:1006–1008, 1954.

Hamilton M: Development of a rating scale for primary depressive illness. *Brit J Soc Clin Psychol* 6:278–296, 1967.

MacLean PD: Psychosomatic disease and the visceral brain: recent developments bearing on the Papez theory of emotion. *Psychosom Med* 11:338–353, 1949.

Seligman MEP: *Helplessness: On Depression, Development, and Death.* San Francisco, CA: Freeman, 1975.

Reviews and Landmark Research Articles

American Psychiatric Association: *Diagnostic and Statistical Manual of Mental Disorders,* 4th revised ed. Washington, DC: American Psychiatric Association, 2000.

Baldessarini RJ: Chapter 17: Drug therapy of depression and anxiety disorders. In: Brunton LL, ed. *Goodman and Gilman's The Pharmacological Basis of Therapeutics,* 11th ed. New York, NY: McGraw-Hill, 2006.

Beauregard M, Leroux JM, Bergman S, Arzoumanian Y, Beaudoin G, Bourgouin P, Stip E: The functional neuroanatomy of major depression: an fMRI study using an emotional activation paradigm. *Neuroreport* 9:3253–3258, 1998.

Brody AL, Saxena S, Stoessel P, Gillies LA, Fairbanks LA, Alborzian S, Phelps ME, Huang SC, Wu HM, Ho ML, Au SC, Maidment K, Baxter LR: Regional brain metabolic changes in patients with major depression treated with either paroxitine or interpersonal therapy: preliminary findings. *Arch Gen Psychiat* 58:631–640, 2001.

Charney DS: Neuroanatomical circuits modulating fear and anxiety behaviors. *Acta Psychiatr Scand* 108 (Suppl 417):38–50, 2003.

Dixon JF, Hokin LE: Lithium acutely inhibits and chronically up-regulates and stabilizes glutamate uptake by presynaptic nerve endings in mouse cerebral cortex. *Proc Natl Acad Sci USA* 95:8363–8368, 1998.

Drevets WC, Videen TO, Price JL, Preskorn SH, Carmichael ST, Raichle ME: A functional anatomical study of unipolar depression. *J Neurosci* 12:3628–3641, 1992.

Gottesman II, Gould TD: The endophenotypic concept in psychiatry: etymology and strategic intentions. *Am J Psychiat* 160:636–645, 2003.

Hasler G, Drevets WC, Manji HK, Charney DS: Discovering endophenotypes for major depression. *Neuropsychopharmacology* 29:1765–1781, 2004.

Hedaya RJ: *Understanding Biological Psychiatry*. New York, NY: WW Norton & Co., 1996.

Heim C, Newport DJ, Bonsall R, Miller AH, Nemeroff CR: Altered pituitary-adrenal axis responses to provocative challenge tests in adult survivors of childhood abuse. *Am J Psychiat* 158:575–581, 2001.

Heim C, Newport DJ, Heit S, Graham YP, Wilcox M, Bonsall R Miller H, Nemeroff CB: Pituitary-adrenal axis responses to stress in women after sexual and physical abuse in childhood. *JAMA* 284:592–597, 2000.

Jacobs BL, Praag H, Gage FH: Adult brain neurogenesis and psychiatry: a novel theory of depression. *Mol Psychiatry* 5:262–269, 2000.

Kalia M: Neurobiological basis of depression: an update. *Metabolism* 54 (Suppl 1):24–27, 2005.

Kelsey JE, Nemeroff CB: Affective disorders. In: Enna SJ, Coyle JT, eds. *Pharmacological Management of Neurological and Psychiatric Disorders*. New York, NY: McGraw-Hill, 1998:95–136.

Kupfer DJ, Frank E, Jarrett DB, Reynolds CF, Thase ME: Interrelationship of electroencephalo-graphic sleep chronobiology and depression. In: Kupfer DJ, Monk TH, Barchas JD, eds. *Biological Rhythms and Mental Disorders.* New York, NY: Guilford, 1988.

Kupfer DJ, Frank E, McEachran AB, Grochocinski VJ: Delta sleep ratio: a biological correlate of early recurrence in unipolar affective disorder. *Arch Gen Psychiat* 47:1100–1105, 1990.

Lauer CJ, Wolfgang S, Holsboer F, Krieg JC: In quest of identifying vulnerability markers for psychiatric disorders by all-night polysomnography. *Arch Gen Psychiat* 52:145–152, 1995.

Malberg JE, Eisch AJ, Nestler EJ, Duman RS: Chronic antidepressant treatment increases neurogenesis in adult rat hippocampus. *J Neurosci* 20:9104–9110, 2000.

Martin SD, Martin E, Rai SS, Richardson MA, Royall R: Brain blood flow changes in depressed patients treated with interpersonal psychotherapy or venlafaxine hydrochloride: preliminary findings. *Arch Gen Psychiat* 58:641–648, 2001.

Mayberg HS, Liotti M, Brannan SK, McGinnis S, Mahurin RK, Jerabek PA, Silova JA, Tekell JL, Martin CC, Lancaster JL, Fox PT: Reciprocal limbic-cortical function and negative mood: converging PET findings in depression and normal sadness. *Am J Psychiat* 156:675–682, 1999.

Nemeroff CB, Heim CM, Thase ME, Klein DN, Rush AJ, Schatzberg AF, Ninan PT, McCullough JP, Weiss PM, Dunner DL, Rothbaum BO, Kornstein S, Keitner G, Keller MN: Differential responses to psychotherapy versus pharmacotherapy in patients with chronic forms of major depression and childhood trauma. *Proc Natl Acad Sci* 100:14293–14296, 2003.

Nemeroff CB, Vale WW: The neurobiology of depression: inroads to treatment and new drug discovery. *J Clin Psychiat* 66 (Suppl 7):5–13, 2005.

Pandy GN, Pandy SC, Dwivedi Y, Sharma RP, Janicak PG, Davis JM: Platelet serotonin-2A receptors: a potential biological marker for suicidal behavior. *Amer J Psychiat* 152:850–855, 1995.

Paradiso S, Robinson R: Depression—structural and functional neuroimaging studies. In: Adelman G, Smith BH, eds. *Encyclopedia of Neuroscience*. New York, NY: Elsevier, 2004.

Roffman JL, Marci CD, Glick DM, Dougherty DD, Rauch SL: Neuroimaging and the functional neuroanatomy of psychotherapy. *Psychol Med* 35:1385–1398, 2005.

Sackeim HA: Functional brain circuits in major depression and remission. *Arch Gen Psychiat* 58:649–650, 2001.

Santarelli L, Saxe M, Gross C, Surget A, Battaglia F, Dulawa S, Weisstaub N, Lee J, Duman R, Arancio O, Belzung C, Hen R: Requirement of hippocampal neurogenesis for the behavioral effects of antidepressants. *Science* 301:805–809, 2003.

Soares JC, Mann JJ : The functional neuroanatomy of mood disorders. *J Psychiatr Res* 31:393–432, 1997.

Souetre E, Salvati E, Wehs T, Sack D, Krebs B, Darcourt G: Twenty-four-hour profiles of body temperature and plasma TSH in bipolar patients during depression and during remission and in normal control subjects. *Amer J Psychiat* 145:1133–1137, 1988.

Strakowski SM, Delbello MP, Adler CM: The functional neuroanatomy of bipolar disorder: a review of neuroimaging findings. *Mol Psychiat* 10:105–116, 2005.

Vataja R, Pohjasvaara T, Leppavuori A, Mantyla R, Aronen HJ, Salonen O, Kaste M, Erkinjuntti T: Magnetic resonance imaging correlates of depression after ischemic stroke. *Arch Gen Psychiat.* 58:925–931, 2001.

Williams LS: Depression and stroke: cause or consequence? *Semin Neurol* 25:396–409, 2005.

Wurtman RJ: Genes, stress, and depression. *Metabolism* 54 (Suppl 1):16–19, 2005.

INTERNET RESOURCES

American Foundation for Suicide Prevention
http://www.afsp.org/

Anxiety Disorders Association of America
http://www.adaa.org/

Anxiety Panic Attack Resource Sites
http://www.anxietypanic.com/

Depression and Bipolar Support Alliance
http://www.dbsalliance.org/

Depression Screening
http://www.depressionscreening.org/

International Foundation for Research and Education on Depression
http://www.ifred.org/index.html

Internet Mental Health by Dr. Phillip Long
http://www.mentalhealth.com/

National Alliance on Mental Illness
http://www.nami.org/

National Center for Posttraumatic Stress Disorder
http://www.ncptsd.va.gov/

National Institute of Mental Health
http://www.nimh.nih.gov/healthinformation/index.cfm

MedlinePlus

Depression
http://www.nlm.nih.gov/medlineplus/depression.html

Antidepressants
http://www.nlm.nih.gov/medlineplus/antidepressants.html

National Mental Health Information Center
http://www.mentalhealth.samhsa.gov/

Mental Health America
http://www.nmha.org/

University of Michigan Depression Center
http://www.med.umich.edu/depression/

Answers and Explanations

Chapter 1

1. The answer is B. A typical neuron has a resting membrane potential of -65 mV. The equilibrium potential for K^+ is nearly -90 mV, and an increase in K^+ conductance allows K^+ to flow out of the cytoplasm and shift the membrane potential to -90 mV. Changes in Cl^- conductance have little effect on resting potential because the equilibrium potential for Cl^- is close to the resting potential. Increasing the conductance of Na^+ or Ca^{2+} would depolarize the membrane. Poisoning the Na^+-K^+ pump would not cause an immediate change in membrane potential, but it would eventually allow the membrane potential to completely dissipate.

2. The answer is E. Myelination causes an increase in membrane resistance but does not alter the internal resistance of the axoplasm. By increasing the membrane resistance, myelination increases the length constant, thereby facilitating the flow of ionic current through the axoplasm. Refractory periods are determined by voltage-gated ion channels, not by myelination. Myelination causes a decrease, not an increase, in membrane capacitance. The equilibrium potential for Na^+ is not affected by myelination.

3. The answer is B. Each action potential is characterized by a large increase in the number of opened voltage-gated sodium channels; hence, sodium conductance is high. The conductance of potassium and chloride channels are generally unaffected at the beginning of the action potential, but potassium conductance will increase during the trailing edge of the action potential. Membrane resistance decreases at the leading edge of the action potential (because the sodium channels open), but axoplasmic conductance is not affected.

4. The answer is D. The biphasic waveform of the action potential is characterized by an influx of sodium followed by an efflux of potassium. Action potentials do not depend on changes in chloride currents. EPSPs and IPSPs are graded potentials that travel in the dendrites and soma but do not propagate into the axon. During an action potential, active depolarization (sodium influx through voltage-gated sodium channels) occurs simultaneously with passive depolarization (sodium current through the axoplasm).

5. The answer is D. While axon terminals may form synapses on dendrites, soma, or axon terminals, they never form synapses on the myelinated part of an axon. In some brain regions such as the substantia nigra, dendrites may form synapses on the dendrites of neighboring neurons.

6. The answer is A. As axon diameter increases, the internal resistance of the axon decreases and this facilitates the axoplasmic flow of Na^+ during an action potential. The decrease in axoplasmic resistance contributes to an increase in both the axon's length constant and its conduction velocity. The time constant is unaffected by a change in axon diameter.

7. The answer is A. Nodes of Ranvier represent regions on the axon where voltage-gated sodium channels are very dense, myelination is minimal, and the membrane is less resistive to ionic current. Ligand-gated channels are not found in the nodes of Ranvier or on any other part of the axon.

8. The answer is C. A long length-constant increases the probability that excitatory postsynaptic potentials will summate and produce an action potential. Although postsynaptic IPSPs may also summate, resting postsynaptic potentials are close to the chloride equilibrium potential; hence, an increase in length constant will facilitate summation of EPSPs to a much greater extent. The magnitude of a neuron's length constant has no bearing on axoplasmic transport, nor does it affect the potassium equilibrium potential.

9. The answer is C. The loss of myelin surrounding multiple tracts of nerve fibers may interfere with a variety of motor and sensory functions. The loss of myelin is the opposite of myelin proliferation, and it involves a decline, not an increase, in the glial cells that produce myelin. Multiple sclerosis is not caused by changes in the brain vasculature or in the relative balance of ion channels.

10. The answer is D. Presynaptic inhibition occurs when a synapse on another axon terminal causes a reduction in neurotransmitter release by the second axon terminal. Feedback inhibition represents a disynaptic circuit of two neurons, the second of which is an inhibitory interneuron that projects to the first neuron. The remaining choices usually involve axosomatic or axodendritic synapses and do not require an axo-axonic synapse.

Chapter 2

1. The answer is C. Mitochondria, dense-core vesicles, and small clear vesicles are frequently seen in the same synaptic terminal. All small molecule neurotransmitters are synthesized in the synaptic terminal, and both dopamine and its rate-limiting enzyme, tyrosine hydroxylase, are co-localized in dopaminergic terminals. Neuropeptides and small-molecule neurotransmitters (e.g., substance P and glutamate) are frequently located in the same synaptic terminal. It is rare, however, for two small-molecule neurotransmitters (e.g., glutamate and ACh) to be synthesized in the same neuron.

2. The answer is A. Calcium is essential for (1) vesicular fusion during synaptic transmission, (2) muscle contraction, and (3) protein synthesis. Membrane depolarization by Na^+ influx activates Ca^{2+} calcium channels to initiate neurotransmitter release, but Na^+ does not participate in muscle contraction or protein synthesis. Changes in Cl^-, K^+, or Mg^{2+} concentrations do not directly participate in these three processes.

3. The answer is A. Excessive glutamate release increases Ca^{2+} influx, which activates Ca^{2+}-dependent proteases and leads to the formation of free radicals. Destruction of GABAergic neurons by free radicals releases glutamatergic neurons from the inhibitory effects of GABA and increases the probability that glutamate will cause further damage. ACh, norepinephrine, and substance P are not strongly implicated in epilepsy.

4. The answer is C. Dopaminergic neurons degenerate in patients with Parkinson's disease, but dopamine cannot be administered systemically because it does not cross the blood-brain barrier. The precursor to dopamine, L-dopa, enters the brain after systemic administration and can be converted into dopamine by all neurons that contain the enzyme AAAD, including those that do not normally release dopamine. There is no evidence that Parkinson disease is caused by a lack of tyrosine hydroxylase or by a defective gene that interferes with tyrosine hydroxylase.

5. The answer is E. Myasthenia gravis occurs when nicotinic receptors at the neuromuscular junction are attacked by antibodies produced by the immune system; the decrease in nicotinic receptors reduces the muscle's response to acetylcholine.

6. The answer is B. All dopamine receptors are metabotropic receptors. Neurotransmitters such as glutamate, acetylcholine, or GABA may stimulate ionotropic or metabotropic receptors. *N*-methyl-D-aspartate is a specific agonist for an ionotropic glutamate receptor.

7. The answer is A. Curare, mustard gas, and α-bungarotoxin produce respiratory paralysis by altering cholinergic transmission at the neuromuscular junction. Their lethal effects are not mediated by altering CNS cholinergic transmission, either by stimulating muscarinic receptors or by enhancing acetylcholine release in the brain and spinal cord. These compounds do not alter dopamine synthesis, nor do they block calcium channels.

Chapter 3

1. The answer is D. Aneurysms are arterial dilatations that bleed into the subarachnoid space. The likelihood of a having an aneurysm in the other sites ranges from unlikely (C, E) to impossible (A, B).

2. The answer is D. Subdural hematomas are usually caused by leakage from veins that bridge the arachnoid space. All of the remaining choices are related to the arterial circulation. Epidural hematomas are caused by rupture of arteries that lie between the periosteal dura and the skull. Strokes, which may be hemorrhagic or embolic, most often interrupt arterial blood flow to part of the nervous system. Aneurysms are defects in the arterial wall that may leak or rupture into the parenchyma or subarachnoid space.

3. The answer is B. The lumbar cistern is used to sample CSF because, done properly, there is little danger of damaging the spinal cord or spinal nerves. The lateral ventricle, subarachnoid space, and cerebellopontine cistern contain CSF, but drawing samples from these areas would be difficult, dangerous, and impractical. The superior sagittal sinus contains venous blood.

4. The answer is D. Whereas most aneurysms are located at branch points of the anterior circulation, arteriovenous malformations are found within the parenchyma. They both must be treated surgically, are potentially life threatening, are prone to hemorrhage, and cause headaches.

5. The answer is A. The proximal part of the internal carotid artery joins the circle of Willis before continuing as the middle cerebral artery. The superior cerebellar artery branches from the basilar artery. The ophthalmic artery is a branch of the middle cerebral artery. The cavernous sinus is a venous reservoir located underneath the circle of Willis.

6. The answer is C. The blood-brain barrier would prevent the blue dye from entering the brain, so the nucleus of the solitary tract would retain its normal color. The choroid plexus would turn blue because it is on the vascular side of the barrier. Because there is no blood-brain barrier at the area postrema or the pineal gland, both would turn blue. The liver, part of the systemic circulation that has fenestrated capillaries, also would be blue.

7. The answer is C. Transient ischemic attacks are by definition nonfatal events, so the survivability is 100%. The survivability of the other cardiovascular accidents depends on many factors, including the size and locus of the stroke, aneurysm, or hematoma, and whether medical assistance is close at hand.

8. The answer is D. Most of the basal ganglia is perfused by the lenticulostriate arteries and thus would be severely impacted by an infarct of the proximal middle cerebral artery. Such a stroke also would affect widespread parts of the frontal, parietal, and temporal lobes. The arterial supply of the thalamus derives from the deep penetrating branches of the posterior communicating artery. Primary visual cortex and the inferior temporal gyrus lie within the vascular territory of the posterior cerebral artery. The long circumferential arteries that originate from the posterior cerebral artery and loop around the brainstem perfuse the superior and inferior colliculi.

9. The vein of Trolard is a superficial vein that drains into the superior sagittal sinus, which collects blood from most of the cerebral cortex. The internal cerebral vein and the basal vein are part of the deep drainage system that flows through the great cerebral vein to the confluens of the sinuses. Blood from both the superficial and deep systems, after passing through the confluens, enters the transverse sinus.

10. The answer is B. Papillomas, tumors of the choroid plexus, cause overproduction of CSF, which in turn produces a communicating hydrocephalus. Meningiomas, gliomas, ependymonas, and pituitary adenomas that interfere with CSF flow through the ventricles or into the subarachnoid space may produce a non-communicating hydrocephalus.

Chapter 4

1. The answer is C. Hyperactive tendon reflexes are a characteristic symptom of spinal cord transection after the patient has recovered from spinal shock. Below the level of the lesion, the patient has no sensations and is unable to exert voluntary motor control. After spinal shock subsides, the deep tendon reflexes become hyperactive.

2. The answer is B. Pain sensations are transmitted by nerve fibers that cross the midline via the commissure of the spinal cord. Hence, damage to the spinal commissure at levels C5-C8 may affect nociceptive fibers of both arms without affecting other neurologic functions.

3. The answer is B. Tabes dorsalis results from the destruction of the dorsal root ganglia and their central processes, especially the myelinated fibers ascending in the fasciculus gracilis. After an initial period of intermittent pain and prickly sensations, the eventual degeneration of the posterior columns impairs the sense of limb position. Normal motor function would be affected (diminished reflexes), but would still be present to some degree. Other conditions such as amyotrophic lateral sclerosis, Brown-Séquard syndrome, or a complete transection of the spinal cord would significantly impair motor function. Syringomyelia involves formation of a cavity in the center of the spinal cord that prevents the transmission of nociceptive information.

4. The answer is B. Weakness, fasciculations, and muscle atrophy are all signs indicating degeneration of the lower motor neurons. The lateral horn innervates the autonomic ganglia, and significant weakness or wasting of the muscle would occur only after degeneration of the α-motor neurons. Loss of upper motor neurons in the corticospinal tracts would produce an increase in resting muscle tone. Structures involved in sensory processes, such as the dorsal root ganglia or the posterior horn, would not be implicated in motor degeneration.

5. The answer is E. The substantia gelatinosa uses enkephalin as a neurotransmitter. Opiate narcotics act as agonists at enkephalin receptors located on the dendritic processes of substantia gelatinosa neurons as well as on the presynaptic terminals of primary afferents entering laminae I and II. Enkephalinergic neurons are not found in any of the other listed areas.

6. The answer is B. The clasp-knife reflex is a pathologic sign resulting from upper motor neuron disease or trauma. Reflexes are not present following spinal shock or the loss of lower motor neurons produced by polio or other diseases.

7. The answer is D. The myotactic reflex is elicited by muscle stretch sensed by muscle spindles. Noxious stimulation of free nerve endings elicits the flexor reflex coupled to the crossed extension reflex. Babinski's sign is elicited by gentle tactile stimulation of mechanoreceptors on the sole of the foot. The clasp-knife reflex is a pathologic form of autogenic inhibition elicited by excessive stimulation of the Golgi tendon organs following loss of upper motor neurons.

8. The answer is D. Spasticity represents an increase in the tone of both flexor and extensor muscles following damage to the upper motor neurons. Such lesions may occur at several locations including the internal capsule, crus cerebri, pyramidal tract, and lateral funiculus of the spinal cord. All of the other symptoms are associated with damage to lower motor neurons in the anterior horn.

9. The answer is A. The fasciculus gracilis is an uncrossed fiber tract that conveys cutaneous sensations from the lower half of the body; damage of the fasciculus gracilis at the level of L1 would block touch sensations from the leg. The fasciculus cuneatus does not exist in the lumbar part of the cord, and the spinothalamic and corticospinal tracts do not convey cutaneous sensations.

10. The answer is E. The cerebral cortex, especially primary motor cortex, sends projections to Rexed lamina IX in the spinal cord to mediate voluntary movements. The dorsal nucleus of Clarke projects to the cerebellum, not to the nucleus gracilis. The substantia gelatinosa, which occupies Rexed lamina II, is interconnected with enkephalinergic neurons in neighboring spinal segments, but it does not project to the spinal cord or brain. Neurons in the dorsal root ganglia project to several parts of the spinal cord and brainstem, but they do not project to the cortex.

Chapter 5

1. The answer is C. The oculomotor nerve innervates the levator palpebrae, the pupillary sphincter, and all extraocular muscles except the lateral rectus and the superior oblique. Hence, oculomotor nerve damage results in a drooping eyelid, pupillary dilation, and lateral deviation of the eyeball. A lesion of the abducens nerve produces internal strabismus, not external strabismus. Trochlear nerve damage impairs downward gaze. Facial nerve injury causes Bell's palsy, whereas a lesion of the optic nerve causes blindness.

2. The answer is B. Bell's palsy is a unilateral facial paralysis caused by damage to the lower motor neurons of the facial nerve. Lateral gaze paralysis causes both eyes to be directed to one side. The alternating hemiplegias involve a contralateral paralysis of the body that is associated with ipsilateral paralysis of muscles controlling the eye or the tongue. Lateral medullary syndrome is characterized by a loss of pain and temperature sensation on the ipsilateral face and the contralateral body.

3. The answer is D. The MLF interconnects the abducens and oculomotor nuclei to coordinate both eyes during changes in horizontal gaze; its damage produces a loss of conjugate eye movements. Lateral gaze paralysis is produced by an abducens nucleus lesion, whereas internal strabismus is produced by an abducens nerve lesion. Convergent eye movements are not impaired by MLF lesions because the medial recti are still innervated by both oculomotor nerves and the motor command for convergent eye movements is not transmitted through the MLF. Ptosis is usually a sign of oculomotor nerve damage.

4. The answer is A. The glossopharyngeal nerve contains the afferent limb of the gag reflex. The trigeminal nerve contains GSA fibers that innervate the anterior two-thirds of the tongue, but only stimulation of the posterior tongue elicits gagging. The nucleus ambiguus and its SVE fibers represent the efferent limb of the gag reflex, but these fibers do not emerge from the facial, spinal accessory, or hypoglossal nerves.

5. The answer is C. Occlusion of the posterior inferior cerebellar artery may cause loss of pain sensitivity on the ipsilateral face and contralateral body as well as dysphonia and nausea. These symptoms correspond to the lateral medullary syndrome, which is associated with damage to the spinal trigeminal nucleus, the spinothalamic tract, the nucleus ambiguus, and the nucleus solitarius. The hypoglossal nucleus and nerve are supplied by the anterior spinal artery.

6. The answer is C. The caudal solitary nucleus receives afferent information concerning blood pressure from baroreceptors located in the aortic arch and the carotid sinus. The rostral solitary nucleus solitarius processes taste information from the oral cavity. The production of saliva is controlled by the inferior and superior salivatory nuclei and their connections to specific parasympathetic ganglia. Vagal nerve fibers emerging from the dorsal motor nucleus of the vagus and the nucleus ambiguus control movements of the esophagus and larynx, respectively.

7. The answer is B. The symptoms are consistent with a central facial palsy, which can be produced by a lesion of corticobulbar fibers descending through the internal capsule.

An intact corneal reflex indicates that the facial nerve has been spared. A lesion of the motor trigeminal nucleus would paralyze the ipsilateral masseter muscle and other muscles of mastication, but would not affect the muscles used for facial expression. The remaining structures do not control the muscles of facial nucleus and would not represent possible lesion sites.

8. The answer is D. The hypoglossal nerve courses just lateral to the medial lemniscus, and a single lesion would affect both structures. The remaining pairs consist of structures that are widely separated and would not be affected by a single focal lesion.

9. The answer is C. Projections from the abducens nucleus cross the midline and ascend the medial longitudinal fasciculus to innervate the contralateral oculomotor complex. All of the remaining choices involve structures that are unrelated to each other.

10. The answer is E. Brainstem reflexes require projections from sensory nuclei to motor nuclei. Thus, projections from the spinal trigeminal nucleus to the nucleus ambiguus mediate the gag reflex. The vestibular and salivatory nuclei represent sensory and motor nuclei, respectively, but do not mediate any clinically relevant reflex. The remaining nuclear pairs are exclusively sensory or motor in function and cannot represent a complete reflex arc.

Chapter 6

1. The answer is C. The hallmark of Wernicke's aphasia is that speech remains fluent. Patients with Wernicke's aphasia lose their ability to comprehend spoken or written language. Damage to Broca's area causes labored, telegraphic speech. The ability to hum a tune is not related to damage in Wernicke's area.

2. The answer is A. Because language functions are located in the left hemisphere of most right-handed individuals, a patient with crossed language dominance would have language located in the right hemisphere. An inability to speak following a barbiturate injection of the right carotid artery would indicate that language was located in the right hemisphere. Paralysis of the right arm would occur following injection of the left carotid artery, but it would not indicate the presence of a crossed language dominance. An inability to speak following injection of the left carotid artery would refute the assertion of a crossed language dominance, not support it. Injection of the left carotid artery would not paralyze the left arm under any circumstances. An inability to sing following injection of the right carotid artery also would suggest that language was located in the left hemisphere.

3. The answer is A. Patients with damage to the prefrontal cortex have flattened affect as well as poor problem-solving skills, memory, and social graces. Patients with prosopagnosia have trouble identifying faces following damage to the lateral and ventral surfaces of the temporal lobe. Nonfluent aphasia is caused by damage to Broca's area. Parietal lobe damage in the nondominant hemisphere may cause sensory neglect or apraxias.

4. The answer is D. The internal medullary lamina is the most useful landmark for understanding the organization of the thalamic nuclei because it (1) divides the nucleus into anterior, medial, and lateral sections, and (2) provides an estimate of the anterior-posterior position. The pulvinar, the VPM nucleus, and the anterior thalamic nuclei are local landmarks that do not organize the thalamus along any dimension. The reticular nucleus is not a useful landmark because its shape remains virtually unchanged from one end of the thalamus to the other.

5. The answer is D. The anterior commissure connects the middle and inferior temporal gyri of the two hemispheres. The superior longitudinal fasciculus, uncinate fasciculus, and cingulum are intrahemispheric association pathways. The internal capsule links the cerebral cortex to multiple subcortical areas.

6. The answer is C. Prosopagnosia is an inability to recognize familiar faces. Patients with Gerstmann's syndrome are unable to perform simple arithmetic calculations, cannot write down their thoughts or name their fingers, and have left-right confusions. Broca's aphasia is a nonfluent aphasia caused by damage to the inferior frontal gyrus of the dominant (typically the left) hemisphere. Lesions of the parietal lobe of the nondominant hemisphere cause asomatognosia—sensory neglect of the left side of the body. Patients with Balint's syndrome are able to make spontaneous eye movements but cannot direct their gaze to a target on command.

7. The answer is C. The arcuate and uncinate fasciculi are intra-hemispheric pathways that connect the temporal and frontal lobes. The uncinate fasciculus does not play a role in language, and neither pathway projects to the hippocampus. Neither is a commissural pathway and, if anything, the arcuate fasciculus has assumed more importance since the advent of language.

8. The answer is E. Language recovery is better in patients who have a bilateral representation of language. Accordingly, left-handed patients have the best prognosis for language recovery following damage to the cortical language areas. Some advantage also would be realized by ambidextrous patients.

9. The answer is A. The mammillothalamic tract connects the mammillary nucleus with the anterior nucleus of the thalamus. Nociceptive information conveyed by the anterolateral system projects to the posterior nucleus. Somatosensory information from brainstem and spinal areas projects to VPL. The pulvinar receives projections from the superior colliculus, and the reticular nucleus has no cortical projections.

10. The answer is C. The optic, auditory, and somesthetic radiations, as well as corticospinal fibers, are located either within or near the posterior part of the internal capsule. Damage to the genu of the internal capsule, the frontal lobe, or the temporal lobe would produce only a subset of the four deficits.

Chapter 7

1. The answer is A. Only Pacinian and Meissner corpuscles respond continuously during vibrotactile stimulation. Pacinian fibers discharge at frequencies as high as 100-300 Hz and become entrained to vibrations in that frequency range. Meissner corpuscles become entrained to vibrations at frequencies of 10-30 Hz. Merkel corpuscles are best activated by punctuate indentations; joint receptors and Golgi tendon organs respond to limb movements.

2. The answer is C. Narcotics administered into the lumbar cistern act specifically at enkephalin receptors in the dorsal horn of the spinal cord, and this suppresses pain transmission from the lower body. Opiate narcotics do not alleviate phantom limb pain or central pain syndromes because these are produced by abnormal patterns of activity in the thalamus and cortex, brain regions that do not have high concentrations of opiate receptors. Trigeminal neuralgia is mediated by excessive or abnormal activity in the trigeminal nerve or spinal trigeminal nucleus; the resulting pain is usually treated with anticonvulsant drugs that inhibit neuronal activity without activating opioid receptors. The exact cause of migraine headache is not well understood but appears to be mediated by paroxsyms of cortical activity that are evoked by ascending inputs from the dorsal raphe nuclei. Antimigraine drugs modulate serotonergic transmission; they do not activate opioid receptors.

3. The answer is D. The SII cortex responds both to light touch and nociceptive inputs. The other regions are activated primarily by nociceptive inputs.

4. The answer is B. The trigeminothalamic tract conveys cutaneous and nociceptive information to the VPM nucleus of the thalamus. The spinal trigeminal tract terminates in the spinal trigeminal nucleus, not in the thalamus. The medial lemniscus conveys cutaneous information from the body to the ventroposterolateral (VPL) nucleus. The central tegmental and lateral spinothalamic tracts transmit nociceptive information from the body to the VPL nucleus and the intralaminar nuclei.

5. The answer is B. Approximately 25% of the fibers in the fasciculus gracilis and fasciculus cuneatus originate from cells in the posterior horn; many of these come from the nucleus proprius. Spinocerebellar and spinothalamic fibers reside in the lateral funiculus. Nociceptive A-δ and C fibers terminate in the posterior horn and do not ascend up the posterior columns.

6. The answer is E. Persons with lesions of the posterior columns cannot distinguish two stimuli that are simultaneously applied to neighboring skin regions, nor can they determine the direction of a stimulus moving across the skin. Although the spinothalamic tract conveys some mechanoreceptive information from the skin, damage to this tract does not impair tactile sensitivity because it responds primarily to intense, noxious stimulation. The remaining structures do not play any role in tactile discrimination.

7. The answer is D. Although not yet approved by the U.S. government, controlled experiments in several countries have shown that electrical stimulation of the periaqueductal gray region can alleviate chronic pain in some patients. Electrical stimulation of other parts of the somatosensory system, including the somatosensory cortex and thalamus, produces tingling or unpleasant, paresthetic sensations. The parabrachial nucleus has not been a target for alleviating chronic pain in humans.

8. The answer is A. The association of visceral pain with intense cutaneous sensations (i.e., referred pain) is mediated by the convergence of visceral and cutaneous nociceptive fibers that project to the posterior horn. Chronic pain, phantom limb pain, and paresthetic sensations are likely to be mediated by changes in the spatiotemporal patterns of activity coursing through the spinal cord and brain. Headache may have many different causes, but none of them involve the convergence of different modalities in the dorsal horn.

9. The answer is E. The fasciculus cuneatus conveys fine tactile sensations with a high degree of spatial resolution. Whereas other pathways may convey some cutaneous information, loss of the fasciculus cuneatus impairs the ability to integrate inputs from adjacent sites on the arm or hand. The spinocerebellar and cuneocerebellar tracts are concerned with inputs from muscles, tendons, and joints. The spinothalamic and spinoreticular tracts are activated by intense, noxious stimulation.

Chapter 8

1. The answer is A. The ventral cochlear nucleus receives projections exclusively from the ipsilateral ear. All of the other choices are located further centrally and process binaural input.

2. The answer is D. Hyperacusis, the perception that sounds are excessively loud, is caused by paralysis of the stapedius muscle coincident with facial nerve or nucleus damage. Paralysis of the tensor tympani muscle, obstruction of the Eustachian tube, and fusion of the ossicles impair hearing.

3. The answer is A. The tonotopic organization of the CNS reflects the orderly arrangement of the acoustic spectrum along the basilar membrane. The tuning properties of the ossicles and peak hearing sensitivity have no bearing on the tonotopic organization of the auditory system. The ability of the superior olivary nuclei to localize sound is based on the timing and phase differences of incoming sounds.

4. The answer is B. When an acoustic neuroma involves the motor branch of the facial nerve, ipsilateral weakness of the face is likely. Paresis of the extremities can be caused by damage to the pyramidal tract, an unlikely result of an acoustic neuroma. Loss of the gag reflex accompanies damage to cranial nerve IX, which is unlikely to be affected by a mass growing in the cerebellopontine angle. The tumor is unlikely to produce enough distortion to affect the somatosensory afferent nuclei or pathways from the contralateral face.

5. The answer is C. The superior olivary nuclei receive bilateral projections from the ventral cochlear nuclei. The dorsal and ventral cochlear nuclei do not receive bilateral projections from the spiral ganglia. The inferior colliculus and the medial geniculate nucleus receive bilateral projections, but all are located further centrally than the superior olive.

6. The answer is E. The tips of the inner hair cells contact the tectorial membrane.

7. The answer is D. Only the cochlear nucleus receives projections exclusively from cranial nerve VIII on the ipsilateral side.

8. The answer is E. Otosclerosis reduces the efficacy of sound transmission through the middle ear. Prolonged exposure to loud noise and streptomycin damage the hair cells of the cochlea. Acoustic neuromas damage cranial nerve VIII. Rupture of the round window by barotrauma would affect transmission through the cochlea.

9. The answer is D. Sound conduction in air is better than through bone in normal individuals as well as in patients with sensorineural hearing loss. Because bone conduction was better than air conduction in this patient, it signaled a deficit in conduction through the outer and/or middle ear. Hair cell damage and acoustic neuromas are two causes of a sensorineural hearing loss.

Chapter 9

1. The answer is C. The ability of the lateral vestibulospinal tract to facilitate extensors is illustrated in cases of decerebrate rigidity. The lateral vestibulospinal tract descends the full length of the spinal cord within the anterior funiculus. The medial vestibulospinal tract, on the other hand, descends within the MLF only as far as the cervical cord and affects posture of the head. The rubrospinal tract facilitates flexors, which is why it normally counteracts the action of the lateral vestibulospinal tract.

2. The answer is D. The doll's eye maneuver tests the integrity of the vestibulo-ocular reflex (VOR) circuit, which includes the vestibular labyrinths, both vestibular nerves, the vestibular nuclei, the MLF, and the motor nuclei and nerves of the extraocular eye muscles. The medial and lateral vestibulospinal tracts, which descend to the spinal cord, are not part of the VOR circuit. The doll's eye maneuver operates without participation from forebrain areas such as the thalamus or cortex. The integrity of the cerebellum cannot be ascertained with the doll's eye maneuver.

3. The answer is A. Although most primary vestibular fibers project to the vestibular nuclei, some enter the juxtarestiform body and course directly to the cerebellar flocculus. The brainstem reticular formation, the abducens nucleus, and the spinal cord all receive secondary vestibular projections. The MLF contains secondary fibers that originate in the vestibular nuclei.

4. The answer is B. Turning the head to the left causes inertial flow of the endolymph to the right. This movement depolarizes the receptors of the left crista ampullaris and hyperpolarizes those on the right side. Inhibitory commissural projections reinforce the complementary output from the opposing semicircular canals. The situation is different during linear acceleration because all otolith organs move in concert. These commissural connections reinforce the output from the opposite side. The ascending projections to the oculomotor nuclei travel within the MLF. The fastigial nucleus activates the vestibular nuclei and increases extensor muscle tone. The superior vestibular nucleus plays a key role in the VOR, not muscle tone. There are no direct projections from the vestibular nuclei to the basal ganglia.

5. The answer is A. Turning the head to the left causes endolymph in the left horizontal semicircular canal to flow from the ampulla into the utricle, which increases neural activity in the ipsilateral vestibulocochlear nerve. On the contralateral side, the endolymph pushes the stereocilia away from the utricle and decreases neural activity on that side.

Rotation of the head triggers compensatory movements of the head and neck, but these adjustments are made by the medial vestibulospinal tract. The medial rectus muscle of the left eye would contract.

6. The answer is E. One of the primary determinants of muscle tone in the extensor muscles is the level of neural activity in the lateral vestibular nuclei. Procedures that increase the activity of the lateral vestibular neurons, such as electrical stimulation of the vestibular nerve, increase extensor tone. Other procedures, such as denervation of the labyrinths or lesioning the lateral vestibular nucleus, have the opposite effect. Sectioning the dorsal roots eliminates sensory input from the annulospiral endings, another source of extensor facilitation. Sectioning the ventral roots denervates the muscles.

7. The answer is A. The posterior semicircular canal and the saccule both influence vertical eye movements. Two other correct choices, not offered, would be the horizontal semicircular canal and the utricle (horizontal eye movements), and the anterior semicircular canal and the saccule (vertical eye movements). The paired structures offered in choices B through E are either mismatched, because their optimal stimuli are orthogonal to each other, or misnamed.

8. The answer is E. Seasickness is caused by the vestibular and visual systems sending discordant messages to the brain. Visual fixation on a stationary object such as the horizon is the best way to "convince" the brain that you are, indeed, moving. Lying down is unlikely to have any effect unless you are able to fall asleep. Staying in the cabin where the air may be stale and there are no stationary objects to visualize is not a wise choice. Reading, working on a computer, or doing any close work while in a car or on a boat will make motion sickness worse. Scopolamine prevents seasickness in many people, but the patch requires several hours to take effect.

9. The answer is C. Hair cells are able to signal the direction of movement because they are arranged in an orderly manner in the ampullae and the maculae. The hair cells in the three semicircular canals are not oriented in the same direction. The hair cells in the horizontal canal are polarized toward the utricle; those in the anterior and posterior canals are polarized away from the utricle. Hair cells depolarize when the stereocilia bend toward the kinocilium. The utricle transduces movement parallel to the substrate, not along the dorsoventral axis. Ototoxicity affects both auditory and vestibular hair cells.

10. The answer is E. An abrupt stop will cause the patient's eyes to move clockwise slowly with quick movements to the left and thus a left nystagmus, making answer C incorrect. Past-pointing would be in the direction of movement (i.e., to the right of the doorway), which makes answers B and D incorrect. Answers A and C are incorrect because the patient would fall in the direction of prior rotation (to the right).

Chapter 10

1. The answer is B. The piriform cortex, the largest division of the primary olfactory cortex, receives direct projections from the olfactory bulb via the lateral olfactory stria. The mediodorsal nucleus of the thalamus, which projects to the orbitofrontal cortex, receives olfactory projections from the entorhinal cortex. The olfactory bulb does not have direct projections to the insula or the NST.

2. The answer is B. Positively charged Na^+ ions enter receptor cell through ion channels located in the apical membrane. Because these positive ions depolarize the taste receptor cell directly, no second messengers are required to complete the transduction process.

3. The answer is E. Regardless of origin, the sensation mediated by the common chemical sense is pain, which is discussed in Chapter 7.

4. The answer is E. Ascending gustatory information ascends from the NST in the medulla to the ipsilateral VPMpc of the thalamus. The MD nucleus is a relay for olfactory information bound for the orbitofrontal cortex. The pontine parabrachial nucleus is an obligatory gustatory relay in nonprimate species only; in humans, the central tegmental tract ascends to the thalamus without synapsing in the pons. All gustatory projections are ipsilateral until they reach cortex.

5. The answer is A. Olfactory receptors are bipolar neurons and are located in the olfactory epithelium. Olfactory receptors are fragile and are replaced every 30–120 days. Pain receptors are free nerve endings.

6. The answer is B. Primary taste cortex in humans is located in the rostral insula. For many years it was believed that primary taste cortex was located near the intraoral somatosensory representation at the base of the postcentral gyrus (Brodmann area 43). If the postcentral gyrus plays a role in taste perception, it is likely to be a minor one, at best. Primary olfactory cortex is located in the piriform cortex, which is part of the uncus.

7. The answer is C. Gustatory and olfactory information converges on individual neurons in the orbitofrontal cortex. The amount of convergence between taste and smell in the rostral insula (primary taste cortex) is unknown, but is presumed to be minimal because olfaction has such a minor presence there. The gustatory system does not project to the entorhinal cortex, and the olfactory system does not project to VPMpc of the thalamus.

8–12. The answers are: 8 = C, 9 = C, 10 = A, 11 = B, 12 = D. Gustatory and olfactory receptor cells regenerate, probably because of the harsh environments they inhabit. Gustatory and olfactory receptors use second messengers for some but not all stimuli. Only olfactory receptors are neurons; the gustatory system uses specialized receptor cells. Taste receptor cells are capped by microvilli; olfactory neurons have tufts of cilia at the apical end. The central projections of the olfactory and gustatory systems are almost exclusively ipsilateral.

Chapter 11

1. The answer is A. Accommodation of the lens is mediated by projections from the Edinger-Westphal nucleus to the ciliary ganglion, which innervates the ciliary body and the pupillary sphincter muscle. Convergence is mediated by contraction of the medial rectus muscles, not the lateral rectus muscles.

2. The answer is B. Bitemporal hemianopsia is a visual field deficit that is usually caused by a lesion in the optic chiasm, and it is not evident from an ophthalmoscopic examination. Papilledema, or swelling of the optic disk, can be determined by a funduscopic examination and is almost always produced by an increase in intracranial pressure. Diabetic retinopathy and hypertension may produce noticeable changes in the appearance of blood vessels of the retina.

3. The answer is C. A bitemporal visual field deficit is a classic finding with a pituitary adenoma. Compression of the nerve fibers coursing through the optic chiasm is likely to affect noncorresponding (heteronymous. parts of the visual fields of both eyes. When more posterior structures in the visual system are affected, the visual field deficit is always homonymous. A lesion of one optic nerve would affect the visual field of only one eye. Increased intracranial pressure or oculomotor nerve lesions do not produce a loss in the visual field.

4. The answer is D. Retinal disparity is an inherent property of binocular vision that provides cues for depth perception. Color vision, visual acuity, motion detection, and saccadic eye movements do not depend on binocular vision.

5. The answer is A. A retinal detachment widens the distance between the photoreceptors and the pigment epithelium and, consequently, interferes with phagocytosis of the membranes sloughed off from the photoreceptor's outer segments. Eventually the photoreceptors deteriorate and phototransduction is impaired. The remaining ocular functions would not be affected by a retinal detachment.

6. The answer is C. Loss of the left visual field in both eyes indicates a lesion in the right hemisphere posterior to the optic chiasm. Quadrantic anopsias usually result from partial damage to the optic radiations or their terminals in the striate cortex. Loss of the superior visual field indicates an injury to Meyer's loop or to the lower bank of the calcarine sulcus, but since the macula was not spared, damage to Meyer's loop is more likely.

7. The answer is A. The lens is not innervated; its ability to change shape is secondary to contractions of the ciliary muscle. The cornea, the most densely innervated part of the body, contains highly branched nociceptive endings. The iris contains two muscles, the pupillary sphincter and the dilator, which receive parasympathetic and sympathetic innervation, respectively. The retina is composed largely of neurons; hence, by definition, it is innervated.

8. The answer is E. Ciliary muscle contraction decreases the tension along the zonal fibers, which allows the lens to bulge to a greater degree because of its innate elasticity. The curvature of the cornea does not change in response to neural activation. In response to parasympathetic activation, the pupil decreases in size; this corresponds to an increase in the size of the iris.

9. The answer is C. If the consensual pupillary reflex is unaffected in response to light shone in the left eye, loss of the direct reflex suggests a defect in the oculomotor nerve on the side of the affected eye (i.e., left). A defect in the optic nerve would interfere with both the consensual and direct reflexes when light is shone in the affected eye. A lesion affecting afferent fibers crossing through the posterior commissure would produce a deficit in the consensual reflex.

10. The answer is B. Horner's syndrome is produced by lesions affecting the sympathetic innervation of the eye and other structures; typically it results in pseudoptosis (slightly drooping eyelid) and miosis (small unchanging pupil). The cause of macular degeneration is unknown. Crocodile tears result from improper regeneration of the facial nerve. A pituitary adenoma may produce a visual field defect such as bitemporal heteronymous hemianopsia. Homonymous hemianopsia is produced by lesions or strokes that damage the central visual pathways posterior to the optic chiasm.

Chapter 12

1. The answer is B. Tremor is an involuntary shaking that appears most often in the hands, lips, and legs, but in advanced cases may involve the trunk. Because these tremors are involuntary and involve excess movements, they are hyperkinetic. Bradykinesia, reptilian stare, lead pipe rigidity, and micrographia are hypokinetic signs caused by pathologic retardation of normal movement by the damaged basal ganglia.

2. The answer is C. Granule cells, the only excitatory neurons in the cerebellar cortex, synapse on the apical dendrites of the Purkinje cells. Basket cells, Purkinje cells, Golgi cells, and stellate cells are inhibitory.

3. The answer is A. Seizures that spread across the motor cortex follow a pattern known as the Jacksonian march, named after the 19th century neurologist who first described the phenomenon. As epileptiform activity spreads across the motor cortex, the seizure progresses across the body following the pattern of the motor homunculus—that is, shoulder, elbow, wrist, fingers, face, and mouth.

4. The answer is B. The subthalamic nucleus contains glutamatergic neurons that increase GPi/SNpr inhibition of the thalamic motor nuclei. Neurons in the neostriatum, SNpc, GPi, and GPe are GABAergic.

5. The answer is B. A tumor in the right cerebellum produces limb incoordination on the ipsilateral side. An infarct of the anterior spinal artery on the left side above the pyramidal decussation would produce a spastic paralysis on the right side. Left-side damage to the subthalamic nucleus would produce ballistic movements of the right limbs, but not incoordination, per se. An infarct of the right crus cerebri would produce a left-sided spastic paralysis. Damage to the lateral funiculus at C5 most likely would affect the α-motor neurons of the anterior horn and cause a flaccid paralysis.

6. The answer is C. The efferent projections of the cerebellum cross and terminate on nuclei whose projections, either directly or indirectly, return to the original side of the brain and control the muscles on that side of the body. For example, the right cerebellum projects to the contralateral red nucleus, the origin of the rubrospinal tract that decussates and terminates on interneurons located in the central gray on the right side of the spinal cord. Cerebellar projections that cross and terminate in the thalamus facilitate neurons in the primary motor cortex that controls muscles on the right side of the body. The cerebellum does not have ipsilateral projections to the thalamus, basal ganglia, or red nucleus, and does not receive sensory information from the contralateral side of the body.

7. The answer is B. Supplementary motor cortex (MII) is active during complicated movements that require rehearsal. Primary motor cortex is more closely aligned with motor execution. Primary somatosensory cortex provides some of the sensory information that the posterior parietal cortex uses to construct the extrapersonal space.

8–13. The answers are 8 = A, 9 = A, 10 = A, 11 = B, 12 = A, 13 = B. Damage to the subthalamic nucleus, by reducing the normal inhibition of the thalamus by the GPi/SNpr, causes hemiballismus. A pallidotomy, by removing GPi inhibition on the thalamus, increases movement in patients with Parkinson's disease. Normally, cholinergic neurons in the neostriatum activate D_2 GABAergic neurons of the indirect pathway, which inhibits movement. Anticholinergic drugs increase movement by suppressing the indirect pathway. Thalamic damage reduces facilitation of the motor cortices. Dopamine precursors (e.g., L-dopa) are effective treatments for Parkinson's disease because they facilitate movement. Dopamine antagonists reduce movement and exacerbate Parkinson's disease.

Chapter 13

1. The answer is D. Both sympathetic and parasympathetic preganglionic neurons use acetylcholine. The postganglionic neurons in the PNS use acetylcholine, and sympathetic postganglionic neurons use norepinephrine.

2. The answer is E. Baroreceptors are found in the carotid sinus, the aortic arch, the atria, and the lateral ventricle. The OVLT contains osmoreceptors that detect changes in serum osmolarity. Receptors in the SFO detect elevated levels of serum angiotensin II associated with hypovolemia. There are no baroreceptors in the nucleus of the solitary tract or the lungs.

3. The answer is D. Low levels of vasopressin cause diabetes insipidus, which causes polyuria and polydipsia. Low levels of TSH reduce T3 and T4 release by the thyroid gland and produce hypothyroidism, which is characterized by sluggishness and obesity. Reduced CRH production decreases adrenocorticotropin hormone release by the adenohypophysis and causes Addison's disease. Reduced insulin production by the pancreas causes diabetes mellitus, whose hallmark symptoms are hyperglycemia and polyuria.

4. The answer is B. Complete transection of the sacral spinal cord produces an atonic bladder. Because the atonic bladder lacks parasympathetic innervation, voluntary urination is not possible; these patients must be catheterized. An automatic bladder, which is caused by a lesion of the spinal cord above the sacral level, empties automatically when it reaches capacity. Patients with frontal lobe damage have an uninhibited bladder and are usually unaware that they are urinating.

5. The answer is E. Visceral afferent projections from the thoracic and abdominal viscera project to the caudal part of the NST. The dorsal motor nucleus of the vagus and the nucleus ambiguus contain parasympathetic preganglionic neurons that provide efferent control of the viscera.

The Edinger-Westphal nucleus (part of the oculomotor complex), the lateral hypothalamus, and the nucleus ambiguus do not receive direct afferent projections from the vagus nerve.

6. The answer is E. The efferent fibers of the PNS emerge from the cranium and the sacral cord. The efferent projections of the SNS emerge from the thoracic and lumbar segments of the spinal cord, a choice not offered.

7. The answer is B. Damage to the ventromedial hypothalamus produces voracious eating (hyperphagia), which ultimately leads to obesity. Damage to the lateral hypothalamus has the opposite effect: starvation in the presence of food. The supraoptic nucleus and anterior and posterior hypothalamus are not involved with feeding.

8. The answer is D. Decreased baroreceptor activity in the carotid sinus triggers a compensatory increase in heart rate. Increased activity in the baroreceptors located in the carotid sinus increases the firing rate of NST neurons and lowers heart rate by increasing the parasympathetic output of the dorsal motor nucleus of the vagus and decreasing sympathetic tone.

9. The answer is C. Separate populations of magnocellular neurons in the supraoptic and paraventricular nuclei synthesize oxytocin and ADH, which are transported to the neurohypophysis and then released into the systemic circulation. The ventromedial and lateral hypothalamic nuclei regulate food intake. Neurons in the anterior hypothalamus contribute to heat dissipation, whereas those in the posterior hypothalamus conserve heat. Hormone-releasing factors are produced by neurons in the medial preoptic area, the arcuate nucleus, periventricular nucleus, and the lateral hypothalamus, but not the supraoptic or paraventricular nuclei. Neither nucleus modulates the neurohypophysis.

10. The answer is A. The suprachiasmatic nucleus receives projections from the retina, projects to the pineal gland, and synchronizes the body's circadian rhythm with the daily light-dark cycle. The areas of the hypothalamus involved either directly or indirectly with thirst and drinking include the medial preoptic nucleus, the SON, and the PVN. Blood pressure is controlled by the brainstem. The anterior and posterior hypothalamus regulate body temperature. The ventromedial and lateral hypothalamic nuclei play integral and opposing roles in feeding.

Chapter 14

1. The answer is A. Agnosia is the most likely symptom of a focal lesion of the amygdaloid complex. This type of lesion produces a constellation of symptoms that resembles the Klüver-Bucy syndrome. Thus, human patients often have difficulty with stimulus recognition and may have visual, auditory, tactile, or olfactory agnosia. Amnesia may develop only if the lesion affects the hippocampal formation. Amygdaloid lesions produce a decrease, not an increase, in fear and anxiety. Aphasia is symptomatic of lesions in Broca's or Wernicke's area. An automatism is a repetitive motor activity that frequently occurs in the midst of an epileptic seizure.

2. The answer is B. Subjective feelings of pleasure, which can be caused by drugs such as cocaine and amphetamine, are increased by the synaptic release of dopamine in the nucleus accumbens. Direct infusions of dopamine antagonists into the nucleus accumbens cause animals to cease self-administration of amphetamine and cocaine. Cholinergic projections from the basal nucleus of Meynert are necessary for attention and other cognitive functions of the cerebral cortex. Diazepam (Valium™) and other anxiolytics cause enhanced GABAergic transmission in the amygdala. Long-term potentiation is mediated by glutamatergic transmission in the hippocampus. Fluoxetine (Prozac™) and other antidepressants increase serotonin release in the amygdala.

3. The answer is D. Fluoxetine (Prozac™) inhibits the reuptake of serotonin at serotonergic terminals throughout the brain, including the amygdaloid complex. Amphetamine and cocaine increase dopaminergic transmission in the basal ganglia and prefrontal cortex. Phenobarbital and diazepam enhance GABAergic inhibition at a number of brain sites.

4. The answer is B. The mediodorsal thalamus and the mammillary bodies are bilaterally damaged in chronic alcoholics who develop Korsakoff's syndrome. Loss of neurons in these areas is associated with amnesia for recent memories. The entorhinal cortex shows degenerative changes in Alzheimer's disease that account, in part, for memory impairment. The nucleus accumbens, the prefrontal cortex, and the septal nucleus are not damaged by disorders that affect memory processing.

5. The answer is C. Choice A is incorrect because the mediodorsal nucleus projects to the prefrontal cortex rather than to the cingulate gyrus. Choice B is incorrect because the prefrontal cortex projects mainly to the basal ganglia and other parts of the motor system, not to the hypothalamus. The pathway in choice D is the reverse of the correct answer. Choice E is incorrect because the subiculum does not project to the cingulate gyrus.

6. The answer is B. Consolidation, the process of converting short-term memory into long-term memory, depends on hippocampal processing. Following damage to the hippocampus, it is still possible to learn a motor task, recognize visual patterns, or retrieve memories acquired previously. Attention is impaired in Alzheimer's disease or following damage to the anterior cingulate gyrus.

7. The answer is D. Memories are stored in areas of the cerebral cortex associated with specific sensory modalities; hence, extensive damage to the cerebral cortex interferes with memory retrieval. The hippocampal formation is necessary for consolidating memory in the cerebral cortex, but long-term memories can be stored and retrieved after the hippocampal formation has been completely removed. The remaining structures play ancillary roles in the formation and retrieval of memory.

8. The answer is A. The stria terminalis conveys information from the amygdaloid complex to the bed nucleus of the stria terminalis, the septal nucleus, and the hypothalamus. The perforant pathway sends output from the entorhinal cortex to the dentate gyrus. The cingulum connects the cingulate gyrus with the entorhinal cortex. The fornix conveys information from the subiculum and hippocampus proper to the septal nucleus. The final choice, cingulate gyrus and subiculum, does not contain a fiber system.

9. The answer is C. Long-term potentiation, which depends on NMDA receptor activation, is a neural mechanism for consolidating short-term memory into long-term storage. Memory retrieval is not completely understood, but it does not depend primarily on NMDA receptor activation. Temporal lobe epilepsy involves glutamatergic transmission but is correlated mainly with an increase in extracellular potassium concentration. Depression is a mood disorder caused by an imbalance in biogenic amines such as norepinephrine or serotonin. Retrograde amnesia represents a deficit in memory retrieval produced by head trauma or global cortical damage.

Chapter 15

1. The answer is E. Large-amplitude delta waves (0.5-4 Hz) indicate a state of deep sleep that occurs in stage 4 of NREM sleep. Stage 2 sleep, which is not as deep as stage 4, contains K spike complexes. Muscle atonia, PGO spikes, and an increase in cerebral metabolism are signs of REM sleep.

2. The answer is A. The pedunculopontine and laterodorsal tegmental nuclei contain REM-on neurons that initiate REM sleep. These REM-on neurons activate effector neurons in the medial pontine reticular formation, which in turn depolarize the thalamus to produce cortical desynchronization during REM sleep. The locus ceruleus and dorsal raphe nuclei contain REM-off neurons that suppress the REM-on neurons toward the end of the REM sleep period. The suprachiasmatic nucleus is not involved in REM sleep.

3. The answer is E. One of the leading causes of coma is extensive damage to the brainstem tegmentum at the pontine-mesencephalic junction. Damage to the medulla usually causes immediate death because of cardiac or respiratory failure. Damage restricted to the cerebral cortex or to the posterior thalamus may result in coma if the damage occurs bilaterally. Extensive damage to the right cerebral hemisphere alone results in coma in less than 10% of the cases. The basal ganglia and the anterior thalamus have not been implicated in coma.

4. The answer is B. Uncal herniation compresses the rostral brainstem and, thus, damages the ascending pathways that regulate consciousness. Except in cases of extensive bilateral cortical damage, cerebral infarction produces paralysis, aphasia, or a sensory deficit but not a loss of consciousness. The medial striate artery supplies the basal ganglia, a structure that has not been implicated in coma. A cerebellar contusion is unlikely to cause coma unless the cerebellum swells or hemorrhages, thereby compressing the underlying brainstem. Coma may result from prolonged ischemia or anoxia but is unlikely to develop from a typical transient ischemic attack, which generally last only 10 minutes.

5. The answer is D. Cerebral blood flow and glucose consumption vary with the periodic changes in EEG activity that accompany REM and NREM sleep. Apnea is associated with abnormal sleep and can cause insomnia. Cataplexy is a defining symptom of narcolepsy. Abnormal latencies in the SEPs and diffuse slowing of EEG activity below 8 Hz are associated with coma.

6. The answer is B. The main symptom of narcolepsy is the prevalence of sleep attacks, many of which are prompted by emotional stimuli. Insomnia is characterized by an inability to sleep. Although OSA may increase sleepiness during the day, it does not provoke sudden sleep attacks. Cognitive death is a term used to describe the lack of awareness and loss of other cortical functions that are observed in patients in a permanent vegetative state. Circadian rhythm disorders are characterized by changes in the onset and duration of sleep with respect to the time of day, not by periodic sleep attacks.

7. The answer is D. Small EEG waves in the beta frequency indicate cortical arousal and suggest that the patient is awake, not anesthetized. Bilateral somatic evoked potentials do not differentiate between awake and anesthetized individuals. Theta and delta wave frequencies would not be expected in a conscious individual. Eye movements appear during normal wakefulness but would not be present during most surgeries because paralytic drugs are administered with general anesthesia to prevent unwanted movements.

8. The answer is B. Benzodiazepines enhance GABAergic transmission from the reticular nucleus to the thalamocortical relay neurons, an effect that increases thalamocortical oscillations in the delta frequency range. Benzodiazepines do not directly affect the activity of the cholinergic projections from the nucleus basalis, nor do they directly affect the cholinergic or adrenergic projections from the brainstem.

Chapter 16

1. The answer is B. Failure of the anterior neuropore to close prevents development of the forebrain. Spina bifida is an incomplete formation of the vertebral arch of the spinal vertebrae caused by faulty closure of the neural tube or posterior neuropore. Syringomyelia is an enlargement of the central canal that is not a development defect, but rather one caused by trauma such as whiplash. Hydrocephalus is an enlargement of the cerebral ventricles caused by excessive production or incomplete resorption of CSF.

2. The answer is A. All neurons in the central nervous system begin as neuroblasts located in the subventricular zone. Neurons of the cranial, dorsal root ganglia, and autonomic ganglia develop from the neural crest. Other neural crest derivatives include neurons of the enteric nervous system, as well as the neurosecretory cells of the adrenal gland, the Schwann cells of the peripheral nervous system, and the meninges. The primitive streak is an embryonic predecessor of the central nervous system. The anterior neuropore is closed by the lamina terminalis on embryonic day 24. Following closure of the anterior neuropore, the rostral half of the neural tube dilates into the three primary brain vesicles: the prosencephalon, the mesencephalon, and the rhombencephalon.

3. The answer is D.

4. The answer is D. Maturation of prefrontal cortex during adolescence plays a key role in the emergence of adult-like behaviors. Most cerebellar maturation takes place during the perinatal period. The somatosensory, motor, and visual cortices undergo important changes during adolescence, but none are as dramatic as those that take place in the prefrontal cortex.

5. The answer is E. Early experience shapes the developing nervous system in many ways, including selective synaptic pruning. Experience does not trigger the critical periods of development, but rather takes place during the critical periods. Primary neurulation and release of cell adhesion molecules are driven by genetic and cellular factors. Most neurogenesis takes place prior to the formation of synapses, and therefore is not guided by the individual's experience.

6. The answer is B. Neurogenesis continues in the hippocampus until we die, but it is insufficient to offset neuronal loss in Alzheimer's disease.

7. The answer is A. Apoptosis or programmed cell death prunes neurons that the nervous system is not actively using. Synaptogenesis, neurogenesis, neural migration, and development of the radial glia lattice are all involved in growth and maintenance of neural tissue.

8. The answer is A. The hippocampus and the entorhinal cortex, two areas of the brain closely linked to memory formation, are severely damaged by Alzheimer's disease. Some loss of myelin, neuron shrinkage, and widened cortical sulci takes place during normal aging. The amygdala, a part of the limbic system, is involved with detection and expression of emotion.

Chapter 17

1. The answer is A. Imaging studies of patients who suffer stroke-induced depression have consistently revealed damage in the prefrontal cortex and basal ganglia, usually in the left hemisphere. Although stroke damage may occur in any region of the brain, including the regions listed in choices B through E, depression is not strongly associated with damage to these regions.

2. The answer is E. There is no definitive diagnostic marker for depression. When depressed patients are compared with healthy control subjects, some physiological parameters are statistically significant, but the magnitude of the variability has prevented the identification of cutoff values that might distinguish depressed and healthy individuals.

3. The answer is C. Imaging studies of depressed patients have consistently reported decreased blood flow to the dorsal lateral prefrontal cortex. The next most consistent finding is an increase, not a decrease, in blood flow to the amygdala and hippocampus. Depression among the elderly is often associated with enlarged ventricles, but this may have other causes and represents only a small portion of depressed patients. Few functional imaging studies have reported blood flow changes in the locus ceruleus.

4. The answer is A. Stress-induced depression causes the HPA axis to become hyperactive, which is evident from an increase in CSF levels of CRH and cortisol, as well as hypertrophy of the adrenal gland. Paradoxically, however, the number of CRH-R1 receptors on the pituitary gland decline in response to elevated levels of CRH. Because the number of CRH receptors is reduced, an intravenous challenge of CRH produces an ACTH response than is smaller in depressed than in non-depressed individuals.

5. The answer is C. The strongest evidence that depression is inheritable comes from twin studies showing that the inheritability factor is 0.33. A family history of mood disorders is a strong predictor of susceptibility to depression but is not conclusive proof of its genetic basis. Although some families show a greater incidence of suicide than others, suicidal behavioral is not always caused by depression. There is no conclusive proof that a faulty serotonin transporter gene is directly linked to depression; instead, the short allele of the SERT gene increases the vulnerability to stress and its influence on depression. The effectiveness of an antidepressant in treating the prior depression of a patient's parent or sibling is often considered in determining an appropriate therapy; it does not provide strong evidence for a genetic basis of depression.

6. The answer is D. Any explanation for the delayed efficacy of antidepressant therapy is speculative, but it is known that monoamines stimulate postsynaptic metabotropic receptors and that prolonged stimulation of these receptors initiates a series of time-dependent mechanisms involved in synaptic remodeling. Autoreceptor desensitization also requires time and may lead to increased neurotransmitter release, but the net effect of this increase is more powerful stimulation of the postsynaptic metabotropic receptors. All of the other choices involve processes that occur within minutes of ingesting either an MAO inhibitor or a reuptake blocker.

Index

NOTE: An "f" after a page number denotes a figure; a "t" after a page number denotes a table; a "b" after a page number denotes boxed material that is not discussed in the text on the same page.

F

G

H

O

Q

R

T

W

Y

Z

CPSIA information can be obtained at www.ICGtesting.com
Printed in the USA
LVOW05s0420010915
452336LV00005B/199/P

9 781593 772000